NURSING ASSISTING

ESSENTIALS FOR LONG-TERM CARE

SECOND EDITION

NURSING ASSISTING

ESSENTIALS FOR LONG-TERM CARE

SECOND EDITION

Barbara Acello, MS, RN

THOMSON

DELMAR LEARNING

Australia Canada Mexico Singapore Spain United Kingdom United States

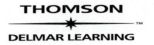

THOMSON

DELMAR LEARNING

Nursing Assisting: Essentials for Long-Term Care, Second Edition
by Barbara Acello

Vice President,
Health Care Business Unit:
William Brottmiller

Editorial Director:
Cathy L. Esperti

Acquisitions Editor:
Marah E. Bellegarde

Developmental Editor:
Sherry Conners

Marketing Director:
Jennifer McAvey

Marketing Channel Manager:
Tamara Caruso

Marketing Coordinator:
Kip Summerlin

Editorial Assistant:
Jennifer McGovern

Project Editor:
Daniel Branagh

Art and Design Coordinator:
Connie Lundberg-Watkins

Production Coordinator:
Jessica McNavich

Library of Congress Cataloging-in-Publication Data

Acello, Barbara.
  Nursing assisting : essentials for long-term care / Barbara Acello.—2nd ed.
    p. ; cm.
  Includes index.
  ISBN 1-4018-2752-7 (pbk.)
  1. Nurses' aides—Training of.
2. Long-term care of the sick.
  [DNLM: 1. Long-Term Care—methods. 2. Chronic Disease—nursing. 3. Nurses' Aides. 4. Nursing Care—methods.   WY 152 A173n 2005]
I. Title.

RT84+

2004049771

NOTICE TO THE READER

CONTENTS

CHAPTER 4   Safety and Emergencies   79

CHAPTER 5   Legal and Ethical Responsibilities   109

CHAPTER 9   Assisting Residents with Mobility   174

CHAPTER 10   Care of the Environment   199

CHAPTER 11   Personal Care Skills   213

CHAPTER 20 Special Behavioral Problems 401

CHAPTER 21 Death and Dying 422

CHAPTER 22 The Nursing Assistant in Home Care 435

LIST OF PROCEDURES

GUIDELINES LISTING

PREFACE

INTRODUCTION

Nursing Assisting: Essentials for Long-Term Care meets the OBRA requirements for nursing assistant education and is designed to prepare the nursing assistant to work in a long-term care facility, hospital skilled unit, or subacute care center. The text emphasizes real-world clinical practice and provides solutions to common problems that nursing assistants encounter. Compliance with current infection control and safety practices and state and federal regulations is emphasized. Long-term care facility surveys are stressful for all facility staff, and the nursing assistant in particular. We have provided information on surviving the long-term care facility survey to help you understand the survey process and make your job easier.

NURSING ASSISTANT CURRICULA

Nursing Assisting: Essentials for Long-Term Care is designed to parallel nursing assistant curricula, as much as possible, in most states. Although the federal requirements for nursing assistant training are standardized, each state has the flexibility to adjust its curriculum to meet regional needs. Hence, there is no "universal curriculum" for OBRA-approved nursing assistant education. Some textbooks organize material by body system. However, most state nursing assistant curricula are organized by subject matter. We have grouped common subjects together in the order presented by many state-approved nursing assistant programs.

FEATURES OF THE TEXT

The nursing assistant has evolved from an unlicensed, untrained individual to an educated, skilled paraprofessional who passes a certification examination and is listed with the state nursing assistant registry. More is expected of the nursing assistant than ever before in the history of long-term care. To help you meet the ever-increasing expectations and demands, this text is designed to assist you in demonstrating responsible, professional employee behavior. We have provided guidelines for keeping your relationships with residents healthy and professional. The text is written according to the Centers for Disease Control and Prevention (CDC) guidelines for standard precautions and describes the CDC criteria for transmission-based precautions. The information presented meets the current Occupational Safety and Health Administration (OSHA) guidelines for health care facilities.

Long-term care facilities are home to individuals from many cultures and of many nationalities, with a variety of chronic illnesses and personal care needs. A chapter is devoted to communicating and interacting with residents who have disabilities. Culture strongly influences the residents' health care preferences. Cultural information is integrated into the text where appropriate. Today's long-term care facility also has residents representing many different age groups. Meeting the needs of this diverse population may be difficult. Information on caring for nontraditional residents, such as infants, children, and young and middle-aged adults, is presented to assist you.

Unfortunately, our society has had increasing episodes of violence over the past decade, and health care facilities are not immune. According to OSHA, health care facilities are one of the leading sites of violence in the workplace. Guidelines for preventing and dealing with incidents of health care facility violence are included in the text. Although we hope you never need them, they are an important part of your basic preparation, and all health care workers must be aware that the potential for violence exists.

Nursing Assisting: Essentials for Long-Term Care uses a practical, reality-oriented approach based on need-to-know information in the long-term care facility. Current trends and issues in health care are emphasized. When appropriate, real-world solutions to problems are presented. The text is designed to assist the student to become a strong clinician. Theory is included when it is necessary to understand the reason for a procedure or to apply the information to other similar clinical situations. In addition to traditional nursing procedures, the text includes lists of general guidelines that describe how to manage many common resident care situations.

Our goal in developing this book was to provide "one-stop shopping" for the nursing assistant and instructor. The book is designed to be all-inclusive, without the need for additional supplements. A review section is included at the end of each chapter. This section contains questions to help the student prepare for state certification testing. Critical thinking questions are included in each chapter to help you become proficient in applying the material.

The second edition of *Nursing Assisting: Essentials for Long-Term Care* has been expanded to better prepare the nursing assistant to meet the needs of an evolving resident base. Each chapter begins with a list of important observations to make and report related to chapter content. New information has been added to reflect current trends in infection control, disease management, and CDC recommendations. Many nursing assistants are required to have basic cardiac life support certification, so basic rescuer procedures have also been added. Additional emphasis has been given to diseases commonly seen in long-term care residents. Preventing pressure ulcers and assisting residents with mobility are discussed in expanded sections. New content has been added to reflect the industry trends in pain recognition and management, as well as general comfort, rest, and sleep measures. Introductory information has been included for working in the home health care industry.

The Instructor's Manual contains a crossword puzzle or word search puzzle for each chapter. Use of puzzles is fun, and assists in mastery of medical terminology and spelling. A comprehensive practice final examination is also provided.

The instructor's manual is filled with resources to augment student learning and retention of the material. It will assist instructors in meeting the needs of various types of learners, while enhancing class quality and improving effectiveness. Using this turnkey package will enhance effectiveness, improve student performance, and help ensure positive results.

A student workbook has been added with this edition to enhance student learning, retention of the material, and ability to use critical thinking. Use of the workbook will assist students in applying the principles learned to a wide variety of resident care situations. A computerized test bank is also available to assist instructors with test and quiz construction. Although the text may be used as a stand alone item, the various teaching aids will meet the needs of a wide variety of programs. Upon class completion, using the Delmar *Nurse Aide Exam Review Cards* (which are available in both English and Spanish) will assist students in studying for the state certification examination.

FINAL THOUGHTS

In the author's opinion, the resident is the most important individual in the long-term care facility. All care is directed to providing the highest possible quality of life for facility residents. This text was written with the belief that the nursing assistant is the most important employee of the facility. Properly trained and motivated nursing assistants are important for the well-being of residents and the overall operation of the long-term care facility. You are an important member of the team and will receive a great deal of personal satisfaction from completing your educational program and working as a nursing assistant. The staff at Delmar Learning is committed to helping you succeed by providing quality educational materials to prepare you for your important responsibilities in the long-term health care delivery system.

ACKNOWLEDGEMENTS

It is always a pleasure to honor the individuals who helped bring a book to fruition. I sincerely appreciate the assistance and support of the following individuals at Delmar Learning: Marah Bellegarde, Acquisitions Editor, and Marge Bruce and Bryan Viggiani, Developmental Editors. I also appreciate the efforts of the many unnamed individuals at Delmar who have contributed to the production team effort. I am always delighted when Brooke Graves edits my books. Thank you, Brooke, for making me look good!

A special thanks to those who contributed to the art manuscript: Patricia King, Tufts University; Arnie Silverman, Skil-Care Corporation; and David Lebovic, Medline Industries. Gathering the art is the most difficult part of the project for me, and your assistance made my job much easier. I also appreciate the help of Brooklyn Fowler, my granddaughter, who took care of many of the tedious details associated with art manuscript preparation.

A team of peer reviewers devoted many hours to reviewing the manuscript, and provided many helpful comments during manuscript development. I can honestly say that this has been the most helpful review team I have ever worked with. Your contributions have made this a better book. Although I was not able to incorporate all your suggestions due to space constraints, I have saved them and will incorporate them into the next revision. Your input has been invaluable, and I sincerely appreciate your dedication, prompt turnaround, and willingness to share your knowledge and suggestions:

Gyl Burkhard, RN
OCM BOCES
Syracuse, NY

Laurie Cochrane, BSN, RN
Director of Patient Care
Girling Health Care, Inc.
Austin, TX

Margaret Connelly, RN
Rochester Community and Technical College
Rochester, MN

Margaret Konieczny, BSN, RN
Nursing Instructor
Western Nevada Community College
Carson City, NV

Margaret Markey, BSN, RN
Director, Training Center
Saint Anne Training Center
Winona, MN

Diann Muzyka, RN
Columbus State Community College
Columbus, OH

Judy Stella, RN
Program Manager Nursing Assistant
Greenville Technical College
Greenville, SC

Linda Sullivan, MS, RN
Associate Professor
Kansas City Kansas Community College
Kansas City, KS

HOW TO USE THIS BOOK

The second edition of *Nursing Assisting: Essentials for Long-Term Care* has been carefully designed and updated to reflect the evolving world of nursing assisting. The major headings and terms that follow and appear in the chapters will help guide readers and focus their learning.

Objectives—state the learning goals of each chapter; help the reader to know the focus of the chapter as they read the text.

Key Terms—focus the reader on the major new vocabulary words to be studied in the chapter. These are important terms readers should be aware of as they study the content in each chapter.

Observations—lists observations about conditions that may be found related to the content of a particular chapter. Quickly identifies content highlighting critical areas. Unless otherwise noted, these should be reported to the nurse.

Key Points—summarizes knowledge learned in the preceding pages.

Guidelines—highlight important points to remember, in an easy-to-use format.

Procedures—contain clinical procedures in a step-by-step format with any notes or cautions about the procedure. The reader is encouraged to practice these procedures until they may be performed correctly and proficiently.

Review—offers multiple-choice, true/false, and fill-in-the-blank questions, as well as Clinical Applications hypotheticals, to reinforce newly acquired knowledge. Offers a hands-on practice to develop specific skills learned in the chapter. After reading a chapter, the reader should try to answer these review questions. If difficulties are encountered, the reader should go back and review the chapter again.

CHAPTER 1

Introduction to Health Care

OBJECTIVES

After reading this chapter, you will be able to:

- Spell and define key terms.
- List five settings in which health care is delivered and describe the function of each.
- Differentiate care given in an acute care hospital, subacute unit, health maintenance organization, private home, and long-term care facility.
- Describe the purpose and function of the interdisciplinary team.
- Explain the chain of command and describe why using the chain of command is important.
- Describe at least five desirable qualities of the nursing assistant.
- Describe responsible behavior and list nine ways to show that you are responsible.

Welcome to the field of health care! You are on the way to becoming a respected health care worker who provides direct care to ill or injured persons in the long-term care facility. The services you provide will be under the direction and supervision of a licensed nurse.

Many titles are used to describe the person who delivers personal care to residents. These include nursing assistant, nurse assistant, nurse aide, patient care technician, patient care associate, attendant or assistant, primary caregiver, and health care technician. This caregiver is very important to resident comfort and well-being. Some health care facilities employ **multiskilled workers.** The multiskilled worker has completed a basic nursing assistant program and has taken advanced classes to be able to provide additional resident care skills. Successfully completing the nursing assistant program is the first step in the health care ladder and will provide you with a secure, rewarding career.

HEALTH CARE DELIVERY

Health care is provided in many settings. Many professional and nonprofessional workers pro-vide patient care in these sites. The type of care given is determined by the types of services the sites deliver, but the basic skills you will learn in this course are used to some degree in all health care settings.

Hospitals

Hospitals are health care agencies that give care to persons with **acute illnesses** and injuries. An acute illness is one that occurs quickly and does not last very long. The person receiving care in the hospital is called a **patient.** Patients usually stay in the hospital for a short period of time. When the patient is medically stable, he or she returns home or is transferred to a facility or unit in which patients are not acutely ill and require a lower level of care. The goal is for the individual eventually to return to his or her own home.

Long-Term Care Facilities

Long-term care facilities are agencies that care for persons with **chronic illnesses** who require **rehabilitation, restorative care,** or assistance with personal care. A chronic illness is one that lasts for a long time, perhaps for life. An example of a chronic illness is heart disease. Sometimes a chronic illness can cause an acute problem. Acute problems related to chronic illnesses are usually treated in the hospital. Rehabilitation and restorative care are individualized programs designed to assist residents to attain and maintain the highest level of function possible in their individual situations. These programs help residents overcome the disabling effects of their illness or injury.

The person receiving care in the long-term care facility is called a **resident** because the facility is considered "home," either temporarily or permanently. Long-term care facilities may be called by many different names. Some of these names are nursing homes, nursing facilities, convalescent homes, rehabilitation centers, care centers, care facilities, and skilled nursing facilities.

Skilled Nursing Facilities

Often the name of the agency describes the type of care that the facility provides. Some hospitals have units called *skilled units*. These units are licensed as long-term care facilities. Some nursing homes are licensed to provide skilled care in all areas of the facility. Others license only specific wings or units to provide skilled care. Residents who require skilled care have illnesses or injuries that require daily services that only a licensed health care professional can provide. These services can involve one or more disciplines within the health care facility. For example, nurses must administer injections and are responsible for complex treatments. The services of a licensed nurse are also required to assess the residents' medical condition and take appropriate action if problems are noted. If the resident has many complex needs, planning and monitoring daily care is considered a skilled service. Licensed therapy personnel provide skilled therapy on a daily basis to rehabilitate the resident. Skilled nursing facilities provide care for residents who have highly specialized medical needs, but who are medically stable and not acutely ill.

Subacute Units

Care may also be given in **subacute** care centers or units. The subacute unit is a transitional step between the hospital and the skilled nursing facility. These units may be part of a hospital or long-term care facility. Residents in subacute units have complex medical needs, but are not critically ill. However, they require close monitoring by health care professionals because their conditions may change at any time. The residents are not ill enough to require the services of the acute care hospital, but still require frequent care. They usually require many services from the nursing assistant. Some facilities call the person receiving care "patient." Others use the term "resident."

Assisted Living Facilities

Assisted living facilities (ALFs) are a rapidly growing segment of the long-term care industry. Other names for assisted living facilities are residential care facilities, personal care facilities, and adult congregate care facilities. Assisted living facilities are designed to meet consumer needs for independence in a safe, homelike, residential setting. They provide housing and personal care support services to residents. Residents are encouraged to remain involved with their families and the community. Some facilities provide specialized services, such as caring for residents with Alzheimer's disease. A resident in an assisted living facility can rent one room or an entire apartment. Each unit has an emergency call system. The services vary somewhat depending on the type of services offered, and state laws. Other services provided by most assisted living facilities are:

- 24-hour security
- 24-hour staff availability
- Three meals a day in a common dining area; some units have limited cooking and refrigeration facilities residents can use to prepare meals and store food
- Assistance with eating, bathing, dressing, toileting, and walking
- Medication management
- Social and recreational activities
- Transportation
- Housekeeping services
- Personal laundry services
- Access to health and medical services; hands-on delivery of health services is not provided in most assisted living facilities
- Exercise and wellness programs

Residents of assisted living facilities may:

- Display signs of mental or emotional disturbance, but are not considered at risk of harm to self or others.
- Need some assistance with movement; residents who are immobile or totally dependent on staff are not appropriate for an ALF.
- Require assistance with bathing, dressing, and grooming.

- Need assistance with routine skin care, such as application of lotions, or treatment of minor cuts and burns.
- Need reminders to use the toilet to prevent incontinence.
- Be incontinent without pressure sores.
- Need assistance with toileting.
- Need assistance with medications, supervision of self-medication, or administration of medication.
- Need special diets.
- Need assistance with meals, or require encouragement to eat, monitoring, or prompting during meals.
- Be hearing-impaired or speech-impaired.
- Need self-help devices.

Assisted living facilities promote the concept of "aging in place," in keeping with state rules and regulations governing resident health and safety. Whenever possible, the facility provides services so the resident does not have to move his or her living space. The assisted living facility provides assistance or supervision with personal care activities, and monitors resident health and safety. The facility coordinates any services by outside health care providers and agencies needed by the resident. Rules and licensing regulations vary from state to state. Some states require special education and certification for staff members. Many nursing assistants work in assisted living facilities.

Home Care

Many health care consumers receive care in the home from qualified caregivers. The person who receives care in the home is called the **client.** Most care is provided by home health agencies. These agencies have many workers who are responsible for care and supervision of clients in the home. Commonly, the nursing assistant is the primary caregiver. In the home care setting, the assistant may be called a home care aide or home care assistant. The home care assistant provides personal care, cares for the client's environment, makes observations, and reports abnormal findings to the registered nurse supervisor (case manager). Home health care is one of the fastest growing segments of health care today.

Some clients receiving home health care are acutely ill and need 24-hour care. Many require only short visits daily or several times a week. A visit usually lasts from 45 minutes to 2 hours. Other workers, such as physical, occupational, speech, or respiratory therapists, may also visit the home to perform services for the client.

The caregiver who works in the home does so without direct supervision. A **registered nurse (RN)** is responsible for planning and supervising the care given in the home, but the RN may not be present when the care is actually given. An RN has completed two to four years of nursing education and has passed a state licensing examination. The personal care given in the home is the same as care provided in other settings. Sometimes you must improvise by using common items in the home to care for the client. Caring for the client in the home may also involve preparing meals, shopping for groceries, doing light housekeeping, and doing laundry. The nursing assistant must follow a plan of care developed by the RN case manager. Because a caregiver may not be in the home at all times, making accurate observations and reporting your findings to your nurse manager by telephone and in writing is important.

Hospice Care

Hospice care may be provided in the home and also in a health care facility. A **hospice** is an organization dedicated to caring for persons with limited life expectancy. In hospice care, the resident and family are considered a single unit. A team of workers ensures that the physical, psychological, and spiritual needs of the entire family are met. Team members provide the resident the opportunity to die with dignity, in comfortable, familiar surroundings. Emphasis is given to keeping the resident pain-free and maintaining the highest quality of life possible. Support is provided so the resident and family members are not left alone in a time of crisis.

Because people are living longer, quality of life has become an important consideration in health care delivery. Many health care decisions are made with the future quality of the individual's life in mind. Quality-of-life policies and requirements focus on creating and maintaining an environment that humanizes and individualizes each person. In some situations, preserving the quality of the resident's life is viewed as more important than the length or duration of life. In any event, assisting each individual to maintain the highest possible quality of life is very important.

Other Types of Health Care Facilities

Health care may also be delivered in many other settings. These include:

- Freestanding clinics and emergency care centers
- Mental health facilities

- Adult day care facilities
- Adult group living centers

FINANCING HEALTH CARE

Health care is paid for in many different ways. Some individuals pay for care out of their personal bank accounts. Others pay premiums to insurance companies. When these people get sick, the insurance company **reimburses,** or pays, the facility for providing medical care. **Medicaid** is a health care program funded by both the state and federal governments that pays for health care for individuals with low incomes. **Medicare** is a federally funded program for individuals who are elderly or disabled. Medicare pays for certain services in hospitals, long-term care facilities, and home health care settings. Although most hospitals accept payment from the Medicare and Medicaid programs, some home health agencies and long-term care facilities do not.

Occasionally, other sources pay for health care. The Veterans Administration has special hospitals to care for veterans with service-related illnesses and injuries. It also pays long-term care facilities for care they provide to veterans in certain circumstances. Private agencies in the community may also help pay the cost of care for certain individuals.

The **health maintenance organization (HMO)** is a group of health care providers and hospitals. An HMO may be funded by Medicare, Medicaid, or the patient's private money. HMO members are given a list of physicians, clinics, offices, and hospitals from which they may receive care. The member must see only certain doctors and go to only designated hospitals, except in certain situations and emergencies. The HMO pays the doctor (or group of doctors) a fee for each member every month. The doctor is paid the fee even if the member does not visit. The doctor or clinic is expected to deliver all care, whenever needed, for this monthly fee. There are no additional payments. Some HMOs have special outpatient clinics in which outpatient surgery, diagnostic testing, patient teaching, and preventive health care are delivered. Medical care may be provided for individuals with acute illness. Usually the patient returns home after treatment in the clinic.

Another common method of paying for health care is through a **preferred provider organization (PPO).** The PPO consists of various doctors, hospitals, and other health care agencies that contract with insurance companies to care for their subscribers. When members are

sick, they can choose a physician or agency on the preferred provider list to care for them. The member's out-of-pocket expenses are reduced as long as the patient uses the physicians and agencies on the list. The patient may go to any other service provider of his or her choosing. However, going to providers who are not on the PPO list will cost the member more.

OBRA LEGISLATION

OBRA is an abbreviation used to describe the *Omnibus Budget Reconciliation Act.* The OBRA legislation of 1987 was designed to improve the quality of life, quality of care, health, and safety of residents in long-term care facilities. Residents' rights are emphasized. Residents in long-term care facilities have the same legal rights as all other citizens. The facility must maintain a homelike environment **(Figure 1-1)** and maintain or improve the quality of the residents' lives.

The OBRA legislation requires that all states follow minimum standards to ensure that nursing assistants working in long-term care facilities are educated and competent to give personal care. The legislation specifies that a nursing assistant must have a minimum of 75 hours of instruction in certain subject matter to work in long-term care. Many states require more than 75 hours of preparation. The skills learned in the nursing assistant program are the basic skills required for entry-level positions in most health care settings.

Before the OBRA legislation, each state decided whether nursing assistants should receive special preparation to work in long-term care.

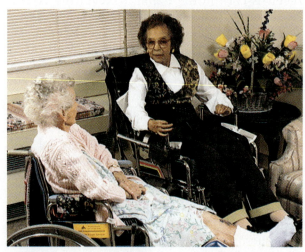

FIGURE 1-1 The long-term care facility is the residents' home. Providing a comfortable, homelike environment enhances quality of life.

Some states had no education requirement. Although many states did require nursing assistant classes prior to OBRA, the content of programs varied widely from state to state. OBRA recognizes that the person receiving care, the health care facility, and the nursing assistant all benefit from the nursing assistant education program. The information learned is useful in many different health care settings and also in the assistant's personal life. The care required by the OBRA legislation translates into good care regardless of the setting. However, the OBRA legislation was specifically designed to improve the quality of care in the long-term care facility and the skilled unit of the hospital.

Benefits of the Nursing Assistant Program

Many people benefit when the nursing assistant understands the responsibilities of the position. Nursing assistant classes are designed to ensure that all care providers understand and are able to provide basic procedures for resident care.

Benefits to the person receiving care. It is comforting to the resident in a long-term care facility to know that the staff is properly prepared to deliver care. When a person is sick, he or she has many worries. The resident is relieved of the burden of worrying about the qualifications of the staff caring for him or her. Additional benefits to the resident are that:

- The care given is safe, effective, and of high quality, because the staff is properly trained.
- Changes in condition are rapidly recognized, reported, and treated.
- Residents are satisfied with the care received.
- Quality of life is improved because the staff has a better understanding of resident needs.
- There are fewer incidents of abuse and neglect because of an understanding of what constitutes abuse and neglect, what causes it, and how to prevent it.
- Facility and personal safety are improved because nursing assistants are aware of how to prevent accidents and injuries.
- The incidence of infection is reduced because nursing assistants know what causes infection, and know and take measures to prevent its spread.

Benefits to the long-term care facility. The long-term care facility has a great responsibility for the health, safety, and welfare of its residents. A large amount of trust is placed in the employees to deliver the highest possible quality of care. Employees understand their duties and responsibilities and provide safe care. Other benefits to the employer are that:

- Staff turnover is decreased. Turnover is costly to the facility and upsetting to residents.
- Quality of care is improved because staff members know how to perform procedures.
- Safety is improved, so residents and workers have fewer accidents.
- Observation and reporting of important changes in condition lead to more timely medical care.
- Nursing assistants have many different skills. This enhances the workers' value to the organization and allows more cost-effective care to residents.
- The image of the facility is enhanced because of the qualified caregivers on staff.
- The image of the long-term care industry is enhanced because all caregivers are prepared and qualified to do their jobs.

Benefits to the licensed nurse manager. The licensed nurse manager may also be called the charge nurse. This individual is responsible for what happens on the unit during each shift. This is a great responsibility. The manager must be able to trust the other workers to take proper care of residents, make observations, and report changes in a timely manner. Benefits of nursing assistant education to the licensed nurse are:

- Observations and reporting of changes in resident condition are improved. This is because nursing assistants have a greater understanding of residents' needs and better ability to recognize problems.
- Improved understanding of the role and responsibilities of the nursing assistant.
- All care providers perform procedures and give care in the same manner. This consistency benefits the resident, and the nurse does not have to worry about variations from standard procedures.
- Improved skill level of the caregiver.

Benefits to the nursing assistant. The nursing assistant benefits greatly from completing the OBRA-required education program. Benefits to the nursing assistant include:

- Information gained is useful in many areas of your life. In addition to teaching you how to care for residents, you will gain information that will help you care for yourself and family members.
- The program gives you an improved understanding of your role and responsibilities as a nursing assistant.

- Your knowledge and skill level are improved so that you can give safe, high-quality personal care.
- Job satisfaction increases because you understand the reason behind what you are doing.
- You become aware of the factors that cause resident and employee accidents and illnesses, so you can prevent injury to yourself and others.
- You develop a sense of accomplishment, pride in what you are doing, and an improved self-image. Completing the nursing assistant program is a great accomplishment and something to be proud of.

Nursing Assistant Certification

After completing the nursing assistant program, you must understand how to get and keep your certification. Some states require the employing long-term care facility to complete a criminal background check on all applicants. This background check will show if the applicant has ever been arrested. In these states, if an individual has been convicted of certain crimes, he or she cannot work in a long-term care facility.

After completing the state-approved course, the nursing assistant must take written and manual competency skills examinations given or sponsored by the state. After passing these examinations, the nursing assistant is entered into the state nursing assistant registry. To keep nursing assistant certification active, you must work in a health care agency for pay every two years. The number of hours you must work in the two-year period varies with the state. If you do not work for 24 months or longer, you must complete another nursing assistant program or refresher course and successfully complete another competency evaluation test to work as a nursing assistant again. Some states will allow you to take the test over without repeating the class. The OBRA legislation requires the nursing assistant to attend a minimum of 12 hours of continuing education each year to remain active. Some states require more than the 12-hour minimum. The facility that you work for will offer these classes. It is your responsibility to attend them to maintain your certification. Your facility is required to evaluate your skills every year to be sure that you can perform your duties in the way you were taught.

Supervision of the Nursing Assistant

In the most health care facilities, you will provide personal care to residents under the supervision of a licensed nurse. The director of nursing in the long-term care facility must be an RN. The nurse who directly supervises you is usually your charge nurse. This person may also be an RN. Some nurses are **licensed practical nurses (LPN).** In Texas and California, these nurses are called **licensed vocational nurses (LVN).** LPNs and LVNs have completed 1 year to 18 months of full-time nursing education and have passed a state licensing examination. The nurse will give you your assignment at the beginning of your shift. You will report your concerns and observations to this nurse.

INTERDISCIPLINARY TEAM

The health care team is also called the **interdisciplinary team.** The interdisciplinary team consists of many individuals who contribute to the care, health, and well-being of residents. The residents and family members that residents want to be included are also members of the team. All team members are important. We need each other, and the residents need us. To be successful, we must work together and cooperate with each other.

Members of the Interdisciplinary Team

Many individuals, both inside and outside the health care agency, are members of the interdisciplinary team. We must use whatever resources are necessary to meet the physical, mental, and emotional needs of residents. The goal of the interdisciplinary team is to assist residents to maintain the highest possible level of physical, mental, emotional, and psychosocial well-being. Team members meet shortly after a new resident admission and periodically after that to develop a **care plan** for that resident **(Figure 1-2).** The care plan is a mutually agreed-upon list of problems, goals, and approaches to help the resident reach his or her highest potential. A system, called **Nursing Interventions Classification (NIC),** is being used by many facilities. This system provides specific approaches that all team members use to deliver care. The effectiveness of the approaches and all care provided is measured by **Nursing Outcomes Classification (NOC).** Using these systems provides consistent care and a method of measuring whether the care is helping the resident meet the goals established by the interdisciplinary team.

All team members must know the information and follow the instructions on the care plan. When everyone follows the care plan, all staff

MARYSVILLE CARE CENTER	CARE PLAN	09/07/20XX
		FORM # 280L

PROBLEM	SHORT TERM GOAL	APPROACH

(1) DEFICIT FLUID VOLUME RELATED TO DECREASED FLUID INTAKE.
 	
    ONSET   TARGET   RESOLVE
    09/06/XX 12/05/XX 00/00/00
	(1) REHYDRATE/ESTABLISH FLUID BALANCE.
	
	    BEGIN TARGET RESOLVE
	    09/06/XX 12/05/XX 00/00/00
		(1) RECORD INTAKE AND OUTPUT EVERY SHIFT.
		    DISC: NSG
		
		(2) CHECK & RECORD B.P. AS ORDERED.
		    DISC: NSG
		
		(3) MONITOR SKIN TURGOR.
		    DISC: NSG
		
		(4) ENCOURAGE ADEQUATE FLUID INTAKE DAILY.
		    DISC: NSG NA D
		
		(5) OFFER FLUIDS OF CHOICE.
		    DISC: ALL
		
		(6) INCREASE AMOUNT OF FLUID INTAKE TO 2500CC DAILY.
		    DISC: NSG
		
		(7) CHECK MUCOUS MEMBRANE MOISTNESS Q SHIFT
		    DISC: NSG
		
		(8) MONITOR VITAL SIGNS Q 4 HOURS AND PRN.
		    DISC: NSG

(2) POTENTIAL FOR IMPAIRED SKIN INTEGRITY DUE TO DECREASED MOBILITY.
 	
    ONSET   TARGET   RESOLVE
    09/06/XX 12/05/XX 00/00/00
	(1) FREE FROM RED OR OPEN AREAS.
	
	    BEGIN TARGET RESOLVE
	    09/06/XX 12/05/XX 00/00/00
	
	(2) MAINTAIN SKIN INTEGRITY.
	
	    BEGIN TARGET RESOLVE
	    09/06/XX 12/05/XX 00/00/00
		(1) HAVE DIETITIAN CONSULT ABOUT DIET.
		    DISC: D
		
		(2) INCREASE AMOUNT OF FLUID INTAKE DAILY.
		    DISC: NSG
		
		(3) INCREASE MEAT/PROTEIN IN DIET.
		    DISC: NSG D

PHYSICIAN / ALT. PHYSICIAN	PHONE NO.	ALLERGIES / NOTES				
SMART, NANCY D.O. KEELEY, SHAWN D.O.	(555) 888-1212					

RESIDENT	STATION / ROOM / BED	ADMISSION NUMBER / DATE		SEX	DATE OF BIRTH	CARE PLAN DATE	PAGE #
MARTIN, FRANK	WEST-322-B	23891	09/22/XX	M	08/04/1918	09/07/XX	1

FIGURE 1-2 The care plan directs and guides resident care. It is updated for changes in condition. Your assignment will reflect care plan goals for each resident.

MARYSVILLE CARE CENTER	CARE PLAN	09/07/20XX
		FORM # 280L

PROBLEM	SHORT TERM GOAL	APPROACH
		(4) KEEP BED LINEN OFF EXTREMITIES. DISC: NSG (5) KEEP EXTREMITIES IN GOOD ALIGNMENT & PROPERLY SUPPORTED. DISC: NSG (6) KEEP LEGS ELEVATED ON PILLOWS SO HEELS ARE OFF THE MATTRESS TO REDUCE PRESSURE. DISC: NSG (7) KEEP DRY AND CHANGE AFTER VOIDING. DISC: NSG (8) KEEP SKIN CLEAN, DRY AND FREE OF PRESSURE. DISC: NSG (9) TURN EVERY 2 HOURS AND PRN. MAINTAIN GOOD BODY ALIGNMENT WITH PILLOWS. DISC: NSG (10) MULTIVITAMINS WITH IRON AND VITAMIN C. DISC: NSG (11) SPENCO MATTRESS TO BED AND CHAIR. DISC: NSG

PROBLEM	SHORT TERM GOAL	APPROACH
(3) CONSTIPATION. ONSET TARGET RESOLVE 09/06/XX 12/05/XX 00/00/00	(1) WILL HAVE A B.M. EVERY OTHER DAY. BEGIN TARGET RESOLVE 09/06/XX 12/05/XX 00/00/00	(1) OFFER PRUNE JUICE AT BREAKFAST. DISC: D NSG (2) MONITOR BOWEL SOUNDS DAILY. DISC: NSG (3) DO DIGITAL BOWEL CHECK IF CONSTIPATION SUSPECTED. DISC: NSG (4) INCREASE FIBER IN DIET AS ALLOWED BY DIET ORDER. DISC: NSG D

PHYSICIAN / ALT. PHYSICIAN	PHONE NO.	ALLERGIES / NOTES				
SMART, NANCY D.O. KEELEY, SHAWN D.O.	(555) 888-1212					
RESIDENT	STATION / ROOM / BED	ADMISSION NUMBER / DATE		SEX	DATE OF BIRTH	CARE PLAN DATE	PAGE #
MARTIN, FRANK	WEST-322-B	23891	09/22/XX	M	08/04/1918	09/07/XX	2

FIGURE 1-2, *Continued*

MARYSVILLE CARE CENTER	CARE PLAN	09/07/19XX FORM # 280L
PROBLEM	SHORT TERM GOAL	APPROACH

Approach column:

(5) ADMINISTER MEDICATIONS AS ORDERED BY NANCY SMART D.O.
   DISC: NSG

(6) ENCOURAGE FLUIDS.
   DISC: NSG

(7) ACTIVITY AS TOLERATED.
   DISC: NSG

(8) OBSERVE FOR MEDICATION EFFECTIVENESS.
   DISC: NSG

(9) MONITOR AND RECORD BOWEL MOVEMENTS.
   DISC: NURSING

Problem column:

*** CURRENT MEDICATIONS ***

*** WEIGHT HISTORY ***

*** CURRENT DIAGNOSIS ***

PHYSICIAN / ALT. PHYSICIAN	PHONE NO.	ALLERGIES / NOTES				
SMART, NANCY D.O. KEELEY, SHAWN D.O.	(555) 888-1212					
RESIDENT	STATION / ROOM / BED	ADMISSION NUMBER / DATE	SEX	DATE OF BIRTH	CARE PLAN DATE	PAGE #
MARTIN, FRANK	WEST-322-B	23891 09/22/XX	M	08/04/1918	09/07/XX	3

FIGURE 1-2, *Continued*

members are using the same approaches and working on the same goals for the benefit of the resident. Team members that provide services to residents are listed in **Table 1-1.**

CHAIN OF COMMAND

The **chain of command** (**Figure 1-3**) is very important to the proper operation of all health care facilities. The chain of command is the line of authority that each department follows in reporting information. You will report your observations, problems, and concerns to the nurse. If you have a problem with another department, you will also report this information to the nurse. The nurse will contact the appropriate person in that department to solve the problem. It is your responsibility to know and follow your facility's chain of command.

TABLE 1-1 Interdisciplinary Health Care Team Members	
Team Member	**Responsibilities**
Provide Most of the Direct Care Services to Residents	
Licensed Nurse (licensed nurses may be either RNs or LPN/LVNs)	Directs the care of residents, administers medications, and performs treatments. Supervises and directs nursing assistant staff.
Nursing Assistant (NA, CNA, or STNA)	Provides most of the personal care to residents under the supervision of the licensed nurse. The nursing assistant spends more time with the residents than other team members.
Medication Aide (MA) (Certified Medication Assistant [CMA]) (Medication Technician [MT])	A certified nursing assistant who has met certain criteria, taken additional classes in medication administration methods, and completed a state certification examination. Allowed to pass medications in skilled nursing facilities, assisted living facilities, and home health care in 25 states.
Restorative Nursing Assistant (RNA)	A certified nursing assistant who has additional education and experience in restorative nursing care. Delivers care designed to assist the resident to attain and maintain his or her highest level of function, and prevent physical deformities.
Dining Assistant (Feeding Assistant, Nutrition Assistant)	A single task worker with at least 8 hours education in nutrition and hydration. Assists stable residents with eating and drinking. May not assist residents with complex feeding problems.
Dietary Staff Member	Prepares meals and is responsible for ordering groceries, washing dishes, and other kitchen duties.
Registered Dietitian (RD)	Writes the menus for meals prepared by the dietary department. Responsible for seeing that residents on special diets receive the right food in the proper amounts. Assesses each resident's individual dietary needs; calculates individual calorie, fluid, and other requirements; and makes recommendations for care of chronic illnesses and complications.
Activities	Provides activities for resident enjoyment. Some activities are done to provide exercise for residents. Other types of activities are designed to provide positive **self-esteem.** Self-esteem is how you feel about yourself. Activities also provide opportunities for residents to socialize with others.
Social Service Worker (LSW or SSD)	Helps meet residents' mental and emotional needs. Coordinates functions with personnel and agencies inside and outside the facility to see that resident needs are met. When it is time for the resident to be discharged home or to another health care agency, the social worker coordinates the resources the resident will need and makes the transition as smooth as possible. An LSW is a licensed social worker. The SSD is a social services designee.
Physical Therapist (PT, LPT)	Helps residents regain strength and physical function lost because of illness or injury. The goal of the therapist is to help the resident achieve the highest possible level of physical function. The physical therapist also teaches residents and staff how to perform physical activities in a safe manner. A physical therapy assistant (PTA) may assist with physical therapy services.

Continues

TABLE 1-1 Interdisciplinary Health Care Team Members, *Continued*

Team Member	Responsibilities
Occupational Therapist (OT, OTR/L)	Helps residents regain strength and physical function lost because of illness or injury. This therapist helps residents to relearn self-care skills, such as feeding, bathing, grooming, and dressing. The goal of care is to help the resident become as independent as possible. Residents who have lost physical function may be able to use adaptive or self-help devices to be independent. The occupational therapist helps residents obtain these devices and learn how to use them. The OT may also fabricate or order splints and other equipment to prevent deformities. An occupational therapy assistant (OTA) may assist in providing occupational therapy services.
Respiratory Care Practitioner (RCP)	Works with residents who have breathing problems and those who need oxygen and other special treatments for their lungs. The goal of the treatment is to see that residents receive enough oxygen to meet their needs.
Speech Language Pathologist (SLP)	Works with residents who have diseases or injuries that have affected their ability to speak properly. This therapist also helps residents who have swallowing problems to learn to eat and drink without choking.
Physician (MD or DO)	Orders the resident's medical plan of care. Medications, diagnostic tests, and treatments must be ordered by the physician.
Clinical Nurse Specialist (CNS)	An advanced-practice registered nurse with a master's degree who focuses on a very specific resident population (e.g., medical, surgical, diabetic, cardiovascular, operating room, emergency room, critical care, geriatric, neonatal, etc.).
Nurse Practitioner (NP)	A registered nurse with advanced academic and clinical experience, which enables him or her to diagnose and manage common acute and chronic illnesses, either independently or as part of a health care team. A nurse practitioner provides some care previously offered only by physicians and in most states is legally permitted to prescribe medications.
Physician Assistant (PA)	A health care professional licensed to practice medicine with physician supervision. PAs conduct physical examinations, diagnose and treat illnesses, order and interpret tests, counsel on preventive health care, assist in surgery, and in most states are permitted to write prescriptions. Because of the close working relationship the PA has with the physician, PAs are educated in the medical model designed to complement physician training.
Provide Less Direct Resident Care	
Clergy	Members of the **clergy** are pastors of churches or other religious workers who help residents meet their spiritual needs.
Bookkeeping or Office Worker	Responsible for answering the telephone, recordkeeping, and taking care of business and financial functions.
Medical Records Worker	Keeps permanent records of residents' care and treatment. Records are an important tool for communication with other members of the health care team. They are legal documents that may be used in court.
Maintenance Worker*	Responsible for seeing that the building and equipment are safe and in good repair at all times.
Laundry Worker*	Washes facility linen and keeps the nursing units supplied with sheets, towels, and other items needed to care for residents. The laundry worker in most long-term care facilities also washes residents' personal clothing.
Housekeeping Personnel*	Keeps the facility clean and sanitary.
Beautician/Barber	Provides haircuts and other services needed to care for residents' hair.

*These departments may be combined into one environmental service department.

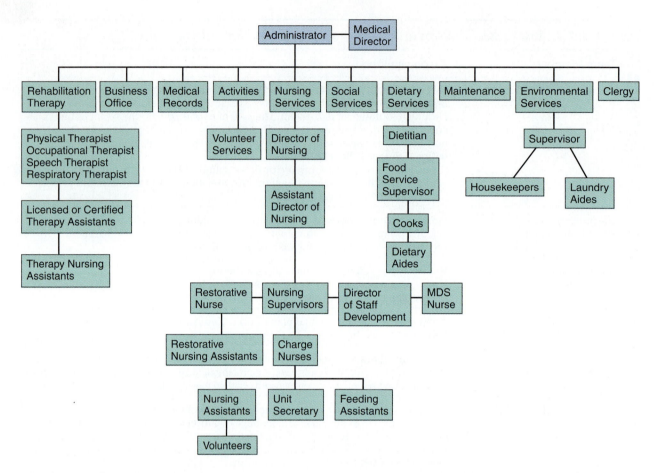

FIGURE 1-3 Following the chain of command for reporting shows respect and enhances communication in the long-term care facility.

DESIRABLE QUALITIES IN THE NURSING ASSISTANT

The nursing assistant is a special person. The successful assistant likes people, takes responsibility seriously, and believes in the importance of the position.

Personal Qualities

A pleasant personality is an important quality for health care workers. You will learn how to communicate and interact with many different people. Being pleasant and polite to everyone is important, even if they have not treated you this way. Treat others with respect and dignity. Show genuine concern for your residents and coworkers. Be available to help others and accept help if you need it. Do not judge other people's feelings. You will become more aware of how to assist residents with their feelings as you learn more about emotional needs. Remember, behavior is influenced by things such as culture, personality,

illness, and emotional health. Understanding why others respond as they do will help you accept and deal with people's behavior.

A positive **attitude** is an important characteristic to bring to your job. Your attitude is the outer reflection of the way you feel. Others can see your attitude by your behavior. The tone of your voice and your body language can change the message you are trying to send. Your attitude will be reflected in your work. Be positive about your job and your contribution to resident care.

You must also learn to work as a team player. This means that you depend on other people to help care for residents. It also means that other people can depend on you. Good resident care cannot be accomplished by one person or department. It takes many people and departments working together to meet the residents' needs.

Practice tact. **Tact** involves the ability to say and do things at the right time. Being tactful means you are considerate, polite, and thoughtful. Be sensitive to the problems and needs of others. Do not judge others or give advice. Treat residents and coworkers with courtesy, respect, and consideration. Do not argue, gossip, criticize your employer or others, or use abusive language.

Be proud of what you do, and feel good about yourself. It takes a special person to provide personal care to other people. The nursing assistant is a very important person to the operation of the long-term care facility. Work to do the best job you can. Others will follow your example.

Professional appearance. You should be clean, neat, and well groomed at all times (Figure 1-4). A **professional** appearance gives others confidence in you and sends a message that you feel good about yourself and the job you do. A professional is a person who is capable, competent, and efficient. Your facility will have a dress code or uniform that you must wear. Be sure to wear the clothing your facility requires. Your uniform must be clean and wrinkle-free each day. The color and design of your undergarments should not be visible beneath your uniform.

A name pin is a very important part of your uniform. The name pin identifies you by name and title. Residents have the right to know the name and position of the person caring for them. Many facilities issue name badges that are also used to electronically scan the time clock. If your facility does not issue a badge, it is your responsibility to obtain a name tag.

Because you will be standing and walking for much of the day, having comfortable, well-fitting shoes is important. Some facilities require athletic shoes or shoes with closed toes that provide good foot support. Your shoes are an important part of your uniform. Keep them clean and in good repair.

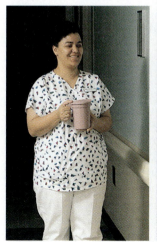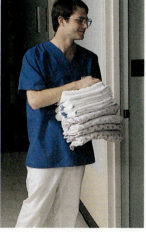

FIGURE 1-4 A professional appearance projects a positive image to residents, families, and other staff.

Good personal hygiene, grooming, and personal health. Staying clean is one way to maintain your personal health. Take a bath or shower every day. Use a deodorant or antiperspirant. Keep your hair clean and neat. If your hair is long, wear it up or pulled back. Your hair is like a magnet for germs. Keeping it short makes it easier to care for. Washing your hair regularly is best. Keeping long hair pulled back reduces the risk of injury from hair becoming entangled in equipment or being inadvertently pulled by a resident. Long fingernails, artificial nails, and chipped nail polish are also good hiding places for germs. Avoid acrylic and artificial nails. Keep your natural nails short and clean.

Jewelry should be kept to a minimum. Jewelry also harbors germs. Sharp stones and settings can injure residents and tear gloves. Only simple jewelry should be worn when on duty. Small stud-type pierced earrings also reduce your risk of injury from an earring being pulled or caught. Many facilities allow only a watch and wedding band. Cologne and aftershave should not be worn when on duty. Some residents have allergies to different fragrances. Residents who are nauseated or have other medical problems may become ill from the scent of cologne. Others with respiratory problems may have difficulty breathing with a heavy fragrance in the room.

Body piercings and tattoos. Residents in the long-term care facility are elderly, and many are offended by, do not understand, or are afraid of employees with piercings and tattoos. In communities with gang activity, residents may associate piercings and tattoos with gang membership. Most facilities do not permit employees to have conspicuous body piercings in areas of the body other than the ears. This includes the tongue. If you have piercings in other areas, cover them with clothing. Conspicuous tattoos are unacceptable in many facilities. A tattoo is considered conspicuous when it is visible. Methods of concealing tattoos, such as makeup and bandages, are usually not permitted in facilities. The only acceptable covering is clothing. Some facilities will not permit employees with visible tattoos to work in resident care positions.

Personal communication devices. Most facilities have policies prohibiting the use of nonwork-related personal communication devices, such as cell phones and pagers. Safety and care of residents is paramount and communication devices distract employees from this purpose. Plan to make and return phone calls during your breaks. Personal communication devices should not be worn in resident care areas. In some facilities, employees may carry electronic pagers or cellular phones set for a silent alert that is imperceptible to others. However, staff are not permitted to respond to calls when on duty. Remember, you are being paid to work, and interrupting care even briefly to make or answer calls is not consistent with your job description. Another great concern is that some radio frequency devices will interfere with medical equipment and may jeopardize resident health and safety, as well as facility operations.

Personal Health and Safety

If you are to do your job well, you must be in good physical and emotional health. You will learn many health and safety principles and practices throughout this course that you can apply to your personal life.

Preventing physical illness. Practice the principles of proper nutrition, good health, and personal hygiene taught in this class. Eat three well-balanced meals each day. Avoid fad diets and junk foods. Avoid using alcohol, tobacco, and drugs. These substances endanger you and others.

Get adequate rest. Most people need eight hours of sleep each night. Exercise for at least 30 minutes three times each week. This is a good way to keep your body healthy, and it helps relieve stress.

See your doctor regularly for checkups and preventive health care. Treat your medical problems early. Do not wait for them to become worse.

Men should perform testicular self-examination monthly. Women should practice breast self-examination each month and have mammograms as recommended by their treating physicians.

Preventing physical illness is very important. You will learn principles of infection prevention in Chapter 3. These principles will help you prevent infection and communicable disease. Avoid going to work if you have a cold, flu, diarrhea, or other illness that may be infectious. Follow your facility policy for reporting your absence. If you think you have been exposed to an illness at work, notify your supervisor and follow his or her instructions.

Immunizations. Immunizations involve the administration of medications to stimulate your immune system to protect you against certain communicable diseases. Some states require health care workers to be immunized against certain diseases. Immunizations will protect you from many diseases. **Table 1-2** lists recommended immunizations for health care workers. The recommendations do not distinguish workers in long-term care facilities from those employed in other settings. However, the likelihood of contracting measles and mumps in a long-term care facility is minimal. Additional immunizations may be necessary in special circumstances.

Health and safety education. Attend classes on health and safety. In addition to learning how to protect residents from illness and injury, you will learn how to protect yourself and family members.

Other methods of preventing illness. Follow your facility policies and procedures for prevention of infection and injury. If you identify health risks, take the proper precautions. It is your responsiblity to learn and follow these practices. Cooperate with your infection control nurse or department during audits, education, investigation of outbreaks and exposure, and review of infection control practices. Sometimes recommendations to prevent infection change. It is your responsibility to learn new techniques and make changes in the way you practice.

Preventing injuries. Safety practices taught in this class will protect both you and the residents you care for. The most common causes of employee injuries in health care facilities are slips, falls, and back injuries caused by improper lifting and moving. Wear a back support for lifting and moving if this is your preference or the policy of your employer. Lifting, moving, and using your body correctly while on duty will be discussed in detail in Chapter 8. Know and follow your facility policies for reporting injuries of residents or employees, and follow them if an accident or injury occurs.

Your Emotional Health

Your feelings and behavior are your responsibility, and you must work to control them. A sign of maturity is your ability to control your emotions. Ask yourself how your behavior will affect others. If you are upset, leave the area and take time out, if necessary. If you feel angry, upset, or impatient, try to understand why you feel this way. Find acceptable ways to cope with these feelings. Do not take negative comments from residents personally. Often the resident is reacting to a situation, not to you. Try to understand why

TABLE 1-2   Immunizations

Vaccine name	Primary booster dose schedule	Indications	Major precautions	Special considerations
Hepatitis B (recombinant vaccine)	Two doses 4 weeks apart. Third dose 5 months after second dose. No booster necessary.	Health care personnel who may be exposed to blood and body fluids.	**Warning: May cause shock in individuals allergic to baker's yeast.**	No apparent adverse effects to developing fetuses. Not contraindicated in pregnancy.
Influenza vaccine (inactivated whole or split virus vaccine)	Annual single-dose vaccine with current virus strain.	Health care personnel who have contact with high-risk residents in long-term care facilities; individuals with high-risk medical conditions.	**Warning: May cause shock in individuals allergic to eggs.**	No evidence of maternal or fetal risk when given to pregnant women with underlying medical conditions that cause high risk for serious influenza complications.
Measles (live virus vaccine)	One dose immediately, second dose 1 month later.	Health care workers born in or after 1957 without documentation of previous vaccine, physician-diagnosed measles, or laboratory evidence of immunity. Vaccine should be considered for all workers born before 1957 who have no proof of immunity.	**Do not use during pregnancy, immunocompromised state,* history of shock following gelatin ingestion, or receipt of neomycin. Do not use if recent recipient of immune globulin.**	A combined measles-mumps-rubella (MMR) vaccine is the vaccine of choice if the health care worker is also susceptible to rubella and/or mumps. Persons vaccinated between 1963 and 1967 or who were treated with a vaccine of unknown type should consider being revaccinated.
Mumps (live virus vaccine)	One dose, no booster.	Health care workers who are believed to be susceptible. Adults born before 1957 can be considered immune.	**Do not use during pregnancy, immunocompromised state,* history of shock following gelatin ingestion or receipt of neomycin.**	MMR is the vaccine of choice if the health care worker is also susceptible to rubella and/or measles.
Rubella (live virus vaccine)	One dose, no booster.	Health care personnel who lack documentation of live vaccine on or after their first birthday, or of laboratory evidence of immunity. Adults born before 1957 can be considered immune except women of childbearing age.	**Do not use during pregnancy, immunocompromised state,* history of shock following receipt of neomycin.**	Risk to fetus if pregnant when vaccinated or if woman becomes pregnant within 3 months of vaccination. MMR is the vaccine of choice if the health care worker is also susceptible to mumps and/or measles.

Continues

		TABLE 1-2 Immunizations, *Continued*		
Vaccine name	**Primary booster dose schedule**	**Indications**	**Major precautions**	**Special considerations**
Varicella zoster (live virus vaccine)	Two doses, 4-8 weeks apart.	Health care workers without reliable history of chickenpox or laboratory evidence of immunity.	**Do not use during pregnancy, immunocompromised state,* history of shock following gelatin ingestion or receipt of neomycin. Salicylate use should be avoided for 6 weeks after vaccination.**	Many individuals without a history of chickenpox are immune. Serologic testing may be cost-effective.
Bacille Calmette Guerin (BCG) vaccine (tuberculosis [TB])	One dose, no booster	Should be considered only in areas where multidrug-resistant TB is prevalent, a strong likelihood of infection exists, and comprehensive TB control precautions have failed to prevent transmission in health care workers.	**Do not use during pregnancy or immunocompromised state.***	In the United States, TB control efforts are aimed at early identification, treatment, and preventive therapy.

Note: *Persons immunocompromised because of immune deficiency diseases, HIV infection (who should normally not receive BCG, OPV, and yellow fever vaccines), leukemia, lymphoma or generalized malignancy, or who are immunosuppressed as a result of therapy with corticosteroids, alkylating drugs, antimetabolites, or radiation.

the resident is acting this way. You must respond with respect and courtesy even if the resident is not kind to you.

Stress in the workplace. **Stress** is emotional and physical tension that can be harmful to your health. Working in a health care facility can be stressful at times. Your job may be physically or emotionally demanding. Stress is sometimes unavoidable when you are helping other people with their problems. If stress goes unchecked, you may feel overwhelmed and out of control. Personal or family problems may also contribute to the stress you feel. If your physical health is not good, stress may seem to worsen. **Burnout** is complete mental and physical exhaustion that occurs as the result of a buildup of stress. Feel good about yourself and the job you are doing. Having good self-esteem helps you cope with stressful situations. Use stress-reducing techniques to help cope with stress or sadness. The goal of stress management is to prevent burnout. Try to think through a problem before you worry about it. Understand that health care is constantly changing, and that to be successful, you must change with it. If stress is caused by

change, resolve to accept it. If you know of a stress-relieving technique that works for you, use it.

Ways of managing stress. Everyone has certain ways of managing stress. Learn which ways work for you and practice them regularly. Some suggestions for controlling stress are:

- Be nice to yourself. Be aware of your own needs. Leave home problems at home and work problems at work.
- Replay the good things that you have done in your mind. Dwell on these things and not on mistakes you have made.
- Do something that you enjoy and have fun.
- Exercise.
- Take a break and relax in a pleasant atmosphere (**Figure 1-5**).
- Sit with your feet up and your eyes closed and relax for a few minutes. Take a few deep breaths. Try to think of a pleasant scene or event. Imagine that you are there.
- Use specific relaxation techniques or audio or videotapes.
- Soak in a warm bath.
- Listen to quiet music or read a book.

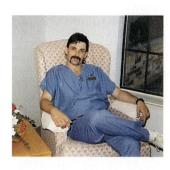

FIGURE 1-5 Taking a break and relaxing in a pleasant, comfortable atmosphere is a good stress reliever.

- Find a hobby that you enjoy.
- Talk with a friend.
- Get in touch with nature. Contact with plants and animals has been proven to reduce stress.
- Watch a funny movie or do something that makes you laugh. Laughing is a good stress reliever.
- Sing. Singing relieves stress.
- Have someone give you a massage.
- Employ spiritual practices, such as prayer, yoga, or meditation.

Proper Equipment

Health care facilities and agencies have different requirements for equipment that you will be expected to provide. By law, the health care facility is required to supply you with well-fitting gloves and other protective equipment. Gloves and personal protective equipment are used when some care is given to prevent the spread of infection. This will be explained in detail in Chapter 3. In most cases you will be expected to furnish your own uniform and name pin. Some facilities expect their employees to provide a **gait belt,** also called a transfer belt. This is a canvas belt used for moving and walking residents. Some facilities also require you to have a back-support belt, blood pressure cuff and stethoscope, watch with second hand, pen, and pocket-sized note pad. Know and follow your facility policies.

Responsible Behavior

Responsible behavior is very important for workers in health care professions. Practicing responsible behavior means being dependable and trustworthy. If a member of the health care team is not responsible, residents and coworkers suffer. Because you care for the health and welfare of human beings, you must take your job duties very seriously. Think of how you would feel if a family member was a resident of a health care facility. You would want the best care possible for your loved one. To deliver the best care, all team members must demonstrate responsible behavior.

Health care facility rules must be followed even if you do not agree with them. Learn and profit from constructive criticism. Responsible behavior includes:

- Honesty in word and behavior.
- Reporting to work on time on the days that you are scheduled.
- Keeping absences to a minimum. If you must be absent, follow your facility policy for reporting your absence. Notify the facility as early as possible so that it can call in a replacement. If the facility does not know you will be absent, care will suffer and your coworkers will have to work much harder than usual.
- Keeping your promises to residents and other staff members.
- Completing tasks that are assigned to you quickly and accurately.
- Demonstrating initiative; this means doing things that you see need to be done without waiting to be told to do them.
- Cooperating with other staff members in all departments.
- Being **dependable,** so that residents and coworkers will trust you to do your job to the best of your ability. A person who is dependable is trustworthy and can be relied upon.
- Reporting safety and infection control problems.
- Reporting mistakes if you make them.
- Giving proper notice of resignation if you must resign from your position. Most facilities require a minimum of two weeks notification.

Organization of Your Work

Practice organizing your work. Organization is not something that can be taught in the classroom. The principles of organization will be taught by your instructor, but it is up to you to learn, practice, and master them. Organizing your work means learning how to set **priorities.** Prioritizing your work means performing tasks in order of importance. It also means that you will anticipate your own supply needs and residents' personal needs. Bring needed items to the room before you begin your care. This will save time and steps. If you can plan and prepare to meet these needs in advance, the quality of care you give will be better and the job will be much easier for you.

Manage your time well. Report for duty at your assigned time. Listen to the report and get your assignment **(Figure 1-6)** from the nurse. Set your priorities to make the most of your day. Setting priorities makes the job easier. Good organization also reduces stress.

When organizing your work, rate each assignment in order of importance. Do not become frustrated if your priorities change or must be adjusted midway through the shift. Priorities are constantly changing in health care because of resident illness and other emergencies.

After you have established your priorities, plan your work for the most efficient use of your time. Identify tasks that you can group together. For example, a well-organized worker can make the bed while the resident is sitting in a chair or washing at the bathroom sink. Plan your schedule around meal times, activities, appointments, and the residents' rehabilitation schedules. Plan for tasks that will require someone else to help you or for which you will need special equipment.

Check on all of your residents before beginning your assignment. Take care of immediate needs. List special procedures that must be done and the time, such as positioning and turning residents according to an assigned schedule. Check to see if residents are scheduled for tests, appointments, or other activities during your shift. Follow your assignment sheet and the resident's care plan.

Remember that while you are at work, you are on duty. You are being paid to work the whole time. Report to the nurse when you go on break. Return from lunch and breaks on time. If you run out of things to do, help your coworkers or perform tasks that need to be done on your unit. Do these things without being told.

Other Qualities of the Successful Nursing Assistant

The successful nursing assistant delivers quality care to the residents in the long-term care facility. Always do things in the manner in which you were taught. Taking shortcuts can be dangerous. Do not perform procedures unless you have been taught to do so and your facility allows nursing assistants to perform the procedure in question. For example, giving medication is not taught in your class, so this is something that you cannot do without additional education. Some states allow specially prepared nursing assistants to pass medications, but in most states the nursing assistant cannot legally give medicine. If you are not sure how to carry out a procedure, consult the nurse or check the procedure manual. Inform the nurse if you will be unable to complete a job.

Conduct yourself as a professional at all times. Being compassionate and empathetic with residents and families shows that you care and sets a good example for others. A nursing assistant who is compassionate treats others with mercy and kindness. Empathy is the art of understanding how someone else feels.

Continue to Learn and Grow

This class is just the beginning of your career. Health care changes daily, and it is your respon-

CNA ASSIGNMENT SHEET 10/12/XX														
Room	Resident Name	Bath	Position Schedule	Range of Motion	Vital Signs	Weight	Toileting	B & B	ADL Program	Ambulate	Transfer or Gait Belt	Restraint or Alternative	Safety	I & O
300A	Mary King	S	X	PROM			X					Wedge in chair	X	
300B	Susan Kowalski	WP	X	PROM			X						X	
301A	June Lee		X	PROM	X				X					
301B	Elena Hernandez	BB	X	PROM	X							Side rails	X	X
302	John Murray			AROM				X	X		X			
303A	Albert Strong	S		AROM	X					X				X
303B	Norman Jones		X	PROM			X					Lap buddy	X	
304	Hazel Urich	TB		AROM		X		X		X	X			

FIGURE 1-6 The nurse will give you an assignment each day based on the problems, goals, and needs listed on the care plan for each resident. (Two examples are shown.) Use the assignment to set priorities for your shift. If you believe you will have trouble completing your assignment, inform the nurse promptly.

sibility to keep up. You can learn much from your coworkers and by reading books and journals. Attend continuing education classes offered by your employer to learn new information and maintain your certification.

There are professional organizations, support groups, and publications available for nursing assistants. Participating in a professional organization or support group will help you learn and grow.

Protect Yourself Legally

Follow your facility policies and procedures even if you do not agree with them. This protects you as an employee and ensures that you will do your job in accordance with the law. Anticipate residents' needs and meet them in a timely manner. Protect the rights of the residents in your health care facility. These rights and your legal responsibilities are discussed in detail in Chapter 5.

Nursing Assistants' Daily Assignments

DATE: __10/12/XX__

UNIT: __3rd Floor__

Everyone must participate in passing food trays and feeding residents so that hot food is served

Cindy	John	Mary	Susan	James	Norma
Res. group 1 300A-304	Res. group 2 305A-309B	Res. group 3 310-314B	Res. group 4 315A-320A	Res. group 5 320B-325	Res. group 6 326A-330B
Break time: 8:30	Break time: 8:45	Break time: 9:00	Break time: 8:30	Break time: 8:45	Break time: 9:00
Meal time: 10:45	Meal time: 11:15	Meal time: 12:30	Meal time: 10:45	Meal time: 11:15	Meal time: 12:30

SPECIAL ASSIGNMENTS
Fresh Water Pass (AM & PMs)

John AM

Norma PM

Mealtime Assignments

James - hall trays

Norma - feeders

Others to main

dining room

Water Pitcher Collection (PM)

Tub Room/Shower Room
Cindy

Utility Rooms/Soiled Linen
Mary

Deliver Nourishments
Susan

Utensil Collection (PMs)

Fill Humidifiers

CHARGE NURSE NOTES:

Bible Study - 10:00

Current Events - 11:00

Bingo - 2:00

All beds made by

10 AM Please

RESIDENT APPOINTMENTS:

304 - Beauty shop 9:30

317B - Daughter picking up 11:00
for lunch

323A - Dentist - 2:00

TREATMENTS:

WEIGHTS:	INTAKE/OUTPUT:
301A -	301B -
321B -	303A -
329 -	312 -
VITAL SIGNS:	317B -
301B -	324B -
316A -	326B -
321A -	329A -

See Routine Equipment Cleaning Assignment Form on clipboard

FIGURE 1-6, *Continued*

KEY POINTS

- Hospitals provide care to patients with acute illnesses.
- Long-term care facilities provide care to residents with chronic illnesses and those who need personal care.
- Subacute care is given to residents who have complex medical or rehabilitation needs.
- Skilled nursing facilities provide care to residents who are medically stable, but require daily skilled services and intervention by licensed health care professionals.
- Home care is provided to clients in their residences by qualified caregivers.
- The OBRA legislation was designed to improve the quality of life for residents of long-term care facilities. This legislation also specifies requirements for nursing assistant education.
- The health care agency, resident, nurse, and nursing assistant all benefit from nursing assistant education and certification.
- The nursing assistant is supervised by a licensed nurse.
- The interdisciplinary team is a group of caregivers who contribute to the care, health, and well-being of residents.
- The chain of command describes the lines of authority used in the health care facility for reporting information.
- Desirable qualities include a professional appearance, good personal hygiene and grooming, good personal health, responsible behavior, dependability, and good organizational skills.

REVIEW

A. Multiple Choice

Select the one best answer.

1. People with acute illnesses are usually cared for in
   a. home care.
   b. hospitals.
   c. long-term care facilities.
   d. physicians' offices.

2. The person who receives care in the long-term care facility is the
   a. client.
   b. patient.
   c. resident.
   d. invalid.

3. The OBRA legislation
   a. is concerned with improving the quality of life for residents in home health care.
   b. describes requirements for nursing assistant education.
   c. describes requirements for professional nurse education.
   d. regulates employee saftey.

4. Benefits of nursing assistant education to the health care facility include all of the following *except*
   a. allowing the nursing assistant to give medicine to residents.
   b. improving the quality of care given to residents.
   c. lowering infection rates because the nursing assistant understands how to prevent infection.
   d. improving the image of the health care facility.

5. According to the OBRA (federal) rules, the minimum number of hours of continuing education that the nursing assistant must have every year is
   a. two.
   b. four.
   c. eight.
   d. twelve.

6. Personal care is provided to residents under the supervision of the
   a. administrator.
   b. clergy.
   c. licensed nurse.
   d. social worker.

7. Your uniform should
   a. be all white.
   b. include a stethoscope.
   c. include well-fitting, comfortable shoes.
   d. identify you as a nurse.

8. Responsible behavior includes
   a. working at least three of every five days that you are scheduled.
   b. calling your facility in advance if you are unable to come to work.
   c. doing only those tasks that you want to do.
   d. not taking breaks.

9. The interdisciplinary team always includes the:
   a. resident.
   b. resident's roommate.
   c. resident's friends.
   d. resident's children.

B. True/False

Answer each statement true (T) or false (F).

10. _____ Everyone involved with the resident's care should follow the care plan.

11. _____ The resident is a member of the interdisciplinary team.

C. Fill in the Blank

Complete each sentence by adding the missing word.

12. A _____ illness is one that lasts for a long time.

13. A _____ employee is one whom residents and coworkers trust.

14. To maintain nursing assistant certification, you must work in a health care facility for pay for a specified period of time every _____ years.

15. The nursing assistant must be compassionate and _____ with residents and families.

16-20. List five members of the interdisciplinary team.

16. _____   19. _____

17. _____   20. _____

18. _____

D. Clinical Applications

Please read the following case study, then answer the questions.

The Meadows Nursing Center has three nursing assistants on the day shift on Wing A. These assistants care for 24 residents. Mary is a 26-year-old CNA. She completed her CNA class two years ago. She works two jobs and states that she "really doesn't like this work, but needs the money." Mary's resident care is fast and thorough. When she is finished caring for her residents, she often sneaks out the back door for a quick cigarette. She frequently complains of being tired and calls in sick at least once every two to four weeks. She tells her friends that she was not really sick, but was just too tired to get up for work. Kevin is 39 years old. He has been a nursing assistant for 15 years. He is well liked by the residents and staff. He is kind to residents and his care is thorough. He does extra tasks without being asked. Kevin is satisfied with his career choice and says he does not think he would be happy doing any other type of work. Lisa is 19 years old. She says she would eventually like to become a nurse. She recently completed her nursing assistant program and has been working at The Meadows for two months. She is having trouble getting all her work done by the end of the shift.

21. Does Mary demonstrate responsible behavior? Why or why not?

22. Instead of sneaking outside to smoke, what should Mary do if her assignment is complete?

23. When Kevin does extra tasks without being asked, what positive trait is he demonstrating?

24. Lisa is frustrated because she cannot get her work done by the end of the shift. What advice can you give to help her?

25. On Saturday, Lisa is assigned to care for Mrs. Straight. Mrs. Straight's daughter will be picking her up at 9:00 a.m. and taking her out for the day. The resident finishes eating breakfast at 8:15. Lisa has seven other residents to care for in her assignment. What advice can you give to help her make sure that Mrs. Straight is ready to leave when her daughter arrives?

CHAPTER 2

Working in Long-Term Care

OBJECTIVES

After reading this chapter, you will be able to:

- Spell and define key terms.
- List the aging changes that occur in each body system.
- Describe the purpose of Maslow's hierarchy of needs and explain why understanding this theory is important to the nursing assistant.
- Recognize declines in the elderly and describe the nursing assistant's role in preventing declines.
- List six general categories of nursing assistant responsibilities in the long-term care facility.
- Describe some ways to establish meaningful relationships with residents.

ELDERLY

Many patients in the hospital, long-term care facility, subacute unit, health maintenance organization, and home care setting are elderly. The elderly are like you in many ways. They have, or have had, families, jobs, homes, and status in the community. Their physical and emotional needs are similar to yours. They may be anxious or frustrated and fear the unknown, their disease, and dependence on others. A basic understanding of the aging process and needs of the elderly are essential to the success of the nursing assistant.

Common Myths and Beliefs About the Elderly

People may believe things about the elderly that are not always true. **Myths** are common beliefs that have no basis in fact. Some common myths and facts about the elderly are listed in **Table 2-1**.

THE HUMAN BODY

The human body consists of millions of *cells*. Cells are the basic building blocks of all living things, including the human body. Cells provide body growth and repair. They use food and convert it to provide energy for their functions. Living depends on the release of energy in every cell of the body. Secretions are also a function of cells. Collectively, all these functions are called body metabolism.

There are different types of cells with many specialized functions. Cells with similar functions are grouped together into four basic types of *tissues:*

- Epithelial tissues are strong tissues whose purpose is protection, secretion, absorption, diffusion, and filtration.
- Muscle tissues are responsible for voluntary and involuntary movement.
- Connective tissues are for connection, support, and protection.
- Nerve tissues are responsible for sending information to and from the brain and body parts.

Similar tissues form larger structures called *organs*. Organs work together. They do not work independently of each other. A group of organs that are needed to perform specific body functions is called a *system*. The human body has 10 systems.

TABLE 2-1	Common Myths and Facts About the Elderly
Myth	**Fact**
All elderly people become senile and confused.	Mental confusion occurs in some people, but not all. Not all elderly people become confused, and mental confusion is not a normal part of the aging process. Many people live to be quite old with their mental abilities intact.
Old people do not like to be touched.	All human beings need to be touched. Touch shows love and respect, and provides comfort to people who are in physical or mental pain.
All old people are irritable and crabby.	Everyone gets upset from time to time. The elderly get upset, too. Elderly people are not more irritable than younger people. Irritability is not determined by age.
Old people are unable to do anything for themselves.	We are all dependent on other people for certain things. The elderly may depend on others for some things, but may be able to do other things for themselves. A person's worth should not be judged by his or her degree of independence.
Old people cannot contribute anything to society.	Many elderly people have contributed a great deal to society. The elderly continue to make contributions. Many presidents of the United States were considered elderly when they were elected to office. They ran the country efficiently. Some societies value and respect the elderly because they have a lifetime of experience to share with others. The elderly can teach us many things if we take the time to listen.

AGING CHANGES

Aging begins at birth and continues throughout life. Some aging changes are visible. Others cannot be seen, but affect the functioning of the body and the way people adapt to their environment. Each system of the body has a specific function. These functions are summarized in **Table 2-2.** Every body system undergoes aging changes.

People age at different rates. Some people seem to age quickly. Others can be quite old, but remarkably healthy. The rate at which people age is determined by factors such as heredity, lifestyle, disease, nutrition, and environment.

Aging Changes in the Cardiovascular System

The cardiovascular system **(Figure 2-1)** is also called the circulatory system. It is the transportation system for the body. The cardiovascular system transports food and oxygen to every cell in the body through the bloodstream. This system consists of the heart **(Figure 2-2),** which pumps blood throughout the body, and a series of blood vessels. **Arteries** are blood vessels that carry freshly oxygenated blood to the body parts. **Veins** are the blood vessels that carry blood from the body parts back to the heart. The **immune system** is the part of the

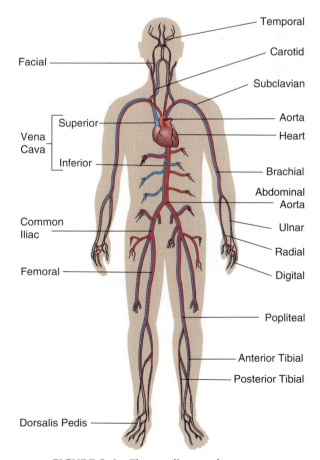

FIGURE 2-1 The cardiovascular system

TABLE 2-2 Body Systems: Components and Functions

System	Function	Organs
Cardiovascular	Carries or transports oxygen and water to the body and eliminates some forms of waste materials.	Heart, blood, arteries, veins, capillaries, spleen, lymph vessels and nodes.
Respiratory	Supplies oxygen to the body and eliminates carbon dioxide.	Lungs, nose, larynx, pharynx, trachea, bronchi.
Urinary	Elimination of liquid body wastes.	Kidneys, ureters, bladder, urethra.
Digestive	Ingestion transports food. Digestion breaks down and absorbs nutrients, and eliminates wastes.	Mouth, teeth, tongue, salivary glands, pharynx, esophagus, liver, gallbladder, stomach, small intestine, appendix, rectum, anus.
Nervous	Regulates body movement and functions. Controls all mental processes.	Brain, spinal cord, nerves.
Muscular	Allows movement of the body.	Muscles, ligaments, tendons.
Skeletal (Musculoskeletal)	Protects vital organs and gives shape and support to the body.	Bones, joints.
Integumentary	Provides protection against infection, aids in the removal of waste, and serves as a vehicle for sensory perception.	Skin, hair, nails, sweat and oil glands.
Endocrine	Produces hormones to regulate body functions (metabolic processes).	Pituitary gland, pineal gland, parathyroid gland, thyroid gland, adrenal glands, thymus glands, testes, ovaries.
Reproductive	Reproduction of the species.	Female: ovaries, uterus, fallopian tubes, vagina. Male: testes, scrotum, penis, prostate gland.

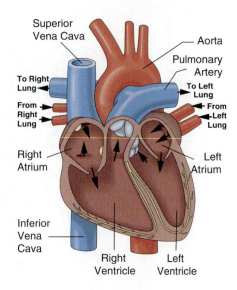

FIGURE 2-2 The heart

circulatory system that recognizes foreign germs in the body and helps fight disease.

As the body ages, the following changes occur in the cardiovascular system:

- The heart rate slows, causing a slower pulse and less efficient circulation.
- Blood vessels lose elasticity and develop calcium deposits, resulting in narrowing.
- Blood pressure increases because of changes to the walls of the blood vessels.
- It takes longer for the heart rate to return to normal after exercise.
- Veins become enlarged, causing the blood vessels near the surface of the skin to become more prominent.

Aging Changes in the Respiratory System

The respiratory system **(Figure 2-3)** consists of organs that make it possible for the body to exchange gases with the air. This exchange of

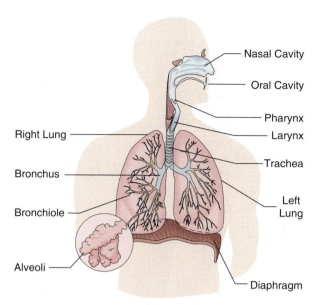

FIGURE 2-3 The respiratory system

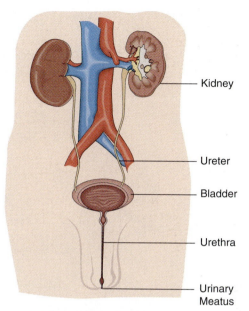

FIGURE 2-4 The urinary system

oxygen and other gases is known as respiration, or breathing. The respiratory system consists of two lungs, the nose, **larynx** or voicebox, **pharynx** or throat, **trachea** or airway, and **bronchi,** which are branches of the airway that extend into the lungs.

Aging changes in the respiratory system include:

- Lung capacity is decreased because of muscular rigidity in the lungs.
- Cough becomes less effective, allowing pooling of secretions and fluid in the lungs, increasing the risk of infection.
- Shortness of breath may occur on exertion.
- Less effective gas exchange takes place in the lungs.

Aging Changes in the Urinary System

The urinary system **(Figure 2-4)** is made up of those organs that produce urine and eliminate it from the body. This system consists of two **kidneys,** two **ureters,** or tubes leading from the kidneys to the **bladder,** one bladder, and the **urethra,** or tube that leads from the bladder to the outside of the body. Urine is produced in the kidneys and travels through the ureters to the bladder, a muscular organ where urine is stored until it is eliminated from the body through the urethra. The urinary system plays a major role in maintaining fluid balance in the body.

Aging changes in the urinary system include:

- Bladder capacity decreases, increasing the frequency of urination.

- Kidney function increases at rest, causing the elderly to get up during the night to urinate.
- Bladder muscles weaken, causing leaking of urine or inadequate emptying of the bladder.
- The **prostate gland** (a tubular gland that encircles the urethra just below the bladder in the male) frequently enlarges, increasing the frequency of urination and causing dribbling, urinary obstruction, and urinary retention.

Aging Changes in the Digestive System

The digestive system **(Figure 2-5)** begins in the mouth and extends all the way through the body to the **anus,** or external outlet of the intestines. Food is taken into the mouth and moves through the **esophagus,** or food tube, to the stomach, where it is mixed with fluids that aid in the digestion process. The food continues to move downward through the **small intestine,** the part of the intestine where digestion is completed. The food is further digested and nutrients are absorbed. The remaining food mass then moves to the **large intestine,** or lower part of the bowel, where water is absorbed. The last 6 to 8 inches of the large intestine is called the **rectum.** This area stores the food mass until it is eliminated from the body as solid waste, or **fecal material.**

Aging changes in the digestive system include:

- Saliva production in the mouth decreases, interfering with digestion of starch.
- Taste buds on the tongue decrease, beginning with sweet and salt.

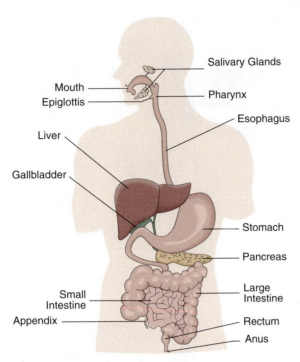

FIGURE 2-5 The digestive system

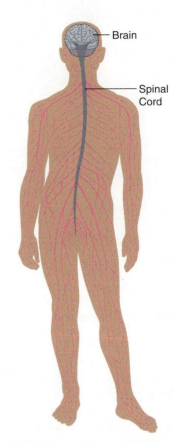

FIGURE 2-6 The nervous system

- The gag reflex in the throat is less effective, increasing the risk of choking.
- Movement of food into the stomach through the esophagus is slower.
- The stomach takes longer to empty into the small intestine, so food remains there longer.
- Fewer digestive enzymes are present in the stomach, causing indigestion and slower absorption of fat.
- Movement of the food mass through the large intestine is slower, resulting in constipation.

Aging Changes in the Nervous System

The nervous system **(Figure 2-6)** is vital to the body's ability to communicate internally, as well as with the environment. The nervous system consists of the brain **(Figure 2-7)**, spinal cord, and all the nerves in the body. Messages travel back and forth from the nerves, spinal cord, and brain. These messages control how the body functions **(Figure 2-8)**. They also tell the body how to react to environmental conditions. For example, if you touch something very hot with your hand, the nerves send a message to the brain **(Figure 2-9)**. The brain sends a message back telling you to pull your hand away.

Aging changes in the nervous system include:

- More time is needed for tasks involving speed, balance, coordination, and fine motor activities, such as those involving the fingers.

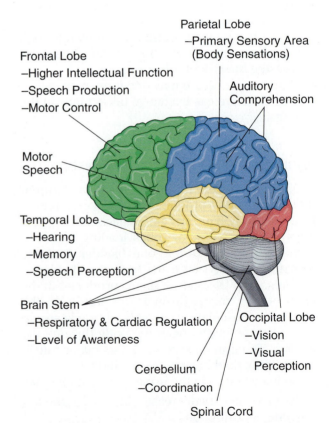

FIGURE 2-7 Functional areas of the brain

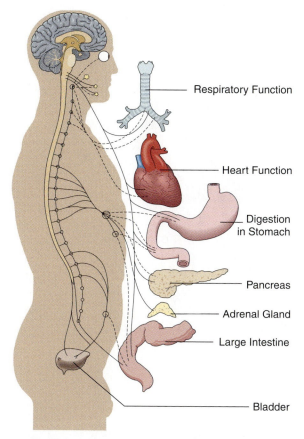

Respiratory Function

Heart Function

Digestion in Stomach

Pancreas

Adrenal Gland

Large Intestine

Bladder

FIGURE 2-8 The brain sends signals to various parts of the body to control their functions.

- Problems develop with balance and coordination as a result of deterioration of the nerve terminals that provide information to the brain on the movement and position of the body.
- The lens in the eye becomes less flexible, causing visual changes.

- Decreased secretion of fluid in the eye causes dryness and itching.
- Nerves and blood supply to the ears decrease, causing difficulty hearing.
- There is a decrease in the ability to feel pressure and temperature, resulting in higher potential for injury.
- Blood flow to the brain decreases, which may result in mental confusion and memory loss.

Aging Changes in the Musculoskeletal System

The **musculoskeletal system** actually consists of two systems, the muscular system **(Figure 2-10A)** and the skeletal system **(Figure 2-10B)**. They function together to move and protect the body and are commonly referred to together. The skeletal system consists of 206 bones; its function is support, movement, protection, blood cell formation, and calcium storage. The muscular system produces body heat, maintains posture, and permits movement.

Aging changes in the musculoskeletal system include:

- A decrease in strength, endurance, muscle tone, and reaction time is caused by loss of elasticity of muscles and decrease in muscle mass.
- Bones lose minerals, become brittle, and break more easily.
- The spine is less stable, less flexible, and more easily injured.
- Posture may become poor because of weakness in back muscles.
- **Degenerative changes,** or deterioration, occur in the joints, resulting in limited movement, stiffness, and pain.

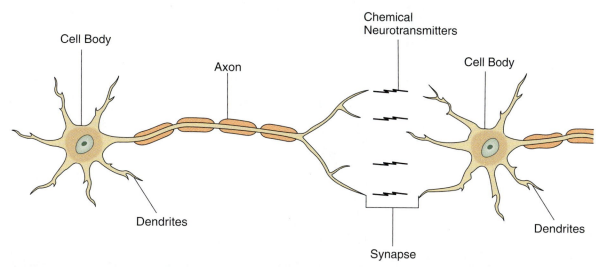

Cell Body

Axon

Chemical Neurotransmitters

Cell Body

Dendrites

Synapse

Dendrites

FIGURE 2-9 Chemicals called neurotransmitters help messages pass across the synapse from one neuron to the next.

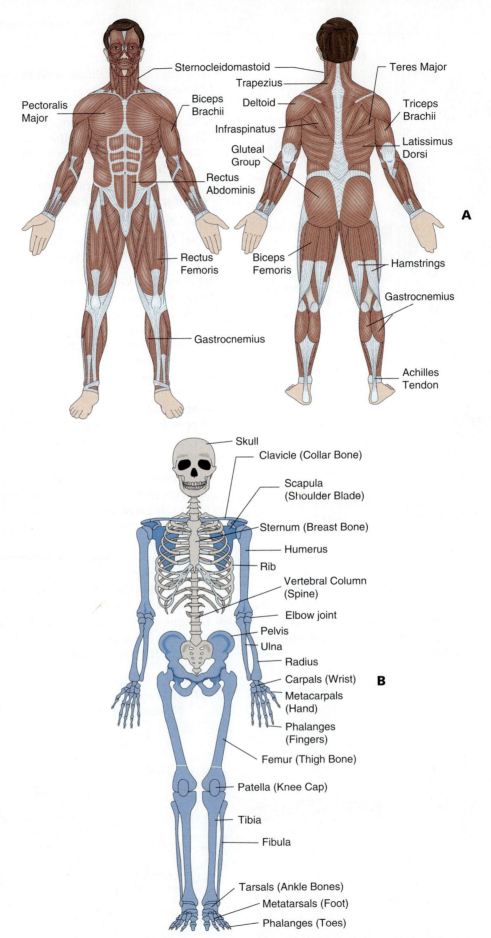

FIGURE 2-10   (A) The muscular system and (B) the skeletal system work together. They are commonly called the musculoskeletal system.

Aging Changes in the Integumentary System

The integumentary system **(Figure 2-11),** or skin system, covers the body. It consists of the skin, hair, and nails. The skin protects against infection, maintains fluid balance in the body, excretes waste products, maintains temperature, and provides sensation for the body. The skin consists of the outer layer, or **epidermis,** and a thicker, inner layer called the **dermis.** Beneath the dermis is a layer of **subcutaneous tissue,** or fat.

Aging changes in the integumentary system include:

- The skin thins and becomes less elastic; wrinkles appear, and the skin becomes irritated and breaks more easily.
- Blood vessels that nourish the skin become more fragile and break more easily, resulting in bruising, **senile purpura,** and **skin tears.** Skin tears are irregular-shaped injuries in which the top layer of the skin peels back. Senile purpura are dark purple bruises that appear on the backs of hands and forearms in the elderly.
- Blood flow in vessels that nourish the skin is reduced, resulting in slower healing.
- Oil glands that supply the skin secrete less, causing drying of the skin and itching.
- Perspiration decreases, and the body's ability to regulate temperature is impaired.
- Subcutaneous fat diminishes.
- Blood supply to the feet and legs is reduced.

- Fingernail and toenail growth slows and nails become brittle.
- Hair thins and turns gray.

Aging Changes in the Endocrine System

The endocrine system **(Figure 2-12)** produces **hormones.** The hormones are released into the bloodstream to all parts of the body. Hormones are chemical messengers responsible for growth and development, reproduction, and stress responses. They play an important role in regulating fluid and energy balance in the body.

Aging changes in the endocrine system include:

- Blood sugar level increases because of delayed release of **insulin,** a hormone that regulates sugar use in the body.
- The amount of calories needed for the body to function normally decreases because of a lower **metabolism rate,** or slower body function.

Diabetes

Diabetes is a chronic disease of the endocrine system, affecting as many as 50 percent of all elderly adults. Diabetes affects the utilization of sugar in the body. Sugar (glucose) production in the body is regulated by insulin, a hormone secreted by the pancreas. Diabetes results from a deficiency of insulin or a resistance to the effects of insulin, causing the body to be unable to properly process food into energy. As the blood sugar level rises, more insulin is secreted to regulate the sugar level in the blood. In a person with diabetes, the output or use of insulin is not adequate. The glu-

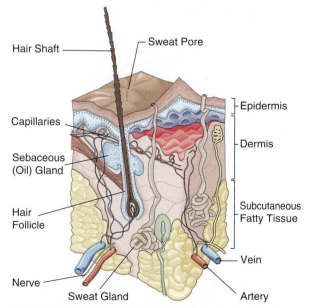

FIGURE 2-11 The skin is the largest organ in the body. It protects the underlying structures, and provides temperature regulation and elimination.

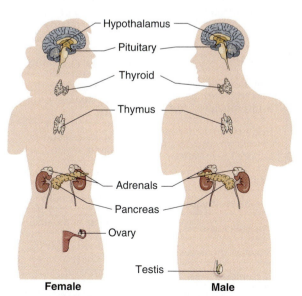

FIGURE 2-12 The endocrine system

cose from the food breakdown remains in the blood, resulting in elevated blood sugar (too much glucose in the blood). Proteins and fats are not broken down correctly. Dehydration and fluid imbalances can result. Indications that the resident has diabetes are extreme thirst, hunger, frequent urination, fatigue, itching, slow healing, infections of the skin, and changes in vision. Overweight and obesity are common. Diabetes is treated with an injection of insulin, or oral drugs that lower the blood sugar level. The resident is placed on a special diet and is not given free sugar or extra snacks. The resident's blood sugar is monitored by a finger stick test in the long-term care facility.

Complications of diabetes.   Diabetes has two very serious complications. **Hyperglycemia,** or too much sugar in the blood, occurs when there is not enough insulin to meet the body's needs. **Hypoglycemia,** or too little sugar in the blood, occurs when the blood sugar level is too low. Both of these conditions can be life threatening. Persistent elevated glucose levels affect the blood vessels and nerves, making the person with diabetes more likely to develop heart attack, stroke, blindness, renal disease, and other serious complications and conditions. If you notice signs of diabetes-related problems developing, report them to the nurse immediately. Signs and symptoms of hyperglycemia and hypoglycemia are listed in **Table 2-3.**

Aging Changes in the Reproductive System

The reproductive system consists of organs whose function is to produce a new individual. Some of the reproductive organs produce hormones. Despite aging changes, the elderly can enjoy an active sex life. Elderly men are able to father children.

The primary reproductive organs in the male **(Figure 2-13)** are the **penis,** which is the male organ used for reproduction and urinary elimination, and the **scrotum,** a small ovoid pouch containing the **testes.** The testes produce **sperm** for reproduction, and male hormones.

Aging changes in the male reproductive system include:

- Hormone production decreases, causing decreased size of testes and a lower sperm count.
- More time is needed for an erection to occur.

The main reproductive organs in the female **(Figure 2-14)** are two **ovaries,** glands that produce hormones and eggs for reproduction; the **uterus,** the organ where a baby grows and receives nourishment; the **vagina,** or birth canal; and the **vulva,** or **external genitalia (Figure 2-15).** The breasts are also part of the female reproductive system.

TABLE 2-3 Signs and Symptoms	
Hyperglycemia	**Hypoglycemia**
Nausea, vomiting	Complaints of hunger, weakness, dizziness, shakiness
Weakness	
Headache	Cold, moist, clammy, or pale skin
Full, bounding pulse	
Fruity smell to breath	Rapid, shallow respirations
Hot, dry, flushed skin	Nervousness and excitement
Labored respirations	
Drowsiness	Rapid pulse
Mental confusion	Unconsciousness
Unconsciousness	No sugar in the urine
Sugar in the urine	Low blood sugar by finger stick
High blood sugar by finger stick	

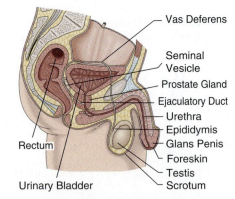

FIGURE 2-13   The male genitourinary system

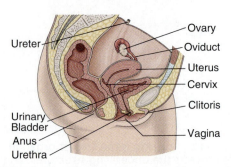

FIGURE 2-14   The female genitourinary system

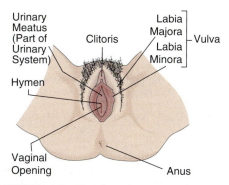

FIGURE 2-15 The female external genitalia

Aging changes in the female reproductive system include:

- Fewer female hormones are produced.
- Menstruation stops.
- The vagina becomes shorter and narrower.
- Vaginal secretions decrease.
- Breast tissue decreases and the muscles supporting the breasts weaken.

Effects of Aging Changes on Functional Status

Normal changes of aging affect the way the human body functions. You must look at each resident holistically. This means to look at the entire person and realize that something that affects one part or system affects the person as a whole. Aging changes in vision and hearing may cause the resident to feel confused and disoriented. Some aging changes cause the resident to feel a loss of control and loss of self-care ability. Changes in the environment may cause confusion, changes in behavior, feelings of loss of control, stress, and sleep disturbances. An acute illness may cause mental confusion, changes in behavior, and loss of self-esteem. The nursing assistant must understand that these changes are beyond the resident's control and help the resident adapt to them as much as possible.

COMMON DISEASES IN LONG-TERM CARE FACILITY RESIDENTS

Because of aging changes, elderly residents are at greater risk of developing chronic diseases. These diseases require a change in lifestyle and a period of time to mentally adjust. Presence of one or more chronic conditions can be frustrat-

ing. In some cases, the diseases make self-care difficult or impossible. Many chronic diseases cause pain, fatigue, or immobility, and limit activity. Some interfere with sexual function. A list of common diseases and conditions in elderly long-term care residents is found in **Table 2-4.**

BASIC HUMAN NEEDS

The nursing assistant has a very important responsibility in helping residents meet their needs. When the resident's needs are not met, you may notice a change in behavior. When needs on a lower level are not met, you will notice physical problems. For example, if the resident needs food and fluids, he or she may be weak and tired. When needs on a higher level are not met, you may notice anger, withdrawal, or other behavior problems. Your care and observations are important to the success of the resident and all team members in meeting the care plan goals. Understanding the nature of human needs will enable you to assist residents in meeting their needs.

The care plan uses a holistic approach and is designed to meet the resident's physical and psychological needs. The interdisciplinary team establishes approaches for all caregivers to use to help residents meet their care plan goals. The team meets periodically to reevaluate whether the resident has met or is making progress toward the goals. You will be required to assist residents to meet needs on many different levels. As the resident's condition improves, he or she will begin to meet more needs on his or her own. This provides a sense of self-satisfaction and accomplishment that aids in meeting psychological needs. Residents who are totally dependent on others for their physical care can still derive mental satisfaction from being in control of their care and making decisions about their routines.

Maslow's Hierarchy of Needs

A psychologist named Abraham Maslow proposed a widely accepted theory about human nature. The theory is based on the belief that all human beings are innately good, and centers around self-actualization. Maslow's theory states that self-actualization, or realizing one's full potential, is the goal of life. If something blocks the path to achieving this goal, the individual becomes frustrated. Normal, healthy development enables people to actualize their own

TABLE 2-4   Common Diseases/Conditions in Elderly Long-Term Care Residents

Disease or Condition	Description
Alzheimer's Disease	A progressive disease of brain cells in which the resident loses mental and physical ability. The disease is incurable and ends in death.
Amputation	Removal of an extremity. Amputation is usually performed because of diabetes, vascular disease, trauma, or gangrene.
Arteriosclerosis	A narrowing of the inside walls of the arteries that makes them rigid and thick. Adequate blood flow cannot pass through the vessel walls to nourish the body. High blood pressure is common because the heart has to work harder to force blood through the blocked vessels. Residents are at high risk of stroke and heart attack.
Arthritis	A painful inflammation of joints that results in limited movement, swelling, and deformities.
Atherosclerosis	A buildup of plaque, calcium, and fat on the walls of the arteries, which makes them rigid and thick. Adequate blood flow cannot pass through the vessel walls to nourish the body. High blood pressure is common because the heart has to work harder to force blood through the narrow vessels. Residents are at high risk of stroke and heart attack.
Cancer	A malignant tumor or new growth anywhere in the body. Cancer may spread slowly or rapidly.
Cerebrovascular Accident (CVA, Brain Attack, or Stroke)	An incident in the brain caused by a blood clot or bursting of blood vessels, allowing blood to spill out into the brain cavity. Common effects of a stroke are paralysis on one side of the body, loss of bowel and bladder control, and speech impairments. The effects may be temporary or permanent.
Congestive Heart Failure	A condition in which the heart is unable to pump sufficient blood to meet the needs of the body. Characterized by high blood pressure and fluid retention.
Diabetes Mellitus	A disorder of the endocrine system in which the body cannot metabolize carbohydrates, proteins, and fat properly.
Emphysema	A disorder in which the air sacs of the lungs have stretched and lost their elasticity, causing them to be unable to contract to remove excess air.
Head Injury	An injury to the brain that results from falls or trauma. Head injuries may affect mental function, physical function, or both. In the elderly, the effects are often permanent because of brain damage.
Hearing Impairment	Difficulty hearing from a number of causes. Impairment may range from being hard of hearing to complete deafness. Some residents may benefit from use of a hearing aid.
Heart Attack (Myocardial Infarction)	A serious medical emergency in which the blood vessels that nourish the heart muscle are blocked or burst, disrupting the normal flow of blood through the heart.
Heart Block	A condition that may require a pacemaker for treatment. Caused by a disruption in the electrical conduction of the heart in which the heart's own internal pacemaker does not beat regularly.
Hip Fracture	A broken hip that is usually the result of a fall but can result from trauma (such as an auto accident) or osteoporosis. The hip must be repaired surgically or by using traction to enable the resident to walk again. This is a serious injury, and there is a known relationship between hip fracture and mortality in the elderly.
Hip Replacement	Removal of the entire hip joint and replacement with a synthetic joint. The resident usually requires skilled therapy and restorative nursing after surgery to enable him or her to return to the former level of function.

Continues

TABLE 2-4 Common Diseases/Conditions in Elderly Long-Term Care Residents, *Continued*

Disease or Condition	Description
Huntington's Disease	A progressive, hereditary disease that results in rapid, involuntary movements and progressive dementia.
Hypertension	High blood pressure. The resident may have no symptoms, or may develop dizziness, headaches, and fatigue. Serious complications can result if hypertension is not treated.
Multiple Sclerosis	A chronic, progressive disease marked by intermittent periods of remission. The resident has loss of muscle control, weakness, incoordination, and speech, visual, and sensory disturbances.
Paraplegia	Paralysis below the waist. The condition is usually caused by trauma, but can be caused by tumors and other conditions.
Parkinson's Disease	A neurological disorder that results in tremors, muscular rigidity, and a shuffling gait.
Peripheral Artery Disease	A condition caused by atherosclerosis that results in insufficient blood flow to the legs. It may result in leg ulcers or necessitate amputation.
Peripheral Vascular Disease	A disorder that is frequently the result of varicose veins. Blood return from the legs is not adequate. The condition commonly results in blood clots and leg ulcers.
Pneumonia and Influenza	Serious infections of the lungs contracted by the droplet method of transmission.
Quadriplegia	Paralysis below the neck. The usual cause is trauma, but can result from tumors, infection, and other conditions.
Transient Ischemic Attack (TIA)	A temporary period of diminished blood flow to the brain. An attack occurs suddenly and usually lasts from 2 to 15 minutes, although it may last longer. Signs and symptoms are similar to those of a stroke but are reversible and temporary. Persons who experience TIA's are at high risk for strokes.
Vision Impairment	Difficulty seeing, caused by any one of a number of causes. Sometimes vision can be improved with glasses or surgery. In some disorders, vision cannot be restored.

true nature and realize their full potential. Aggressive behavior may result from frustration because the individual's needs are not met.

Maslow writes that all human beings have the same basic needs. **Maslow's hierarchy of needs** is shown in **Figure 2-16.** The most basic needs are at the bottom of the figure. The needs at one level must be satisfied before the needs at the next level become important. The most urgent needs are the physical needs that are important for survival. As the physical needs are met, the psychological needs become important. Psychological needs must be met for a person to be emotionally healthy. Maslow believes that as more needs are fulfilled, the quality of a person's life improves.

Physiological needs. Basic physical needs for survival are at the bottom of the Maslow hierarchy. They include the need for food, water, sleep, rest, physical activity, elimination, and oxygen. When these needs are met, needs at the next level become important. We may take these

things for granted, but some residents may have diseases or conditions that make it difficult to meet the needs on this level. Think about the resident who is struggling to breathe. The resident is using all of his or her energy to fulfill this one

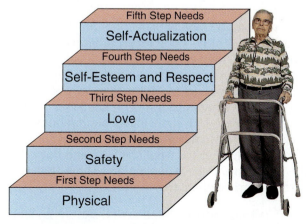

FIGURE 2-16 Maslow's hierarchy of needs

basic need. Until the resident's breathing problem is resolved, other needs are not important.

Safety and security needs. When the resident's basic survival needs are met, safety and security become important. The resident must feel safe and protected from harm in the environment. The resident must also feel personal security in his or her family and relationships. Financial security is important. If the illness causes the resident to worry about how he or she will pay the medical bills, the resident's security needs are not met. The social worker and other team members may be called to assist in meeting these needs.

Love and belonging needs. You will notice that the first two levels of Maslow's hierarchy involve physical needs. After physical needs are satisfied, emotional needs become important. The most basic emotional need is the need to give love and receive love from others. If the resident has a strong family unit, this will help meet the need for love. The nursing assistant also helps to meet this need by showing a sincere interest in the resident. Show the resident that you care and accept him or her, regardless of disability, condition, appearance, or behavior. Providing privacy during care, treatments, and procedures, and respecting the resident's dignity will also help you to meet this need.

Self-esteem. Everyone has the need to feel important and worthwhile. Our self-esteem involves the mental image of ourselves that we believe we project to others. Residents may respond negatively when they feel their self-images are threatened. They may not know or understand why they feel this way. Often they are reacting out of fear. A resident who has had a body part, such as a breast, removed may believe that she is ugly and disfigured. This has a negative effect on self-esteem. She may be angry and complain about your care and many other things. The resident is not mad at you. She is upset about her situation. She is afraid of how she looks, what will happen to her, and how she will manage. This threat to her self-esteem makes her react with anger. Other residents may react in different ways. Assist the resident with her appearance. If she looks attractive **(Figure 2-17)**, she will feel better about herself. Allow her to talk about what is bothering her. Do not judge her for what she says and does. Be aware of what she is feeling and show that you are concerned about her.

Self-actualization. Self-actualization is feeling a sense of accomplishment and success. You

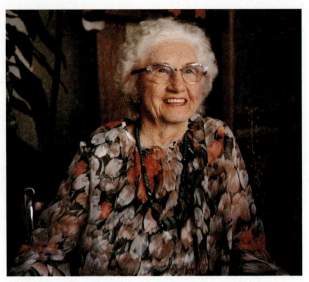

FIGURE 2-17 Assisting residents to maintain an attractive appearance is an important nursing assistant responsibility.

can help the resident meet this need by recognizing improvements and assisting him or her to return to self-care. Sincerely compliment residents for these accomplishments. If the resident feels that he or she is overcoming a disease or disability, this will promote self-actualization.

OBRA REQUIREMENTS

The OBRA law requires facilities to maintain or improve the resident's condition. Declines are deteriorations in condition that are not allowed unless they are medically unavoidable. The resident's condition is assessed on admission by licensed facility staff, and a record is made of this assessment. The facility is expected to maintain or improve the resident's condition compared with how the resident was at the time of admission. For example, if the skin was free from injury on admission, the facility is expected to keep the skin free from injury. If the skin was injured at the time of admission, the facility is expected to take steps to heal the injured area. Although this is a simple example, it is important to remember that the resident should not have declines in any area of life.

The long-term care facility must help the resident function at the highest level possible for his or her individual situation. To do this, long-term care facilities use a written tool developed by the government to assess residents. This tool is called the Minimum Data Set 2.0 (MDS), part of which is shown in **Figure 2-18**. Risk

SECTION D. VISION PATTERNS

1.	VISION	(Ability to see in adequate light and with glasses if used) 0. *ADEQUATE*—sees fine detail, including regular print in newspapers/books 1. *IMPAIRED*—sees large print, but not regular print in newspapers/books 2. *MODERATELY IMPAIRED*—limited vision; not able to see newspaper headlines, but can identify objects 3. *HIGHLY IMPAIRED*—object identification in question, but eyes appear to follow objects 4. *SEVERELY IMPAIRED*—no vision or sees only light, colors, or shapes; eyes do not appear to follow objects	
2.	VISUAL LIMITATIONS/ DIFFICULTIES	Side vision problems—decreased peripheral vision (e.g., leaves food on one side of tray, difficulty traveling, bumps into people and objects, misjudges placement of chair when seating self)	a.
		Experiences any of following: sees halos or rings around lights; sees flashes of light; sees "curtains" over eyes	b.
		NONE OF ABOVE	c.
3.	VISUAL APPLIANCES	Glasses; contact lenses; magnifying glass 0. No 1. Yes	

SECTION E. MOOD AND BEHAVIOR PATTERNS

1.	INDICATORS OF DEPRES- SION, ANXIETY, SAD MOOD	(*Code for indicators observed in last 30 days, irrespective of the assumed cause*) 0. Indicator not exhibited in last 30 days 1. Indicator of this type exhibited up to five days a week 2. Indicator of this type exhibited daily or almost daily (6, 7 days a week)				

VERBAL EXPRESSIONS OF DISTRESS

a. Resident made negative statements—e.g., *"Nothing matters; Would rather be dead; What's the use; Regrets having lived so long; Let me die"*

b. Repetitive questions—e.g., *"Where do I go; What do I do?"*

c. Repetitive verbalizations— e.g., calling out for help, (*"God help me"*)

d. Persistent anger with self or others—e.g., easily annoyed, anger at placement in nursing home; anger at care received

e. Self deprecation—e.g., *"I am nothing; I am of no use to anyone"*

f. Expressions of what appear to be unrealistic fears—e.g., fear of being abandoned, left alone, being with others

g. Recurrent statements that something terrible is about to happen—e.g., believes he or she is about to die, have a heart attack

h. Repetitive health complaints—e.g., persistently seeks medical attention, obsessive concern with body functions

i. Repetitive anxious complaints/concerns (non-health related) e.g., persistently seeks attention/reassurance regarding schedules, meals, laundry, clothing, relationship issues

SLEEP-CYCLE ISSUES

j. Unpleasant mood in morning

k. Insomnia/change in usual sleep pattern

SAD, APATHETIC, ANXIOUS APPEARANCE

l. Sad, pained, worried facial expressions—e.g., furrowed brows

m. Crying, tearfulness

n. Repetitive physical movements—e.g., pacing, hand wringing, restlessness, fidgeting, picking

LOSS OF INTEREST

o. Withdrawal from activities of interest—e.g., no interest in long standing activities or being with family/friends

p. Reduced social interaction

2.	MOOD PERSIS- TENCE	**One or more indicators** of depressed, sad or anxious mood **were not easily altered by attempts to "cheer up", console, or reassure the resident over last 7 days** 0. No mood indicators 1. Indicators present, easily altered 2. Indicators present, not easily altered	
3.	CHANGE IN MOOD	Resident's mood status has changed as compared to status of **90 days ago** (or since last assessment if less than 90 days) 0. No change 1. Improved 2. Deteriorated	

4.	BEHAVIORAL SYMPTOMS	(A) *Behavioral symptom frequency in last 7 days*
		    0. Behavior not exhibited in last 7 days
		    1. Behavior of this type occurred 1 to 3 days in last 7 days
		    2. Behavior of this type occurred 4 to 6 days, but less than daily
		    3. Behavior of this type occurred daily
		
		(B) *Behavioral symptom alterability in last 7 days*
		    0. Behavior not present OR behavior was easily altered
		    1. Behavior was not easily altered
			(A)	(B)

		a. WANDERING (moved with no rational purpose, seemingly oblivious to needs or safety)		
		b. VERBALLY ABUSIVE BEHAVIORAL SYMPTOMS (others were threatened, screamed at, cursed at)		
		c. PHYSICALLY ABUSIVE BEHAVIORAL SYMPTOMS (others were hit, shoved, scratched, sexually abused)		
		d. SOCIALLY INAPPROPRIATE/DISRUPTIVE BEHAVIORAL SYMPTOMS (made disruptive sounds, noisiness, screaming, self-abusive acts, sexual behavior or disrobing in public, smeared/threw food/feces, hoarding, rummaged through others' belongings)		
		e. RESISTS CARE (resisted taking medications/ injections, ADL assistance, or eating)		

5.	CHANGE IN BEHAVIORAL SYMPTOMS	Resident's behavior status has changed as compared to **status of 90 days ago** (or since last assessment if less than 90 days) 0. No change 1. Improved 2. Deteriorated	

SECTION F. PSYCHOSOCIAL WELL-BEING

1.	SENSE OF INITIATIVE/ INVOLVE- MENT	At ease interacting with others	a.
		At ease doing planned or structured activities	b.
		At ease doing self-initiated activities	c.
		Establishes own goals	d.
		Pursues involvement in life of facility (e.g., makes/keeps friends; involved in group activities; responds positively to new activities; assists at religious services)	e.
		Accepts invitations into most group activities	f.
		NONE OF ABOVE	g.
2.	UNSETTLED RELATION- SHIPS	Covert/open conflict with or repeated criticism of staff	a.
		Unhappy with roommate	b.
		Unhappy with residents other than roommate	c.
		Openly expresses conflict/anger with family/friends	d.
		Absence of personal contact with family/friends	e.
		Recent loss of close family member/friend	f.
		Does not adjust easily to change in routines	g.
		NONE OF ABOVE	h.
3.	PAST ROLES	Strong identification with past roles and life status	a.
		Expresses sadness/anger/empty feeling over lost roles/status	b.
		Resident perceives that daily routine (customary routine, activities) is very different from prior pattern in the community	c.
		NONE OF ABOVE	d.

SECTION G. PHYSICAL FUNCTIONING AND STRUCTURAL PROBLEMS

1.	(A) ADL SELF-PERFORMANCE—(*Code for resident's PERFORMANCE OVER ALL SHIFTS during last 7 days—Not including setup*) 0. *INDEPENDENT*—No help or oversight —OR— Help/oversight provided only 1 or 2 times during last 7 days 1. *SUPERVISION*—Oversight, encouragement or cueing provided 3 or more times during last 7 days —OR— Supervision (3 or more times) plus physical assistance provided only 1 or 2 times during last 7 days 2. *LIMITED ASSISTANCE*—Resident highly involved in activity; received physical help in guided maneuvering of limbs or other nonweight bearing assistance 3 or more times — OR—More help provided only 1 or 2 times during last 7 days 3. *EXTENSIVE ASSISTANCE*—While resident performed part of activity, over last 7-day period, help of following type(s) provided 3 or more times: — Weight-bearing support — Full staff performance during part (but not all) of last 7 days 4. *TOTAL DEPENDENCE*—Full staff performance of activity during entire 7 days 8. *ACTIVITY DID NOT OCCUR* during entire 7 days

			(A)	(B)
	(B) ADL SUPPORT PROVIDED—(*Code for MOST SUPPORT PROVIDED OVER ALL SHIFTS during last 7 days; code regardless of resident's self-performance classification*) 0. No setup or physical help from staff 1. Setup help only 2. One person physical assist 8. ADL activity itself did not 3. Two+ persons physical assist occur during entire 7 days		SELF-PERF	SUPPORT
a.	BED MOBILITY	How resident moves to and from lying position, turns side to side, and positions body while in bed		
b.	TRANSFER	How resident moves between surfaces—to/from: bed, chair, wheelchair, standing position (EXCLUDE to/from bath/toilet)		
c.	WALK IN ROOM	How resident walks between locations in his/her room		
d.	WALK IN CORRIDOR	How resident walks in corridor on unit		
e.	LOCOMO- TION ON UNIT	How resident moves between locations in his/her room and adjacent corridor on same floor. If in wheelchair, self-sufficiency once in chair		
f.	LOCOMO- TION OFF UNIT	How resident moves to and returns from off unit locations (e.g., areas set aside for dining, activities, or treatments). **If facility has only one floor,** how resident moves to and from distant areas on the floor. If in wheelchair, self-sufficiency once in chair		
g.	DRESSING	How resident puts on, fastens, and takes off all items of **street clothing,** including donning/removing prosthesis		
h.	EATING	How resident eats and drinks (regardless of skill). Includes intake of nourishment by other means (e.g., tube feeding, total parenteral nutrition)		
i.	TOILET USE	How resident uses the toilet room (or commode, bedpan, urinal); transfer on/off toilet, cleanses, changes pad, manages ostomy or catheter, adjusts clothes		
j.	PERSONAL HYGIENE	How resident maintains personal hygiene, including combing hair, brushing teeth, shaving, applying makeup, washing/drying face, hands, and perineum (EXCLUDE baths and showers)		

FIGURE 2-18 The Minimum Data Set is an important assessment tool used to evaluate the residents' most common problems and needs. (Page 2 is shown.)

factors are conditions that could cause the resident's health to worsen. The MDS assists facility personnel in identifying risk factors in advance, so a plan of care can be developed to prevent the resident's condition from worsening. For example, a resident who is in bed all the time is at risk of skin breakdown and other problems. If the resident does not have bowel and bladder control, the risk of skin problems increases. The MDS identifies the resident's risk of skin breakdown, and the facility is expected to take steps to prevent it. The MDS is the basic assessment on which the care plan is built. However, additional assessment tools may also be used, and many factors are considered when planning resident care. When the interdisciplinary team reevaluates the resident's care plan goals, they will look for signs of decline and plan ways to avoid them. Declines will be addressed in other chapters of the book, but understanding what declines are and how to prevent them is important. Preventing declines is a good practice in all health care settings.

The OBRA laws require caregivers to look at the resident in the long-term care facility holistically. We are not to look at the medical problems alone. Needs in one area of life can affect the resident's entire life and well-being. For example, a resident may need help to overcome problems with sadness and depression. If this need is not met, the resident may stop eating, refuse therapy, and eventually give up on living entirely. Many people can be taught to use their own strengths to meet their needs.

THE LONG-TERM CARE FACILITY

Long-term care facilities employ many nursing assistants. Some long-term facilities provide general care to all types of residents with chronic diseases and personal care needs. Some facilities offer care to residents with special needs, such as those with Alzheimer's disease, or those who depend on ventilators and other special equipment.

Long-term care facilities are regulated and inspected by government agencies. Agency representatives visit the facility unannounced to inspect resident care and facility cleanliness. Facilities that are not in compliance with the law must pay penalties and fines according to the nature and severity of the problems surveyors observe. The nursing assistant has an important responsibility to follow all laws, rules, and facility policies. If you follow facility policies and do your job in the way that you were taught, you will stay in compliance with the law.

Skilled nursing units in hospitals must follow the same laws as long-term care facilities. They follow requirements listed in the OBRA legislation. Inspections in hospital skilled units are done by state or federal surveyors who use the same survey tool that is completed in long-term care facilities. The survey process is discussed in detail in Chapter 24.

Types of Residents in Long-Term Care Facilities

Long-term care facilities are home for many types of residents. Some will spend the rest of their lives in the facility. Others come to the facility for a short time for rehabilitation and restoration, which help residents regain strength after an acute illness or injury. These residents then return to their own homes or a less intensive care setting. Regardless of discharge plans, remember that the quality of the resident's life is as important as the length of the resident's life. As a nursing assistant, you should try to give all residents the highest quality of life possible.

All humans have developmental tasks that must be completed throughout each stage of life. These are intellectual, social, and emotional skills that a person must master at a certain age level. The tasks are simple in early childhood, and become more complex as a person ages. Developmental tasks are described in **Table 2-5.** Residents in the long-term care facility, like everyone else, have developmental tasks that they must complete while living in the nursing facility.

Geriatrics. Many residents in the long-term care facility are *geriatric*, or elderly. Geriatrics refers to the care of the elderly. Some residents of long-term care facilities have a physical or mental condition, or disability, that prevents them from taking care of themselves in the community.

Residents who are mentally retarded. Some residents may be mentally retarded. These residents have lower-than-average intelligence that prevents them from caring for themselves or living independently. Most can learn new things, but learning may take a long time.

Residents with developmental disability. Some residents have a developmental disability. People with a developmental disability developed this condition before the age of 22. They may have a physical impairment, mental impair-

Age	Stage of Development	Developmental Tasks
Birth to 1 Year	Infant	Learns to trust self and others
Toddler	1–3 years	Learns to differentiate self from other people
Preschool	3–5 years	Develops initiative and is able to plan and initiate tasks
School Age	6–11 years	Develops physical and mental ability; develops relationships with others
Adolescence	12–18 years	Develops a sense of identity and sexuality
Young Adulthood	19–25 years	Establishes intimate relationships with a spouse or significant other
Middle Adulthood	26–50 years	Self-realization in marriage and family, establishes a career
Late Adulthood	51–65 years	Adjusts to the aging process, helps adult children
Old Age	65+ years	Critical review of the events and circumstances of life, develops feelings of fulfillment, acceptance, and self-worth

TABLE 2-5 Developmental Tasks

ment, or a combination of both. Individuals with mental retardation or developmental disabilities may not be admitted to skilled nursing facilities unless their medical needs require skilled nursing care. If they do not require skilled care, they are usually admitted to special facilities that provide services to meet their highly individual needs and teach skills to make them as independent as possible.

Young and middle-aged adults. Not all residents in the long-term care facility are elderly. Some are young and middle-aged adults who have chronic diseases or have suffered severe trauma and cannot live independently. Still others have infectious diseases, such as AIDS.

Making the transition from living in the community to life in a long-term care facility may be very difficult for this population. Over the course of a lifetime, our experiences teach us flexibility. Elderly individuals gradually learn to cope with losses of friends, family, and health. They understand the vulnerability that comes with age and chronic illness, although they do not necessarily like it. Younger residents do not always have the benefit of learning to cope with losses gradually. Many are admitted into the facility as a result of sudden illness or trauma. They have not had a lifetime to adjust to their losses. They are often learning to accept and cope with their physical losses at the same time they are trying to adjust to living in a facility. They may fear what the

future holds for them. This is a difficult and frustrating time for the resident. They may view staff as their peer group because they are closer in age than the geriatric residents. By empathizing with the resident and understanding the frustration he or she feels, the nursing assistant can help to make the transition easier.

Infants and children. Some specialized long-term care facilities care for infants and young children. The laws vary among the states with regard to children in nursing facilities. Some facilities are licensed strictly for children. In other facilities, children are mixed into the adult population.

INFANTS, CHILDREN, YOUNG, AND MIDDLE–AGED ADULTS IN THE LONG-TERM CARE FACILITY

Some long-term care facilities have a mixed population, with residents of all ages. It is very difficult for facility staff to meet the needs of all age groups at the same time. Each group has different needs. Young individuals admitted to long-term care must complete the developmental tasks for their age group while they are residents of the facility. If they fail to complete the developmental tasks because of illness or facility admission, their emotional growth slows or stops at the point where it was before their illness.

Long-term care facilities that accept younger residents find they must adapt their activity programs to the needs of the younger population. The videotapes that the geriatric residents watch are of no interest to children and younger adults. More out-of-facility shopping trips and outings are often planned. The menu must be adapted to meet the nutritional needs and preferences of younger residents. Children and young and middle-aged adults may want yogurt, pizza, tacos, or Chinese stir-fry recipes. These foods are not normally on the nursing home menu. However, younger populations want and need the same foods they would eat if they were living in the community. They may also need larger portions than the geriatric residents. This population also looks for the same social and intellectual stimulation they had in the community.

Infants and Children

Children are often admitted to the long-term care facility as a result of problems occurring at birth or in early childhood. They often have complex medical problems and needs. Children in long-term care facilities attend school, if they are able. Infants and children must be able to trust the people who care for them. They will develop a sense of autonomy from reassurance and support. Understanding what these tasks are and helping children achieve them is an important responsibility.

Young Adults

Young adults are commonly admitted to the long-term care facility because of trauma and severe injuries. They may feel a sense of great loss when they are admitted to long-term care. Their lives have been disrupted. Their relationships frequently fall apart, which is emotionally trying. Friends and loved ones go on with their lives, leaving the young adult resident behind. Behavior problems, including drug and alcohol abuse, are not uncommon in this age group. Young adult residents are in the same age group as many of the staff members. They attempt to form relationships with staff that are not always healthy. They are frequently manipulative and play staff members against each other, because their coping skills are not well developed. The manipulation often causes them to be labeled as "problem residents." Their behavior often interferes with their care. Young adult residents often feel misplaced in the long-term care facility because there are very few residents in their age group.

Middle-Aged Adults

Middle-aged adults are commonly admitted to the long-term care facility as a result of chronic illnesses, such as multiple sclerosis. Middle-aged adults often are in the prime of their lives and careers. They have great worries about their children's education and their families' security and future. They are often frustrated by the effects of their illnesses, and feel a great sense of loss. Spouses may feel guilty over placing their loved ones in a nursing facility. They may distance themselves, visiting less often and for shorter periods of time. They may have difficulty managing their homes and families alone. Some become lonely and seek other companionship. The emotional effects of the injury or illness and separation can be devastating to both the resident and the spouse.

Helping Special Resident Populations

Meeting the needs of special populations in the facility is not difficult. The most important thing to remember is that not all residents fit into one mold. All are individuals, with both physical and emotional needs. Staff must be realistic about the resident's conditions and abilities. Avoid becoming friends with residents. Viewing them as friends causes you to lose objectivity as a caregiver and may violate professional ethics. Likewise, avoid viewing yourself as a savior of the residents. Many will not get better. They may spend their lives in a facility. Your personal goal should be to contribute to providing the highest possible quality of life for each resident in your assignment. Because we are all different, what constitutes quality of life will vary with the individual. Follow the care plan and strive to give personalized care that meets each resident's needs.

Infants and Children. The nursing assistant who provides long-term care to infants and children should strive to keep routines as normal, consistent, and secure as possible for the child. Children often fear separation from their parents. Facility staff become parent figures to the child. Staff must not get so caught up in physical caregiving that they forget about the child's emotional needs. Helping the youngest residents to live as normally as possible and master their developmental tasks are important goals.

Young and Middle-Aged Adults. Adjusting to life in a long-term care facility may be difficult for young and middle-aged adults. These residents often prefer to stay up late at night, then sleep in the morning. Many elderly residents prefer to live by the adage, "early to bed, early to rise." The movies, music, food, and television shows that young adults prefer are different from those enjoyed by the geriatric age group. Young and middle-aged residents cannot relate to residents with dementia.

The interdisciplinary team will involve residents in developing their plans of care. If the resident establishes and agrees to the goals, he or she is more likely to work toward meeting them. Give residents as much control over their daily routines as possible. Make eye contact and use good communication skills. Avoid labeling the resident as a "behavior problem" or "uncooperative." Show the resident that he or she can depend on you. If a resident will not cooperate, ask if there would be a better time. Or say, "I want to give you the care you need, but cannot do so if you call me names. I will return in five minutes." When you leave the room, inform the nurse of the problem and your actions. When you return, start fresh and forget the problems that occurred previously. Set limits on the resident's behavior. Compliment the resident for positive behavior.

RESPONSIBILITIES OF THE NURSING ASSISTANT

The nursing assistant is an important member of the health care team. You will spend more time with residents than any other caregiver and perform many valuable services to assist residents and other team members.

Responsibilities for Providing Personal Care

You will help residents with bathing, personal hygiene, and grooming. You may need to help residents with dressing and undressing. Some residents may need assistance turning and positioning in bed or moving from one place to another. Some require help with toileting and elimination needs.

Providing Food Service and Mealtime Assistance

An important responsibility of the nursing assistant is to provide food and fluids. You are responsible for delivering food trays, special supplements, and snacks. There may be times when you will help residents eat, or even feed them.

You are also responsible for passing fresh drinking water and encouraging residents to drink enough liquid.

Caring for the Resident's Unit and Belongings

The resident's room is called the **unit.** The unit consists of a bed, chair, overbed table, nightstand, dresser, wastebasket, and closet. You are responsible for keeping the unit tidy and safe. You will make beds and handle the residents' clothing and belongings. Treating personal items with care shows respect for the residents. Many residents bring only their most important possessions with them to the health care facility. It is your responsibility to see that these items are kept safe.

Observation and Reporting

A very important responsibility of the nursing assistant is to make observations of resident conditions and report changes to the nurse. The nursing assistant spends more time with the resident than any other caregiver. This puts you in an ideal position to get to know how the resident is most of the time. Because of this close contact, you may be the first person to recognize a variation from the resident's normal condition. All changes, even if they seem minor, may be important and should be reported to the nurse. Observation and reporting are discussed in detail in Chapter 7.

Caring for Equipment and Supplies

Many different pieces of equipment are used in the health care facility. Some are used once and thrown away. Others are used for one resident only. Some pieces of equipment are used for many residents. They are cleaned and disinfected after each use. You will learn how to safely care for and use the equipment found in the health care facility. Take this responsibility very seriously.

Recordkeeping, Communication, and Messenger Duties

We communicate in many different ways in the health care facility. These will be discussed in more detail in Chapter 6. You will be responsible for keeping accurate records in writing and for communicating information to others verbally.

You will report changes in resident condition to your supervisor. There will be times when you will be asked to inform other departments and staff members of pertinent information.

RELATIONSHIPS WITH RESIDENTS

Learning how to establish meaningful relationships with residents is important. Always be kind, empathetic, and professional with residents. Health care workers must always be **tactful,** or considerate and thoughtful, with residents and families. Find ways to control your emotions if you are angry or upset. Allow residents to express their thoughts, feelings, and emotions without judging them. Try to understand the residents' concerns, even if you do not agree with them. Do not criticize residents to other staff members. Avoid criticizing your coworkers to residents. Leave your personal problems at home, and do not discuss them with residents.

Professional Boundaries

As a nursing assistant, you must stay within certain **professional boundaries** in the care of residents. Boundaries are unspoken limits on physical and emotional relationships. They limit and define how a health care worker acts. Respecting boundaries involves using your best behavior, ethical practices, and good judgment when caring for residents. Respecting boundaries is one way that you will act appropriately on the job.

You see boundary lines when looking at a map. However, when you drive down the road, you do not see the boundaries when you cross from one city or state to the next. Professional boundaries are the same way. They exist, but you cannot see them. You must be aware of boundaries and avoid crossing them. You may cross them inadvertently or deliberately, thinking that you are meeting a resident's need. It takes good judgment and experience to identify boundaries and keep from crossing them.

Being aware of boundaries is especially important when caring for residents with emotional stress. To avoid crossing boundaries, strive to act professionally, as you were taught in class. Avoid putting yourself in a position in which you think and act as a family member or friend. Use good judgment and determine the amount of contact and assistance that are right for the resident. Too much or too little contact can be unhealthy for both the assistant and the resident. Treat all residents professionally. Consult the nurse if you are uncertain.

Ethical behavior with residents and families. Because you are a nursing assistant, residents expect you to act in their best interests and to treat them with dignity. Ways in which you do this are not taking advantage of a resident's situation and avoiding inappropriate involvement in the resident's personal and family relationships. Some relationships with residents and families are not healthy for the resident or the nursing assistant. It is not always easy to recognize unhealthy relationships until it is too late. Once you have crossed over a boundary line, it is difficult to turn back. Be aware of boundaries at all times, and strive to keep your relationships professional.

Try to find a balance in your relationships with residents and families. If any of the following occur, you are probably crossing professional boundaries and may be in a relationship danger zone:

- Discussing your personal problems with the resident or family members.
- Being flirtatious with a resident, including making sexual innuendos, telling jokes that are sexual in nature, or using offensive language.
- Discussing your feelings of sexual attraction with a resident.
- Feeling that you may become involved in a sexual relationship with the resident.
- Keeping secrets with a resident and becoming defensive when someone questions your relationship or involvement with the resident's personal life.
- Thinking you are immune from having an unhealthy relationship with a resident.
- Believing that you are the only nursing assistant who can meet the resident's needs.
- Spending an inappropriate amount of time with the resident, including off-duty visits or trading assignments with others so you can be with the resident.
- Reporting only partial information about the resident to the nurse because you fear disclosing unfavorable information or secrets the resident has told you.
- Feeling that you must protect the resident from other health care workers and always siding with the resident's position.

If you have trouble staying objective, or think you may cross a boundary, seek help from the nurse, clergy, or another professional person whom you trust.

Consequences of boundary violations. Boundary violations lead to inappropriate relationships with residents or families. These cloud your clinical judgment, and may lead to serious consequences, such as inappropriate sexual relationships. They often carry over into your personal life. The improper relationship may cause you to do things that you would not ordinarily do (such as stealing from the employer). There are many serious personal, legal, and professional consequences to inappropriate relationships. For your own well-being, be aware that professional boundaries exist, and work to keep from crossing them.

KEY POINTS IN CHAPTER

- Quality of life is very important for residents of a long-term care facility.
- Residents in long-term care facilities are like you in many ways.
- Aging affects the function of the entire body.
- All human beings have the same basic needs, which are described in Maslow's hierarchy of needs.
- The OBRA legislation states that declines in residents' conditions are not permitted unless they are medically unavoidable.
- It is important to look at the resident holistically, as a complex person with many strengths and needs.
- Basic resident care skills include providing personal care, providing food service and mealtime assistance, observation and reporting, caring for the resident's unit and belongings, caring for equipment and supplies, recordkeeping, and messenger duties.
- Developing good relationships with residents is important.
- Professional boundaries are unspoken limits on physical and emotional relationships that limit and define how a health care worker acts. Respecting boundaries involves using your best behavior, ethical practices, and good judgment when caring for residents.

REVIEW

A. Multiple Choice

Select the one best answer.

1. The term *geriatrics* means
   a. care of residents in the hospital
   b. care of the elderly.
   c. care of the client in the home.
   d. care of middle-aged adults.

2. Needs on the lowest level of Maslow's hierarchy include
   a. love.
   b. safety.
   c. food.
   d. self-esteem.

3. According to Maslow's theory
   a. the needs at one level must be satisfied before needs at the next level become important.
   b. the need for self-esteem is the most important of all.
   c. self-actualization is the feeling of love from your family members.
   d. satisfying emotional needs is most important.

4. An example of an aging change in the cardiovascular system is
   a. lung capacity increases due to muscular rigidity.
   b. blood pressure increases.
   c. the heart rate increases.
   d. reaction time slows down.

5. An example of an aging change in the urinary system is
   a. bladder capacity decreases.
   b. kidney function increases during the day.
   c. fewer hormones are secreted.
   d. kidney stones are common.

6. An example of an aging change in the digestive system is
   a. movement of food through the stomach increases.
   b. the stomach stretches, enabling it to hold more food.
   c. the gag reflex is less effective.
   d. waste travels through the colon more rapidly.

7. An example of an aging change in the musculoskeletal system is
   a. the ability to feel pressure and temperature increases.
   b. bones become more porous and break easily.
   c. endurance increases.
   d. muscles become more elastic.

8. The outer layer of the skin is called the
   a. dermis.
   b. epidermis.
   c. subcutaneous layer.
   d. external membrane.

9. Aging changes in the integumentary system include
   a. the skin thins and becomes less elastic.
   b. oil glands secrete more.
   c. blood vessels no longer nourish the skin.
   d. the skin no longer provides protection.

10. The prostate gland
    a. is not affected by aging.
    b. controls urination.
    c. may enlarge and obstruct the urethra.
    d. shrinks and becomes less effective.

B.   True/False

Answer each statement true (T) or false (F).

11. _____ All old people become senile and confused.

12. _____ Old people are always very crabby.

13. _____ It is important to understand what the OBRA laws require regarding resident declines.

14. _____ All people age at the same rate.

15. _____ The way people age is determined, in part, by their lifestyle.

C.   Fill in the Blank

Complete each sentence by adding the missing word or words.

16. The OBRA laws require long-term care facilities to maintain or _____ residents.

17. _____ care focuses on the whole person, with many strengths and needs.

18. _____ _____ are conditions with the potential to cause a person's health to worsen.

19. The hormone secreted by the pancreas that regulates glucose metabolism is _____.

20. Dark purple bruises on the back of the hands and forearms are _____ _____.

21. Young adult residents may act manipulative because their _____ _____ are not well developed.

22. One way the nursing assistant acts appropriately on the job is by respecting professional _____.

23. Your personal goal should be to provide the highest possible quality of _____ for each resident in your assignment.

D.   Clinical Applications

Please read the following case study, then answer the questions.

Mr. Hoover is a 78-year-old resident with a diagnosis of arteriosclerosis. He is mentally confused, but pleasant. He spends most of the day sitting in his armchair, watching television. Mr. Hoover walks with a walker from his chair to the bathroom. He uses a wheelchair for longer distances. You are assigned to walk him 50 feet in the hallway each day using a gait belt and his walker. He accomplishes this well. Mr. Hoover's skin is very dry. If he accidentally bumps his arms or legs, they bruise easily. Mr. Hoover's appetite is good. He uses three packages of sugar in his coffee. His son tells you that he used to use only one package of sugar in his coffee when he was younger. The care plan states to monitor and make sure Mr. Hoover has a bowel movement daily. If he does not, report to the nurse. Mr. Hoover urinates frequently. The care plan states that he has an enlarged prostate gland. Mr. Hoover takes pride in his appearance and likes to receive compliments about how nice he looks.

24. Which of the conditions listed in this case study are related to the normal aging process?

25. When you compliment Mr. Hoover on his appearance, you are fulfilling needs on which level of Maslow's hierarchy?

26. Mr. Hoover is able to walk in his room with a walker. Why is it important to walk him a longer distance in the hallway each day?

27. If the nursing assistant does not walk Mr. Hoover in the hallway and the resident loses the ability to walk 50 feet, is this a decline as defined by the OBRA legislation? Why or why not?

28. Why does Mr. Hoover use three packages of sugar in his coffee when he formerly used only one?

29. What is a potential explanation for Mr. Hoover's frequent urination?

30. At the end of your shift, you realize that you forgot to see if Mr. Hoover had a bowel movement today. The care plan states that the nursing assistant should monitor for a BM each day and report to the nurse if the patient does not have one. The resident's memory is poor, so he cannot tell you. What action should you take?

CHAPTER 3

Infection Control

OBJECTIVES

After reading this chapter, you will be able to:

- Spell and define key terms.
- Define medical asepsis and describe how it is used to prevent the spread of infection.
- List three ways that infection is spread.
- List eleven things you can do to prevent the spread of infection.
- Describe how bloodborne pathogens are spread and list measures to take to prevent the spread of bloodborne pathogens to yourself and others.
- Describe the three types of transmission-based precautions and explain when each type is used.
- Discuss infectious conditions that are seen in long-term care facilities.
- Describe how pathogens become drug resistant and explain why this is a problem.
- Describe how to recognize head lice and scabies and explain how each is treated.
- Define bioterrorism.
- Demonstrate procedures related to infection control.

OBSERVATIONS TO MAKE AND REPORT RELATED TO SIGNS AND SYMPTOMS OF INFECTION

New mental confusion or worsening mental confusion (may be the first sign of infection in elderly individuals)

Elevated temperature (elderly persons can be very ill, but have a normal or below-normal temperature; they do not always have a fever because of aging changes to the immune system)

Rapid pulse

Rapid respirations

Noisy respirations

Abnormally low blood pressure

Sweating

Chills

Skin hot or cold to touch

Skin color abnormal (flushed, red, gray, or blue)

Inflammation of skin (redness, swelling, heat, pain)

Drainage from any skin opening or body cavity

Any unusual body discharge, such as mucus or pus

Rash

MEDICAL ASEPSIS

Infection is a state of illness caused by foreign organisms in the body. Preventing the spread of infection is an important responsibility. **Medical asepsis** is also called **infection control.** It involves practices that prevent the spread of infection in the long-term care facility. Infection control practices prevent the spread of infection to many people. These practices protect you and your family members, residents and their family members, other staff members, and visitors to the health care facility.

Nosocomial infection is a serious risk for health care facility workers and residents. A nosocomial infection is one that originates in the health care facility. Some infections are **localized,** or confined to one area of the body. Signs of a localized infection are redness, swelling, and drainage at the site of the infection. An infection can also be **generalized.** A generalized infection is spread throughout the body. Signs of a generalized infection are fever, chills, pain, disorientation, fatigue, and nausea. Report any signs or symptoms of infection to the nurse.

The **immune system** is part of the circulatory system. It recognizes invading germs and works to eliminate them from the body. If the immune system recognizes a harmful microbe, the body's natural defenses are stimulated. The body then works to eliminate the organism and prevent infection. Some diseases weaken and destroy the immune system. **Susceptibility** is the body's ability to resist infection and is determined by age, presence of an underlying disease, health, nutritional state, and certain medications. When the immune system is weakened, the resident's body cannot defend well against invading organisms, and infection may occur. Elderly residents, those receiving cancer treatments, and others with certain diseases often have weakened immune systems.

Microorganisms are also called *microbes* **(Figure 3-1).** They are living organisms that cannot be seen with the eye. They are present everywhere in the environment. Some are harmless and do not cause disease. **Normal flora** are microbes that are helpful to the function of the body. For example, the normal flora in the digestive tract help break down food and turn it into waste products. However, when these organisms gain access to an area of the body where they do not belong, they may cause disease.

Pathogens are microbes that cause disease. **Bacteria** are microorganisms that can be elimi-

nated with **antibiotics. Viruses** are tiny pathogens that cause many diseases and cannot be eliminated by antibiotics. However, many viral infections can be prevented by vaccines. We can destroy many pathogens in the environment by a process known as **disinfection.** This commonly involves scrubbing or soaking an item with a special chemical or cleaning agent. The item is then rinsed to remove all traces of the chemical. **Sterilization** eliminates all microbes and can be done by using heat, gas, or chemicals. An **antiseptic** is a product used to cleanse the skin and as a scrub to remove microorganisms before certain invasive procedures. Antiseptics should not be used on equipment or for cleaning environmental surfaces.

SPREAD OF INFECTION

Infection is spread by many methods. The most common methods are by contact and in the air. The spread of infection by contact occurs in two different ways. Infections spread by **direct contact** are caused by touching a resident or person who has the infection. A handshake is an example of direct contact. Your hands pick up the pathogen when you shake hands. If the pathogen can enter your body through broken skin or the mucous membranes of your eyes, nose, mouth, or genital area, an infection may develop. Pathogens may also be spread by **indirect contact.** This involves touching environmental surfaces and **fomites** such as linen, supplies, or equipment that have pathogens on them **(Figure 3-2).** You pick up the pathogen on your hands and spread it to the inside of your body through nonintact skin or by touching your mucous membranes.

Infection may also be spread by the **airborne** route. Pathogens spread by this method are very

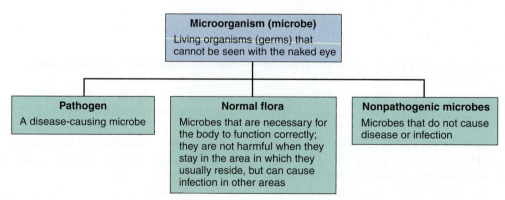

FIGURE 3-1 Various types of microbes

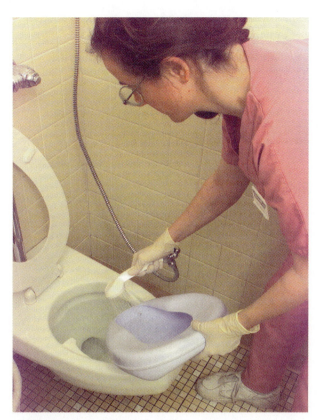

FIGURE 3-2 Your hands pick up unseen pathogens from many objects and environmental surfaces. Likewise, you can transfer these pathogens to humans and nonhuman items by touching them with your hands or gloves.

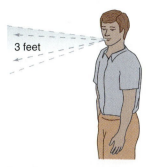

3 feet

FIGURE 3-3 Droplets generated by sneezing do not usually spread more than three feet from the carrier (source of the infection).

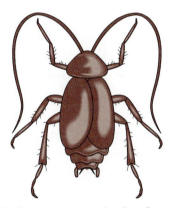

FIGURE 3-4 Vectors carry microbes from one place to another.

tiny and lightweight. They enter the air in respiratory **secretions.** Secretions are drainage from the body. In this case, mucus from the nose and mouth contains the pathogens. A cough or sneeze expels the pathogens into the air. Because they are so light, they travel long distances in the ventilation system, in dust, or on moisture particles in the air. Because of their weight, these pathogens do not drop to the ground quickly and are easily inhaled by others.

Pathogens may also enter the air and spread infection by the **droplet** method. Droplets are also respiratory secretions, such as those produced by sneezing or coughing. Pathogens spread by droplets are larger and heavier than those spread by the airborne method. Because of their size and weight, they usually do not spread beyond three feet from the **host** (**Figure 3-3**). Understanding the difference between the airborne and droplet methods of transmission is important so you can follow proper procedures to prevent infection from spreading.

Infections can also be spread by a **common vehicle.** Examples of common vehicles are food, water, or medication containing pathogens. The pathogens are taken into the body by eating and drinking.

Vectors (**Figure 3-4**) are insects and small animals that can carry pathogens.

Table 3-1 lists common ways microbes are spread.

Chain of Infection

The **chain of infection** (**Figure 3-5**) describes six factors necessary for an infection to develop. The **causative agent** is the germ that causes disease. The **mode of transmission** is the way in which the pathogen is spread. The **susceptible host** is the person who can become infected. Persons at the greatest risk for infection are the very young, the very old, persons with chronic diseases or weakened immune systems, people who are exposed to large numbers of pathogens, and

TABLE 3-1 Modes of Transmission of Microbes

Airborne	Tiny microbes are carried by moisture or dust particles in air and are inhaled
Droplet	*Droplets spread* within approximately three feet (no personal contact). Droplets are larger and heavier than airborne microbes, so they cannot travel as far. Droplet nuclei are inhaled: • Coughing • Laughing • Sneezing • Singing • Talking
Contact	*Direct contact* of health care provider with resident: • Touching • Rubbing • Toileting (urine and feces) • Blood, body fluid, mucous membranes, • Bathing or nonintact skin • Secretions or excretions from patient
	Indirect contact of health care provider with objects used by residents: • Clothing • Dressings • Bed linens • Diagnostic equipment • Personal belongings • Permanent or disposable • Personal care equipment health care equipment • Instruments and supplies used in • Environmental surfaces such as treatments counters, faucets, and doorknobs
Common Vehicle	Spread to many people through contact with items such as: • Food • Medication • Water • Contaminated blood products
Vector-Borne	Intermediate hosts such as: • Flies • Fleas • Rats • Ticks • Mice • Roaches

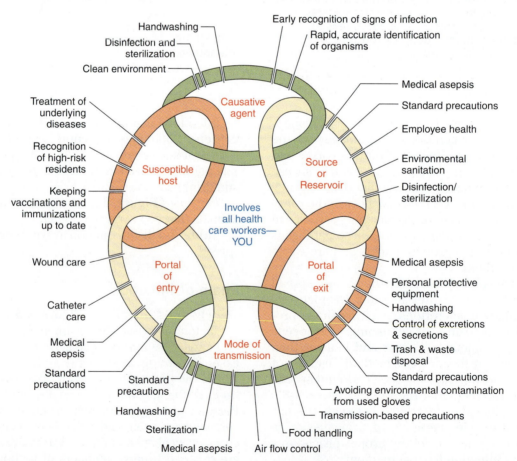

FIGURE 3-5 If one link in the chain is broken, the infection cannot be spread to others. This diagram shows the chain of infection, with examples of how health care workers can break each link of the chain.

TABLE 3-2 Elements in the Chain of Infection

Causative Agent	Source or Reservoir	Portal of Exit	Mode of Transmission	Portal of Entry	Susceptible Host
Bacteria	People	Blood	Direct contact	Mucous membranes	Chronic diseases
Fungi	Medicine	Moist body fluid	Indirect contact	Nonintact skin	Immuno-suppression
Viruses	Food	Droplets	Airborne	Urinary tract	Surgery
Parasites	Water	Secretions	Droplet	GI tract	Diabetes
	Equipment	Excretions	Fomites	Respiratory tract	Elderly residents
		Skin	Common vehicle	Blood	Burns
			Vectors	Body fluid	Cardiopulmonary disease

individuals who do not use good hygiene or infection control practices. The **source** or **reservoir** is the place where the pathogen can grow. A **carrier** is a person who is infected with a disease that can be spread to others. The carrier may not know that he or she is infected. The **portal of entry** is where the microbe enters the body. Pathogens can enter through any opening, such as a tiny cut or crack in the skin. They can also enter through the mucous membranes of the eyes, nose, mouth, or genital area. The **portal of exit** is the way pathogens leave the body. This may be in excretions, secretions, or body fluids, such as urine, feces, saliva, tears, drainage from open wounds, blood, mucus, or respiratory fluids. If any part of the chain of infection is broken, the disease will not spread. Figure 3-5 shows breaks in each link of the chain of infection. Using one of the methods listed next to any link will break the chain and prevent an infection from developing. **Table 3-2** lists some common elements in each link of the chain.

PREVENTING THE SPREAD OF INFECTION

You have learned that infective organisms are everywhere in the environment. You have an important responsibility to prevent the spread of infection. This is done in many ways.

Separation of Clean and Soiled Items and Equipment

To prevent infection, clean and soiled items must be kept separate. Clean items are either new, wrapped articles or reusable articles that have been washed or cleaned by staff. Soiled items are things that have been used by a resident or brought into a resident's room. The items are considered soiled even if they were not used to care for the resident. They must be cleaned or disinfected when they are removed from the room. For

GUIDELINES FOR
Reducing the Spread of Infection

- Wash your hands or use alcohol-based cleaners often.
- Keep the resident's unit neat, tidy, and sanitary.
- Clean equipment after each use. This includes small items used in the resident's room and larger, permanent items such as the bathtub and shower chair.
- Handle and dispose of soiled material properly.
- Assist residents to bathe and maintain personal cleanliness.

- Practice good personal hygiene.
- Handle food properly.
- Handle clean and soiled linen correctly.
- Keep clean and soiled items separate from one another.
- Perform procedures in the way you were taught, without taking shortcuts.

GUIDELINES FOR
Separating Clean and Soiled Items

• Keep the food cart and clean linen cart separated from the housekeeping cart and soiled linen hamper by at least one room's width **(Figure 3-6)**. The food cart and clean linen cart are clean items. The housekeeping cart and linen hamper are contaminated items.

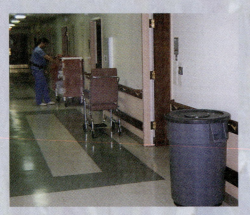

FIGURE 3-6 Keep clean and soiled items separated by at least one room's width in the hallway.

• Remove the housekeeping cart from the hallway when food trays are being served. Many facilities also remove soiled linen hampers from the hallway when food is being served.
• Many long-term care facilities have pets. They should not enter areas where food is being prepared or served. Wash your hands after you touch a pet.
• Wash soiled items in the soiled utility room. After cleaning, move them to the clean utility room for storage. Be sure that items are dry before storing them.
• Bring only necessary linen and supplies into the resident's room. Avoid carrying these items next to your uniform.
• Avoid carrying trash, linen, or other contaminated items next to your uniform.
• Dispose of trash contaminated with blood or body fluid according to facility policy in covered containers in a special storage area.
• Wear gloves if needed to apply the principles of standard precautions when caring for residents. Wash your hands before applying gloves. Use gloves for the care of one resident only. After each resident, remove the gloves and wash your hands again.
• Gloves are contaminated after resident contact. Avoid contaminating clean supplies, linen, equipment, or environmental surfaces with them. You can do this by removing one glove and using your ungloved hand for touching other items or by placing a clean paper towel under one glove and contacting environmental surfaces with the towel.
• Dispose of used gloves according to facility policy. Generally they are not discarded in the open wastebasket in the resident's room. Some facilities place extra plastic bags in the bottom of the wastebasket. If you must put soiled gloves and other contaminated items into the wastebasket, remove the bag containing the contaminated items, tie it, and take it with you when you leave the room. Replace it with a new bag from the bottom of the wastebasket.
• Follow facility policy for covering soiled items in the hallway during transport. If use of gloves is necessary, remove one glove. Carry the soiled item in the gloved hand **(Figure 3-7)**. Use the ungloved hand to turn on faucets, open doors, and touch items considered clean. Follow the same procedure when emptying bedpans and urinals in resident

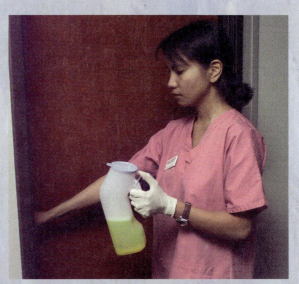

FIGURE 3-7 The one-glove technique is used for disposing of contaminated items and avoiding environmental contact with and contamination from used gloves. Remove the glove from one hand and carry it in the other hand with the soiled item. Use the ungloved hand to open doors, turn on faucets, pull up side rails, and so forth. If you cannot remove one glove, hold a paper towel under your gloved hand to contact environmental surfaces.

Continues

Separating Clean and Soiled Items, *Continued*

bathrooms. Use the ungloved hand to open the door, turn on faucets, and flush the toilet.

- Cover bedpans and urinals when you are carrying them.
- Lab specimens are never stored in the refrigerator with food or beverages. A separate, specially marked refrigerator or cooler should be used.
- Follow your assignment and facility cleaning schedule for washing and disinfecting resident care items. Special cleaners are used to disinfect reusable items. The friction created by wiping is important to remove microorganisms. Make sure supplies are completely dry before storing them. Store clean supplies in an area designated for clean items. You may be asked to date and initial items after they are cleaned.
- When working in rooms with two or more beds, clearly mark each resident's drinking glass and water

pitcher, bedpan, urinal, emesis basin, and personal care items so that they are not accidentally mixed up.
- Use liquid soap whenever possible. Keep residents' individual bars of soap separated. Soap should be stored in a container that allows water to drain away from the bottom of the bar.
- Cover food and beverages when you carry them in the hallway.
- Monitor resident rooms for snacks and other food items, which should be stored in a sealed package or covered container. Make sure the items can be safely stored unrefrigerated.
- Additional guidelines for handling of clean and soiled linen are listed in Chapter 10.
- Additional guidelines for handling food and beverages are listed in Chapter 13.

example, linen is brought into a resident's room, but is not needed. It cannot be removed from the room and used in the care of another resident. The linen is placed in the soiled linen hamper and must be washed before it is used.

HAND HYGIENE

In the health care facility, many infections are spread on the hands **(Figures 3-8A** and **B).** Because of this, special attention is given to hand hygiene. Keep the skin on your hands in good condition. Outside of the facility, wear gloves when performing tasks, such as gardening or washing dishes, that put the hands at risk of injury. Use hand lotion in moderation to keep the skin supple and prevent drying and irritation. Many facilities do not permit caregivers to wear artificial fingernails of any type, including nail tips, overlays, silk wraps, gels, sculptured, or acrylic nails. Long nails (beyond the fingertips) are also not usually permitted. Keep natural nail tips less than $\frac{1}{4}$-inch long. Long and artificial nails have been proven to hold microbes and increase the risk of infection. They are difficult to clean and may cause gloves to tear. Avoid chipped nail polish as well. Chips and cracks in nail polish also hide germs. Wear only simple rings, such as a plain wedding band. Rings with many stones and elaborate settings can also hold

harmful pathogens, and are difficult to clean. Microbes may also hide under the rings. The stones and settings on rings may also tear gloves.

Handwashing is the most important method used to prevent the spread of infection. You can pick up microbes on your hands and introduce them to your own body. You can also transfer the microbes on your hands to residents. If your hands touch a clean object, the microbes on your hands may be transferred there. This is a potential source of indirect contact transmission.

Quickly rinsing the hands with water, then drying them on a towel, does not remove germs. Oils on your skin must be washed away, along with attached germs. This can be done only by using warm water, soap, and friction. You must spend enough time to wash the germs away. The purpose of handwashing is to clean the hands and prevent microorganisms from spreading. Handwashing should take a minimum of 15 seconds. If your hands are visibly soiled, you will need to take longer. The longer the handwashing, the more microbes are eliminated. The most important part of the handwashing procedure is the friction caused by rubbing your hands together. The friction removes the microbes from your hands.

Rules for Handwashing

Never wash your gloved hands. Handwashing damages the gloves so that they will not protect

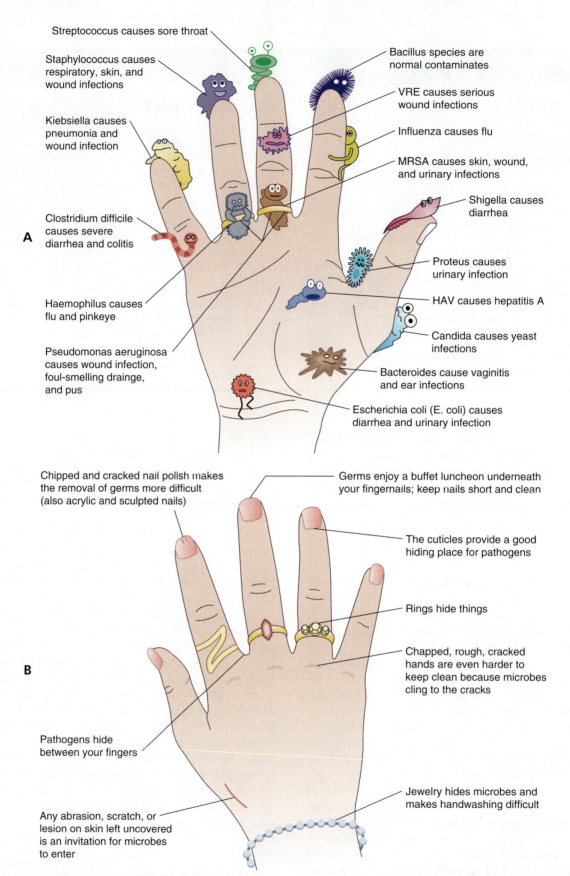

Streptococcus causes sore throat

Staphylococcus causes respiratory, skin, and wound infections

Klebsiella causes pneumonia and wound infection

Clostridium difficile causes severe diarrhea and colitis

Haemophilus causes flu and pinkeye

Pseudomonas aeruginosa causes wound infection, foul-smelling drainge, and pus

Bacillus species are normal contaminates

VRE causes serious wound infections

Influenza causes flu

MRSA causes skin, wound, and urinary infections

Shigella causes diarrhea

Proteus causes urinary infection

HAV causes hepatitis A

Candida causes yeast infections

Bacteroides cause vaginitis and ear infections

Escherichia coli (E. coli) causes diarrhea and urinary infection

A

Chipped and cracked nail polish makes the removal of germs more difficult (also acrylic and sculpted nails)

Germs enjoy a buffet luncheon underneath your fingernails; keep nails short and clean

The cuticles provide a good hiding place for pathogens

Rings hide things

Chapped, rough, cracked hands are even harder to keep clean because microbes cling to the cracks

Pathogens hide between your fingers

Jewelry hides microbes and makes handwashing difficult

Any abrasion, scratch, or lesion on skin left uncovered is an invitation for microbes to enter

B

FIGURE 3-8   (A) Many infections are spread on the hands, so health care workers must pay close attention to good hand hygiene and eliminating areas where pathogens can hide. (B) Jewelry with many stones or complicated settings provides a hiding place for pathogens. Long fingernails, chipped nail polish, and acrylic nails also provide hiding places for microbes. Chapped, cut, cracked hands increase the risk of contracting an infection.

Times when Handwashing Should Be Done

- When coming on duty.
- After picking up anything from the floor.
- Before and after caring for each resident.
- Before applying and after removing gloves.
- After personal use of the toilet or using a tissue to blow your nose.
- After you cough or sneeze.
- Before and after applying lip balm.
- Before and after manipulating contact lenses.
- Before and after eating, drinking, or smoking.
- Before handling a resident's food and drink.
- After contact with anything considered soiled or contaminated.
- Before handling any supply considered clean.
- Before treating a cut or break on your own skin.
- After handling uncooked foods, particularly raw meat, poultry, or fish.
- After changing an infant's diaper or adult incontinence brief.
- After touching an animal (especially a reptile).

- After handling trash or garbage.
- Immediately before touching **nonintact skin** (skin that is broken, chapped, cut, or cracked); if you are already wearing gloves, change them.
- Immediately before touching **mucous membranes** (tissues of the body that secrete mucus; these tissues are open to the outside of the body); if you are already wearing gloves, change them.
- After touching nonintact skin, mucous membranes, blood, or any moist body fluid, secretions, or **excretions** (human waste products eliminated from the body), even if gloves were worn during the contact.
- Whenever your hands are visibly soiled.
- After touching equipment or environmental surfaces that might be contaminated.
- After touching anything that many people have handled.
- Any time your gloves become torn.
- Before you go on break and at the end of your shift before you leave the facility.

PROCEDURE 1

Handwashing

1. Turn on warm water using a paper towel.
2. Wet your hands. Keep your fingertips pointed down.
3. Apply soap from the dispenser.
4. Rub your hands together vigorously to create a lather. Rub the hands together in a circular motion for at least 15 seconds. Rub all surfaces of the hands. Pay particular attention to the area between your fingers. Keep your fingertips pointed down **(Figure 3-9)**.
5. Rub the fingernails against the palm of the opposite hand. Clean the nails with a brush or an orange stick if they are soiled.

6. Rinse your hands from the wrist to the fingertips. Keep the fingers pointed down.
7. Dry your hands with a paper towel.
8. Use a clean, dry paper towel to turn off the faucet **(Figure 3-10)**. Do not touch the faucet handle with your hand.
9. Discard the paper towel.
   Note: Avoid touching the sink with your body or clothing during this procedure. Avoid splashing water onto your clothing.

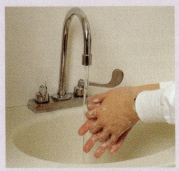

FIGURE 3-9 Keep your fingertips pointed down to prevent contaminants from rolling down your hands and arms.

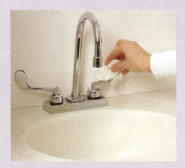

FIGURE 3-10 The faucet is contaminated with microbes deposited when people with unclean hands turned the water on. Use a paper towel to turn it off, to avoid picking up unwelcome guests on your clean hands.

you. Remove gloves, wash your hands, and then reapply a clean pair of gloves.

1. Avoid leaning against the sink during the handwashing procedure. The inside of the sink and the faucet handles are contaminated. The outside of the sink may contaminate your uniform.
2. Avoid splashing your uniform when washing your hands.
3. Keep your fingertips pointed down during the handwashing procedure.
4. Bar soap can hold microorganisms on its surface. Use liquid soap whenever possible.
5. Turn the faucets on and off with a clean, dry paper towel.

Waterless Hand Cleaners

Many facilities provide dispensers containing waterless hand cleaners **(Figure 3-11)** in various locations in the facility. The hand cleaners contain an alcohol-based gel, lotion, or foam that is dispensed in small dime- to quarter-sized por-

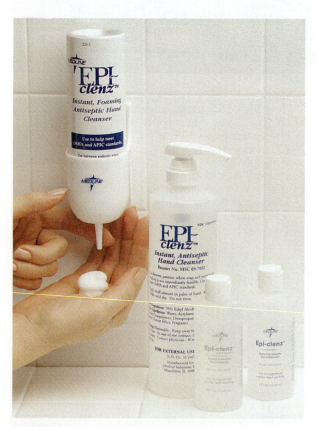

FIGURE 3-11 Alcohol-based hand cleaners may safely be used instead of washing at the sink unless your hands are contaminated with a protein substance. *(Courtesy of Medline, Industries, Inc. 1-800-MEDLINE)*

tions (approximately 2 to 3 mL). Alcohol-based products are often less irritating to the hands than washing repeatedly with soap. Most alcohol solutions contain moisturizers that prevent drying of the skin. In addition, paper towels are not necessary when alcohol products are used. Paper towels contain wood fibers that can be very irritating to sensitive skin.

Each facility has directions for using waterless hand cleaners and policies and procedures for when the product may be used. A waterless hand cleaner may safely be used instead of handwashing during routine resident care. However, washing at the sink should be done any time the hands are visibly soiled.

To use the waterless cleaning product, dispense the proper amount into the palm of your hand. Rub the product into the hands until it dries, making sure to rub all areas and surfaces, including the nail beds and between the fingers. This should take at least 15 seconds. Become familiar with the products used by your facility and their applications. They are very effective in reducing infection and eliminating pathogens from the hands.

BLOODBORNE PATHOGENS

Bloodborne pathogens are microbes that cause disease through contact with blood, nonintact skin, mucous membranes, secretions, excretions, or any moist body fluid except sweat. Many diseases can be transmitted by contact with these substances. **Hepatitis B, hepatitis C, human immunodeficiency virus (HIV) disease,** and **acquired immune deficiency syndrome (AIDS)** are diseases that are commonly spread through contact with blood and body fluids.

Hepatitis

Hepatitis means "inflammation of the liver." It can be caused by a number of factors, including drugs, toxins, autoimmune disease, and infectious agents (viruses). Six main types of viral hepatitis are prevalent in the United States. **Table 3-3** summarizes the various types of hepatitis.

Hepatitis B. Hepatitis B is a virus that causes an infection of the liver. This disease can cause liver damage, liver cancer, and death. Individuals with hepatitis B may have no symptoms at all, but may still be infectious. These people are carriers of the disease. The presence of the hepatitis

TABLE 3-3 Types of Hepatitis

Type	Mode of Transmission	Signs & Symptoms	Vaccine	U.S. statistics	Treatment	Comments
Hepatitis A	Oral/fecal; on hands or transferred to food	Abdominal pain, loss of appetite, fatigue, nausea, diarrhea, dark urine, jaundice	Vaccine available; immune globulin used for short-term immunity	125,000 to 200,000 cases and approximately 100 deaths annually	Bed rest and limited activity for up to 30 days	Usually lasts less than 2 months; not a chronic condition
Hepatitis B	Blood and body fluid; mother to fetus	Abdominal pain, loss of appetite, fatigue, nausea, diarrhea, dark urine, jaundice	Vaccine available	140,000 to 320,000 total infections; approximately 5,000 to 6,000 deaths annually	Most recover within 6 months; for chronic cases, interferon	More than 1 million chronically infected; can lead to cirrhosis or liver cancer
Hepatitis C	Blood and body fluid; mother to fetus	Most asymptomatic; abdominal pain, loss of appetite, fatigue, nausea, diarrhea, dark urine, jaundice	None	28,000 to 180,000 total infections; approximately 10,000 deaths annually	Interferon; effective in approximately 33% of patients	Approximately 4 million chronically infected; can lead to cirrhosis or liver cancer. Leading cause of liver transplant in U.S. Many carriers are asymptomatic for years before learning of infection
Hepatitis D	Blood and body fluid	Abdominal pain, loss of appetite, fatigue, nausea, diarrhea, dark urine, jaundice	Hepatitis B vaccine	Approximately 5,000 infections annually	Interferon may be effective in some patients	Develops only in the presence of hepatitis B or acquired simultaneously with HBV; few chronic cases. 70% to 80% develop cirrhosis
Hepatitis E	Oral/fecal; contaminated water	Abdominal pain, loss of appetite, fatigue, nausea, diarrhea, dark urine, jaundice	None	Rare in U.S.	Rest, limited activity for 2 weeks	Almost all U.S. cases are in travelers returning from high-risk areas (primarily Mexico, Asia, Africa); few chronic cases
Hepatitis G	Blood	Most patients are asymptomatic	None	900 to 2,000 cases annually	Rest	Serious disease rare

B virus (HBV) can be diagnosed only by a blood test. You probably cannot tell that the carrier is sick by his or her appearance. Some people may be sick with mild symptoms that mimic the flu. Common symptoms of hepatitis B are fever, aches and pains, nausea, and fatigue. Urine may turn dark in color. The skin, mucous membranes, and white area of the eyes may appear jaundiced, or yellow in color. A person can transmit the disease even after recovering from the symptoms. Many people who have had hepatitis B have permanent liver damage and are disabled for life.

Hepatitis C.   Hepatitis C is transmitted in the same manner as HIV and hepatitis B. There are also documented cases of transmission from unclean medical instruments. Hepatitis C is primarily a disease of the liver, but can also affect the white blood cells. At first, hepatitis C may be mistaken for the flu. Common signs and symptoms are extreme fatigue, depression, fever, mood changes, and weakness. There are many other signs and symptoms, ranging from pain to loss of appetite. Hepatitis C may cause liver cancer and liver failure. People with hepatitis C may have the disease for years and not know it. Even though the infected person is unaware of it, the disease is silently destroying the liver. The hepatitis C virus (HCV) changes constantly, so finding a treatment is difficult. Presently there is only one approved treatment for hepatitis C in the United States, and it does not work for all patients. Hepatitis C is the leading cause of the need for liver transplants in the United States. Many patients die waiting for a transplant.

Human Immunodeficiency Virus Disease

Human immunodeficiency virus is the virus that causes HIV disease and AIDS. An infected person is called "HIV-positive," or "HIV+." A newer term for this is to say that the individual has HIV disease. Most, but not all, people with HIV disease develop AIDS over time. After exposure to HIV, a person may have no symptoms at all. Sometime between one week and six months later, the exposed person may develop fever and flu-like symptoms. When this occurs, the blood converts from HIV-negative to HIV-positive. This can be very confusing, because some individuals can go for longer periods before the blood converts from negative to positive. Some people convert from negative to positive, but do not experience the flu-like symptoms. These people do not know that they are HIV-positive. The only way to know for sure is to get a blood test. Once a person converts to HIV-positive, it may take six to ten years or more for AIDS to develop. The HIV-positive person becomes a lifelong carrier and can spread the virus to others.

Acquired Immune Deficiency Syndrome

As HIV disease progresses, the immune system is destroyed. When the blood count reaches a certain level, the individual develops AIDS. People with AIDS contract many illnesses and infections because of the immune system destruction. Normally the immune system would prevent these infections from causing illness. A person with AIDS may have a chronic fever and swelling of the lymph nodes, particularly in the neck, armpits, and groin. Weight loss, diarrhea, extreme fatigue, and night sweats are common. White patches called thrush **(Figure 3-12)** may form inside the mouth and throat. Occasionally, Kaposi's sarcoma develops **(Figure 3-13)**. This is a form of cancer in which raised, purple spots appear on the skin and internal organs. Many individuals develop chronic herpes **(Figure 3-14)**. People with advanced AIDS may develop mental confusion, emotional problems, and loss of motor control. When these individuals enter the long-term care facility, they are often in the end stage of the disease. Caring for them may be emotionally trying because many are young adults. Staff may feel that these individuals are too young to die and have not had a chance at life. Some have young families and children. When caring for residents with AIDS, the staff must support each other and may need outside resources to help them deal with their feelings

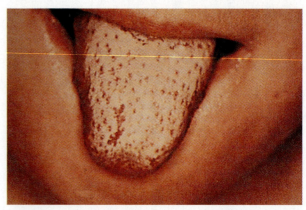

FIGURE 3-12   Oral thrush in an AIDS patient. *(Courtesy of Daniel J. Barbaro, MD, Fort Worth, Texas)*

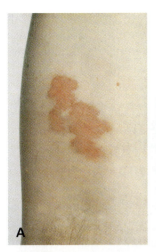
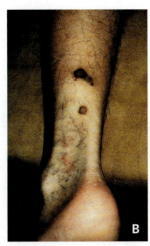

FIGURE 3-13 (A) Typical purple lesions caused by Kaposi's sarcoma. (B) Raised Kaposi's sarcoma lesions. *(Courtesy of Daniel J. Barbaro, MD, Fort Worth, Texas)*

about the disease. AIDS was previously the main cause of death in males between the ages of 25 and 44. With new advances in care and treatment, it is now the second-leading cause of death in this age group. Nevertheless, AIDS continues to take a great many lives and remains a very serious public health concern.

AIDS is seen in all races and socioeconomic groups. State and federal laws prohibit discrimination against people with AIDS. Some health care workers have contracted the HIV virus at work, but the total number of work-related cases is small. Estimating the number of new AIDS cases each year is very difficult. In 2001, a total of 43,158 new cases had been reported. An estimated 344,178 persons with HIV were living in the United States. Remember that AIDS is *not the same* as HIV disease. The best way to prevent HIV disease and AIDS is to know how the

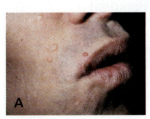
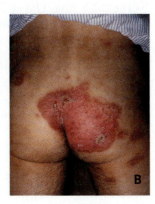

FIGURE 3-14 (A) Oral herpes simplex molluscum in an AIDS patient. (B) Chronic herpes in an AIDS patient. *(Courtesy of Daniel J. Barbaro, MD, Fort Worth, Texas)*

disease is transmitted. Hepatitis B, hepatitis C, and HIV are transmitted in the same manner. Methods of transmission are listed in **Table 3-4.** Take measures to protect yourself both at work and in your personal life.

Treatment

Over the past few years, great strides have been made in treating HIV disease and AIDS. A laboratory test called the viral load is used as an indicator of when and how to medicate. By monitoring the viral load, the physician knows when to begin medications and when to change the drug regimen. Several different types of drugs are used in combination to treat the HIV virus in the body. These drugs do not eliminate the disease. Treatment is geared to controlling symptoms. The combination drug therapy is effective in many individuals because each drug works on a different part of the HIV virus in the body. The drugs control new virus that is produced in the body each day. They do not reverse damage that was done before drug therapy was started. Taking the drugs exactly as ordered is important because the HIV virus can become drug resistant in a very short time. Following directions exactly increases the time the individual will benefit from the drugs, before resistance develops. Because of the progress in treating the HIV virus, HIV disease and AIDS are now viewed as chronic, manageable diseases rather than fatal illnesses.

TABLE 3-4 Methods of HIV, HBV, and HCV Transmission
Heterosexual and homosexual sexual intercourse
Sharing needles and other paraphernalia with IV drug users
Occupational exposure through direct or indirect contact with blood and body fluids of an infected person
Transfusion with contaminated blood or blood products
Mother-to-infant transmission, prenatally or through breastfeeding
Tattooing and body piercing with unclean instruments
Sharing household items such as razors and toothbrushes with infected individuals

Risk Factors for Diseases Spread by Bloodborne Pathogens

Because hepatitis B, hepatitis C, and HIV are spread by blood and body fluid contact, the diseases are seen in heterosexual, homosexual, and bisexual individuals. People who use intravenous drugs and share needles are at particularly high risk. Children born to mothers who are infected may also develop the disease. People who received blood between 1978 and 1984 may have contracted HIV from the blood transfusion. Since 1984, donor blood has been routinely tested for HIV. You cannot contract HIV by donating blood at a blood bank or hospital.

You can contract HIV, HBV, and HCV by contacting the virus through your nonintact skin. This means that cut or chapped skin touches blood, body fluid, secretions, excretions, or nonintact skin containing the virus. The virus can also be passed by contact with the mucous membranes of the eyes, nose, mouth, and genital area. You cannot contract the virus through casual contact or airborne transmission.

HBV is much more contagious than HIV. Imagine that $\frac{1}{4}$ teaspoon of HBV is mixed into a 24,000-gallon swimming pool of water. Someone draws a quarter teaspoon of that water into a syringe and injects you with it. Although the virus is extremely diluted, you will become HBV-positive. Now imagine that 10 people are in the room. Someone takes $\frac{1}{4}$ teaspoon of HIV and mixes it into a quart of water. Each person is injected with $\frac{1}{4}$ teaspoon of this solution. Only one person in the room will become HIV-positive. Hepatitis B, then, is a much greater threat to health care workers than HIV. We now know that some people do not contract HIV because of certain elements within their cells. These elements are not easy to identify, however, so everyone must assume that they can contract the disease and take the proper precautions. A vaccine is available to prevent hepatitis B. If your job involves handling blood or body fluids routinely, your employer is required to provide you with the vaccination free of charge. The vaccine is given in a series of three injections over several months. Presently, there is no vaccine to prevent hepatitis C, HIV disease, or AIDS.

Each health care facility is required to have an **exposure control plan,** which is a written program that describes what to do if you contact blood or body fluid. Immediately wash the area thoroughly. Report accidental contact with blood or body fluid to the nurse immediately. You will be treated according to the established plan, have blood samples taken, and may begin drug therapy to prevent a bloodborne disease from developing. Medical care and monitoring will continue over a long period of time.

PROTECTING YOURSELF AND OTHERS FROM EXPOSURE TO BLOODBORNE PATHOGENS BY USING STANDARD PRECAUTIONS

Health care workers can take measures to prevent the spread of infection to themselves and others. These measures are called **standard precautions (Figure 3-15).** The purpose of using standard precautions is to prevent the spread of infection. We cannot tell whether someone has a disease or infection by appearance, so standard precautions are used in the care of all residents regardless of their disease or diagnosis. Standard precautions are based on the assumption that all blood and body fluids are potentially infectious. Many individual infection factors are very difficult to control. Standard precautions are directed mainly at preventing the transmission of microbes. Standard precautions effectively prevent the spread of many diseases besides HIV disease, AIDS, and hepatitis B and C.

Standard precautions include the use of **personal protective equipment (PPE)** when performing certain tasks. Personal protective equipment consists of garments and apparel that protect the health care worker from contracting a disease from a resident. It also protects the resident from contracting a disease from a microbe passed from the worker's hands.

Selection and Use of Personal Protective Equipment

Standard precautions are used anytime the health care worker anticipates contact with blood or any moist body fluid (except sweat), secretions, or excretions. They are also used anytime you will have mucous membrane contact. Mucous membranes are found in the eyes, nose, mouth, and genital area. If either you or the resident has nonintact or broken skin, PPE is also used. There are many variables in resident care situations, so there are no absolute rules for the use of PPE. The nursing assistant must think about the situation and use good judgment. You are responsibile for applying the principles of

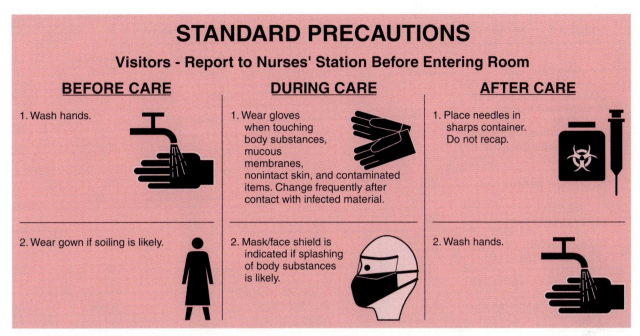

STANDARD PRECAUTIONS

Visitors - Report to Nurses' Station Before Entering Room

BEFORE CARE	DURING CARE	AFTER CARE
1. Wash hands.	1. Wear gloves when touching body substances, mucous membranes, nonintact skin, and contaminated items. Change frequently after contact with infected material.	1. Place needles in sharps container. Do not recap.
2. Wear gown if soiling is likely.	2. Mask/face shield is indicated if splashing of body substances is likely.	2. Wash hands.

FIGURE 3-15 Standard precautions are used in the care of all residents, regardless of disease or diagnosis. *(Courtesy of Briggs Corporation, Des Moines, IA 800-247-2343)*

standard precautions and selecting the PPE according to the task to be done. Equipment is worn during some direct resident care activities. **Table 3-5** will guide you in selecting PPE for common tasks. Personal protective equipment is also worn during cleaning procedures when contact with blood, body fluids, secretions, or excretions is likely.

Personal protective equipment will protect you only if it fits properly, if it is free from defects, and if you use it regularly in the way you were taught. Never use equipment that is torn or has defects. You must study and learn the principles of standard precautions so you can apply them correctly. It is your responsibility to use standard precautions to protect yourself and facility residents. Always follow the infection control policies and procedures for your facility.

Rules for Standard Precautions

Certain common procedures apply to using standard precautions in resident care. You must anticipate and select the correct type of PPE and use handwashing before and after every procedure.

Handwashing. Handwashing or use of alcohol-based hand cleaners must be done before all resident care and procedures. It is also done before applying and after removing gloves. It is possible to pick up a microbe on your hands even when you are wearing gloves. Sometimes this occurs because of microscopic defects in the gloves. It is also possible to unknowingly contact microbes when your gloves are removed. Handwashing is also done immediately if your hands contact blood or any moist body fluid except sweat. Handwashing is performed at the end of each procedure, after gloves are removed.

Barrier precautions. Personal protective equipment is also called *barrier equipment.* Using barrier precautions involves wearing gloves for handling or touching blood, any moist body fluid (except sweat), secretions, excretions, mucous membranes, or nonintact skin. If your gloves become visibly soiled, you should remove them, wash your hands, and apply a clean pair of gloves. When using barrier precautions, you should remove your gloves, wash your hands, and reapply clean gloves *immediately* before contact with mucous membranes and nonintact skin. You may have to change your gloves and wash your hands several times during the care of one resident. Change gloves:

- Before each resident contact
- After each resident contact
- *Immediately before* touching mucous membranes
- *Immediately before* touching nonintact skin
- After you touch a resident's secretions or excretions, before moving to care for another part of the body

TABLE 3-5	Examples of Personal Protective Equipment in Basic Resident Care			
Resident Care Task	**Gloves**	**Gown**	**Goggles/ Face Sheild**	**Surgical Mask**
Controlling bleeding when blood is squirting	Yes	Yes	Yes	Yes
Wiping a wheelchair, shower chair, or bathtub with disinfectant solution	Yes	No	No	No
Emptying a catheter bag	Yes	Yes, if facility policy	Yes, if facility policy	Yes, if facility policy
Serving a meal tray	No	No	No	No
Giving a back rub to a resident who has intact skin	No	No	No	No
Brushing a resident's teeth	Yes	No	No	No
Helping the dentist with a procedure	Yes	Yes, if facility policy	Yes	Yes
Cleaning a resident and changing the bed after an episode of diarrhea	Yes	Yes	No	No
Changing a bed in which the linen is not visibly soiled	No, or follow facility policy. If gloves are worn for removing soiled linen, remove and wash hands before handling clean linen	No	No	No
Taking an oral temperature with a glass thermometer (gloves are not necessary with an electronic thermometer)	Yes	No	No	No
Taking a rectal temperature	Yes	No	No	No
Taking a blood pressure	No	No	No	No
Cleaning soiled utensils, such as bedpans	Yes	Yes, if splashing is likely	Yes, if splashing is likely	Yes, if splashing is likely
Shaving a resident with a disposable razor	Yes, because of the high risk of this procedure for contact with blood	No	No	No
Giving eye care	Yes	No	No	No
Giving special mouth care to an unconscious resident	Yes	No, unless coughing is likely	No, unless coughing is likely	No, unless coughing is likely
Washing the resident's genital area	Yes	No	No	No
Washing the resident's arms and legs when the skin is not broken	No	No	No	No

Note: There are exceptions to every rule. Use this chart as a guideline only. Add personal protective equipment if special situations, such as possible splashing, exist. Follow your facility policies on use of PPE routine tasks.

- After touching blood or body fluids, before moving to care for another part of the body
- After touching contaminated environmental surfaces or equipment
- Anytime your gloves become visibly soiled
- If your gloves become torn

Your facility is required to have barrier equipment available in a variety of sizes in locations where use can be reasonably anticipated. Gloves **(Figure 3-16)** are also worn for touching dressings, tissues, infective items, and contaminated surfaces or equipment. Do not carry glove use to extremes. Use gloves when necessary, but do not use them for all resident contact. Using gloves at all times sends a negative message. It says that the resident is untouchable. Touching is very important to all human beings. Gloves should be used only when contact with blood, body fluids, secretions, excretions, mucous membranes, or nonintact skin is likely. Gloves are also worn for resident contact if the skin on your hands is cut, cracked, or chapped. Be very careful not to contaminate clean equipment, supplies, or environmental surfaces with used gloves.

A gown **(Figure 3-17)** is worn anytime your clothing may contact blood or any of the body fluids mentioned. The gown may be cloth or paper, but must be fluid resistant. Many gowns are specially treated so they will resist fluid.

A face shield **(Figure 3-18A)** or goggles **(Figure 3-18B)** and a mask are worn during procedures when body fluids or secretions may splash into your face. A good rule to follow is that you can wear a mask without eye protection, but you should never wear eye protection without a mask.

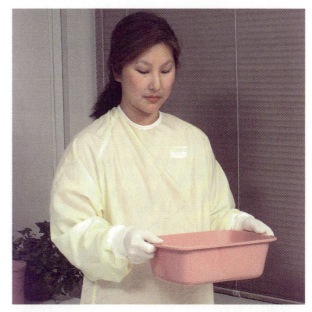

FIGURE 3-17 Gowns are specially treated to resist fluid.

An alternate type of mask with a plastic eye shield attached may also be used **(Figure 3-18C)**. The facial barriers protect the mucous membranes in your eyes, nose, and mouth. It is your responsibility to anticipate what you will need and apply it before you begin a procedure. Check the equipment before you use it. If it is cut or torn, it will not protect you and should be replaced. If you tear your gloves during a procedure, remove them as soon

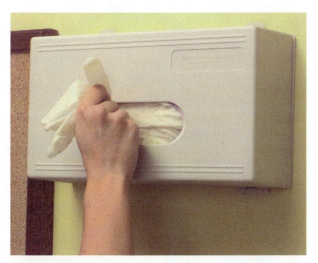

FIGURE 3-16 Gloves are stored in convenient locations near areas where they are likely to be used.

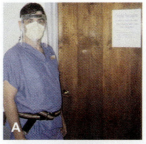
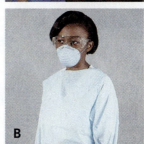
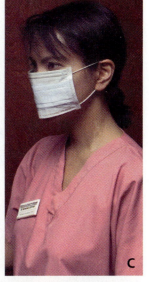

FIGURE 3-18 (A) A mask should always be worn with a regular face shield. (B) Goggles are always worn with a mask. (C) This mask has a protective eye shield attached.

as possible. Wash your hands and put on a new pair of gloves before continuing.

Personal protective equipment is discarded, laundered, or decontaminated according to facility policy after use. Be sure to replace what you have used so it is available the next time it is needed. Wash protective eyewear with soap and water after each use.

Handling needles and sharps.   Needle and sharp precautions are also used. Handle needles, razors, and other sharp objects with care. Needles should never be cut, bent, broken, or recapped by hand. After using a sharp object, dispose of it in a puncture-resistant "sharps" container **(Figure 3-19).** The sharps container should not be overfilled. The cap is placed on the container when it is three-quarters full. The cap is designed so it cannot be snapped back off after it is closed. The sealed sharps container is stored until it can be picked up with the **biohazardous waste.** The biohazardous waste disposal area is used for discarding items contaminated with blood or body fluids. Special precautions are taken to contain waste in this area.

If you must clean up broken glass, always wear gloves. Do not pick up glass with your hands. Use a broom and dustpan **(Figure 3-20),** forceps, or other mechanical method. Protect your hands from being cut. Dispose of the broken glass in a puncture-resistant container.

Cleaning blood and body fluid spills.   Follow your facility policy for cleaning up spills of blood or body fluid. Many facilities use an absorbent powder to soak up the fluid. After the fluid has been absorbed, sweep it up **(Figure 3-21).** Wipe the area with a facility-approved disinfectant. If your facility uses bleach as a disinfectant, it should be mixed in a container using one part bleach to ten parts of water. Some facilities are now using a different concentration of bleach solution for cleaning blood spills. Research has shown that a much lower concentration (1:100) is needed to eliminate bloodborne pathogens. Know and follow your facility policy. The container should be labeled with the contents and the date it was mixed.

Disposing of biohazardous waste.   Items that have contacted blood or body fluids are biohazardous waste. Dispose of linen and trash contaminated with blood or body fluids according to your facility policy. Contaminated trash is discarded in containers marked with the biohaz-

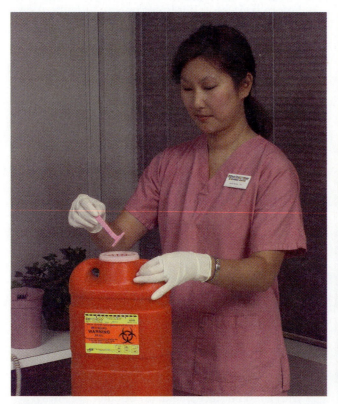 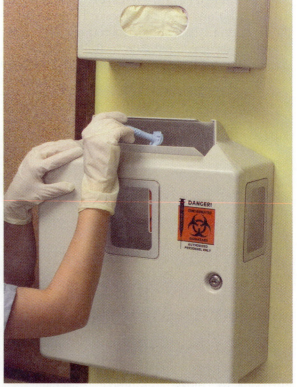

FIGURE 3-19   Razors, needles, blades, broken glass, and other potentially hazardous sharp objects are discarded promptly after use in the puncture-resistant sharps container.

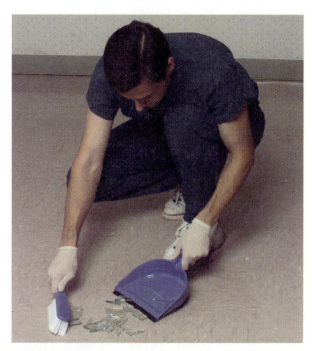

FIGURE 3-20 Never pick up broken glass with your bare hands. Always wear gloves and use an instrument to clean broken glass, even if the amount is small.

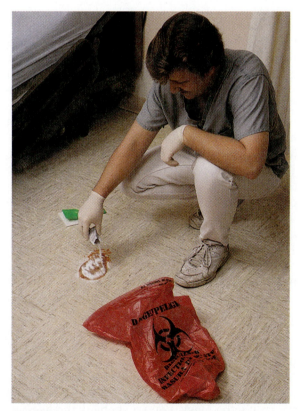

FIGURE 3-21 The absorbent powder turns the body fluid spill into a solid material for easy cleanup. The floor must be disinfected after the powder is removed.

ardous waste emblem **(Figure 3-22).** The biohazard emblem has a red or orange background with a black biohazard symbol. Biohazardous waste requires special handling when it is removed from the facility. Having biohazardous waste removed is very expensive, so do not place nonbiohazardous materials into this trash container. Biohazardous trash is stored in a special holding area until it can be safely removed.

Body fluids such as urine can safely be disposed of in a drain connected to a sanitary sewer. Your instructor will teach you facility policies for handling and disposing of biohazardous waste.

Laboratory specimens. Laboratory specimens are always considered potentially infectious. They are collected in covered containers. The containers are placed in sealed plastic transport bags with a biohazard emblem on them before they are transported to the lab. If a specimen must be refrigerated, it should not be stored in a refrigerator with food or beverages. A separate refrigerator or cooler, marked with a biohazard emblem, is used.

Cleaning equipment. Each facility has policies and procedures for cleaning equipment that will be reused for resident care. If the equipment may have been contaminated with blood or body fluid, always use personal protective equipment. Utility gloves are better for cleaning duties than the disposable gloves used in resident care. The chemicals used for cleaning make the pores of the disposable gloves too large. Although you probably cannot see this defect, the large pores allow microbes to pass through the gloves to your hands. Follow your facility policy for the use of gloves.

Latex allergies. Some health care workers develop allergies to latex because of repeated exposure to latex gloves and other supplies. Avoiding powdered gloves can decrease the risk of latex sensitivity. The powder in the gloves absorbs

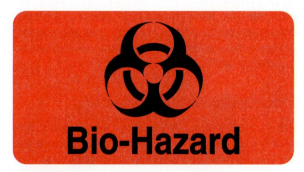

FIGURE 3-22 The biohazard emblem has a red or orange background with a black symbol.

latex proteins. When the gloves are removed, the particles are inhaled, increasing sensitivity. If you are allergic to latex, your facility will provide you with another type of glove. Glove liners and topical barrier products are also available to individuals who are allergic to latex. The liner or topical product forms a barrier and prevents the latex from touching the skin.

ISOLATION MEASURES

Isolation measures are used when certain pathogens are present in a resident. Isolation is used to prevent others from becoming infected. Some facilities place residents with diseases of the immune system in reverse or protective isolation. Residents in protective isolation do not have a contagious disease. Because of their immune system disorder, they can catch diseases easily. They are isolated to prevent them from contracting pathogens from others and from the environment. Residents with other conditions, such as burns, and those receiving cancer treatment may also be placed in protective isolation. Some facilities do not use this category of isolation.

When caring for a resident in isolation, remember that you are isolating the pathogen and not the person. Isolation can be emotionally difficult for a resident. The resident may feel unclean, unwanted, and untouchable. He or she may not like being confined to a room and separated from others. Staff and visitors must wear personal protective equipment when they are in the room. Sometimes this is upsetting to the resident. A confused resident may be very frightened of staff wearing isolation garments. Because of the difficulty involved in putting on PPE, staff may not visit residents as often. This, too, can be difficult for the resident. Do everything you can to teach the resident about the purpose of the isolation. Check on residents in isolation frequently, and avoid making them feel unclean, unwanted, and unloved. The least amount of isolation possible to contain the pathogen is used. It is unnecessary to use extra precautions beyond those that are required to prevent the spread of disease.

Transmission-Based Precautions

The Centers for Disease Control and Prevention (CDC) is a governmental agency that studies infectious diseases and makes recommendations to prevent their spread. The CDC recommends three types of transmission-based precautions. These are isolation categories designed to interrupt the mode of transmission so the pathogen cannot spread. Standard precautions are always used in addition to transmission-based precautions. The type of precautions used is selected by the nurse manager and physician according to how the disease is spread. Transmission-based precautions are used because ordinary cleanliness and standard precautions may not protect you or others from the spread of certain pathogens. Residents with the same disease may share a room. Otherwise, a private room is used to confine the pathogen to the resident's unit.

Airborne precautions. Airborne precautions (Figure 3-23) are used for residents whose disease is spread by the airborne method of transmission. The type of pathogen involved is very tiny and light. It can be suspended on dust and moisture in the air and travel for long distances in the ventilation system. Because of the mode of transmission, special precautions are taken to contain the microbe. A private room is necessary. This room must have a special ventilation system that prevents the pathogen from escaping into the rest of the facility. In a normal health care facility room, the air is forced downward from the ventilation system. In an airborne precautions room, the ventilation is reversed so that room air is drawn upward into the vents. This creates a negative pressure environment. The ventilation is either specially filtered or exhausted directly to the outside of the building. This room has six to twelve complete changes of air per hour. The door to the room is always kept closed.

Some long-term care facilities do not have the special ventilation required for airborne precautions rooms. These facilities use portable units that are placed in the room to filter the air and create a negative pressure environment. They are slightly noisier than the ventilation system, but are effective in eliminating airborne pathogens.

Staff entering the room must wear a special mask, called a high efficiency particulate air (HEPA) respirator (Figure 3-24). This mask has very small pores that prevent the tiny pathogen from entering. The mask must be fit-tested by a professional to be sure it fits the employee properly and does not leak. Each time you apply the mask, you must check the fit yourself. After the HEPA mask is professionally fit-tested, the employee must also have a medical

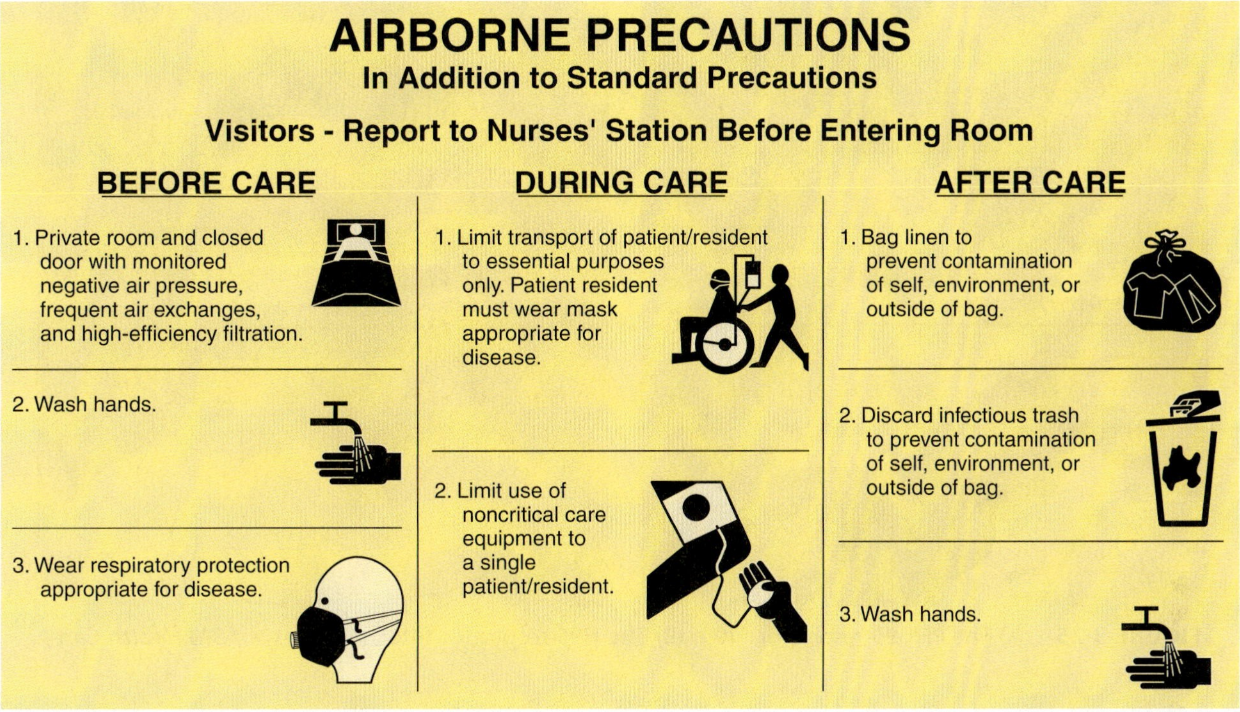

AIRBORNE PRECAUTIONS
In Addition to Standard Precautions

Visitors - Report to Nurses' Station Before Entering Room

BEFORE CARE	DURING CARE	AFTER CARE
1. Private room and closed door with monitored negative air pressure, frequent air exchanges, and high-efficiency filtration.	1. Limit transport of patient/resident to essential purposes only. Patient resident must wear mask appropriate for disease.	1. Bag linen to prevent contamination of self, environment, or outside of bag.
2. Wash hands.	2. Limit use of noncritical care equipment to a single patient/resident.	2. Discard infectious trash to prevent contamination of self, environment, or outside of bag.
3. Wear respiratory protection appropriate for disease.		3. Wash hands.

FIGURE 3-23 Airborne precautions. *(Courtesy of Briggs Corporation, Des Moines, IA 800-247-2343)*

exam to be sure that use of the HEPA mask is not dangerous to his or her health. The medical examination is done because some individuals have underlying diseases that make working in such a mask difficult or impossible. Men with facial hair cannot wear the HEPA mask because the facial hair prevents a tight seal. If a man with facial hair must enter the room, a special hood is

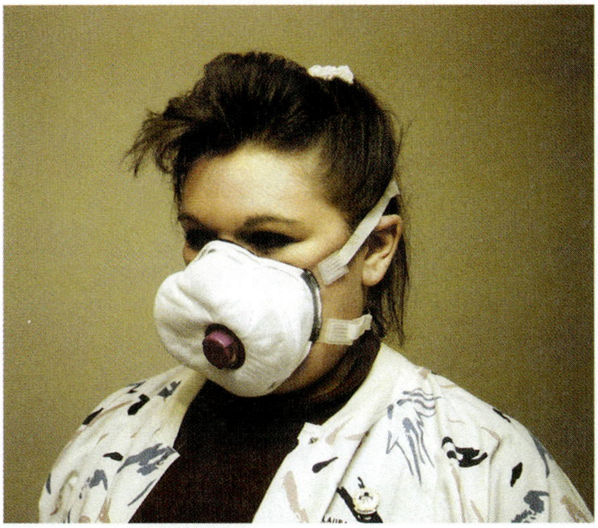

FIGURE 3-24 The HEPA respirator filter

worn. Because of the fit-testing and health examination requirements, facilities may select only certain employees to work in rooms where airborne precautions are used. When working in an airborne precautions room, no other personal protective equipment is necessary unless it is needed to apply the principles of standard precautions.

A **PFR95 respirator** (**Figure 3-25A**) or **N95 respirator** (**Figure 3-25B**) may be worn instead of the HEPA mask. Some health care workers prefer these masks because they are lighter in weight and more comfortable to wear. As with the HEPA mask, there are fit-testing and health examination requirements. These masks are also fit-tested by the worker each time they are worn (**Figure 3-26**).

Droplet precautions. **Droplet precautions** (**Figure 3-27**) are used for some residents whose infections are spread in the air. An example of a disease for which droplet precautions are used is influenza. The pathogen is spread by the droplets in mucus from oral, nasal, and respiratory secretions. The droplets usually remain within three feet of the resident. The secretions containing the pathogen are too large and heavy to be carried in the air currents. A private room is necessary, but special ventilation is not used. Regular surgical masks are worn. The pathogen

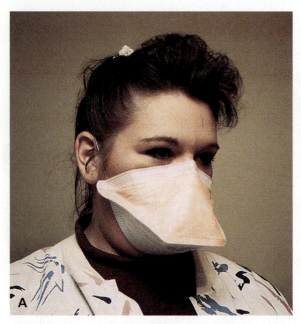
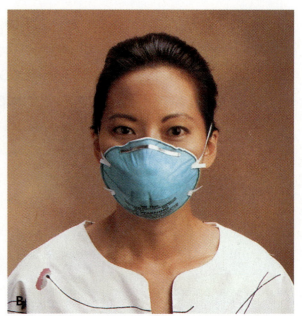

FIGURE 3-25 (A) The PFR-95 respirator filter. (B) The N95 respirator filter. *(Courtesy of 3M Health Care)*

Donning instructions (to be followed each time product is worn):

1 Cup the respirator in your hand with the nosepiece at fingertips, allowing the headbands to hang freely below hands.

2 Position the respirator under your chin with the nosepiece up.

3 Pull the top strap over your head so it rests high on the back of head.

4 Pull the bottom strap over your head and position it around neck below ears.

5 Using two hands, mold the nosepiece to the shape of your nose by pushing inward while moving fingertips down both sides of the nosepiece. Pinching the nosepiece using one hand may result in less effective respirator performance.

6 FACE FIT CHECK
The respirator seal should be checked before each use. To check fit, place both hands completely over the respirator and exhale. If air leaks around your nose, adjust the nosepiece as described in step 5. If air leaks at respirator edges, adjust the straps back along the sides of your head. Recheck.

NOTE: If you cannot achieve proper fit, do not enter the isolation or treatment area. See your supervisor.

Removal instructions:

1 Cup the respirator in your hand to maintain position on face. Pull bottom strap over head.

2 Still holding respirator in position, pull top strap over head.

3 Remove respirator from face and discard or store according to your facility's policy.

FIGURE 3-26 All respirators must be fit-tested by the employee each time he or she wears one. *(Courtesy of 3M Health Care)*

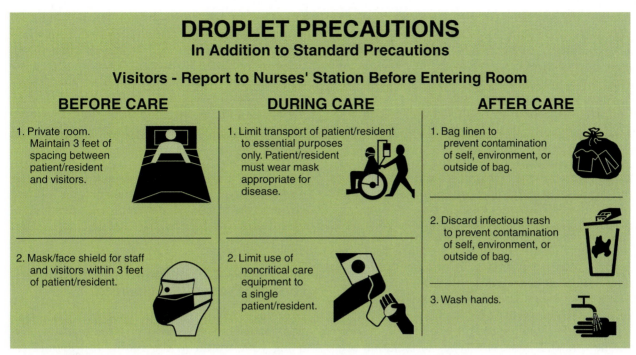

FIGURE 3-27   Droplet precautions. *(Courtesy of Briggs Corporation, Des Moines, IA 800-247-2343)*

is too large to fit between the pores of the surgical mask. The door to the room does not have to be kept closed unless direct care is being performed, because the organism stays within three feet of the resident. No other personal protective equipment is necessary unless it is needed to apply standard precautions.

Contact precautions.   Contact precautions **(Figure 3-28)** are used to contain pathogens that are spread by direct or indirect contact. The microbes that spread the disease in residents in contact precautions are usually found in infections of the skin, urine, and fecal material. Standard precautions are used in addition to

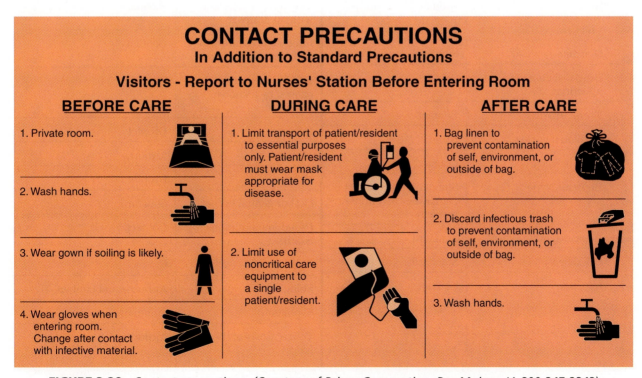

FIGURE 3-28   Contact precautions. *(Courtesy of Briggs Corporation, Des Moines, IA 800-247-2343)*

contact precautions. Gloves are worn anytime you enter the room. No other personal protective equipment is necessary unless you anticipate having direct contact with the resident or with environmental surfaces. When contact is expected, you must wear a gown to cover your uniform. Additional PPE is used only if you anticipate splashing of secretions. If you think this may happen, you will need a face shield or goggles and a surgical mask to protect the mucous membranes in your eyes, nose, and mouth. The principles of standard precautions are also used for residents in contact precautions.

Special circumstances. Residents may have infections that are transmitted by more than one method. A resident may have an infection, such as a cold, that is spread by the droplet method. The resident may also have a separate infection of the skin. Some diseases, such as chickenpox, and shingles, are spread by more than one method. In this case, two types of isolation are used in addition to standard precautions. **Table 3-6** lists common diseases and the type of transmission-based precautions used for each.

Identifying residents in isolation. Most facilities post signs on the door to the room when a resident is in isolation. The sign provides directions on personal protective equipment to wear and describes precautions to take. Some facilities feel that posting signs on the door of the resident's room is an invasion of privacy. These facilities usually post a stop sign on the door that advises you to check with the nurse before entering the room. Before caring for these residents, you must get verbal directions from the nurse or look for specific instructions on the cover of the resident's chart or other designated location.

Sequence for Applying and Removing Personal Protective Equipment

There are times when you must wear full isolation garments in a resident's room. If you will be using your watch in the room, you should remove it first and place it on a clean paper towel. You will carry the watch on the towel. The sequence in which you apply and remove your per-

TABLE 3-6 Diseases Requiring Transmission-Based Precautions

Disease or Condition	Type of Precautions	Disease or Condition	Type of Precautions
AIDS	Standard	Infected pressure sore with no drainage	Standard
Chickenpox	Airborne and contact	Infected pressure sore with heavy drainage	Contact
Diarrhea	Standard		
Drug-resistant skin infections	Contact	Infectious diarrhea caused by a known pathogen	Contact
E. coli 0157:H7	Contact	Influenza	Droplet
German measles	Droplet	Measles	Airborne
Head or body lice	Contact	Mumps	Droplet
Hepatitis, type A	Standard. Use contact if diarrhea or incontinent resident.	Oral or genital herpes	Standard
		Pseudomembranous colititis	Contact
Hepatitis, other types	Standard	Scabies	Contact
HIV disease	Standard	Shingles	Airborne and contact
Impetigo	Contact	Syphilis	Standard
		Tuberculosis of the lungs	Airborne

Note: Use standard precautions in addition to other types of precautions listed.

GUIDELINES FOR

Isolation Handwashing

- Roll your sleeves up to your elbows.
- Wash your hands and forearms following the procedural guidelines for handwashing.
  - Wash your hands:
  - Before entering an isolation room.
  - After removing the isolation gown and gloves.
  - Before and after removing an isolation mask.

- Immediately before leaving the isolation room. Use a paper towel to turn the doorknob when leaving the room; discard the towel in the room.
- Any other time that handwashing is required to practice standard precautions.
- Any time your hands touch a contaminated or potentially contaminated surface.

PROCEDURE

2

Applying and Removing Personal Protective Equipment (Disposable Gloves, Gown, Surgical Mask, Protective Eyewear)

Applying Disposable Isolation Gloves

1. Wash your hands.
2. Remove clean gloves from the box.
3. Put hands into the gloves, adjusting the fingers for comfort and fit.
4. Pull the cuff of the gloves over the sleeve of the gown, if worn.

Removing Disposable Isolation Gloves

1. Grasp the outside of the glove on the nondominant hand at the cuff. Pull the glove off so that the inside of the glove faces outward (**Figures 3-29A** and **B**). Avoid touching the skin of your wrist with the fingers of the glove.
2. Place this glove into the palm of the hand that is still gloved.

3. Put the fingers of the ungloved hand inside the cuff of the gloved hand. Pull the glove off (**Figure 3-29C**) inside out. The first glove removed should be inside the second glove (**Figure 3-29D**).
4. Discard the gloves into a covered container or isolation trash, according to facility policy.
5. Wash your hands.

Putting On an Isolation Gown

1. Wash your hands.
2. Hold the clean gown by the neck in front of you, letting it unfold. Do not let the gown touch the floor.
3. Place your arms in the sleeves and slide the gown up to your shoulders.
4. Slip your hands inside the neck band and grasp the ties. Tie them at the neck.

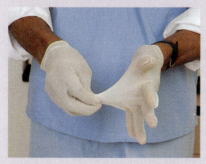

FIGURE 3-29A Grasp the outside cuff or center of the palm of the glove without touching your hand.

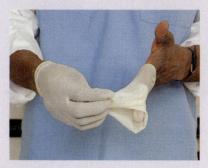

FIGURE 3-29B Pull the glove off inside out.

Continues

PROCEDURE

2

Applying and Removing Personal Protective Equipment (Disposable Gloves, Gown, Surgical Mask, Protective Eyewear), *Continued*

5. Cover your uniform at the back with the gown and tie the ties at the waist. The gown must completely cover your clothing.

Removing the Isolation Gown

1. Untie the waist ties of the gown.
2. Remove gloves.
3. Wash your hands.
4. If a mask is worn, untie the bottom ties of the mask, then the top ties.
5. Discard the mask, holding it only by the ties.
6. Untie the neck ties of the gown and loosen it at the shoulders, touching only the inside of the gown.
7. Grasp the neck ties and pull the gown off inside out.
8. Roll the gown away from your body. Touch only the inside. Discard according to facility policy.
9. Wash your hands.

Applying the Surgical Mask

1. Wash your hands. Remove a mask from the box by holding the ties.
2. Cover your nose and mouth with the mask.
3. Pinch the metal nose piece over the bridge of your nose until it fits comfortably.
4. Tie the top tie or stretch the elastic over the top of your head or ears, depending on the type of mask used.

5. Tie the bottom tie.
6. Wash your hands.

Removing the Isolation Mask

1. Remove gloves.
2. Wash your hands.
3. Untie the neck tie of the mask.
4. Untie the upper tie.
5. Remove the mask by touching only the ties.
6. Discard according to facility policy.
7. Wash your hands.

Applying Protective Eyewear

1. Wash your hands and apply the surgical or HEPA mask.
2. Apply the goggles and secure the elastic strap around the back of your head, or apply the face shield.
3. Wash your hands.

Removing Protective Eyewear

1. Remove your gloves and wash your hands.
2. Lift the protective goggles or face shield away from your face.
3. Remove your surgical or HEPA mask.
4. Wash your hands.

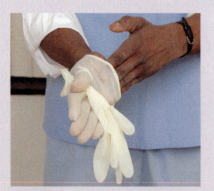

FIGURE 3-29C Hold the glove in your hand.

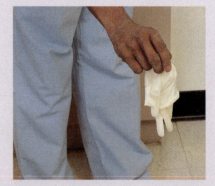

FIGURE 3-29D Remove the opposite glove inside out.

sonal protective equipment is important. Follow the guidelines on page 69.

Exiting the Isolation Room

If you used your watch in the isolation room, pick it up after removing your personal protec-

tive equipment and put it on your wrist. Holding the clean upper side of the paper towel, pick up the towel and discard it in the trash. Obtain a clean paper towel from the dispenser and use it to open the door of the room. After the door is open, discard the towel inside the room. The door may be left open in contact and droplet

GUIDELINES FOR
Putting on Personal Protective Equipment

1. Wash your hands.
2. Put on the isolation gown.
3. Put on the isolation mask.

4. Apply goggles or face shield, if needed.
5. Put on the isolation gloves.

GUIDELINES FOR
Removing Personal Protective Equipment

1. Remove gloves.
2. Wash your hands.
3. Remove protective eyewear, if worn.
4. Wash your hands.
5. Untie the waist tie of the isolation gown.

6. Untie the neck tie of the gown and remove it carefully.
7. Wash your hands.
8. Remove your mask.
9. Wash your hands.

precautions if this is the resident's preference. It is a good idea to wash your hands again after leaving the room.

PROBLEMATIC PATHOGENS

Escherichia Coli

Escherichia coli (E. coli) is a type of bacteria that normally resides in the intestines. Outside of the intestines, it can cause serious problems. This bacterium sometimes causes urinary tract infections. Another strain, **E. coli 0157:H7,** has caused outbreaks resulting in serious illness and death. This is a nonhuman strain that is found in the intestines of some cattle. A small amount of this bacteria can contaminate a large amount of meat, particularly ground beef. It is transmitted in contaminated and undercooked meat, by produce that has been rinsed in water contaminated with feces, or by a person who has been handling contaminated food. It has been found on cutting boards and utensils. The bacteria have been found in unpasteurized milk and apple juice, and in pools and lakes contaminated with fecal matter. The best way to prevent its spread is to use good handwashing and food preparation practices. Ground beef (hamburger) should be cooked until it is well done in the center. The high temperature required to cook meat to well done will kill the pathogen.

Signs and Symptoms. When E. coli 0157:H7 enters the human intestinal tract, it multiplies rapidly, producing large amounts of toxins. One to two days later, the person develops watery diarrhea, nausea, vomiting, and cramping. In another day or two, the diarrhea becomes bloody. The abdomen becomes **distended** (enlarged) and very tender. The resident may show signs of dehydration, swelling, and **petechiae,** small purplish spots on the body surface, caused by minute hemorrhages. The diarrhea may subside in five to seven days, but the condition injures the mucous membranes, causing the pathogen to escape into the bloodstream. This creates a situation in which bloodflow to the brain, kidneys, and other organs is endangered. The resident develops signs and symptoms of serious illness, such as:

- Decreased urine output that may progress to complete renal failure
- Mental confusion
- Seizures (convulsions)
- Muscle weakness
- Pain and numbness of the feet and legs

Treatment. In some conditions, the risk of transmitting infection is highest before the diagnosis is made. Because of this, many facilities place residents in contact precautions if one of these conditions is suspected. Diapered and incontinent residents remain in contact precautions for the duration of the illness. Standard precautions may safely be used for other residents. E. coli 0157:H7 can be deadly, particularly in elderly adults and persons with conditions that weaken the immune system. Care is supportive, and the resident must be carefully monitored. Unfortunately, many drugs increase the risk of kidney damage. Water intake is very important, but liquid intake must be observed closely because of the potential for kidney damage. Careful monitoring of the resident's vital signs is required.

Pseudomembranous Colitis

Many bacteria live in the bowel of a healthy person. Most of them are harmless, and some friendly bacteria help with digestion. A few of these have the potential to be troublemakers if they get out of control. Most of the time, the bad bacteria are outnumbered by the good bacteria, and no harm comes to the person. Taking antibiotics can upset the balance in the colon. Many people experience a brief bout of diarrhea because the balance is upset, but the condition resolves quickly on its own.

Pseudomembranous colitis is a very serious condition in which the diarrhea is caused by a bacterium called Clostridium difficile (C. difficile). It is often called by its nickname, "C. diff." This condition develops in residents who have been on antibiotic therapy. The friendly (good) bacteria die as a result of the antibiotic, and the harmful (bad) bacteria grow out of control. Without the other friendly bacteria to keep it in check, C. difficile breeds rapidly, producing toxins that cause serious illness.

C. difficile is very common in health care facilities. It is picked up on the hands from bedpans, bedside commodes, toilets, sinks, countertops, bed rails, doorknobs, and other surfaces that have been contaminated by stool. It spreads into the body (most commonly the mouth) by unwashed hands.

Signs and Symptoms. Pseudomembranous colitis may occur several weeks or months after the resident has completed the course of antibiotics, so it can be difficult to diagnose. C. difficile produces a toxin that causes inflammation of the intestine. This results in sudden, severe, foul-smelling, watery diarrhea. Stopping the antibiotic will not stop the diarrhea. The diarrhea may be so frequent and severe that the resident becomes dehydrated rapidly and develops other serious imbalances within the body. Other signs and symptoms are:

- Cramping and pain in the lower abdomen; sometimes this begins several days before the diarrhea starts

- Fever
- Mucus, pus, or blood in the stool
- Abdomen very tender to touch
- In severe cases, low blood pressure and signs of shock

If the condition is not promptly treated, it can cause ruptured bowel and a condition in which the bowel becomes severely distended and retains stool.

Diagnosis and Treatment. If pseudomembranous colitis is suspected, the doctor will order laboratory tests on one or more stool specimens. The laboratory will identify the bacteria that are causing the illness. The antibiotic suspected of causing the problem is stopped, if possible. Another drug is used to eliminate the harmful bacteria in the colon. The resident may be given yogurt to eat and several other medications to increase the balance of healthful flora in the bowel. Although drug therapy usually eliminates the condition, it sometimes recurs, making a second course of therapy necessary. The resident is placed in contact precautions until 72 hours after the appearance and frequency of stools return to normal, or as ordered by the physician. Use good handwashing techniques with antibacterial soap and water. Do not use alcohol-based hand cleaners. This disease is spread by spores, and alcohol will not eliminate them. The friction and running water will remove them from your hands during handwashing.

Hantavirus

In May 1993, a cluster of unexplained deaths occurred among young Native Americans in the southwestern United States. An investigation revealed a virus that was previously unknown. This situation attracted a great deal of media attention. Several additional outbreaks have been reported since 1993. This strange disease is called **hantavirus.** It is spread by contact with rodents (rats and mice) or their excretions, including urine and stool. Once disturbed, viral particles in the excretions become airborne and are inhaled by the susceptible host. Signs and symptoms appear one to five weeks later. They include high fever, chills, muscle aches, cough, nausea, vomiting, diarrhea, dizziness, and feeling very tired. As the disease progresses, the resident becomes very short of breath. When this occurs, the disease progresses rapidly, and the resident becomes seriously ill. The resident may be transferred to the hospital for respiratory support. Hantavirus is not transmitted from person to person. Spread of this condition can be reduced by taking steps to prevent rodents from entering the facility or home, and eliminating them if they are present.

Shingles

Shingles (herpes zoster) is a condition that occurs only in people who have had chickenpox. Although the person recovered from the chickenpox, the virus that caused the condition remained hidden in the nervous system. The immune system kept it in an inactive state. The immune system weakens with age. In some people, it is no longer able to contain the virus. The resident develops blister-like lesions on the torso that are often mistaken for a rash. The lesions follow the nerve pathways, and are extremely painful. Health care workers who have not had chickenpox should not enter the room, if other immune caregivers are available. Inhaling airborne viruses will cause chickenpox in workers who are not immune. The lesions are infectious in the blister state. Airborne precautions may be used for residents if there is a widespread outbreak, and for those who are immune-compromised. Contact precautions are also used, at least until all blisters have burst and crusted over. For a minor, localized outbreak, standard precautions may be used.

DRUG-RESISTANT ORGANISMS

Drug-resistant organisms are pathogens that cannot be eliminated by the usual antibiotics. These microbes have become a problem because eliminating them may be difficult or impossible. If antibiotics are available to eliminate the pathogen, they are often very expensive and have toxic side effects such as kidney, liver, and hearing damage. The elderly are very vulnerable to the side effects of antibiotics. The pathogens have become drug resistant for several reasons:

1. People took antibiotics for minor conditions for which antibiotics were not necessary. Over the years, many unnecessary antibiotics have been prescribed.
2. People who were taking antibiotics stopped taking them when they felt better, but before finishing the prescription. The pathogens were still in the body and built up resistance to the antibiotic. The next time the pathogen was exposed to the antibiotic, the drug had no effect.

Methicillin-Resistant *Staphylococcus Aureus*

Methicillin-resistant Staphylococcus aureus (MRSA), is a common drug-resistant organism found in health care facilities. MRSA is very difficult to control and treat. It causes many different types of infections. Skin and urinary infections caused by this pathogen are common. Occasionally, a resident will develop respiratory MRSA. As with the other pathogens discussed earlier, you cannot always tell that the person has an infection. MRSA is spread primarily by direct and indirect contact. Use of standard precautions will prevent the spread of MRSA, particularly in urine and skin infections. Contact precautions are used if the resident is known to have MRSA in a wound or urine. Droplet precautions are used when a resident is known to have MRSA in the respiratory tract.

Vancomycin-Resistant *Enterococcus*

Vancomycin-resistant Enterococcus (VRE), is a newer drug-resistant organism. It originates in the colon, but can cause severe infections in other parts of the body. This organism is spread by contact. Standard precautions and contact precautions are used to prevent the spread of this pathogen.

TUBERCULOSIS

Tuberculosis (TB) is a disease that has been with us for many years. The incidence of tuberculosis was steadily declining until the 1980s, when it began increasing. Many cases of tuberculosis that we see today are drug resistant. TB is spread only through the airborne method. The organism is very small and can travel long distances in the air. Tuberculosis can occur in many different sites in the body, but it is always spread by the airborne method and not through contact.

Signs and Symptoms of Tuberculosis

Signs and symptoms of tuberculosis include feeling tired and sleepy all the time, fever, night sweats, weight loss, cough, coughing up blood-tinged mucus, chest pain, and shortness of breath. When a resident has tuberculosis, airborne precautions are used. A HEPA mask is worn, and the room must have negative pressure ventilation. A resident can usually be removed from isolation after two to three weeks of antibiotics, but treatment will continue for six months to a year.

Testing for Tuberculosis

Health care facilities are required to test residents and employees periodically for the presence of the organism that causes TB. Skin testing is done. Health care facilities are using a two-step test for the initial testing. A one-step test is used thereafter. Employees are tested upon employment and every 3 to 12 months thereafter. The frequency of the testing is determined by how high the risk of infection is in your health care facility and community. If the skin test is positive, the employee is referred to a physician or public health agency for follow-up. A chest x-ray and other lab tests are done. If the tests are negative, another x-ray will be required if the employee later develops symptoms suggestive of tuberculosis. A positive skin test does not mean that an individual has TB. It indicates exposure to the pathogen that causes tuberculosis, and further testing and treatment may be indicated. Individuals over the age of 35 are not always treated because the drugs used to treat the infection could cause complications in persons of this age. The decision on whether to treat is left to the individual, the personal physician, and the local health authority.

Treating Tuberculosis

Tuberculosis is treated with a combination of antibiotics. It is very important to take the antibiotics exactly as ordered, and for as long as directed, to prevent drug resistance. If the individual is not treated, the TB germ can remain in the body for many years. It may become active sometime in the future. In some people it never becomes active.

Tuberculosis in the Long–Term Care Facility

Tuberculosis should be taken very seriously in long-term care facilities. Many elderly residents were exposed to tuberculosis years ago when the disease was common. Their skin tests are positive, indicating that the microbe is in the body and that they were not treated. The immune systems weaken with age. It is possible for the tuberculosis microbe to become active because the weakened immune system is no longer able to contain it. Fatigue is often the only sign of tuberculosis in the elderly, so a number of people can be infected before the disease is detected.

HEAD LICE

Head lice are **parasites.** Parasites are tiny animals that survive by feeding off humans or other animals. Fleas and ticks are examples of common parasites.

Head lice are spread primarily by direct contact with an infected person. You cannot contract head lice from pets and animals. They are spread by sharing personal belongings such as brushes, combs, ribbons, caps, clothing, and bedding with others. Head lice **(Figure 3-30)** do not hop, jump, or fly, but they can crawl very quickly. When performing hair care, check residents for **nits (Figure 3-31A).** Nits are tiny, oval shaped eggs that are yellow-white. They look like dandruff, but are firmly attached to the hair and are usually very difficult to remove. Empty nit cases are shown in **Figure 3-31B.** These nits have hatched into live lice. *Lice* are tiny brown insects about the size of a sesame seed. They move away from light quickly. **Figure 3-31C** shows how hair spray drops appear on the hair. **Figure 3-31D** is a magnified picture of dandruff. **Figure 3-31E** shows hair casts. Casts and plugs occur when oil glands in the scalp are overactive. They are easily removed. It may be difficult to differentiate nits from other conditions of the scalp. Notify the nurse for further assessment if you notice any abnormalities.

Treatment for Head Lice

If you suspect that nits or lice are present, notify the nurse immediately. You will be directed to wear gloves for further resident contact. You must also wear gloves and a gown when handling the resident's clothing or linen. The physician will be contacted for an order for a special medicated shampoo to kill the parasite. The resident's hair must be washed with this shampoo. Shampoos containing the chemical lindane have proven to be toxic to some people, and are not

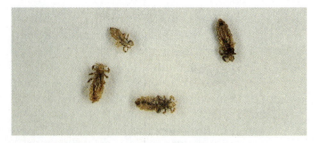

FIGURE 3-30 Head lice are tiny and run very quickly. They do not jump, hop, or fly.

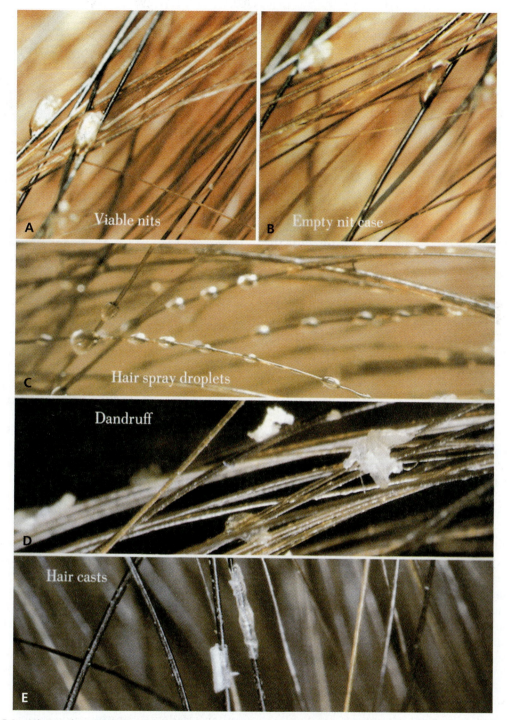

FIGURE 3-31 Nits and eggs that attach firmly to the hair shaft are very difficult to remove. Differentiating one condition from another may be difficult. *(Courtesy of Hogil Pharmaceutical)*

recommended. Contact precautions will be used for 24 hours after the resident is treated. A special comb is used to remove nits from the hair. If the nits cannot be removed by combing, it may be necessary to snip the hair with eggs attached with a pair of safety scissors. The nurse will inspect the resident's scalp the day after the medicated shampoo to look for additional lice and nits. It is important to remove all of the nits, as the shampoo may not kill them. They may be difficult to remove, and this is a time-consuming task. You may be directed to check other residents for the presence of head lice, because the parasite is highly contagious.

As with other diseases, some head lice have become resistant to the medicated shampoos used to eliminate them. If the lice cannot be eliminated with a shampoo, the only way to remove them is by checking the head and eliminating them manually. Manual removal of lice and nits is done using a comb, tweezers, or double-sided tape. It may be necessary for two people to check the head simultaneously, because the lice can run very quickly. Shining a flashlight on the head may be helpful, as the lice move away from the light source. Always wear gloves when caring for the hair of a resident with known or suspected head lice.

All clothing and linen must be bagged and sent to the laundry for washing. Furniture and personal items in the room must be vacuumed to eliminate lice in the environment. Vacuuming is safer and more effective than using pesticide sprays, which leave a toxic residue. After vacuuming, wipe environmental surfaces with a facility-approved disinfectant to eliminate microbes left from the outside of the vacuum cleaner. Previously, toxic sprays were used to eliminate lice from environmental surfaces and personal belongings, but this is no longer recommended.

SCABIES

Scabies is a skin condition caused by a parasite called a mite (Figure 3-32). A mite is a microscopic organism that cannot be seen with the eye. Scabies is highly contagious and is spread by direct and indirect contact. It causes a rash (Figure 3-33A) and severe itching of the skin. The rash may be seen in the webs of the fingers, inside the wrists, outside the elbows, in the underarm, or on the waist and nipple area. It is also sometimes seen in the genital area in men and around the knees (Figure 3-33B) and lower buttocks. One type of scabies causes scaling of the skin on the palms of hands and soles of feet. If you notice a rash, notify the nurse immediately. As with head lice, you will be directed to wear a gown and gloves for further resident contact.

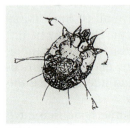

FIGURE 3-32 The scabies mite is microscopic and cannot be seen without a microscope. *(Courtesy of L.E. Morris and Donna J. Lewis, Management of Chronic, Resistive Scabies: A Case Study,* Geriatric Nursing *16 [Sept/Oct 1995]: 230–37)*

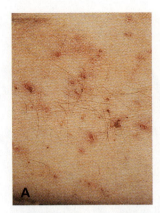 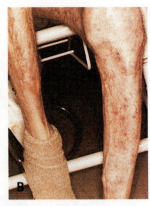

FIGURE 3-33 (A) Typical rash of scabies on the back. (B) Typical rash of scabies on the legs and knees. *(Courtesy of L.E. Morris and Donna J. Lewis, Management of Chronic, Resistive Scabies: A Case Study,* Geriatric Nursing *16 [Sept/Oct 1995]: 230–37)*

Treatment for Scabies

Special medicated creams and lotions are used to kill the mites. Products containing the chemical lindane are toxic and are not recommended. Some strains of scabies have become resistant to commonly used treatments. The resident's nails should be clipped before beginning the procedure. The medicated treatment is worked into and around the fingernail area with a cotton swab. The resident must not be bathed before or after the lotion is applied. You may be directed to apply the lotion to the resident's entire body, not just the rash area. It is not applied to the eyelids or lips. Wear a gown and gloves when applying this treatment. The lotion remains on the resident's skin for 12 to 24 hours, then is washed off in the tub or shower. If the resident's hands are washed during this period, reapply the lotion. Depending on the solution used, another treatment may be required several days to several weeks later. It takes about a month from the first treatment for the rash to disappear. The resident may experience itching even after the scabies are eliminated. You may be directed to check other residents for the appearance of a rash. Facility personnel who have had direct contact with the host resident may also be treated to prevent the spread of the mite.

The resident's room, clothing, and linen must also be cleaned. Wear a gown and gloves when you are assigned to this task. The room and furnishings should be vacuumed thoroughly to capture mites in the environment. Check the mattress and furniture for cracks, as the mite often crawls into the foam padding. If items cannot be vacuumed, they are bagged in a sealed plastic bag for 14 days. The mite cannot live beyond this time without food. Some facilities expose the bags to extreme heat or cold to kill the mite more quickly. The mattress is turned and vacuumed, then wiped with a facility-approved disinfectant to remove microbes left from the outside of the vacuum cleaner. Contact precautions are used for 24 hours after the resident is treated. If the resident requires a second treatment, the cleaning procedure is repeated for clothing, linen, and furnishings.

Drug resistance. As with other microbes, lice and scabies have become resistant to some of the common pesticides used in shampoos and body lotions. When treating for head lice or scabies, it is important to use the products exactly as directed. If live parasites are noted after a resident has been properly treated, it is recommended that the treatment product be changed or discontinued. Products for treating lice and scabies are pesticides and repeated use can cause toxicity and other serious complications.

BIOTERRORISM

Bioterrorism is the use of biological agents, such as pathogenic organisms or agricultural pests, for terrorist purposes. Since October 2001, state, local, and governmental public health authorities have been investigating cases of bioterrorism-related illness in the United States. Some individuals died from inhalation anthrax, a condition that was spread by a powdery substance sent through the mail. A number of other individuals developed the cutaneous (skin) version of this disease. Cutaneous anthrax is not fatal. Anthrax cannot be passed from one person to the next. It is transmitted only through contact with spores. Fortunately, the number of workplaces and individuals contaminated was small, but it raised concerns regarding future terrorist attacks. Many individuals could be infected by a biological weapon before the exposure is detected and diagnosed. Some of the diseases that can potentially be used as biological weapons have been eradicated for years and today's health care professionals have never seen or treated them. Thus, bioterrorism potentially represents a significant threat.

Many health care facilities have developed disaster plans to address bioterrorism. The plans outline the steps necessary for responding to bioterrorism with the most common agents, including smallpox, botulism, anthrax, and plague. The disaster plan covers information for residents, employees, and visitors, and lists public health precautions and protocols to follow in the event of an emergency. Unfortunatedly, health care facilities must be prepared for potential terrorist actions in the future.

KEY POINTS

- Medical asepsis refers to practices used in health care facilities to prevent the spread of infection.
- Microorganisms are everywhere. Pathogens are microorganisms that cause disease.
- The most common methods for spread of infection are airborne, droplet, direct contact, and indirect contact.
- The nursing assistant plays an important role in preventing the spread of infection.
- The nursing assistant must know which items are considered clean and which are considered soiled. These items must be separated to prevent the spread of infection.
- Handwashing is the most important method used to prevent the spread of infection.
- Bloodborne pathogens are microbes that cause disease through contact with blood, any moist body fluid except sweat, secretions, excretions, nonintact skin, and mucous membranes.
- HIV disease, hepatitis B, and hepatitis C are examples of diseases that are spread by contact with bloodborne pathogens.
- Hepatitis B is a greater threat to health care workers than HIV.
- Standard precautions are measures used in the care of all residents to prevent the spread of disease.
- The nursing assistant is responsible for selecting and using the correct personal protective equipment for the procedure being performed.
- Needles, razors, and other sharps are disposed of in puncture-resistant biohazardous waste containers.
- Trash and linen that have contacted blood or body fluids are biohazardous waste.
- Transmission-based precautions are isolation categories designed to interrupt the mode of transmission so the pathogen cannot spread.

- Isolation can be emotionally difficult for the resident.
- A HEPA mask is used when a resident is in airborne precautions. A PFR95 or N95 respirator may be worn instead.
- A surgical mask is used when a resident is in droplet precautions.
- A gown and gloves are used when a resident is in contact precautions.
- Standard precautions are used in addition to transmission-based precautions.
- Escherichia coli is a type of bacteria that normally resides in the intestines. It can cause serious illness outside the intestinal tract.
- E. coli 0157:H7 is a nonhuman strain that is found in the intestines of some cattle. It is most commonly spread in undercooked hamburger, and has caused outbreaks resulting in serious illness and death.
- Pseudomembranous colitis occurs when antibiotics destroy the normal, helpful bowel flora, except for C. difficile. Without the other friendly bacteria to keep it in check, C. difficile breeds rapidly, producing toxins that cause diarrhea and serious illness.
- Hantavirus causes serious respiratory illness. It is spread by contact with rodents or their excretions, including urine and stool.
- Shingles develop only in individuals who have had chickenpox. The resident develops painful, blister-like lesions on the torso that are often mistaken for a rash.
- Health care workers who have not had chickenpox should not enter the room of a resident who has shingles, if other immune caregivers are available.
- Drug-resistant organisms are a problem in health care facilities. Their spread can be prevented by medical asepsis and use of standard precautions.
- Tuberculosis is a growing public health problem that is detected by a skin test and treated with antibiotics.
- Head lice and scabies are highly contagious and require the use of contact precautions for 24 hours after the resident is treated.
- Bioterrorism is the use of biological agents, such as pathogenic organisms or agricultural pests, for terrorist purposes.

REVIEW

A. Multiple Choice

Select the one best answer.

1. Medical asepsis is
   a. a surgical technique.
   b. practices used to prevent the spread of infection.
   c. of concern only to licensed personnel.
   d. part of the chain of infection.

2. An infection that develops when a person is a resident in a health care facility is called a/an
   a. facility infection.
   b. acquired infection.
   c. nosocomial infection.
   d. delayed infection.

3. Some factors that affect the body's natural ability to resist disease are
   a. height.
   b. nutritional status and presence of other diseases.
   c. range of motion.
   d. a heater in the room to prevent chilling.

4. The system that detects pathogens in the body and stimulates the body's defenses to prevent disease is the
   a. immune system.
   b. nervous system.
   c. genitourinary system.
   d. respiratory system.

5. Infections can be spread by
   a. direct contact.
   b. inhaling a microbe.
   c. vectors.
   d. all of the above.

6. An example of common vehicle method of transmission is
   a. touching a contaminated object.
   b. eating contaminated food.
   c. inhaling droplets in the air.
   d. shaking hands.

7. Droplets usually are confined to a space within
   a. 3 feet of the resident.
   b. 6 feet of the resident.
   c. 12 feet of the resident.
   d. 24 feet of the resident.

8. Pathogens spread by the airborne method:
   a. are confined to a space within three feet of the resident.
   b. pose no threat to others.
   c. travel long distances in the ventilation system.
   d. are contracted in a negative-pressure room.

9. The six factors necessary for an infection to spread are called the
   a. mode of transmission.
   b. reservoir of infection.
   c. portal of exit.
   d. chain of infection.

10. _____ must be used in the care of all residents.
    a. Standard precautions
    b. Substance isolation
    c. Skin precautions
    d. Isolation precautions

11. The most important measure health care workers use to prevent the spread of infection is
    a. wearing a mask.
    b. handwashing.
    c. surgical asepsis.
    d. wearing a gown.

12. Handwashing should be performed
    a. at least three times a day.
    b. after work only.
    c. before applying and after removing gloves.
    d. before visiting with a resident.

13. Handwashing should be done for a minimum of
    a. 3 seconds.
    b. 5 seconds.
    c. 15 seconds.
    d. 60 seconds.

14. A vaccination is available to protect health care workers from
    a. AIDS.
    b. hepatitis B.
    c. herpes.
    d. MRSA.

15. Hepatitis B, hepatitis C, and AIDS are spread by
    a. blood and body fluid contact.
    b. the inhalation method.
    c. casual contact.
    d. using the same bathroom.

16. Gloves should be worn when
    a. combing a resident's hair.
    b. entering a resident's room.
    c. taking a blood pressure.
    d. brushing a resident's teeth.

17. The transmission-based precautions category in which a gown is routinely worn during close resident care is
    a. airborne precautions.
    b. contact precautions.
    c. droplet precautions.
    d. standard precautions.

18. When working in an airborne precautions room, you should wear a
    a. HEPA mask (or equivalent).
    b. surgical mask (or equivalent).
    c. gown.
    d. face shield.

19. Trash that is contaminated with blood or body fluids is identified by
    a. using a black bag.
    b. a circle with a slash through it.
    c. the biohazard emblem.
    d. a pink label.

20. Apply personal protective equipment in this order
    a. gloves, gown, mask.
    b. mask, gown, gloves.
    c. gown, mask, gloves.
    d. gloves, mask, gown.

21. Drug-resistant organisms
    a. are of no concern to the nursing assistant.
    b. can be eliminated easily with most antibiotics.
    c. are a threat to residents and health care workers.
    d. are very uncommon.

22. Tuberculosis is
    a. a growing public health concern.
    b. a disease that was eliminated in the 1960s.
    c. easily treated.
    d. a vector-borne respiratory illness.

23. Head lice and scabies are
    a. the same as nits.
    b. fomites.
    c. parasites.
    d. viruses.

24. When a resident has scabies, he or she will be placed in
    a. airborne precautions.
    b. contact precautions.
    c. droplet precautions.
    d. secretion precautions.

25. Alcohol-based hand cleansers
    a. should not be used during resident care.
    b. may be used unless hands are visibly soiled.
    c. are used only when a sink is not available.
    d. may be used only by nurses during medication pass.

26. After removing gloves
    a. wash your hands or use an alcohol-based cleanser.
    b. quickly rinse your hands with cool water and dry them.
    c. scrub your hands with disinfectant solution.
    d. handwashing is not necessary.

27. Pseudomembranous colitis
    a. occurs only in infants wearing diapers.
    b. is spread by rats and other rodents.
    c. is contracted by the airborne method.
    d. is diarrhea caused by antibiotics.

28. Shingles
    a. occurs only in residents who have had measles.
    b. does not readily spread to others.
    c. follows the nerve pathways, causing pain.
    d. is spread by vectors and fomites.

29. Petechiae are
    a. small, purple spots on the skin.
    b. swollen and painful.
    c. breaks in the skin surface.
    d. immune factors.

30. The use of biological agents for terrorist purposes is
    a. bioterrorism.
    b. chemical warfare.
    c. biology.
    d. biomedical warfare.

B. True/False

Answer each statement true (T) or false (F).

31. _____ The term infection control refers to practices that reduce the spread of infection in the health care facility.

32. _____ Susceptibility is the ability of the body to resist disease.

33. _____ Hepatitis B destroys the immune system.

34. _____ A handshake is an example of the spread of infection through indirect contact.

35. _____ A microbe that is capable of causing disease is a pathogen.

36. _____ The objective of using medical asepsis is to break the chain of infection.

37. _____ Always wear gloves on both hands when carrying contaminated items in the hallway.

38. _____ It is not necessary to wash your hands after gloves are removed.

39. _____ Standard precautions are used in the care of all residents.

40. _____ Gloves should be changed immediately before contact with mucous membranes.

41. _____ Artificial fingernails may be worn when on duty, as long as they are kept short.

42. _____ Rings may hide pathogens.

43. _____ Flora are microbes that inhabit the internal and external surfaces of healthy individuals.

C. Fill in the Blanks

44–49. List six times when you should wash your hands.

44. _____   47. _____

45. _____   48. _____

46. _____   49. _____

D. Clinical Applications

Answer the following questions.

50. David Long, a nursing assistant, has just completed caring for Mr. Brent. The resident had a loose bowel movement in a bedpan. David must carry the bedpan to the bathroom and clean it. David has BM on his gloves. How does David pull up the side rail and open the bathroom door without contaminating the environment with his soiled gloves?

51. Sam and John have been roommates for years. Both are mentally confused and walk around in the room. You are assigned to pass fresh water to the residents on Hall C. When you get to Sam and John's room, you find two water pitchers and two cups sitting side by side on the counter in the bathroom. You do not know which pitcher and cup belong to which resident. What should you do?

52. Susan Lange is a 37-year-old resident with AIDS. She has bumped her leg on the side rail and is bleeding. You accidentally get some blood on your hand. What should you do?

53. You are assigned to care for Mr. Jefferson, who is in contact precautions for an MRSA infection of a surgical wound. Mr. Jefferson is alert, oriented, and cooperative. He feeds himself. What personal protective equipment will you wear when you
    a. Serve the meal tray?
    b. Change the linen on the bed?

54. While caring for Mr. Jefferson, your gloves become soiled. You are not through with giving care. What should you do?

CHAPTER 4

Safety and Emergencies

OBJECTIVES

After reading this chapter, you will be able to:

- Spell and define key terms.
- Describe measures to take to keep the environment safe.
- List three measures to take to prevent burns.
- Describe safety factors to consider when using heat and cold applications.
- Describe safety factors to use when caring for a resident who is using oxygen.
- List the three elements necessary to start a fire.
- Describe your responsibilities if there is a fire, tornado, hurricane, earthquake, or bomb threat.
- Describe what to do if you find a resident in an emergency situation.
- List seven guidelines to follow in an emergency.
- State the purpose of early access defibrillation.
- Demonstrate procedures related to safety and emergencies.

OBSERVATIONS TO MAKE AND REPORT RELATED TO SAFETY AND EMERGENCIES

Chest pain
Shortness of breath
Difficulty breathing
Weakness or dizziness
Headache
Pain or body language suggesting pain
Nausea or vomiting
Diarrhea (multiple loose stools; one loose stool is not diarrhea)
Cough
Cyanosis or change in color

Change in mental status
Excessive thirst
Lethargy
Unusual drainage from the skin, a wound, or a body cavity
Abnormal appearance of urine or feces
Inability to hear blood pressure or palpate pulse
Changes in vital signs
Abnormal behavior, including crying
Requests for medication for an acute problem

IMPORTANCE OF SAFETY IN THE LONG-TERM CARE FACILITY

Safety is everyone's concern. Special safety measures are described throughout this text. Every employee is responsible for keeping the environ-ment safe and preventing **accidents.** However, because of their close and consistent contact with the residents, much of the burden for maintaining a safe environment rests with the nursing assistants.

Accidents are unexpected events that often result in injuries, which can range from minor to serious. An **incident** is an occurrence that disrupts the normal procedures and routine of the facility. It may be the result of an accident. A fall is an accident, but it is also an incident. If a confused resident wanders away, but is returned unharmed, an incident has occurred. An **incident report** (**Figure 4-1**) is completed by the charge nurse on all accidents and incidents. The incident report states what happened, describes injuries, lists witnesses, and records special notifications of the doctor and resident's family. Information written on the incident report is al-

ways **factual.** This is information that you *know* is true, not what you *think* may have happened. You may be asked to do extra monitoring of the resident until the signs of the incident are **resolved.** An incident is resolved when the charge nurse is certain that problems related to the incident are over and the resident is stable and out of danger.

Most accidents can be prevented. Accidents can occur to residents, visitors, and employees. Everyone benefits from a safe environment. The

RESIDENT INCIDENT REPORT

IF INJURY SERIOUS, GIVE IMMEDIATE NOTICE TO THE ADMINISTRATOR AND DIRECTOR OF NURSING SERVICE   NOTE: PLEASE COMPLETE IN DETAIL

INSTRUCTIONS: Completed report to D.O.N. for review and filing in Administrator's Office. Make detailed report in Nurses Notes/Resident Records.

DATE OF OCCURRENCE _1/4/XX_   PLACE _Room 304_   TIME _4³⁰_   AM (PM)

NAME _Jane Walther_   TEMP _98⁴_   BLOOD PRESSURE _134/88_   PULSE _80_   RESPIRATIONS _16_

ASSISTANCE NEEDED (Partial or Total)	FUNCTIONING (Partial or Total)	MENTAL STATUS*** Yes No	BEHAVIOR PROBLEMS 1-Minimum 2-Moderate 3-Maximum
P T Ambulation	P T Bedfast	(Y) N Lucid	2 Confused
P T Amb. w/Cane, Crutch, Walker	P T Fecal Incontinent	Y (N) Labile	0 Withdrawn
(P) T Transferring	(P) T Urinary Incontinent	(Y) N Disoriented	0 Hyperactive
(P) T Wheelchair Mobility	(P) T Blindness	Y (N) Comatose	0 Wanders
P T Bedside Chair	P T Deafness	Y (N) Semi-Comatose	0 Suspicious
(P) T Bathing	P T Aphasia	(Y) N Forgetful	0 Combative
(P) T Dressing	P T Speech Problem	Y (N) Controlled with Medication	2 Supervised for Safety
P T Grooming			0 Causes Mgt. Problems

RESTRAINTS ORDERED: ☐ YES   ☑ NO   ☐ NOT APPLICABLE   ***Complete this section *ONLY IF* mental status contributed to incident/accident

IF NOT USED, WHY? _____

WAS PRN MEDICATION ADMINISTERED BEFORE INCIDENT?   ☐ YES   ☑ NO   ☐ NOT APPLICABLE

NAME OF DRUG ADMINISTERED & TIME ADMINISTERED _____

DESCRIPTION OF INCIDENT (include circumstances under which incident occurred): _Resident attempted to transfer self from bed to w/c unassisted. No witnesses to incident. Res. was found on floor. Brakes to w/c were not locked. Footrests to w/c were in down position. Res. had socks on feet, but no shoes. States "I slipped"._

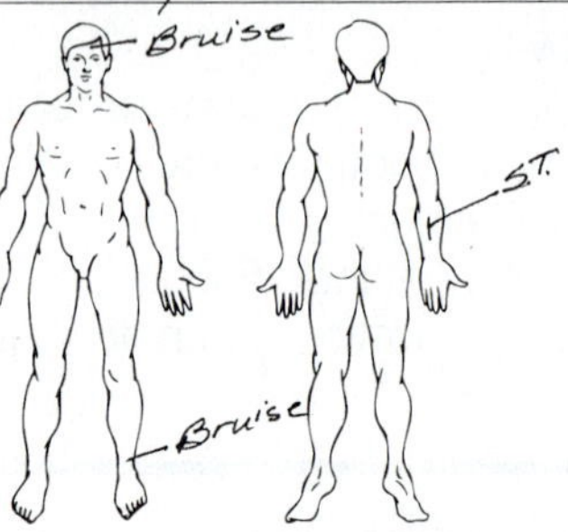

INDICATE ON FIGURES PART OF BODY AFFECTED AND DESCRIBE EXTENT OF INJURY:

Bruise (L) temple
Skin tear (R) forearm
Bruise (L) ankle

PHYSICIAN'S NAME _John Dennis, D.O._

PHYSICIAN NOTIFIED: DATE _1/4/XX_   TIME _450/_   AM (PM)

PHYSICIAN'S ORDERS, TREATMENT OR STATEMENT: _Cleanse skin tear + apply dry dressing._

HOSPITALIZED: ☐ YES   ☑ NO   NAME OF HOSPITAL _____

FIGURE 4-1   An incident report is completed on all incidents and accidents.

most common accidents in long-term care facilities are falls and burns.

Physical and Mental Changes in Disease and Aging that Increase the Risk of Incidents

Physical and mental changes occur with aging and with certain diseases. Many of these changes affect the resident's awareness of hazards in the environment, and thus increase the risk of incidents. Factors that influence resident safety include:

- Changes in vision affect the resident's ability to see unsafe conditions. Other changes in vision may cause residents to be unable to judge distance.
- Changes in hearing may affect the resident's ability to hear warnings, or approaching carts or equipment.
- Some diseases cause **tremors,** or shaking that the resident cannot control. Tremors affect the resident's balance and increase the risk of falls.
- Changes in the blood vessels may cause residents to become dizzy when they stand up.
- **Reflexes** are slower in the elderly and in people with certain diseases. Reflexes are automatic, involuntary reactions that cause us to pull away from danger. Because some individuals react more slowly, they cannot move away quickly. For example, if you place your hand under very hot water, you quickly pull away. If a resident with impaired reflexes placed a hand under hot water, he or she would remove it more slowly, and could be burned.
- Some residents have mental changes that cause them to be confused and forgetful. These residents may not use good judgment and may not be aware of common dangers.
- Some residents may be weak because of an illness or injury. This may cause them to fall.
- Some medications have side effects that can cause dizziness, visual disturbances, blood pressure changes, and other problems that increase the risk of injury.

Some residents may not be aware that their activities can be harmful to them. They may resent the staff's efforts to protect them. They feel that they can protect themselves. Residents may also be in **denial.** When a person is in denial, he or she is afraid to admit that something is true. Residents may be afraid that if they admit to having a need, they will no longer be independent. Speak with residents about safety. Explain what you are doing to keep the environment safe. Explain safety to residents during the proce-

dures that you do. Always be alert to safety factors when you enter and leave a room.

Providing a Safe Environment

You can do many things to make the long-term care facility safe. If you notice an unsafe condition that you can correct, you should do so immediately. Report unsafe conditions that you cannot correct to the nurse or the proper person in your facility. Warn others of safety hazards. Follow facility policies and procedures. Set a good example for others by using safe practices. Attend classes on health and safety issues and practice what you are taught.

Safety in the hallways. Everyone is responsible for keeping the hallways safe. If you notice a spill on the floor, wipe it up immediately and place a "wet floor" sign **(Figure 4-2)**. Keep all equipment and supplies on the same side of the hallway. Your goal is to have one side of the hallway free so that residents can walk safely without having to go around large pieces of equipment or the wheelchairs of others. Follow your facility policy for separating items considered clean or soiled. Pick up any items, papers, or equipment dropped on the floor.

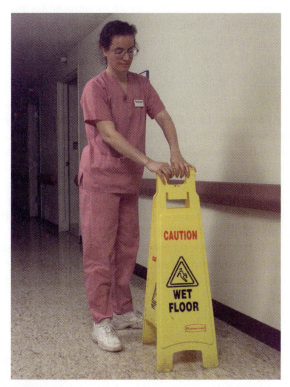

FIGURE 4-2 A wet floor sign warns others of slippery spots.

Never run in the hallways. Teach residents to use the handrails when they walk in the hallway. If you are transporting residents or equipment in the hall, watch where you are going. Approach corners slowly and look before you go around them. Take care when approaching or going through swinging doors. Avoid blocking exit doors or automatic fire doors with equipment or furnishings. Back wheelchairs and stretchers in and out of elevators, down ramps, and over thresholds in doorways.

Safety in the resident's room. Be sure there is enough light in residents' rooms. Visual changes as a result of aging and disease make it difficult to see in dim lighting. However, avoid bright lights that shine directly into the residents' eyes. Remove any items that have fallen on the floor. Arrange the furniture so it is against the walls, not in the middle of the room. Other safety considerations for the resident's room are described in Chapter 10.

Avoid dressing residents in long clothing that may cause them to trip. Avoid clothing or linen that may get caught in the wheels of a wheelchair. If residents will be walking or transferring from a bed to a wheelchair, make sure their footwear is appropriate for the floor surface. In facilities with tile floors, nonslip footwear is best. On carpeted floors, leather or plastic soles may work better. Nonslip soles may catch on carpeting, causing the resident to stumble. Residents should not walk or transfer in socks or with bare feet, because of the risk of falls.

Follow your facility policy for use of electrical appliances, such as televisions, radios, heating pads, and hair dryers in resident rooms. Most facilities require that appliances brought in from home be checked by the maintenance department for safety before they are used. Extension cords are not permitted. If you observe an electrical hazard, notify the proper person immediately. Follow your facility policy for removing it from service.

Perform procedures in the way you were taught and avoid taking shortcuts. Taking shortcuts in your work may cause injury to yourself and others.

All residents should have a call signal within reach at all times. Residents who are mentally confused must also have a call signal available. Answer all call signals as soon as possible. If residents are unable to get up from their beds or chairs, make sure that needed personal items are within reach. If residents have to bend or stretch to reach items they need, they may lose their balance and fall.

If you notice items in a room that you think are unsafe, follow your facility policy for removing them, or ask the nurse for advice. Common items, such as nail polish remover and denture cleaning tablets, can be harmful if swallowed by a confused resident.

Safety in the bathroom. Many accidents occur in the bathroom. Residents may be in a hurry to get to the bathroom. They may lose their balance, slip, trip, and fall. Sometimes they slip on a wet floor. Always check the bathroom for safety. Leave a nightlight on for residents who get up at night to use the bathroom.

Check hot water temperatures with a thermometer before bathing residents. If a thermometer is not available, check the temperature on the inside of your wrist or forearm. Water temperatures are regulated in long-term care facilities to keep the water from getting too hot. Sometimes the regulators fail. If you have to add cold water to wash your hands, the water may be too hot. Ask the proper person in your facility to check the temperature. The hottest temperature allowed by law may be too hot for some residents. Use a thermometer so that you know the exact temperature of the water. Turn hot water on last and off first. Some whirlpool and bathing units have built-in thermometers. These thermometers are checked by the maintenance department regularly. However, the thermometers sometimes fail. Use common sense. If the built-in thermometer on the whirlpool shows a low reading, but the water feels hot to touch, or is steaming, do not put the resident in the tub until you have checked the temperature with another thermometer. Follow your facility policy for using bath oil. It is not used in some facilities because it makes the tub very slippery. Use shower chairs in the shower. Do not leave residents alone in the bathtub, whirlpool, or shower.

Safe use of chemicals. Many different types of chemicals are used in long-term care facilities. Chemicals are substances that may be harmful if they touch the skin or mucous membranes. They are usually harmful if swallowed or inhaled. Most cleaning products are chemicals. Keep all chemicals in their original containers. All chemicals must be labeled. Never pour them into unmarked containers. Never use the contents of an unmarked container. If you think the label on a container is incorrect, do not use the product. The label on the package of cleaning products will have a warning if the chemical is dangerous. Some cosmetics, such as nail polish remover, also contain harmful chemicals. Cosmetic manufacturers are not required to provide as much information on the label as other chemical manufacturers. Use each chemical according to the directions on the package. Cleaning products should be stored in a locked area when not in use. Avoid storing them in the same area as food or beverages. If you are using a cleaning product in a resident care area, you must be able to see it at all times. Never put a bottle down and turn your back on it. If you suspect that a resident has swallowed a chemical product, take the container to the nurse immediately.

The Hazardous Communication Right to Know program is designed to make employees aware of the correct use and hazards of chemicals used in the workplace. The long-term care facility is required to keep **material safety data sheets (MSDS)** **(Figure 4-3)** for all chemicals used. Know the location of these information sheets in your department. The MSDS will provide information and instructions for safe use, identify health risks, and describe first aid and safety precautions.

Safety with mentally confused residents. Besides the safety practices already discussed, keep sharp objects and plants away from residents who are mentally confused. If you are not sure about the safety of an item, check with the nurse.

Equipment safety. Use equipment only according to manufacturers' directions. If you have not been taught to use electrical or mechanical equipment, do not use it. If you feel that a piece of equipment is unsafe, follow your facility policy for notifying the proper person. Many facilities use a **lockout-tagout** system. Under this program, a locking device is placed on the equipment in a way that prevents the equipment from being used. A special tag identifies the equipment as broken and warns others not to use it **(Figure 4-4).** Always follow your facility policy for reporting and removing unsafe or broken equipment from service.

Answering Call Signals

Your facility will have policies for staff to follow for answering call signals. The call signal may be the only way that the resident has to get help in an emergency. Remember, all residents should have a call signal available at all times.

Most facilities require all staff to answer residents' call signals, whether or not they are assigned to care for that resident. Facilities usually have two types of call signals. One type is the regular signal used in resident rooms **(Figure 4-5A).** The other type is an emergency signal **(Figure 4-5B)** used in bathrooms, tubs, and shower rooms. Become familiar with both types of signals. Regular call signals should be answered as soon as possible, usually within three minutes or less. Emergency call signals should be answered immediately.

When you answer a call signal, knock on the resident's door and wait for a response before entering. Identify yourself and ask how you can help. Turn the call signal off. Do what the resident asks, or notify the proper person of the resident's request.

Resident Identification Systems

Many types of identification systems are used by health care facilities. The most common type is the **identification band** system. The identification band is a plastic band, placed around the resident's wrist or ankle, that contains identifying information. Some facilities use color-coded identification bands for specific purposes. For example, many facilities use pink or red bands to identify residents with diabetes. Residents at risk of wandering outside may have a special color band. Some facilities use self-adhesive colored dots on the identification band. These dots have special meanings. For example, a resident who needs extra liquids may have a blue dot on the identification band. Some facilities place a dot on the identification band with the resident's "code" status. This tells staff at a glance if CPR should be performed if the resident experiences a cardiac arrest. Facilities use color-coded bands and dots for many different conditions. Find out the meaning of these systems, if used by your facility.

Many long-term care facilities place the resident's name on the door of the room. Some also place the resident's picture by the door. The resident or responsible party must give permission to list the resident on a roster, or to post the name by the door of the room. The facility cannot disclose the names of residents without consent. Sometimes special decorations, such as bows or decorated hats, are placed on the doors to help confused residents find their rooms. They are

Material Safety Data Sheet

PRODUCT CODE NUMBERS:
MSC5300

SECTION 1

ISSUE DATE: 9-21-96
IDENTITY: **Exuderm Hydrocolloid Ultra Dressing**

MARKETED OR DISTRIBUTED BY:
Medline Industries, Inc.
One Medline Place
Mundelein, IL 60060
1.800.MEDLINE

Emergency Telephone Number:
Contact Your Regional Poison Control Center

SECTION 2 - HAZARDOUS INGREDIENTS/IDENTITY INFORMATION

HAZARDOUS COMPONENTS (SPECIFIC CHEMICAL IDENTITY, COMMON NAME(S)	CAS#	OSHA PEL	ACGIH TLV	OTHER LIMITS RECOMMENDED	% (OPTIONAL)
None					

SECTION 3 - PHYSICAL/CHEMICAL CHARACTERISTICS

BOILING POINT: N/A	SP GRAVITY (WATER=1): N/A
VAPOR PRESSURE (MM HG): N/A	MELTING POINT: N/A
VAPOR DENSITY (AIR=1): N/A	EVAPORATION RATE(BUTYL ACETATE=1): N/A
SOLUBILITY IN WATER: N/A	
APPEARANCE AND ODOR: Light caramel in color and no odor	

SECTION 4 - FIRE AND EXPLOSION HAZARD DATA

FLASH POINT (METHOD USED): N/A		
FLAMMABLE LIMITS: N/A	LEL: N/A	UEL: N/A
EXTINGUISHING MEDIA: Water, dry chemical or foam		
SPECIAL FIRE FIGHTING PROCEDURES: None		
UNUSUAL FIRE AND EXPLOSIVE HAZARDS: None		

SECTION 5 - REACTIVITY DATA

STABILITY: Stable
CONDITIONS TO AVOID: Avoid overheating and freezing.
INCOMPATIBILITY (MATERIALS TO AVOID): N/A
HAZARDOUS DECOMPOSITION OR BYPRODUCTS: N/A
HAZARDOUS POLYMERIZATION: Will not Occur
CONDITIONS TO AVOID: N/A

SECTION 6 - HEALTH HAZARD DATA

ROUTE(S) OF ENTRY: INHALATION: N/A	SKIN: N/A	INGESTION: N/A
HEALTH HAZARDS (ACUTE AND CHRONIC): None		

CARCINOGENICITY? N/A	NTP? N/A	IARC? N/A	OSHA REGULATED? N/A

SIGNS AND SYMPTOMS OF EXPOSURE: May cause moderate irritation in eyes
MEDICAL CONDITIONS GENERALLY AGGRAVATED BY EXPOSURE: N/A
EMERGENCY AND FIRST AID PROCEDURES: Eye contact: Flush.
Excessive Ingestion: Induce vomiting and consult physician.

SECTION 7 - SPILL, LEAK, AND WASTE DISPOSAL PROCEDURES

STEPS TO BE TAKEN IN CASE MATERIAL IS RELEASED OR SPILLED: N/A
WASTE DISPOSAL METHOD: In accordance with all local, state and federal regulations.
PRECAUTIONS TO BE TAKEN IN HANDLING AND STORING: N/A
OTHER PRECAUTIONS: N/A

SECTION 8 - CONTROL MEASURES

RESPIRATORY PROTECTION (SPECIFY TYPE): N/A		
VENTILATION:	LOCAL EXHAUST: N.A.	SPECIAL: N/A
	MECHANICAL (GENERAL): N/A	OTHER: N/A
PROTECTIVE GLOVES: N/A		EYE PROTECTION: N/A
SPECIAL CLOTHING: N/A		
WORK/HYGIENIC PRACTICES: None		

SECTION 9 - SPECIAL PRECAUTIONS

None

SECTION 10 - ADDITIONAL INFORMATION

Exuderm Hydrocolloid Dressing has passed all testing required for medical devices as outlined in the FDA Biocompatibility Guidelines for short term devices in contact with breached or compromised skin.

The information provided in this Material Safety Data Sheet has been obtained from sources believed to be reliable.

Medline Industries, Inc. provides no warranties, either expressed or implied and assumes no responsibility for the accuracy or completeness of the data contained herein.

ISSUE DATE: 9-21-96
Revised: 10/31/01 Updated telephone information

FIGURE 4-3 Material Safety Data Sheets provide important information and instructions on chemical use, health risks, first aid, and safety precautions. *(Courtesy of Medline Industries, Inc., 1-800-MEDLNE)*

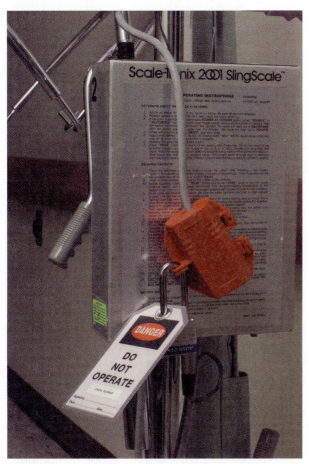

FIGURE 4-4 A tag is locked to a broken piece of electrical or mechanical equipment, to warn others not to use it.

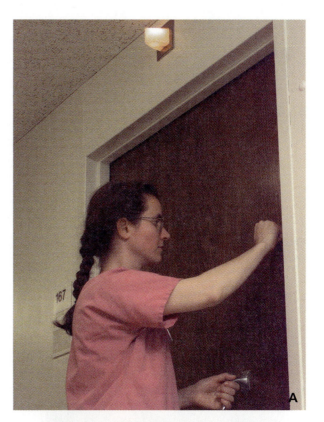

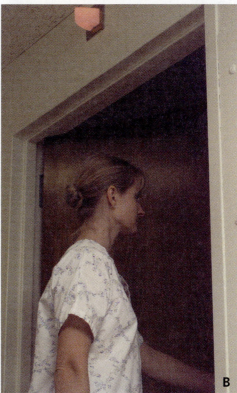

FIGURE 4-5 (A) The regular call signal is white and does not blink. (B) The emergency call signal is red and blinks, indicating that the resident needs immediate attention.

directed to find the "blue bow" or the "straw hat" when they are looking for their rooms.

Some long-term care facilities use special identification systems for residents who may be in danger if they wander away. These devices are discussed in detail in Chapter 15. However, the visual appearance of the device is distinct, so you can assume that if a resident is wearing one, he or she is at high risk of leaving the facility and will require close monitoring. Commonly, these are bracelets with magnetic sensors in them **(Figure 4-6)**. The sensors are similar to the devices used in stores to prevent shoplifting. Use of the sensor allows the resident to move freely about the facility. If the resident tries to leave through an outside door, an alarm will sound. The bracelets are usually put on the wrist of the dominant hand to make them difficult to remove.

Always identify residents before giving care. Check the resident's identification band and call the resident by name. Some residents will answer to any name they are called, so make sure that you have the right resident before giving

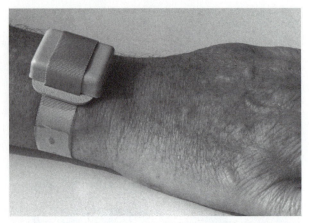

FIGURE 4-6 The magnetic sensor band is used in addition to the facility identification band. The sensor sets off an alarm if the resident tries to leave through an exit door, or enter a dangerous area, such as the stairwell. (© 1996 RF Technologies. Used by permission)

care. Do not be embarrassed if you have to ask a resident his or her name. It is better to ask than to provide care to the wrong resident.

Burn Prevention

Burns are a leading cause of injury. Residents with some diseases do not feel heat as acutely as healthy people. Hot water may burn them during bathing or treatments. Occasionally, hot liquids are spilled on residents, resulting in burns. Unsafe cigarette smoking is also a leading cause of burns.

Cigarette smoking. Know and follow your facility policy for cigarette smoking. If you smoke, do so only in designated areas. Some facilities allow smoking outside. Others do not allow smoking anywhere on the property. Some facilities do not allow residents to keep smoking materials. Most require that residents be supervised when they smoke. Residents are not allowed to smoke in their rooms except in special circumstances, and then only with direct supervision. Provide large, deep ashtrays for residents to use. Empty ashtrays only into metal cans with lids.

Thermal burns. Thermal burns are common injuries in long-term care facilities. Thermal burns are caused by contact with a hot substance or object, or an open flame. Be sure that you do not serve very hot food or liquids to residents. Help residents who are confused or who have poor hand control. Thermal burns are also caused by water that is too hot and careless smoking.

HEAT AND COLD APPLICATIONS

Heat and cold applications are used for many different purposes. Moist applications can be hot or cold. In this type of application, water touches the skin. Dry applications are those in which no water touches the skin. Some dry applications have water inside them, such as hot water bottles. However, the outside of the application stays dry, and the skin does not get wet. Sometimes dry applications are used to maintain the temperature of moist applications.

A localized application is used to apply heat or cold to a specific area of the body. An example of this type of application is an ice bag applied to a swollen ankle. A generalized application is used to apply heat or cold to the resident's entire body. An example of this type of application is the cooling or tepid sponge bath to reduce a resident's temperature. Many facilities use cooling blankets for this purpose.

General Principles for Using Heat and Cold Applications

Localized heat and cold applications that touch the resident's skin should have a protective cover. Covers are usually made of flannel. Pillowcases and towels are also used. Some facilities use a thin layer of protective foam. Check with the nurse for the type of cover to use. If the device you are using, such as a hot water bottle or ice collar, has a metal cap, face the cap away from the resident. The metal in the cap can conduct heat or cold and cause injury to the resident.

Check the resident's skin under the application every 10 minutes. If the skin under a heat application appears very red, or if a dark area

GUIDELINES FOR
Using Heat and Cold Applications

Before using a heat or cold application, you should know the:
- Type of application
- Area of the resident's body to be treated
- Length of time the application is to stay in place
- Proper temperature of the application
- Safety precautions to use
- Side effects to watch for

appears, stop the application and notify the nurse. When using a cold application, stop the application and notify the nurse immediately if the resident's skin appears blue, pale, white, or bright red. If the resident is shivering and cold, remove the application, cover the resident with a blanket, and notify the nurse.

Applying Heat and Cold

Heat applications **dilate** or enlarge the blood vessels to bring oxygen and nutrients to an area. Heat may be used to relieve pain and speed healing. Local cold applications are used to relieve pain and prevent or relieve **edema.** Edema, or swelling, is common after an injury. Cold applications can also be used to stop or control bleeding. Cooling reduces the blood flow to the area and **constricts** blood vessels (makes them smaller). Generalized cooling may be used to reduce body temperature. This is done by cooling the entire body. The elderly may be very sensitive to heat and cold. When performing heat and cold treatments, assist the resident into a comfortable position that he or she can maintain for the duration of the treatment. Expose only the part of the body that you will be treating.

Follow all safety rules to prevent spills and falls. If the resident has a dressing covering the area to be treated, ask the nurse for assistance. Wear gloves if your hands will contact blood, moist body fluids (except sweat), secretions, excretions, nonintact skin, or mucous membranes. Always check the temperature of the solution to be used with a thermometer. You may need to add more liquid to the solution during the treatment to maintain the temperature. When you are done with the treatment, pat the skin dry. Make the resident comfortable. Clean and put away used equipment. Remove gloves, if worn, and dispose of them according to facility policy. Wash your hands. Report to the nurse that the procedure was completed, and also report the resident's reaction.

OXYGEN SAFETY

Oxygen is necessary for life. We take in oxygen from the air when we breathe. Some diseases and conditions cause the resident to be unable to take in enough oxygen. In these cases, the doctor will usually order additional oxygen to be given by an oxygen delivery system. The doctor will order how much oxygen is to be used, the method of oxygen delivery, and the

length of time it is to be applied. You should not start, stop, or change the flow rate of oxygen. However, you must know how to check the flow rate and know general safety measures to take when oxygen is in use. You must also be aware of where oxygen is stored in your facility, because the nurse may send you for the oxygen supply in an emergency. In many facilities, the nursing assistant is also responsible for cleaning oxygen equipment. Know and follow your facility policy.

Usually, the resident who is receiving oxygen will need the head of the bed elevated. Elevating the head of the bed makes breathing easier. Follow the instructions on your assignment sheet and the resident's care plan.

Oxygen Delivery Systems

Several types of oxygen delivery systems **(Figure 4-7)** are used in long-term care facilities. Oxygen may be piped in through the wall. Most facilities use oxygen tanks or concentrators. The oxygen concentrator converts room air to oxygen and delivers it to the resident. Oxygen also comes in a liquid canister **(Figure 4-8).** This canister delivers a higher concentration of oxygen than a concentrator, but is portable and convenient. It does not require electricity to operate. The canister is quiet compared with a concentrator, which has an electric motor and

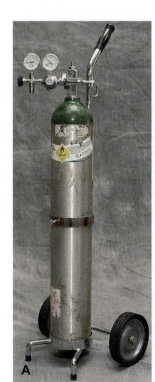
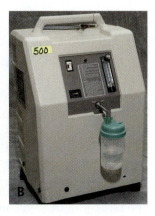

FIGURE 4-7 Most long-term care facilities use oxygen in (A) tanks and (B) concentrators.

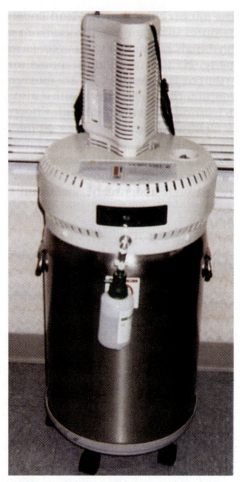

FIGURE 4-8 Liquid oxygen is portable and convenient. The small upper tank can be filled from the larger lower tank.

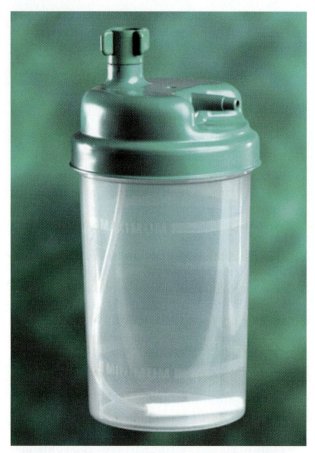

FIGURE 4-9A Humidification is not necessary for residents receiving low liter flows of oxygen, but some facilities use humidifiers to provide extra moisture and comfort. *(Courtesty of Hudson RCI, Temecula, CA, USA)*

makes a humming noise. It is also more economical for the resident.

Oxygen can be very drying and uncomfortable for the resident. Dry oxygen thickens the respiratory secretions, making breathing more difficult. The oxygen may pass through a **humidifier** before it reaches the resident. The humidifier is a water bottle that moistens the oxygen for comfort and prevents drying of the mucous membranes in the nose, mouth, and lungs. Use of oxygen humidifiers is a controversial subject. Humidification is not necessary in liter flows below 5. Humidifiers are not used at all in some facilities.

The humidifier bottle **(Figure 4-9A)** screws into a male adapter on the flow meter. Oxygen passes through the water in the humidifier, picking up moisture, before it reaches the resident. The delivery device plugs into a male adapter on the side of the humidifier. Checking and changing the humidifier is a nursing assistant responsi-

bility in some facilities. Sterile distilled water is always used. Avoid tap water. Inhalation of tap water is associated with an increased incidence of Legionnaire's disease. The water level in the humidifier should always be at or above the "minimum fill" line on the bottle. When the oxygen delivery system is functioning correctly, the water in the humidifier will bubble. Oxygen will not exit the tubing into the mask or cannula if the tubing is kinked or obstructed. If this occurs, pressure builds up in the unit and discharges through a pressure relief valve.

Two types of humidifiers are used. The *prefilled* type of humidifier is disposable. This unit is usually changed once a week, when it is empty, or according to manufacturers' directions or facility policies. Discard the bottle after replacing it with a new one. Your facility may require you to attach a sticker to the bottle listing the date and time it was changed, and your initials.

Refillable humidifiers are washed, rinsed, and sterilized every 24 to 48 hours, or according to

Flow meter

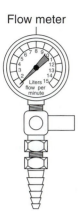

FIGURE 4-9B The flow meter shows how much oxygen the resident is receiving.

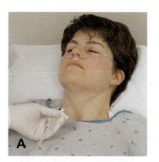

FIGURE 4-11 Oxygen is usually delivered through (A) a cannula for liter flows of five or less and (B) a mask for high liter flows.

facility infection control policies. Refill the sterile bottle with sterile distilled water. Never add water to a partially filled humidifier. A sticker may be attached to this bottle showing the date and time it was changed.

Oxygen is given through a flow meter (**Figure 4-9B**) that shows how many liters of oxygen are being delivered to the resident each minute. Although you will not be responsible for adjusting this meter, you should check it each time you are in the room to be sure it is set at the proper rate. If you notice a difference from the ordered rate, report this important information to the nurse. The gauge on the oxygen tank also shows how much oxygen is left in the tank (**Figure 4-10**). Oxygen is measured in pounds. Follow your facility policy for checking this gauge, and notify the nurse before the tank is empty. Many facilities consider tanks to be empty when the pressure reaches 500 pounds. The tanks are changed when this pressure is reached.

Oxygen delivery equipment. Many different types of oxygen delivery equipment are used.

Liter flow   Amount of O₂ in tank

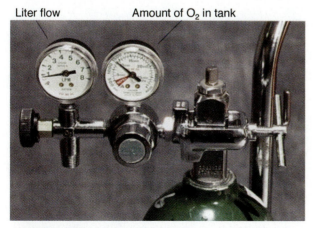

FIGURE 4-10 One gauge shows the liter flow the resident receives. The other indicates how much oxygen is in the tank.

The most common devices are cannulas and masks (**Figure 4-11**). The doctor will order the type of equipment to use. You must observe the skin under the device to be sure that it does not become red or irritated from the elastic that holds it in place. Report any skin problems to the nurse. Residents receiving oxygen may need extra liquids to drink. They will also need frequent care of the mouth and nose. Sometimes residents feel warm when receiving oxygen and will perspire heavily. Extra bathing and linen changes may be necessary. You may need to adjust the temperature in the room and help the resident change into lightweight clothes. The care plan and your assignment sheet will provide information on how and when to perform these procedures.

Being unable to breathe is very frightening. Residents who are receiving oxygen may need reassurance and emotional support. Check on the resident frequently and spend as much time in the room as possible. Difficulty in breathing makes it hard to talk, so the resident may be unable to carry on a normal conversation. Just being with the resident without talking is very reassuring.

Use of Oxygen in an Emergency

There are several differences between routine oxygen use and use of oxygen in an emergency. In an emergency, high concentrations of oxygen are necessary. Tanks, liquid oxygen, or oxygen piped in through the wall are used. Oxygen is usually delivered through a mask for emergency purposes. A mask should not be used with liter flows of less than 5 because it has a smothering effect.

A concentrator will not deliver an adequate amount of oxygen for emergencies. Concentrators cannot deliver liter flows over 5. Most facilities use small, portable tanks for emergency purposes. In an emergency, oxygen may be delivered dry if necessary, until sterile distilled

GUIDELINES FOR
Safe Use of Oxygen

Extra oxygen in the air may cause objects to burn or explode. By itself, oxygen is not explosive. The resident's gown and linen on the bed absorb extra oxygen from the air. Special precautions should be taken when oxygen is in use.

- Before initiating oxygen therapy, check the resident's room to make sure it is safe for oxygen delivery.
- When using tank oxygen, identify the contents of the cylinder. Oxygen cylinders are always green. Read the label listing the contents as a double-check.
- Never use grease or oil on oxygen tank connections.
- Post "Oxygen in Use" signs over the bed and on the door of the room, or according to facility policy. The sign should list warnings, such as not smoking.
- Teach the resident and visitors the precautions to take.
- Do not force the flow meter into the wall or tank when assembling an oxygen unit. Forcing the flow meter may cause a valve to stick in an open position, allowing oxygen to leak out.
- Some electrical appliances can cause a spark. Check with the nurse before using a hair dryer, electric shaver, fan, radio, or television.
- Never use **flammable** liquids such as nail polish remover or adhesive tape remover. Avoid using alcohol-based aftershave, colognes, perfumes, or other products on residents receiving oxygen. Flammable liquids are combustible and will burn readily.
- Tank oxygen should be secured in a base or chained to a carrier or the wall.
- Smoking is not allowed in the room when oxygen is in use.
- Cover the resident with a cotton blanket. Avoid using wool and synthetic blankets and clothing.
- Some facilities remove the call signal and replace it with a bell that is used manually. The call signal may cause a spark.
- Avoid sparks. Static electricity can start a fire.

- Residents receiving oxygen receive frequent oral and nasal care because the oxygen dries the mucous membranes. Avoid using petroleum jelly or other petroleum products as a lubricant. Consult the nurse for a water-soluble lubricant.
- Make sure the tubing is not kinked or obstructed.
- Respond to equipment alarms, including oxygen equipment, immediately. Take corrective action or notify the appropriate person.
- If oxygen equipment makes an unusual noise, take corrective action or notify the appropriate person. If you suspect that a tank is leaking, remove the resident from the room and close the door.
- Learn how to turn off oxygen in case of a fire emergency. Piped-in oxygen may be turned off at a zone valve in the hallway. Tanks, canisters, and concentrators must be turned off at the unit.
- Learn facility policies for emergency transportation and evacuaton of residents who need continuous oxygen.
- Follow infection control precautions when caring for residents receiving oxygen, such as keeping the cannula covered when not in use. Keep the oxygen cannula and tubing off the floor.
- Learn facility policies for using liquid oxygen. When liquid oxygen is used, high concentrations of oxygen build up quickly. Some materials are very flammable when saturated with oxygen. Follow all safety precautions for preventing sparks and fires.
- Liquid oxygen is nontoxic, but will cause severe burns upon direct contact. Avoid opening, touching, or spilling the container. If your skin or clothing contacts the liquid oxygen, flush the area immediately with a large amount of water. Never seal the cap or vent port on the liquid oxygen. Doing so will increase the pressure within the system, creating a potentially dangerous situation. If a bottle falls or tips, evacuate yourself and the resident from the room and close the door. Follow facility policies for getting assistance in this type of emergency.

water is available. Avoid using tap water, because it increases the resident's risk of contracting Legionnaire's disease.

FIRE SAFETY

Long-term care facilities are built with safety features that will prevent fires from spreading. These safety features include doors that close automatically when the fire alarm sounds, an automatic sprinkler system, smoke detectors, and fire exits. Fire alarms and fire extinguishers are located on

the walls in the hallways. The facility will have an evacuation plan posted **(Figure 4-12).** Many materials used on the floors, doors, walls, and furnishings are fire rated. This means that they will take longer to burn. Nevertheless, fire prevention is an important responsibility. Despite the built-in safety features, long-term care facilities can catch fire. Many lives can be lost.

Your facility will have periodic fire drills. Take these drills seriously and follow instructions. Your actions in a fire drill must become automatic, so that if a real fire starts you will react properly. Find the evacuation plan on your unit

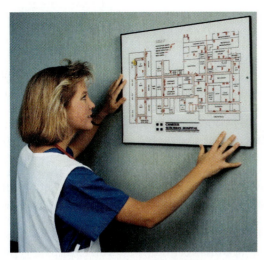

FIGURE 4-12 Become familiar with your facility evacuation plan. Commit it to memory so that you will be prepared in an emergency.

and become familiar with the escape routes. Know the location of fire alarms and fire extinguishers. Your facility may conduct inservices to teach you how to use the fire extinguisher.

Three elements are necessary for a fire to start. These are oxygen, fuel, and a spark or source of ignition **(Figure 4-13).** Oxygen is in

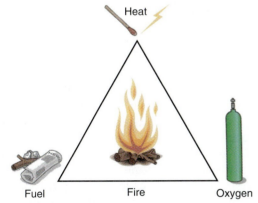

FIGURE 4-13 The three elements necessary to start a fire

the air. Wood, paper, linens, and other materials provide fuel. Because two of the three elements necessary for fires are everywhere, the only thing missing is the spark, or source of ignition.

Careless and unsupervised smoking is a major cause of fire in long-term care facilities. Follow facility smoking policies. Check for and remove smoking materials from resident rooms, if this is your facility policy. Another common cause of fire is electrical problems. Avoid overloading electrical outlets. Report frayed wires or other problems with electrical equipment to the proper person. Lock and tag this equipment out if this is your facility policy.

Other steps you should take to prevent fires are to store flammable materials correctly, and dispose of trash and other wastes in the proper location.

Steps to Take in a Fire Emergency

In a fire emergency, remain calm and do not panic. Most facilities use the **RACE System** **(Figure 4-14).** The resident is removed from immediate danger. After the alarm is sounded, the fire is contained by closing doors and windows. Residents are moved behind closed doors to keep them safe. Closing doors and windows slows the spread of fire. The hallways are cleared of residents and pieces of equipment that will burn. If the fire is large and spreading rapidly, residents may be evacuated from the building. If the fire is small, use a fire extinguisher to put it out. Fire extinguishers are rated A, B, C, or according to the type of fire they are used on.

- A is used for trash, wood, and paper fires.
- B is used for flammable liquids, such as grease and oil.
- C is used for electrical fires.
- ABC is used on any type of fire.

Fire extinguishers are used by aiming the spray at the base of the fire. Remembering the word

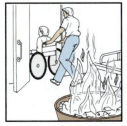
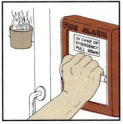
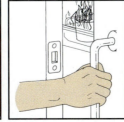
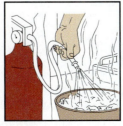
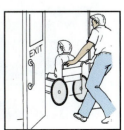

Remove   **A**ctivate   **C**ontain or   **E**xtinguish or   **E**vacuate

FIGURE 4-14 The RACE system

PASS will help you remember how to use the fire extinguisher:

P—Pull the pin out of the upper extinguisher handle.

A—Aim the extinguisher at the base of the fire.

S—Squeeze the handle to discharge the contents of the extinguisher.

S—Sweep the extinguisher from side to side while keeping it aimed at the base of the fire. Hold the hose securely when spraying.

In a fire, smoke is very dangerous. If you are in a smoke-filled area, stay as close to the floor as possible. If you can crawl to an exit, cover your mouth and stay on your knees. The floor has the most oxygen available, because smoke rises. Before entering a room, touch the door with the *back* of your hand **(Figure 4-15).** *If the door is hot to touch, do not open it.* If you are trapped in a room and the door is hot to touch, stay in the room and place wet blankets or towels under the door to keep the smoke out. Opening the door could cause the fire to enter explosively.

Never use the elevator in a fire emergency. If you are instructed to evacuate, you must use the stairs.

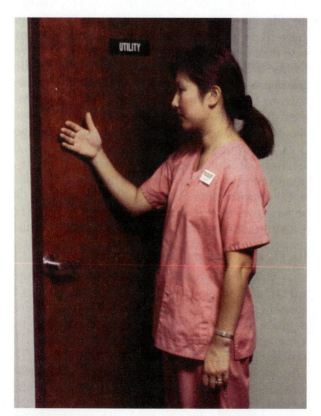

FIGURE 4-15 If you suspect a fire, touch the door with the back of your hand. Do not open the door if it feels hot.

OTHER TYPES OF EMERGENCIES

When a natural disaster occurs, many people can be injured in a short period of time. Know what natural disasters are possible in your area and find out what evacuation or safety measures are used by your facility. If evacuation is anticipated, you may be instructed to tell ambulatory residents to stay out of bed and to get bedfast residents up in wheelchairs so that they can be moved quickly. You will evacuate ambulatory residents first, followed by residents in wheelchairs. Evacuate bedfast residents last. Your facility will have a disaster plan that describes what actions to take. Regardless of the type of emergency, remaining calm is very important.

Tornado Safety

Although rare in some parts of the country, a tornado can occur anywhere. All facilities have specific policies for natural disasters. Your community may be placed under a **tornado watch** or **tornado warning.** A tornado watch means that conditions are favorable for a tornado to develop. A tornado warning means that a tornado is actually in the area. Residents are not evacuated during a tornado watch. Someone is designated to monitor the weather in case the situation changes.

During a tornado warning, you will help with the evacuation of residents. This means that all residents will be moved to the basement, if the facility has one. In multiple-story buildings, residents are moved to the lowest level. Frequently, residents are moved to a strong area in the center of the building. Residents should not be moved to areas where there are windows, because flying glass may cause serious injuries. Evacuation must be done very quickly, because tornadoes strike with little warning. If residents cannot walk, they are moved in wheelchairs or beds. You may be instructed to cover residents with blankets to protect them from flying debris. You may also be required to close the room doors, fire doors, windows, and curtains facing the direction of the oncoming tornado. Remove items from window sills, such as plants and pictures. Put sharp or heavy objects away in drawers or closets. If there is time, check the outside of the facility. Bring lawn furniture, tools, and other objects inside the building. Locate and carry a flashlight to use in case of a power failure. Do not go near the windows during the storm. Follow the nurse's directions until the tornado has left the area.

GUIDELINES FOR

Tornado Safety

Tornado Watch

The nurse will monitor the weather. During the watch, you may be instructed to:

- Remove nonessential items from hallways.
- Close windows and drapes. Remove items from window sills.
- Put sharp or heavy objects away in drawers or closets.
- Clear desks and countertops of nonessential items.
- Ask residents to return to their rooms or units.
- Remove or secure outdoor furniture or other objects.
- Turn on lights if the sky darkens.
- Locate and verify working order of flashlights and battery radios.
- Locate extra wheelchairs and small oxygen tanks and bring them to a central area in case they are needed for resident evacuation.
- Account for all residents on the unit; you may be asked to tape a list to the desk, or give it to the nurse.
- Instruct residents not to leave the building.

Tornado Warning (Severe Thunderstorm Warning)

- You may be asked to move residents before an official warning is issued.

- If a warning is announced, return to your assigned unit.
- Help move residents to the designated area(s). Move ambulatory residents first, followed by residents in wheelchairs. Evacuate bedfast residents last. Cover residents' heads with blankets. Be calm and reassuring.
- After each room is evacuated, close the door. You may be instructed to place a paper or the corner of the privacy curtain out of the door to signify that the room has been evacuated.
- If a resident refuses to move, move other residents, then return and try to persuade the resident. If he or she continues to refuse, inform the nurse. If the resident is in a potentially life-threatening situation, the nurse may instruct you to move the resident against his or her will.
- Instruct visitors and residents not to leave the building.
- If there is no time to evacuate, cover residents with blankets, push beds away from windows, and pull privacy curtains. (Window drapes should already be closed and window sills cleared.) If time allows, protect the side of the bed closest to the window by padding it with pillows or other soft materials. Begin in the area of the building where the storm is approaching.

Hurricanes

Some facilities in coastal areas are at risk for hurricanes. Hurricanes are not like other emergencies because they can be predicted in advance and there is adequate time to evacuate residents before the hurricane strikes. If a hurricane warning occurs, facility management may give the order to evacuate residents to an area farther inland. Residents, medications, and residents' charts are also moved. Follow the directions of facility management during the evacuation procedure.

If residents are not evacuated, you may be instructed to move them into interior rooms or hallways. As with a tornado, residents should be protected from flying glass and other debris. Close the doors to rooms and fire doors. Avoid blocking the emergency exits.

Earthquakes

During an earthquake, the ground shakes. It may cause building destruction and fires. Windows may break and objects may fly around. Earth-

quakes occur suddenly and without warning. If an earthquake strikes, remain calm. Cover or protect your head from flying debris. Take cover under a large heavy object, or in a door frame, if possible.

After the earthquake, check residents for injuries. Avoid moving injured residents unless they are in danger. Clean up spills on the floor to prevent falls. Do not smoke or use candles, matches, or open flames. Earthquakes can rupture gas lines and cause chemicals to spill, creating fire hazards. Be prepared for aftershocks. Avoid using electrical appliances. Use a flashlight for light, if needed. Listen to a battery-powered radio for emergency information.

Bomb Threats

Occasionally a long-term care facility will receive a phone call warning of a bomb. A bomb threat should be taken seriously. Facility management may order the building to be evacuated quickly. Law enforcement and fire officials will be notified. They will search the facility for a bomb, and may help with the evacuation. If you answer the telephone and the caller tells you there is a bomb in the building, stay on the line for as long as possible and obtain as much information as possible **(Figure 4-16).** Be polite and remain calm. Ask where the bomb is, or where it will explode and at what time. Be alert to the sound of the caller's voice, and try to determine the age, sex, and other identifying factors such as an accent. Listen for any background noise such as music, church bells, or machinery. This information will be useful to the police later in trying to identify the caller. Follow the nurse's directions in evacuating the facility. Law enforcement authorities will advise facility management when it is safe to return.

Bomb Threat Checklist

Questions to ask the caller:

• Where is the bomb right now? _____

• Did you place the bomb? _____

• Why did you place the bomb? _____

• When is the bomb going to explode? _____

• What will cause the bomb to explode? _____

• What kind of bomb is it? _____

• Where are you? _____

• What is your name? _____

Exact wording of the call:

_____

_____

_____

Date and time of the call: _____

Length of the call: _____

Caller's gender (sex): _____ Approximate age: _____ Accent: _____

Caller's Voice; Circle all that apply

calm	nasal	loud	distinct	lisp	clearing throat
angry	slow	laughing	slurred	raspy	coughing
agitated	rapid	crying	ethnic	deep	deep breathing
excited	soft	normal	stutter	ragged	cracking
disguised	foreign	accent	familiar		

If the voice sounded familiar, whose voice did it sound like? _____

Language; Circle all that apply

Well-spoken (educated)	Irrational	Message read by caller
Foul	Incoherent	Accent or dialect (specify) _____
	Taped message	

Background Sounds

Street (cars, buses, etc.)	Motor (fan, air conditioning)	Local call	Other (specify)
Airplanes	Church bells	Phone booth	_____
PA system	Animal noises	Office machinery	_____
Music	Clear	Video games, pinball, bowling, etc.	
House (dishes, TV, radio)	Static	Factory machinery	
Construction			

FIGURE 4-16 A bomb threat information checklist is available in some facilities. Using the checklist helps obtain essential information.

Other Types of Emergencies

Facilities have many policies and procedures for disasters. If your facility is in a flood plain, you will have a policy and procedure to be used in the event of high water. There may also be policies and procedures for other types of disasters, such as interruptions in food and water supplies, loss of gas and electricity, ice and snow emergencies, and chemical spills. Your facility will teach you how to respond to the appropriate disasters in your community.

OTHER SAFETY REQUIREMENTS

Many governmental agencies regulate safety in health care facilities. These agencies routinely inspect health care agencies and respond to complaints about unsafe conditions. Some laws pertain to the nursing assistant. Facilities receive citations and fines if unsafe conditions exist, or if workers are not following safe practices, so take your responsibilities for safe practices very seriously.

Occupational Safety and Health Administration

The **Occupational Safety and Health Administration (OSHA)** is an agency of the federal government that is responsible for overseeing employee safety in the workplace. Government statistics show that long-term care facilities have the third highest rate of injuries of all workplaces. In 2002, nursing assistants and truck drivers had more back injuries than any other workers. OSHA's role is to see that the workers are protected. Other agencies deal with resident safety. For years, OSHA inspected other types of businesses regularly, but did not inspect health care facilities. This has changed, however, and in recent years, OSHA has become one of the agencies that actively inspects and has regulatory authority over health care facilities.

OSHA inspects facilities to see if they are following governmental safety requirements. Facilities must have an eyewash station and total body wash station within a reasonable distance of areas where chemicals are used. This is to protect employees in case chemicals are splashed into their eyes or spilled on their bodies. Most facilities designate the shower or tub rooms for this purpose. OSHA also monitors the MSDS. The inspectors monitor the use of infection control precautions and isolation procedures and check to see that the facility is following guidelines to prevent the spread of tuberculosis and other infectious diseases. Your facility will teach you the OSHA requirements. It is your responsibility to attend class, learn the material, and apply it to the job you do in the long-term care facility.

Take safety very seriously. This will keep your facility in compliance with the various agencies that inspect it, and protect employees and residents from illness and injury.

GUIDELINES FOR
Violence Prevention

The nursing assistant should follow all facility policies and procedures involving safety and security. Other things you can do to prevent potential incidents are:
- Report suspicious individuals or other potential safety hazards to the nurse.
- If you are responsible for a secured area, control access to the area and keep it locked.
- Follow facility policy for locking all entrance doors at a designated time each evening. If your facility has a doorbell, respond to it quickly so oncoming workers are not outside alone in the dark.
- Participate in continuing education programs to learn how to recognize and manage escalating agitation, assaultive behavior, or criminal intent.
- Attend classes on cultural diversity that teach sensitivity on racial and ethnic issues and differences.

- Report assaults or threats of assaults to the nurse immediately.
- Avoid wearing scarves, necklaces, earrings, and other jewelry that could cause injury if a resident or other individual attacks you.
- Avoid remote, dark areas when you are alone.
- Exercise caution in elevators, stairwells, and unfamiliar areas. Immediately leave the area if you believe a hazard exists.
- If your facility has security personnel, request that they escort you in dark or potentially dangerous areas. If no security personnel are on duty, ask other staff members to accompany you.
- Use the "buddy system" if personal safety may be threatened.
- If a resident or other person is "acting out," or you believe you may be assaulted, do not let the person come between you and the exit.

GUIDELINES FOR
Dealing with a Violent Individual

- Remain calm and avoid raising your voice, which may agitate the perpetrator.
- Speak slowly, softly, and clearly.
- Call for help, if possible, or send someone to get help. Pull the call light from the wall to activate the emergency signal.
- Move away from heavy or sharp objects that might be used as weapons.
- Monitor your body language and avoid movements that could be challenging, such as placing your hands on your hips, moving toward the perpetrator, pointing your finger, or staring directly at the person. However, focus your attention on the person so you know what he or she is doing at all times.
- Position yourself at right angles to the perpetrator. Avoid standing directly in front of him or her.
- Maintain a distance of three to six feet from the perpetrator.
- Position yourself so that an exit is accessible.
- Avoid making sudden movements.

- Listen to what the person is saying. Encourage the person to talk, and communicate that you care and will genuinely try to help. Acknowledge that you understand he or she is upset. Break big problems into smaller, manageable ones.
- Avoid arguing and defensive statements. Accept criticism in a positive way. If you sincerely feel that criticism is unwarranted, ask clarifying questions.
- Ask the person to leave and return when more calm.
- Ask questions to help regain control of the conversation.
- Avoid challenging, bargaining, or making promises you cannot keep.
- Describe the consequences of abusive behavior.
- Avoid touching an angry person.
- If a weapon is involved, ask the person to place it in a neutral location while you continue talking. Avoid trying to disarm the person, which may put you in danger.
- Follow facility policies for subduing or restraining the individual.

Safe Medical Devices Act

The Safe Medical Devices Act of 1991 requires the health care facility to notify the United States Food and Drug Administration of death or serious injury caused by any medical device or equipment. This federal agency investigates all reports of serious injury and death. Using medical equipment according to manufacturers' directions is important to prevent injury. Do not use electrical or mechanical equipment unless you have been taught how to use it safely.

Concealed Handgun Laws

Some states allow citizens to carry concealed weapons. In these states guns *may not* be carried into a health care facility. Law enforcement personnel are exempt from this requirement. If a visitor is carrying a concealed handgun, he or she must leave it in the trunk of the car before entering the facility. If you notice any individual carrying a gun, notify the nurse immediately.

Violence in the Health Care Facility

Episodes of violence in the workplace are increasing in our society. Long-term care facilities are not exempt from violence. Serious episodes have occurred in both rural and urban communities. Many facilities have violence prevention education programs. The goal is to eliminate or reduce worker exposure to conditions that can lead to injury. OSHA has developed guidelines for preventing violence in the health care facility, and many employers use these guidelines to implement safety programs and teach their employees.

Potential reasons for violence in the health care facility include:

- The prevalence of handguns and other weapons
- Acute and chronically mentally ill residents
- Individuals, including coworkers, who abuse alcohol and drugs
- Overwhelming personal or financial stress
- The availability of drugs in the facility, making it a likely robbery target
- The increasing number of gangs and gang members in many communities
- Unrestricted movement of the public in health care facilities
- Distraught family members and other individuals who become angry and frustrated
- Low staffing levels during meals and at other times when staff is busy caring for residents and unable to observe activity in the hallways
- Poorly lighted parking lots, garages, and ramps
- Lack of staff awareness of risk factors, such as locking doors and reporting suspicious individuals
- Residents with dementia
- Residents who are incontinent and nonverbal

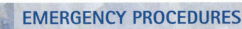
EMERGENCY PROCEDURES

When an emergency occurs in a long-term care facility, the licensed nurse is responsible for treatment of the resident. Follow the nurse's directions. Sometimes, however, you must act before the nurse arrives, to keep the resident from serious harm.

Caring for a Resident Who Has Fainted

Syncope, or fainting, occurs when the blood supply to the brain is not adequate. This sometimes

---

GUIDELINES TO
Follow in All Emergencies

- If you discover a resident who is ill or injured, stay with the resident and call for help. Your facility will teach you the procedure for getting help. Some facilities instruct employees to call out. Others instruct you to pull the call signal or bathroom emergency signal.
- Do not move residents who have fallen to the floor unless they are in immediate danger. Moving the resident may worsen an injury. The nurse will check the resident and give permission for the move.
- Stay calm and do not panic.
- Start emergency measures that you are permitted to do while you are waiting for help to arrive.

- Once the nurse arrives, do as he or she directs.
- Know facility procedures and phone numbers for reporting emergencies and completing incident reports.
- Know the location of emergency equipment and supplies on your unit. You may be instructed to get emergency supplies.
- Many emergencies involve bleeding. Remember that the potential for contact with blood, body fluid, secretions (except sweat), excretions, mucous membranes, and nonintact skin exists. Always remember and apply the principles of standard precautions. Know where personal protective equipment is kept.

PROCEDURE 3

Emergency Care for the Resident Who Has Fainted

1. Stay with the resident and call for help.
2. Lowering the resident's head will increase the blood supply to the brain.
   - If the resident is standing, help him or her sit or lie down.
   - If the resident is sitting, have him or her lean forward and place the head between his or her knees.
   - Once the resident is lying down, elevate his or her legs. Elevate them on pillows, if possible to increase blood flow to the brain. Keep the resident's head flat.
3. If the resident is nauseated, or is vomiting, position him or her on the side. If this is not possible, turn the resident's head to the side.
4. Loosen any tight or restrictive clothing.
5. Apply a cool, wet towel to the forehead.
6. Check the vital signs as directed by the nurse. You may be asked to monitor them at 5- to 15-minute intervals until the resident's condition is stable.
7. Keep the resident quiet, with the head lowered, until directed by the nurse.
8. Help the resident sit up gradually. Be prepared to act if the resident faints again.
9. Leave the resident in a position of comfort and safety. Usually, the resident is returned to bed with the side rails up until he or she has recovered. Leave the call signal and needed personal items within reach.
10. Wash your hands.
11. Report to the nurse:
    - The time the resident fainted, and how long he or she was unconscious.
    - A description of the resident's appearance when the incident occurred.
    - Any measures that you took to assist the resident and the results.
    - Visual problems, change in color, or excessive perspiration.
    - Presence of nausea, vomiting, changes in color or temperature of the skin, and changes in the resident's **level of consciousness,** which is determined by how responsive and alert the resident is. The level of consciousness is the resident's degree of awareness, which ranges from fully awake and alert to confusion or unconsciousness.
    - Vital signs.

occurs as a result of medical problems when residents sit or stand too quickly. The medical condition causes a temporary decrease in the blood flow to the brain, and the resident may lose consciousness. The purpose of emergency treatment for this condition is to restore the blood supply to the resident's brain and prevent injury. During this procedure, you will be required to take the resident's **vital signs,** or temperature, pulse, respiration, and blood pressure. You will learn these procedures in Chapter 16.

Caring for a Resident Who Is Having a Seizure

A **seizure** or convulsion is caused by a disturbance of the impulses in the brain. It is seen in epilepsy and other diseases. It is usually charac-terized by jerking and shaking of the body. Injuries, medication, fever, and infection can also cause seizures. Residents have different types of seizures. Some appear mild, whereas others appear severe. The most common types of seizures are related to epilepsy. These are de-scribed in **Table 4-1.** A seizure is a serious med-ical emergency. The goal of seizure care is to prevent injury. Some residents have a sensation called an **aura** immediately before a seizure. An aura is a sensation, smell, taste, or a bright light that precedes the onset of a seizure.

Caring for a Resident Who Has Fallen and Has a Suspected Fracture

Falls are common emergencies in health care facilities. Bones become more brittle and lose

TABLE 4-1 Characteristics of Common Types of Seizures

Type of Seizure	Signs of Seizure Activity	Comment
Generalized tonic-clonic seizure (Grand mal seizure)	May be proceded by an aura. Loss of con-sciousness, convulsive activity, character-ized by rigid stiffening of muscles and jerking movement of the arms and legs. Saliva runs from the mouth. Resident's color may change because of lack of oxy-gen. Incontinence of bowel and bladder.	Usually lasts three to four minutes. The resident may be very tired after the seizure and may have a headache. The resident may be mentally confused, have slurred speech, and be very weak. The resident will not remember the seizure.
Absence seizure (Petit mal seizure)	Staring, blinking, or stopping what the resident is doing. The resident may stare blankly. One muscle group may twitch or jerk.	Petit mal seizures usually last less than a minute, but may occur many times a day.
Simple-Partial (Jacksonian)	Muscle spasms of the face, hands, or feet. Starts at one extremity, such as an arm or leg, and progressively moves upward on that side of the body.	May spread to other areas in the brain, re-sulting in a grand mal seizure.
Complex-Partial (Psychomotor)	Abnormal acts, irrational behavior, or loss of judgment due to a temporary change in consciousness. Automatic be-havior, such as typing or eating, may con-tinue normally. The resident may uncon-trollably smack his or her lips, wander aimlessly, or uncontrollably twitch part of his or her body.	Usually lasts only a few seconds. The res-ident usually does not remember the seizure.
Myoclonic	Consists of one or more myoclonic jerks. The resident remains conscious but can-not control the muscle movement.	The resident is aware that an extremity is jerking but is unable to stop it. The resi-dent remains conscious throughout and can remember the seizure activity.
Status epilepticus	Multiple seizures occurring simultane-ously with no break between seizures.	Status epilepticus may be precipitated by sudden withdrawal of antiseizure medica-tions, fever, and infection. This type of seizure is dangerous and can lead to de-creased mental function, neurological im-pairment, and death.

calcium during the aging process. Joints are not as flexible as they were when the resident was younger. Because of these aging changes, **fractures,** or broken bones, occur more readily in the elderly. Sometimes fractures are obvious right away. An area of the body may appear swollen or deformed. If the fracture occurs in a hip, the leg on the affected side may appear shorter than the other and rotate outward. Injuries may bleed. The purpose of emergency treatment for falls is to prevent injuries and to assist residents who have suspected fractures.

Head Injury

A resident with a known or suspected head injury always requires close observation and monitoring. Bleeding inside the skull commonly occurs when the head strikes a broad, hard object, such as the floor. Some serious complications of head injuries may not be apparent until 72 hours or longer after a head injury. This is particularly true in the elderly. As people age, the brain shrinks. This does not affect the resident mentally. The space between the brain and the skull allows extra room for swelling and bleeding. Signs and symptoms of an acute bleeding problem may not be apparent for several days until the problem progresses to a point where it increases pressure on the brain. A very tiny bleed can take up to six weeks to show symptoms. This may be long after the original injury has been forgotten. Signs and symptoms of head injury are:

- Change in the resident's alertness or consciousness
- Change in orientation (ability to recognize time, place, person)
- Memory loss
- Unequal pupils
- Visual disturbances
- Blood or clear fluid leaking from ears or nose
- Change in ability to speak or make self understood

PROCEDURE 4
Emergency Care for the Resident Who Is Having a Seizure

1. Stay with the resident and call for help.
2. Use standard precautions if contact with blood, moist body fluids (except sweat), mucous membranes, secretions, excretions, or nonintact skin is likely.
3. If the resident is in bed, remove the pillow and raise the side rails.
4. If the resident is not in bed, gently lower the resident to the floor, protecting the head. Pad the head with a soft, flat object, such as a towel.
5. Turn the resident on the side. If this is not possible, turn the head to the side. This allows secretions to drain from the resident's mouth.
6. Move any hard objects, or pad objects that may injure the resident with pillows, blankets, or other available items, such as chair cushions.
7. Loosen tight and restrictive clothing.
8. Provide privacy by asking onlookers to leave, closing the door to the resident's room, and pulling the privacy curtain.
9. Avoid restraining the resident in any way.
10. Do not try to place any object in the resident's mouth. Doing this could break teeth and cause injury to the resident and yourself.
11. Check the resident's vital signs as requested by the nurse. You may be instructed to check vital signs frequently until the resident is stable.
12. Assist the nurse as directed. The nurse may need to suction the resident, administer oxygen, or give medication to stop the seizure.
13. When the seizure stops, tell the resident where he or she is and what happened. Assist the resident to bed. The resident will be very tired. Allow him or her to sleep.
14. Leave the resident in a position of comfort and safety. Leave the call signal and needed personal items within reach.
15. Remove gloves, if worn, and dispose of them according to facility policy.
16. Wash your hands.
17. Report to the nurse:
    - Any change in the resident before the seizure, such as an aura, confusion, or change in behavior
    - Loss of control of bowel or bladder, eyes rolling upward, rapid blinking, biting tongue
    - Time the seizure started and stopped
    - A description of the way the seizure looked, including the body parts involved
    - Condition of the resident after the seizure
    - Vital signs

PROCEDURE 5

Emergency Care for Falls and Suspected Fractures

If you are walking with a resident who starts to fall, you should:

1. Keep your back straight, your feet about 12 inches apart, and your knees bent.
2. If the resident is wearing a gait belt **(Figure 4-17),** hold the center back of the belt firmly with an underhand grasp. Ease the resident down your legs to the floor. Protect the head from hitting the floor. Guide the resident so that he or she does not hit hard objects in the area.

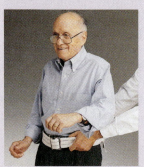

FIGURE 4-17   A gait belt is a safety device used for transfers and ambulation. *(Courtesy of Skil-Care Corporation, Yonkers, NY, 1-800-431-2972)*

3. If the resident is not wearing a gait belt, move close to the resident and wrap your arms around the resident's waist.
4. Pull the resident close to your body, sliding him or her down your leg and easing him or her to the floor. Protect the resident from hitting the head. Guide the resident so that he or she does not hit any hard objects.

Assisting the Resident after a Fall

1. Stay with the resident and call for help. Reassure the resident.
2. Use standard precautions if contact with blood or moist body fluids (except sweat) is likely.
3. Do not move the resident until the nurse has examined him or her and gives approval.
4. Check the resident's vital signs, and assist him or her to bed as instructed by the nurse.
5. Leave the resident in a position of comfort and safety. Place the call signal and needed personal items within reach.
6. Wash your hands.

7. The nurse may direct you to monitor the resident's vital signs frequently until the resident is stable.

Assisting the Resident with a Suspected Fracture

1. Stay with the resident and call for help. Reassure the resident.
2. Use standard precautions if contact with blood or moist body fluids (except sweat) is likely.
3. Do not move the resident until the nurse has examined him or her and gives approval.
4. Keep the resident as quiet as possible.
5. Immobilize the injured area by supporting it to prevent movement. If the area appears out of shape, bent, or deformed, do not attempt to straighten it.
6. Check the resident's vital signs, and assist him or her to bed as instructed by the nurse.
7. If a fracture is suspected, several staff members must assist the resident to bed. One staff member is assigned to move the injured extremity. If possible, splint it with a rigid object, such as a rolled magazine. Other staff members will move the rest of the resident's body. A sheet or other lifting device may be used to move the resident.
8. Leave the resident in a position of comfort and safety. Leave the call signal and needed personal items within reach.
9. Wash your hands.
10. The nurse may direct you to monitor the resident's vital signs frequently until he or she is stable.
11. You may also be directed to apply a cold treatment to the injured area.
12. Observe for and report:
    - The time of the fall
    - The cause of the fall, if known; avoid guessing and report only what you know to be true
    - Measures taken to break the fall
    - Measures taken to assist the resident
    - Known injuries, such as bleeding, deformities, bruises, or changes in the resident's level of consciousness
    - Circulatory problems and abnormal color of the injured extremity
    - Appearance of the injured area and steps taken to immobilize it
    - Witnesses to the fall
    - Vital signs
    - Any additional information needed to fill out the incident report

- Change in ability to follow directions
- No response to verbal stimulation
- Weakness of arms or legs, difficulty maintaining balance
- Complaint of headache
- Nausea and/or vomiting

Remember that signs and symptoms of a problem may not occur for several days. If you notice any of these, you should:

- Stay with the resident and call for help.
- Monitor the pulse and respirations while waiting for the nurse to arrive.

PROCEDURE 6

Application of Cold Packs to Strains and Bruises

1. Notify the nurse of the injury.
2. If the resident is on the floor, stay with him or her and call for help.
3. Do not move the resident until the nurse examines him or her.
4. Wash your hands.
5. Position the resident in a comfortable position.
6. Use standard precautions if contact with blood or moist body fluids (except sweat) is likely.
7. Prepare the cold pack as directed by the nurse and according to facility policy:
   - Place a cloth or flannel cover over the cold pack.
   - Apply the cold pack above or on top of the injured area, as directed. If the resident complains that the cold pack increases the pain, remove it and consult the nurse.
   - Secure the cold pack in place if necessary. You may need to prop it or tie it in place with a gauze bandage.
   - Check the area under the cold pack every 10 minutes and remove it if numbness or discoloration of the skin occurs.
   - Remove the cold pack after 20 minutes.
   - Reapply the cold pack as directed.
8. Wash your hands.
9. Leave the resident in a position of comfort and safety. Leave the call signal and needed personal items within reach.
10. Observe for and report:
    - The time and description of the injured area
    - Edema, deformities, or other injuries
    - Cause of the injury, if known
    - The type of cold pack applied and time
    - Response to the cold pack

PROCEDURE 7

Emergency Care for a Resident with Burns

1. Stay with the resident and call for help. Reassure the resident.
2. Use standard precautions, because contact with body fluids and nonintact skin is likely.
3. Keep the resident's airway open, if necessary, by tilting the head back with one hand while gently lifting the chin with the other hand. Make sure that the resident is breathing.
4. Remove the source of heat, if present.
5. If the burn is minor and the skin is not broken:
   - Remove the resident's clothing from the burned area. Do not remove clothing stuck to the skin.
   - Immerse the burned area in cool water. Do not use ice or ice water.
6. If the burn is very large or deep, do not get the area wet. Do not try to remove clothing stuck to the skin.
7. Cover the burned area with a clean pad, gauze, or cloth.
8. Keep the resident as quiet as possible.
9. Cover the resident to maintain body temperature.
10. Check the resident's vital signs as directed. You may be instructed to check the vital signs frequently until the resident is stable. If the resident's upper arms are burned, do not take the blood pressure. Check with the nurse for further instructions.
11. Do not give the resident food or fluids.
12. Remove gloves, if worn, and dispose of them according to facility policy.
13. Wash your hands.
14. Leave the resident in a position of comfort and safety. Leave the call signal and needed personal items within reach.
15. Observe for and report:
    - Time the resident was discovered
    - Cause of the burn, if known
    - Appearance of the burned area
    - Emergency measures taken
    - Other observations or resident response
    - Witnesses to the incident
    - Vital signs
    - Any additional information needed by the nurse to complete the incident report

- If you suspect a spinal cord injury, instruct the resident not to move. Immobilize the head, neck, and trunk as much as possible.
- Keep the environment quiet and calm.
- Avoid giving the resident anything to drink.
- Reassure and orient the resident.
- Elevate the head on a pillow.
- Avoid moving the resident if he or she is on the floor; wait for the nurse's instructions.
- Cover the resident with a blanket to maintain body temperature.
- Monitor vital signs regularly after the injury, as instructed.

Caring for a Resident with Strains and Bruises

Strains are injuries that occur from overstretching or overusing a muscle. **Bruises** are injuries to the skin caused by hitting, bumping, or striking. The bruised area usually turns black and blue in color. The medical term for a bruise is **ecchymosis.** These injuries are painful, and edema may occur. Cold packs are commonly used to decrease pain and swelling. You should apply cold packs only if you are instructed to do so by the nurse. Cold packs are usually left in place for 20 minutes and then removed to avoid tissue damage.

Caring for a Resident with Burns

Burns are commonly caused by hot water or other hot liquids and careless cigarette smoking. *Thermal burns* are caused by flame and hot objects. *Chemical burns* are caused by harmful chemicals contacting the skin, eyes, or mucous membranes. Burns can range from minor to severe. Severe burns can lead to loss of skin, damage to the muscle, infection, and death. Even small burns can be very painful. The purpose of burn care is to relieve pain, prevent infection and other complications, and promote healing.

Caring for a Resident Who Is Hemorrhaging

Hemorrhage, or severe bleeding, can occur inside or outside the body. Bleeding inside the body cannot be seen or treated by the nursing assistant. This section discusses bleeding on the outside of the body. Many different injuries can cause bleeding. If bleeding is not controlled quickly, serious complications can result. One serious complication is **shock.** Shock is the result of blood loss and causes inadequate blood flow to the heart and brain. If shock is untreated, it can lead to death. The purpose of these guidelines is to control bleeding and prevent shock.

Caring for a Resident with Vomiting and Aspiration

Food and air are both taken into the body through the mouth. The passageway by which food and air enter is shared **(Figure 4-18).** The passage branches into two divisions in the throat. Food goes into the esophagus, then to the stomach. Air goes into the trachea, then the lungs. A small flap, called the **epiglottis,** covers the trachea when you swallow. This flap prevents food and liquid from running into the lungs. The ability to swallow is less efficient in people with some diseases and in the elderly. Occasionally food, water, or other objects accidentally go down the trachea and into the lungs. This is called **aspiration,** and can occur when a resident is vomiting, bleeding, eating, or drinking. Sometimes thick secretions from the mouth enter the lungs. Aspiration can cause serious complications. It can be prevented by turning the resident's body to the side if he or she is vomiting while lying down. If turning the resident's body is not possible, turn the head to the side. Fluid cannot enter the lungs in this position. The purpose of this procedure is to prevent aspiration of food, fluids, secretions, blood, or vomitus.

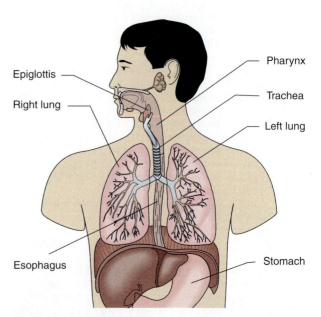

FIGURE 4-18 The trachea and esophagus share a common passage in the throat through which food and air pass.

PROCEDURE 8

Emergency Care for Controlling Bleeding

1. Stay with the resident and call for help.
2. Apply the principles of standard precautions and select personal protective equipment appropriate to the procedure.
3. If the hemorrhage is visible:
   - Apply direct pressure over the site of bleeding with a clean pad or towel and your *gloved* hand.
   - Increase the pressure if the bleeding continues.
   - Do not remove the pad to check the injury. If the pad becomes soaked, add extra padding.
   - Continue direct pressure until you are given further instructions by the nurse.
4. Keep the resident warm and quiet. Have the resident lie flat. Elevate the feet, if possible.
5. Take the blood pressure, pulse, and respirations as directed. You may be instructed to monitor the vital signs frequently until the resident is stable.
6. Do not give the resident anything to eat or drink. The resident may complain of being very thirsty. Thirst is a sign of shock. Notify the nurse of this complaint.
7. Leave the resident in a position of comfort and safety. Leave the call signal and needed personal items within reach.
8. Dispose of items containing blood according to facility policy.
9. Remove gloves and other PPE and dispose of them according to facility policy.
10. Wash your hands.
11. Observe for and report to the nurse:
    - Time the bleeding was discovered
    - Cause of the bleeding, if known
    - Location of the bleeding
    - Emergency measures taken
    - Blood pressure, pulse, and respirations
    - Any additional information required for the incident report
    - Witnesses to the injury
    - Other observations and resident response

PROCEDURE 9

Emergency Care for Vomiting and Aspiration

1. Stay with the resident and call for help.
2. Use standard precautions and select personal protective equipment appropriate to the procedure.
3. Keep the resident's head elevated if possible.
4. Keep the resident's body or head turned to the side to allow fluids to drain from the mouth.
5. Provide an emesis basin if the resident is vomiting.
6. Notify the nurse immediately if the resident:
   - Is choking or is unable to swallow
   - Is unable to spit out the vomitus, blood, or secretions in the mouth
7. The nurse may need to suction the resident or notify the doctor.
8. If the resident begins choking and an airway obstruction occurs, follow the procedure for clearing the obstructed airway (see Procedure 10).
9. After the episode, assist the resident with mouth care.
10. Leave the resident in a position of comfort and safety. Leave the call signal and needed personal items within reach.
11. Dispose of items containing blood or other body secretions according to facility policy.
12. Remove gloves and dispose of them according to facility policy.
13. Wash your hands.
14. Observe for and report to the nurse:
    - Difficulty swallowing, bleeding, vomiting, choking, or aspiration.
    - The color and odor of the vomitus, and the presence of undigested food, blood, or coffee-ground appearance (coffee-ground appearance suggests blood in the stomach).
    - Measure or estimate the amount of vomitus or blood, and record on the intake and output record.
    - Do not discard the vomitus or blood until it is seen by the nurse and a specimen obtained, if needed.

Caring for a Resident with an Obstructed Airway

Sometimes food or a foreign object is aspirated into the windpipe, or trachea. This causes an **obstructed airway,** which is a serious emergency. The obstruction must be removed immediately, or the resident will die. When a person is choking, putting one or both hands about the throat is instinctive. This is known as the **universal choking sign (Figure 4-19).** If you see a resident with hands on the throat, ask if he or she can speak or cough. If the resident can speak, the airway is not obstructed. Stay with the resident and see if he or she can expel the foreign body on his or her own. If the resident is unable to speak, cough, or breathe, you must take immediate action by performing the obstructed airway procedure. The purpose of this procedure is to remove a foreign object from the airway of an adult. The procedure is different for infants, small children, and pregnant women.

Cardiopulmonary resuscitation.   Cardiopulmonary resuscitation (CPR) is an emergency

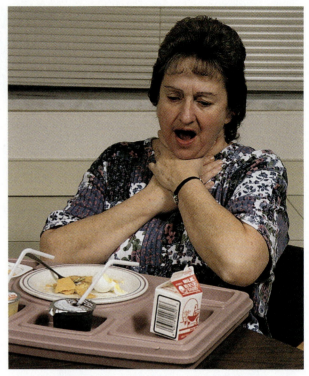

FIGURE 4-19   The universal choking sign.

| PROCEDURE **10** | Emergency Care for Clearing the Obstructed Airway in a Conscious Adult Who Is Sitting or Standing | OBRA |

1. Ask the resident, "Are you choking?" or "Can you speak?"
2. If the resident can speak or cough, leave him or her alone and see if he or she can cough the obstruction out. Assist the resident if the cough is weak and ineffective and the resident is in obvious distress.
3. Stay with the resident and call for help.
4. Tell the resident that you will help.
5. Stand behind the resident and wrap your arms around his or her waist **(Figure 4-20A).**

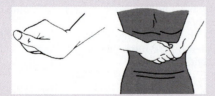

FIGURE 4-20A   Place your arms around the abdomen, slightly above the waist. Avoid resting your forearms on the ribs.

6. Make a fist with one hand and place the thumb side of the fist against the abdomen, just above the navel **(Figure 4-20B).**

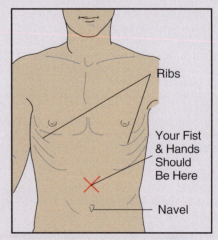

Ribs

Your Fist & Hands Should Be Here

Navel

FIGURE 4-20B   Turn your thumb inward.

Continues

7. Grasp your fist with the other hand. Do not put pressure on the ribs or breastbone with your forearms.
8. Quickly squeeze inward and upward **(Figure 4-20C).** Each thrust should be a separate and distinct movement done with the intent of removing the obstruction. You are trying to push the diaphragm up to force out the air behind the foreign body. As the air is expelled, it will push the object out.
9. If the resident does not expel the foreign body, continue the inward, upward thrusts. If the resident begins to cough forcefully, wait and see if the object can be expelled.
10. Continue until the foreign body is expelled or the resident loses consciousness.
11. When the foreign body is expelled, stay with the resident, and follow the nurse's directions.
12. Leave the resident in a position of comfort and safety. Leave the call signal and needed personal items within reach. The nurse may instruct you to monitor the resident's vital signs periodically.
13. Wash your hands.

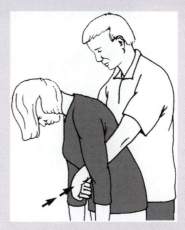

FIGURE 4-20C Squeeze in and up.

 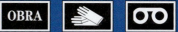
1. Perform abdominal thrusts (see Procedure 10) until the resident loses consciousness. Activate the emergency response system, if this has not already been done. Send someone else, if possible. Remain with the resident and continue to try to relieve the obstruction.
2. Wear gloves during this procedure and use standard precautions.
3. Position the resident on his or her back on the floor, with his or her head facing up.
4. Kneel beside the resident and open the airway by tilting the head back with one hand while gently lifting the chin and tongue with the other hand. Perform a finger sweep with two fingers of your gloved hand to see if you can feel and remove a foreign body. If you feel an object, take care to avoid pushing it farther into the resident's throat.
5. Open the airway by placing one hand on the forehead. Apply firm, backward pressure to tilt the head back. With your other hand, position your fingers in the bony part of the jaw, under the chin. Avoid pressure on the soft tissue of the neck. Lift the jaw forward so the teeth are in good alignment with the upper jaw.
6. Attempt to give a breath into the resident's mouth through a ventilation barrier device **(Figure 4-21).** If the air does not go in, reposition the head and attempt to breathe into the resident's mouth again.

Note: Follow your facility policy for mouth-to-mouth ventilation. To prevent the transmission of disease, standard precautions should be used. This means that a ventilation barrier mask (Figure 4-21) with a valve that prevents the backflow of secretions or resuscitation face shield should be placed between your mouth and the resident's mouth. Familiarize yourself with the devices in your facility. CPR classes are offered to teach you

Continues

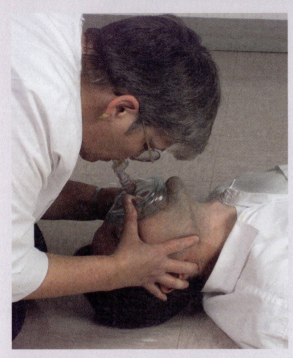

FIGURE 4-21   A pocket mask with a one-way valve is a barrier device for artificial ventilation. You must receive special education in the use of this device.

how to use ventilation devices correctly. Attending a CPR class will benefit you personally and professionally.

7. If no air enters the resident after the second attempt at ventilations, straddle the resident's hips.
8. Place the heel of one hand on the resident's abdomen, immediately above the navel. Your fingers should be pointing up toward the head. Do not place your hand on the ribs or breastbone.
9. Place your other hand on top. Position your shoulders directly above the resident's abdomen.
10. Press your hands inward and upward five times.
11. Open the airway by doing a tongue/jaw lift. Check the resident's mouth and perform another finger sweep.
12. Attempt to ventilate.
13. Repeat steps 5 through 12 until the object is expelled.
14. Assist the nurse, code team, or **EMS** (emergency medical services), as appropriate.
15. Dispose of gloves and face shield according to facility policy.
16. Wash your hands.
17. Observe and report to the nurse:
    - Exact time the choking and unconsciousness started and stopped
    - The procedures done and the time that you started and stopped
    - The resident's response
    - Factors related to the cause of choking, if known

procedure used in health care facilities if the resident's heart and breathing have stopped. CPR is used to keep the resident alive until more advanced life support can be obtained. It is recommended that you attend a CPR course and learn this valuable lifesaving technique. Your facility might require you to become certified in CPR. Additional emergency procedures are listed in Appendix A.

EARLY DEFIBRILLATION

Public access to **defibrillation** has proven to be highly successful. Defibrillation is a method of treatment that uses an electric shock to reverse disorganized activity in the heart during cardiac arrest. Early defibrillation has proven to be critical to survival in cardiac arrest. Defibrillators are

placed in various locations in the community and are used by trained rescuers in the event of cardiac arrest. Some studies have shown that the chance of survival doubles when early access to defibrillation is available. The speed with which defibrillation is performed is the key to success. Early defibrillation (within five minutes) is a high-priority goal in the community. In health care facilities, the goal is to defibrillate within three minutes.

Automatic external defibrillators (AEDs) are computerized devices that are simple to learn to use and operate. The AED is used *only* when a resident is unresponsive, not breathing, and pulseless. When the device is attached to the victim's chest, the unit determines if an electrical shock is necessary to reestablish or regulate the heartbeat. Several different models are available, and the operating instructions are slightly different for each. The four basic steps to using an AED are:

1. Turn the power to the unit on.
2. Apply the electrode pads to the resident's chest.
3. All rescuers stand back to allow the machine to analyze the heart rhythm.
4. All rescuers continue to stand back; the operator of the unit presses the shock button and/or follows the unit's instructions, which are usually audible through a voice-synthesized message.

Hospitals normally use manual, portable defibrillators for caring for resident victims of cardiac arrest. These defibrillators are operated by qualified licensed personnel. The AED is not routinely used in the hospital. However, some long-term care facilities have AEDs available in strategic locations. If your facility purchases an AED, employees will be instructed in its use. Although the AED is simple to operate, only those who are properly trained may use it. CPR and use of the AED are included in basic life support classes for health care professionals.

KEY POINTS IN CHAPTER

- Every employee of the health care facility is responsible for keeping the environment safe.
- Changes in vision, hearing, blood vessels, and reflexes put some residents at high risk for accidents.
- You should correct unsafe conditions, if possible, or report them to the proper person.
- Material safety data sheets give instructions for safe use of chemicals, identify health risks of chemicals, and describe first aid and safety precautions.
- You should answer the call lights of all residents, whether you are assigned to care for the resident or not.
- Identify the resident before giving care.
- Before applying a heat or cold application, know the type of application, area to be treated, length of time the application is to be used, proper temperature, safety precautions, and side effects to watch for.
- The nursing assistant must know and practice oxygen safety.
- Oxygen, fuel, and a spark are necessary to start a fire.
- In a fire emergency, the RACE system is used to remove residents from danger, activate the alarm, and contain and extinguish the fire.
- Know and follow facility policies for tornado, hurricane, earthquake, and bomb threat emergencies.
- The Occupational Safety and Health Administration is an agency that is responsible for overseeing employee safety in the workplace.
- If you discover a resident who is having a medical emergency or is injured, stay with the resident and call for help.
- The universal sign for choking is one or both hands on the throat.
- The speed with which defibrillation is performed is the key to success in cardiac arrest. In the community, defibrillation within five minutes is a goal; in health care facilities, defibrillation within three minutes is the goal.

REVIEW

A. Multiple Choice

Select the one best answer.

1. Safety is the responsibility of the
   a. director of nursing.
   b. housekeeping department.
   c. maintenance department.
   d. entire staff.

2. Physical changes in aging and disease that increase the risk of incidents are
   a. changes in vision, hearing, and reflexes.
   b. chest pain and shortness of breath.
   c. nausea, vomiting, and diarrhea.
   d. hair loss, diabetes, and cancer.

3. When placing the resident's call signal, you should
   a. place the call signal by alert residents only when they are in bed.
   b. never place the call signal near a confused resident.
   c. place the call signal near all residents at all times.
   d. give the resident the call signal only if requested.

4. Chemicals:
   a. are used only in the laundry.
   b. are stored in the clean utility room.
   c. should be kept in their original containers.
   d. are not permitted in the long-term care facility.

5. When using heat and cold applications, you should know
   a. the type of application and area to be treated.
   b. the resident's medical diagnoses.
   c. whether the resident is at risk of heart attack.
   d. the precise temperature preferred by the resident.

6. The three elements necessary to start a fire are
   a. oxygen, fuel, and a spark.
   b. oxygen, chemicals, and fuel.
   c. matches, cigarettes, and chemicals.
   d. matches, candles, and fuel.

7. You answer the facility telephone and the caller advises you that there is a bomb in the nursing home. You should
   a. ask the caller to hold while you get the nurse.
   b. hang up and call the police immediately.
   c. keep the caller on the line and get as much information as you can.
   d. tell the caller not to play silly games with the nursing facility.

8. If you find a resident who is ill or injured, you should
   a. run and get the nurse.
   b. stay with the resident and call for help.
   c. go to the phone and call an ambulance immediately.
   d. leave the room and pretend that you did not see the resident.

9. If you find a resident who has fallen on the floor next to the bed, you should
   a. help the resident back to bed.
   b. go to the desk and fill out an incident report.
   c. tell the resident he or she should have called for help.
   d. reassure the resident while waiting for help to arrive.

10. You find a resident who is having a seizure. You should do all of the following *except*
    a. place an object in the resident's mouth so he or she doesn't swallow the tongue.
    b. stay with the resident and call for help.
    c. loosen tight and restrictive clothing.
    d. move any objects that could harm the resident.

11. A serious complication of hemorrhage is
    a. bleeding.
    b. swelling.
    c. fractures.
    d. shock.

12. The universal choking sign is
    a. waving your hands in the air.
    b. coughing and gagging.
    c. one or both hands on the throat.
    d. clutching the chest.

B. True/False

Answer each statement true (T) or false (F).

13. _____ Most accidents cannot be prevented.

14. _____ Residents in wheelchairs should be parked across the hall from the linen cart.

15. _____ Aging changes in vision make it difficult to see in dim lighting.

16. _____ When answering a resident's call signal, you should knock on the door before entering the room.

17. _____ Thermal burns are caused by chemicals touching the skin.

18. _____ An example of a generalized cold application is an ice bag placed on a swollen ankle.

19. _____ Heat applications dilate the blood vessels.

20. _____ Oxygen is necessary for life.

21. _____ The first step in the RACE system is to run for help.

22. _____ OSHA is responsible for employee safety in the workplace.

C. Fill in the Blanks

Complete each sentence by adding the missing word or words.

23. Syncope is the medical word for _____.

24. The major cause of fire in a health care facility is _____.

25-27. List three safety precautions to take when a resident is using oxygen.

25. _____   27. _____

26. _____

D. Clinical Applications

Answer the following questions:

28. Laura Tyler is walking in her room. She has only nylon stockings on her feet. What should you do?

29. You are assigned to bathe Mrs. Lincoln in the whirlpool tub. The tub has a built-in thermometer that reads 85°. The water is steaming and appears very hot. What should you do?

30. When you go around the corner in Wing A, you notice a large puddle on the floor. The housekeeper is off the unit taking her lunch break. Other personnel are busy passing trays and transporting residents to the dining room. What should you do?

31. Mr. Lake's oxygen concentrator is supposed to be set at two liters per minute. When you check it, you observe that it has been turned up to five liters per minute. Mr. Lake admits that he turned it up so he could "breathe easier." What action should you take?

32. Your facility requires residents to be supervised when smoking. Residents may not keep smoking materials. You enter Mrs. Rose's room and find her smoking a cigarette. She has burn holes in her clothing. How should you handle this situation?

Read the following case study, then answer the questions.

Mrs. Coxon fell three days ago. She has a skin tear on her left forearm, a bruise behind her right ear, and a bump on her head. The resident is normally alert and independent. You enter her room to serve breakfast and find that she is not dressed, which is unusual for this resident. Mrs. Coxon is mentally confused. She asks you to get her mother. She says she feels sick and begins to vomit.

33. How will you respond to the resident's request to get her mother?

34. What action should you take first?

35. What should you do next?

36. What do you think is causing the problem?

CHAPTER 5

Legal and Ethical Responsibilities

OBJECTIVES

After reading this chapter, you will be able to:

- Spell and define key terms.
- Define the purpose of the residents' rights document.
- State the purpose of the advance directive.
- Describe how to assist residents who are physically or mentally unable to exercise their legal rights.
- Define resident abuse and neglect and give one example of each.
- List six other legal considerations of concern to the nursing assistant.
- Explain why understanding the resident's culture is important to the nursing assistant.
- Describe how to promote resident independence and explain why this is important.

LEGAL CONSIDERATIONS FOR THE NURSING ASSISTANT

Long-term care facilities operate under state, federal, and local laws. Some companies and accrediting organizations have additional requirements. All nursing assistants must operate within the scope of these rules. Each facility has policies and procedures governing employee conduct and resident care within the institution. These policies and procedures are designed to maintain compliance with the various bodies that govern the agency.

RIGHTS OF THE RESIDENT

The resident has certain legal rights to safe care. Institutional policies vary regarding how residents are informed of these rights. Some facilities present a copy of the rights to residents upon admission and have them sign an acknowledgment that they have received them. Other agencies post copies of the rights in prominent locations throughout the facility. The bill of rights is written in very simple language that all residents can understand. In some communities with large groups of non–English-speaking residents, the bill of rights is translated into the prevalent language in the community. Health care workers must be aware of what the rights of the resident are. All health care providers are obligated to uphold and protect these rights for all residents. The nursing assistant must assist mentally confused residents to exercise their rights.

Residents' Bill of Rights

Residents in long-term care facilities have the same rights as other citizens of the United States. The Omnibus Budget Reconciliation Act (OBRA) of 1987 guarantees residents of nursing facilities certain legal rights. These rights are listed in a document called the **Residents' Bill of Rights.** The nursing assistant must be familiar with, respect, and assist residents to exercise their rights. The rights of residents who are mentally confused are no different from the rights of others. The nursing assistant must protect the rights of mentally confused residents. Resident rights are summarized in **Table 5-1.**

Privacy. Residents have the right to privacy. Always knock on the door **(Figure 5-1)** and allow time for a response before entering the

TABLE 5-1   Residents' Rights

- Residents have the right to exercise all their rights as citizens of the state and citizens of the United States, as well as any other rights given them by law.
- The facility must explain the rights to residents both verbally and in writing in a language that the residents understand.
- Residents cannot be discriminated against because of age, sex, race, ethnic origin, religion, or disability.

Privacy, Dignity, and Respect

- Residents have a right to privacy.
- Residents will be treated with consideration, dignity, and respect.
- The resident's likes, dislikes, and special needs and preferences must be considered in the services provided by the facility. This is called **reasonable accommodation.**
- Personal and clinical records must be kept confidential. Residents have the right to refuse to allow others to see these records. Permission to release records is given in writing.
- Residents have the right to communicate both verbally and in writing with anyone of their choosing. This includes family members, other visitors, the ombudsman, attorneys, and representatives of governmental agencies.
- Residents have the right to send and receive personal mail unopened. Residents may request that staff assist them to open and read their mail when it arrives.

Safety and Security

- Residents have the right to a safe environment.
- Residents have the right to care that is free from **misappropriation of property** (theft).

Medical Care and Treatment

- Residents have the right to choose their own physicians. They have the right to be informed of matters affecting their care and to make decisions regarding their care.
- Medical problems must be explained to residents in a language they understand.
- Residents may refuse treatment. If they do refuse treatment, they have the right to be informed of the consequences of their refusal.
- Residents have a right to voice problems and complaints about their care without fear of **reprisal,** or retaliation. The facility is required to respond to these complaints.
- Residents have the right to make choices to withhold life-sustaining treatment in the event of terminal illness.
- Residents may designate someone else to make treatment decisions for them in the event they become unable to make these decisions themselves.

Freedom from Restraint, Abuse, Neglect, and Misappropriation of Property

- Residents have the right to be free from abuse, neglect, and misappropriation of property. The facility is responsible for caring for the resident's health, well-being, and personal possessions.
- Drugs cannot be given for discipline or convenience of the nursing home staff. Any mood-altering drugs given must be required for the treatment of a medical condition.
- Residents cannot be punished, scolded, abused, neglected, or secluded. Their privileges cannot be taken away and they cannot be physically, mentally, or sexually abused.
- Residents cannot be restrained by physical means except for their own safety, the safety of others, during certain medical procedures, or in an emergency.

Financial Matters

- Residents have the right to manage their own financial affairs or may choose another person to manage their money.
- Facilities must account for and properly manage resident money deposited with them.

Freedom of Association

- Residents have the right to have visitors at any reasonable hour.
- Residents do not have to talk to or see anyone they do not want to visit.
- Residents may make and receive private phone calls.
- Married couples have the right to share a room.
- Residents have the right to organize and participate in resident and family councils.
- Residents may meet with others outside the facility.
- Residents may leave the facility for visits or shopping trips.
- Family members may meet with families of other residents in the nursing home.
- Residents have the right to plan and execute their daily activities.
- Residents have the right to vote in elections.

Work

- Residents may choose to work in the facility as part of their activity plan. They have the right to be paid the prevailing rate for the same type of work in the community. Residents may also perform certain duties without pay, if they choose to do so.

Personal Possessions

- Residents may wear their own clothing.
- Residents may bring in furnishings and personal belongings from their own homes.

Continues

TABLE 5-1 Residents' Rights, *Continued*	
Grievance	• Residents may not be asked to give up their rights to benefits under Medicaid or Medicare.
• If residents have problems or complaints, they have the right to speak to those in charge. The complaints may be about care or failure to receive expected services. Residents have the right to a response.	• The facility is required to have the same policies and practices regarding services, transfer, or discharge for all individuals, regardless of the source of payment.
• Residents have the right to contact the **ombudsman** for the facility and the state survey and certification agency. The ombudsman is a resident advocate. He or she can provide information on how to find a facility and how to get quality care. An ombudsman can help solve problems and will assist the resident to file a **grievance,** or complaint, if requested.	• The facility may be required to hold the resident's bed for a specified period if the resident is hospitalized or goes on a therapeutic pass.
	• The facility cannot make the resident leave or move to another room unless:
	• The health and safety of the resident or others are affected.
	• The facility cannot meet the resident's needs.
• The facility may not retaliate against residents who have complained.	• The resident's condition has improved so that services are no longer required.
Admission, Transfer, and Discharge	• The resident has not paid the bill and the facility has given the resident reasonable notice of discharge.
• The facility must advise residents about eligibility for Medicaid. If Medicaid or Medicare pays for any items or services, the resident cannot be charged additional money for these services.	• Residents must be given a 30-day written notice before they can be transferred unless there are medical reasons, or the life, safety, and health of the resident or others is endangered. Residents may waive the right to the 30-day waiting period if they choose.
• In the event of the resident's death, the facility must give an accounting of money in the resident's personal account to the person responsible for the estate.	

resident's room. When providing care or performing procedures, close the door to the room, the privacy curtain, and the window curtains. The privacy curtain and window curtains must be closed even if the door to the room is closed and no one else is in the room. The nursing assistant must not unnecessarily expose residents when giving care. To protect dignity

and prevent embarrassment, drape the resident's body so that only the part you are working on is exposed. A bath blanket is used for draping the body during examinations, treatments, and personal care.

Confidentiality. The law guarantees residents **confidentiality** in their medical care and treatment. This means that unauthorized persons may not read the residents' medical records. It also means that health care workers cannot discuss personal information about the residents or their conditions with others. Information about residents should be discussed only in private areas. Do not discuss residents in hallways, on elevators, in the break room, or with others outside the long-term care facility. If a resident tells you something in confidence, you should not tell anyone else unless the information affects the resident's condition or medical care. For example, if a resident tells you something about a private financial matter, you should not tell anyone else. However, if a resident tells you that he or she is secretly spitting out his or her medication, this information should be reported to the nurse. If a visitor asks you for information about a resident, refer the visitor to the nurse for information.

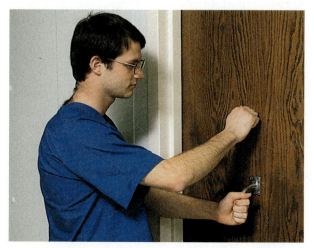

FIGURE 5-1 Knocking on the door and awaiting a response shows respect for the resident's privacy.

Assisting Residents Who Cannot Exercise Their Rights

The nursing assistant is responsible for helping residents exercise their rights if they are physically or mentally unable to do so on their own. This involves using a good deal of common sense. For example, a resident with a physical or mental impairment may not be able to cover her body if it is exposed. It is your responsibility to cover the resident. Offer to help residents who cannot do things for themselves. You may notice an unopened card on the resident's table. Offer to open and read the card to the resident. Do not open the card without the resident's permission.

Give residents as much control over care and daily routines as possible. Always explain what you are going to do and how it will be done. Although the resident may be physically incapable of performing certain tasks, he or she may be able to tell you how and when he or she wants them done **(Figure 5-2)**. Giving residents control and offering choices about care and routines is an excellent way to help residents exercise their rights, and promotes healthy self-esteem. It sends a message to residents that you value them as people and respect their opinions. Inform residents of facility practices, policies, and procedures that affect them.

Although residents are guaranteed many legal rights, they are not allowed to infringe upon the rights of others. If the rights of one resident are interfering with the rights of others, try to find a compromise. If you are unable to resolve the situation, consult the nurse.

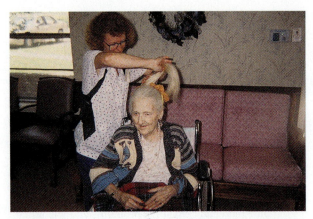

FIGURE 5-2 The resident is mentally alert and able to tell the nursing assistant how she wants her hair styled.

ABUSE AND NEGLECT

Abuse is the willful infliction of injury, unreasonable confinement, intimidation, or punishment that results in physical harm, pain, or mental anguish. Abuse can be physical, verbal, sexual, or mental. **Neglect** is failure to provide needed care or services. It can be deliberate or accidental. An example of neglect is forgetting that you have been assigned to care for a resident and not providing care. All states have laws concerning abuse and neglect of residents in the long-term care facility. You are legally responsible for reporting suspected or actual abuse and neglect of residents. The health care agency must always report abuse to law enforcement authorities and state agencies. This is the nurse manager's responsibility. There are severe penalties for abusing or neglecting residents. Health care workers who witness abuse or neglect and do not report it may be held equally responsible for the situation. If you suspect that a resident has been abused or neglected by a staff member, family, or any other individual, report this information to the nurse immediately.

Abuse and neglect may occur because a nursing assistant or other individual is feeling stressed. Residents may say things that are hurtful or upsetting to you. Remain calm and do not take a resident's behavior or negative remarks personally. Abuse often occurs when a worker is feeling tired, experiencing personal problems, or losing control. If you feel overwhelmed with your duties or with a resident, discuss it with the nurse. Arrange to take a break and compose yourself.

Types of Abuse

Abuse can take many different forms. Sometimes the abuser is not even aware that the behavior or action toward a resident is abusive. The different types of abuse are described in **Table 5-2**.

Recognizing signs of abuse. New bruises, pain, swelling, or other unexplained injuries to a resident may be an indication of abuse and should be reported to the nurse. Other signs of possible abuse include residents responding to the nursing assistant or others with fear and anxiety. Residents who have been abused may show sudden changes in their personality or behavior. You are not required to determine whether the changes in the resident are the result of abuse. Your responsibility is to report the observations to the nurse for further investigation.

TABLE 5-2	Types of Abuse
Type of abuse	**Description**
Physical abuse	Willful, nonaccidental injury, such as handling a resident roughly or striking, slapping, or hitting a resident
Verbal abuse	Swearing, using demeaning terms to talk to a resident, or embarrassing a resident
Mental abuse	Threatening to harm a resident or threatening to withhold food, fluid, or care as a form of punishment
Sexual abuse	• Physical force or verbal threats are used to force a resident to perform a sexual act • Touching or fondling a resident inappropriately • Any behavior that is seductive, sexually demeaning, harassing, or reasonably interpreted as sexual by the resident

ADVANCE DIRECTIVES

A resident of a long-term care facility has the right to execute an **advance directive.** An advance directive is a document that designates the resident's wishes if he or she cannot speak for himself or herself. Advance directives can be in the form of a **living will,** which designates the resident's wishes if he or she is in a terminal condition. The resident also has the right to designate a surrogate decision maker, often called a **health care proxy.** The document that the resident signs is called a **durable power of attorney for health care.** This document allows the health care proxy to make medical decisions on behalf of the resident. State laws vary on how advance directives are implemented, but residents in all states have the right to execute these documents. The long-term care facility informs the resident of this right upon admission. The facility is obligated to follow the written directions of the resident on these documents.

OTHER LEGAL CONSIDERATIONS

Consent means giving permission for treatment when a person is conscious and alert **(Figure 5-3).** Residents have the right to refuse treatment for any reason. They also have the right to have the consequences of the refusal explained to them. Spouses or legal guardians have the right to give consent or refuse treatment for residents who are mentally confused. Report to the nurse for further directions if a resident or guardian refuses care.

Consent and the resident's right to refuse treatment can create a dilemma for the nursing

assistant if the resident is mentally confused. For example, a confused resident may refuse bathing, grooming, or change of clothing. Residents who are confused have legally appointed guardians or family members who make medical decisions on the residents' behalf. These individuals have consented to nursing facility treatment, including the provision of personal hygienic care. In a refusal situation, gaining the resident's cooperation is always best. Avoid forcing a confused resident. Try different techniques, such as leaving and returning later, or making a fun activity of the procedure by singing, laughing, or joking with the resident. Use good communication skills. If the confused resident persists in the refusal, consult the nurse. Additional methods of working with mentally confused residents are described in Chapter 20.

Negligence and malpractice. **Negligence** involves breaching the standard of care. This

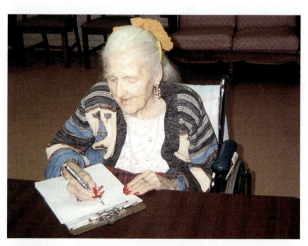

FIGURE 5-3 This alert resident understands her treatment and is able to give permission by signing a consent.

means that a health care worker fails to provide services to residents in the same manner as a reasonably prudent person with the same education would do. An example of negligence is telling a resident it is all right to get up unsupervised even though you know the resident is dizzy and weak. The resident falls and is injured. An attorney can argue that the reasonably prudent nursing assistant should have known that the resident was at risk of injury. The proper course of action would be to instruct the resident to call for help before getting up, and remaining with the resident to assist while he or she was out of bed. To avoid negligence, always perform procedures in the manner in which you were taught, and use good judgment. If you are in doubt about what to do, consult the nurse. Follow your facility policies even if you do not agree with them. **Malpractice** is negligence that results in harm to the resident. For example, the care plan states that the resident's side rails are to be up at all times when in bed. The nursing assistant forgets to put the rails up and the resident falls from the bed, breaking a hip.

Making False Statements

Defamation of character is making false or slanderous statements about another person. An example is to tell others that your neighbor was admitted to the long-term care facility for treatment for AIDS. The neighbor was actually admitted for recovery after hospital treatment for pneumonia and does not have AIDS. Discussing a resident with someone outside the facility is also a serious breach of the resident's right to confidentiality. Discussions about residents should be limited to only those persons who have a legal right to know the information. **Slander** is a negatively spoken statement. **Libel** is a derogatory written statement.

Abandonment

Abandonment means leaving or walking off the premises. If the nursing assistant must leave the facility for any reason, the nurse should be notified. Before you leave, an equally qualified person must be available to care for your assigned residents. An example of abandonment is leaving the facility before a qualified person has been secured to replace you. You can be accused of abandonment, even if other staff is on duty, if no one else has been assigned to care for your residents.

False Imprisonment and Involuntary Seclusion

False imprisonment means holding or restraining residents against their will. Use of physical restraints and side rails can be considered methods of false imprisonment. To avoid this situation, follow all facility policies about the use of restraints. Consult the care plan before using any restraining device. **Involuntary seclusion** is a form of abuse if used as punishment for the resident. This involves separating the resident from others against his or her will. For example, Mrs. Long swears at Mrs. King in the dining room. Mrs. King is upset. To punish Mrs. Long, the nursing assistant removes her from the dining room and takes her to her room to finish eating lunch alone. Involuntary seclusion can be used in certain circumstances as part of the therapeutic plan of care, but this determination is not made by the nursing assistant.

Standards of Care

Although health care is delivered in many different settings, the legal requirements for nursing assistants are similar in all settings. **Standards of care** are common health care practices based on laws, facility policies, information learned in your classes, and information published in textbooks and journals for nursing assistants. Standards are defined by community, state, and national practices. They are used to measure the worker's performance and permit you to be judged based on what is expected of a nursing assistant with your education and experience. All long-term care facilities have standards of performance that you must follow in your job. In legal situations, you will be held to the same standard of care and judgment as the average worker in your job.

Good Samaritan Laws

All states have **Good Samaritan laws** to protect health care workers who provide emergency care outside their place of employment. If you assist someone at the scene of an emergency, you are protected under these laws if you deliver care that you are qualified to provide. These laws do not apply to workers providing emergency care in the long-term care facility.

ETHICAL BEHAVIOR WITH RESIDENTS AND FAMILIES

Professional boundaries are limits on how a health care worker acts with residents. Compare these boundaries to the borders between states on a map. They exist, but you cannot see the boundary lines when you are driving down the highway. Professional boundaries are the same way. They exist, but you do not always know when you cross them. Boundaries are lines that define the best behavior of nursing assistants when caring for residents and meeting their needs. The nursing assistant must act professionally, not personally as a family member or friend. Professional boundaries help the nursing assistant act appropriately. You do not want to have too much or too little contact. You must use good judgment and determine the amount of contact that is right for the resident. Consult the nurse if you are uncertain.

The nursing assistant must treat all residents professionally. Residents expect you to act in their best interests and to treat them with dignity. This means you must not take advantage of a resident's situation, and must avoid becoming inappropriately involved in the resident's personal and family relationships. Some relationships with residents and families are not healthy for the resident or the nursing assistant. Unfortunately, it is not always easy to recognize unhealthy relationships until it is too late. Strive to find a balance in your relationships. If any of the situations in the following list have occurred, you have probably crossed boundary lines and are in a relationship danger zone. Seek help from your nurse, pastor, or another professional person with whom you are comfortable speaking.

- Discussing your personal problems with the resident or the resident's family members
- Discussing your feelings of sexual attraction with a resident
- Keeping secrets with a resident and becoming defensive when someone questions your relationship or involvement with the resident's personal life
- Thinking you are immune from having an unhealthy relationship with a resident
- Believing that you are the only nursing assistant who can meet the resident's needs
- Spending an inappropriate amount of time with the resident, including off-duty visits or trading assignments with others to be with the resident
- Reporting only partial information about the resident to the nurse because you fear disclosing unfavorable information or secrets the resident has told you
- Being flirtatious with a resident, including sexual innuendos, jokes that are sexual in nature, or using offensive language
- Feeling that you must protect the resident from other health care workers and always siding with the resident's position
- Feeling that you may become involved in a sexual relationship with the resident

Discussing Facility Business with Others

Discussing facility business with residents, family members, and others outside the facility is not ethical. You must be tactful and professional in disclosing information. For example, it is inappropriate to tell residents or family members that you are "short of staff," or to discuss working conditions, salary, benefits, or other information about the operation of the facility. It is also inappropriate to discuss this information or complain to others in the community. A common expression is "The long-term care facilities' employees are their worst enemies." When employees make negative comments and disclose private information, it sends a negative message about all parties involved. You have a moral and ethical obligation to your employer. Complaining to others does not solve problems. In fact, it can make problems worse. If you have concerns about staffing, working conditions, or other situations, use the chain of command within the facility to resolve them.

CULTURAL INFLUENCES ON HEALTH CARE DELIVERY

Health care workers care for residents from many different **cultures.** A culture is a pattern or lifestyle of a group of people. Residents may come from other countries or communities **(Figure 5-4)**. Their backgrounds, beliefs, values, religions, hygiene, and health care practices may be very different from your own. Do not judge them for their beliefs. Look at this as an opportunity to learn more about others. If you can learn about the resident's culture, you will be in a better position to meet his or her needs. Cultural background may influence the residents'

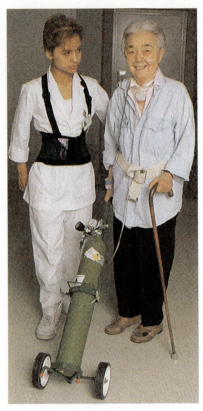

FIGURE 5-4 The resident and nursing assistant are from different cultural backgrounds.

beliefs about illness and preferences in health care. The best way to find out about these preferences is to ask the resident or the family. Asking is not offensive. It shows that you are sensitive, have a sincere desire to learn, and are trying to find ways to help the resident. There is no one good way to meet the needs of an entire cultural group. Trying to place members of a cultural group in a specific category and thinking that they are all alike is called **stereotyping.** Every person is an individual with different wants and needs. Different cultural groups have different beliefs and different ways of meeting their needs. Treat all residents as worthwhile human beings and recognize their individuality!

Language Barriers

Always address each resident in English. Speak slowly, gently, and in a respectful manner. If you determine that the resident does not speak English, ask if the resident has a bilingual dictionary. If not, try using gestures or writing. Some residents learn to read English before they learn to speak it. Use simple terms. Drawing pictures may be useful. If you must perform a procedure on a resident, use gestures and a demonstration to make the resident understand. Always ask the

resident if he or she understands, or say "Okay?". Do not assume that the resident understands because he or she smiles. A smile may be a polite gesture, indicating a lack of understanding. Be prepared to spend extra time with a resident who does not speak English.

Cultural Influences on Personal Space

Personal space is a comfortable distance for communication. The amount of space necessary varies in different cultures. In the United States, personal space is about 18 to 36 inches. People from other cultures may believe that this distance is too great or too small. In some cultures, personal space is much smaller. Be sensitive to residents' discomfort when you are working closely with them. Their beliefs about personal space may be different from yours. People from some cultures will not permit members of the opposite gender to care for them. Saudi Arabians, for example, will not permit a male caregiver to enter the room if a female resident is alone.

Use of Gestures and Eye Contact

The use of gestures and eye contact are not universal. In some cultures, making eye contact when you speak is offensive. Gestures that are acceptable to residents in the United States may be offensive to those from other countries. In India, the head motions used for "yes" and "no" are the direct opposite of the motions used in the United States. Monitor your body language, use of eye contact, and gestures carefully. If something appears to make the resident uncomfortable, don't do it.

Cultural Influences on Pain

Residents from different cultures react differently to pain. Residents from some cultures are very emotional and react very dramatically to pain. In others, the pain can be severe, but the resident will not show any response. In China and Japan, for example, displaying pain in public is unacceptable. In these cultures, pain is considered a sign of weakness.

Cultural Influences on Hygienic Practices

Some countries have different beliefs about bathing, personal hygiene, and the use of deodorant. They may not bathe regularly or use deodorant to eliminate odor. In the United States, it is normal to bathe and use deodorant daily. Women remove hair from their legs and underarms. This is not true of women in some other cultures. Do not be offended if the resident's hygienic practices differ from yours. This may be a difficult problem for you to deal with. Consult the nurse if you are having difficulty with cultural differences.

Cultural Influences on Clothing

Various pieces of clothing may have cultural or religious significance. Some religions require men to keep their heads covered. Others require women to keep their heads covered. In some cultures, women may not show any skin besides their face and/or hands. All other skin must be covered. A resident from such a culture will be very uncomfortable in a bed wearing only a hospital gown, because of the difference in cultural beliefs. Learning about the resident's culture and trying to make accommodations show that you care and will be greatly appreciated by the resident.

Cultural Influence and Home Remedies

People in some cultures have home remedies that they believe will cure their illness or relieve symptoms. These remedies may consist of wraps, rubs, teas, or inhaling herbs and spices. Friends and family members may practice these remedies on residents in the long-term care facility. In some cases, the remedies may actually interfere with the resident's treatment. Consult the nurse for advice if you observe residents practicing home remedies.

Cultural Influence on Food Preferences

Residents may refuse to eat foods served to them because of their cultural and religious beliefs. Some residents eat certain foods because of beliefs that the food has a healing effect on the body. Other residents will refuse certain foods or food combinations because of their religious beliefs. People of some religions have days during which they fast and do not eat. The dietitian and nurse may be able to arrange to have special foods served to residents to meet their needs.

PROMOTING INDEPENDENCE

The OBRA legislation requires long-term care facilities to maintain or improve the residents' condition and to promote independence. This is because being independent promotes healthy self-esteem. Restorative care is care designed to assist residents to function at their highest level in light of their individual situations. This is a very important part of the OBRA philosophy and is used to help residents attain maximum independence. Restorative care is simply good resident care. It is helpful to all residents and makes them feel good about themselves.

There is a common expression, "If you don't use it, you lose it." This is particularly true of self-help skills. We are not doing residents any favors by performing skills that they are able to complete. If the resident does not use the skill, eventually he or she will lose the ability to perform it. Some residents have low self-esteem because of their inability to care for themselves. Do not underestimate confused residents' abilities to do self-care. Test their ability. Provide support and direction, if needed. You may be surprised to find that they can do a great deal of self-care. Allowing them to do so will help maintain their ability.

The sensitive nursing assistant will give residents every opportunity to perform daily life skills independently. Provide support and encouragement. Set the resident up with the needed materials. Allow as much time as necessary to complete the task. If the resident is unable to complete a task independently, offer to finish it and provide positive feedback for what the resident was able to accomplish. Avoid making residents feel like failures. Always stress the ability and not the disability.

KEY POINTS

- Residents in long-term care facilities have specific legal rights that are guaranteed by the federal government.
- Nursing assistants must respect and protect the residents' rights. If the residents are unable to exercise these rights, the nursing assistant should assist.
- Professional boundaries are limits on how a health care worker acts with residents.
- The residents' culture and religion influence your ability to provide care.
- Restorative care is given to assist the resident to attain and maintain the highest level of independence possible.

REVIEW

A. Multiple Choice

Select the one best answer.

1. An advance directive is a document that
   a. gives consent for treatment and procedures while the resident is hospitalized.
   b. states the resident's wishes for care if the resident cannot speak for himself or herself.
   c. gives the health care worker the right to act in the resident's best interest.
   d. designates another person to make medical, legal, and financial decisions.

2. A health care proxy is
   a. a person who makes health care decisions on behalf of the resident.
   b. the health care worker responsible for diagnostic testing.
   c. the individual who prescribes the resident's medical treatment.
   d. another term for the licensed nurse.

3. The Residents' Bill of Rights guarantee residents treatment that is
   a. negligent.
   b. confidential.
   c. libelous.
   d. above the standard of care.

4. When providing care to a resident,
   a. leave the door open so others will know you are in the room.
   b. closing the door is the only step necessary if the resident is alone in the room.
   c. close the door, privacy curtain, and window curtains.
   d. you may leave the door open if the privacy curtain is pulled.

5. It is acceptable to discuss a resident's condition
   a. at the nurses' station or another private area.
   b. in the elevator.
   c. in the cafeteria.
   d. with your family at home.

6. A visitor asks you what is wrong with Mr. Stone, the resident in room 402. You know that Mr. Stone was recently diagnosed with pneumonia related to AIDS. Your best response is:
   a. "He has AIDS. For further information, consult administration."
   b. "He has pneumonia."
   c. "I'm sorry, but I cannot give you that information."
   d. "Ask the doctor."

7. Mr. Stephens is an alert 24-year-old male resident who is unable to move his arms and legs. He was admitted to the long-term care facility for rehabilitation after a serious automobile accident. He is able to communicate with you. The nurse has instructed you to bathe and shave the resident. You should
   a. ask the resident what time he would like the bath.
   b. encourage the resident to be independent.
   c. set up the supplies and ask the resident to try hard.
   d. bathe the resident when it is most convenient for you.

8. You cared for Mrs. King, a 92-year-old confused resident, on Monday. Mrs. King speaks, but does not make sense. You were off on Tuesday. When you return to work on Wednesday, you are assigned to care for Mrs. King again. When you remove her gown to bathe her, you notice bruises on her upper arms. You should
   a. say nothing, as the bruises must have occurred on your day off.
   b. report your findings to the nurse.
   c. ask Mrs. King why she has bruises.
   d. tell the nurse that Mrs. King was neglected on your day off.

9. Mr. Murray is a 72-year-old confused resident. You are assigned to care for him on the 3 p.m. to 11 p.m. shift. When you make your first round to check your residents, you discover that Mr. Murray is in bed. His sheets are wrinkled and soaking wet. There are brown rings of urine on the bottom sheet, indicating that Mr. Murray's linen has not been changed in quite a while. There is food in the bed, and the resident's face and hands are dirty. It appears that someone forgot to care for this resident. This may be an example of
   a. neglect.
   b. abuse.
   c. false imprisonment.
   d. involuntary seclusion.

10. Signs of abuse may include
    a. nausea and vomiting.
    b. unexplained injuries.
    c. fever.
    d. mental confusion.

11. Negligence that results in harm to the resident is
    a. involuntary seclusion.
    b. slander.
    c. malpractice.
    d. defamation.

12. Walking off duty before a suitable replacement can be obtained is
    a. libel.
    b. abandonment.
    c. neglect.
    d. abuse.

13. Good Samaritan laws are designed to protect
    a. health care workers from liability for care provided at the scene of an emergency outside the place of employment.
    b. licensed personnel who provide emergency care as part of their job responsibility.
    c. health care workers on duty in the nursing facility.
    d. physicians only.

14. Standards of care are based on
    a. information in books, journals, and laws.
    b. what the nurse says.
    c. what the doctor would do.
    d. information provided by other assistants.

15. People who come from other cultures
    a. have incorrect beliefs and values.
    b. may have different beliefs than your own.
    c. are all the same.
    d. have different needs.

16. Mrs. Hernandez is a 64-year-old Hispanic female with ovarian cancer. She is in the last stage of her illness, and her family members are at her bedside. When you are making the bed, you notice a raw egg in a cup under the bed. You should
    a. throw the egg away immediately, because it is unsanitary.
    b. tell the family to remove the egg.
    c. ask the resident or family the purpose of the egg.
    d. tell the resident she cannot have raw eggs.

17. Personal space is
    a. a comfortable distance in which to communicate.
    b. a private area used for dressing.
    c. the bathroom.
    d. the resident's room.

18. When caring for residents, you should
    a. provide all care needed even if the residents can do the care themselves.
    b. practice restorative care.
    c. force the residents to do as much as possible.
    d. always consult the doctor for advice.

B. Fill in the Blanks

Complete each sentence by adding the missing word or words.

19. One way of showing that you respect the resident as a person is to offer _____.

20. Residents in the long-term care facility have the right to _____ during personal care procedures.

21. Something that is personal and not known to other people is _____.

22. _____ is a spoken statement that maligns the resident.

23. _____ is treating residents with honor and esteem.

24. _____ _____ are used to measure nursing assistant performance.

25. Failure to provide services that results in harm to residents is _____.

C. Clinical Applications

Answer the following questions.

26. Your friend John is a CNA at another long-term care facility. John tells you that there are much faster ways to do your work than the way you were taught in class. John says that he always gets through with his work early because he has learned all the shortcuts, and offers to teach you what they are. How will you handle this situation?

27. Mary Gray is a mentally confused resident. She goes on an overnight pass with her son and returns after supper the next day. When you are undressing her for bed, you notice bruises on her upper arms and chest. Mary says, "I don't know how I got them." How will you handle this situation?

28. Mr. King is very ill. He has chronic respiratory disease. Mr. King has an advance directive that states that CPR and lifesaving measures will be performed in the event of cardiac arrest or emergency. The resident tells you that he is tired of fighting his illness and has changed his mind. He states he would like to revoke his advance directive. What should you do?

29. You are working the 10 p.m. to 6 a.m. shift. There are two nursing assistants on duty. The other CNA, Mary, has been a close personal friend for a long time. Your friend is upset with the nurse, who corrected her earlier in the shift. She tells you that you should both walk off duty to get back at the nurse. How will you handle this situation?

30. Mrs. Hall is a newly admitted resident. She walks with a strong, steady gait. The nurse instructs you to walk Mrs. Hall to the dining room for supper. Mrs. Hall says, "All the others have wheelchairs, and I want to use a wheelchair, too. I'm paying for it." What should you tell Mrs. Hall?

CHAPTER 6

Communication and Interpersonal Skills

OBJECTIVES

After reading this chapter, you will be able to:

- Spell and define key terms.
- List five methods of communicating with others and give an example of each.
- Describe the four elements of communication.
- List eight barriers to communication and give an example of each.
- Describe goal-oriented communication.
- List six communication styles.
- Explain why listening is an important part of communication.
- Describe how to communicate with residents who have physical disabilities, vision loss, or hearing impairments, residents who are mentally confused, and those who are unable to speak.

OBSERVATIONS TO MAKE AND REPORT RELATED TO COMMUNICATION AND INTERPERSONAL SKILLS

Change in consciousness, awareness, or alertness
Changes in mood, behavior, or emotional status
Changes in orientation to person, place, time, season
Change in communication
Changes in memory

Excessive drowsiness
Changes in ability to respond verbally or nonverbally
Sleepiness for no apparent reason
Sudden onset of mental confusion
Threats of suicide or harm to self or others

COMMUNICATION

Communication involves sending and receiving messages to exchange information with others. Verbal communication is the most common method, but many forms of communication are used in health care. You will communicate verbally, in writing, through gestures, and through use of your body. To be successful, you must understand and practice effective communication. You will communicate with residents, families, visitors, coworkers, and managers. The messages you send and receive must be interpreted accurately. Communication is more than saying words. It is showing honest concern and care for other people.

Factors that Influence Communication with Residents

Sickness, medication, anesthesia, pain, aging, culture, and disease can affect the resident's ability to communicate. Some residents may have trouble seeing, hearing, or speaking. Some residents have language barriers and do not speak English well or at all. When residents have difficulty communicating, the nursing assistant must always practice empathy. This involves putting yourself

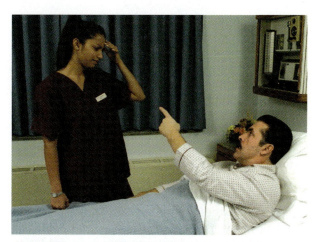

FIGURE 6-1 This resident's body language is sending a message that he is angry.

in the resident's shoes and understanding how he or she feels. Empathy is a positive quality. **Sympathy** is feeling sorry for someone because of his or her physical condition or situation. Avoid feeling sympathy for residents. Sympathy is not healthy for you or the resident. Feeling sympathetic can cause you to cross professional boundaries and enter the relationship danger zone.

Imagine how frustrating it would be if you were unable to make your needs known and communicate with others! Be patient and show empathy when communicating with residents who have physical and mental impairments. Do not assume that residents who are unable to speak are mentally confused. Residents who cannot speak often understand what is said to them. Treat all residents with dignity and respect.

Posture, appearance, and body language also affect communication. All of us use our bodies to communicate **(Figure 6-1).** You must become sensitive to the body language of others and monitor your own body language to be sure that it sends the correct message. Your words and body language should both say the same thing. You may be surprised to learn that whenever there is a conflict between spoken words and body language, the body language is most accurate.

ELEMENTS OF COMMUNICATION

Understanding the elements of communication will help you communicate effectively. Each message has four parts:

1. *Sender*—the person who originates the communication

2. *Message*—the information the sender wants to communicate
3. *Receiver*—the person for whom the communication is intended
4. *Feedback*—confirmation that the message was received as intended

Feedback may be verbal or nonverbal. An example of verbal feedback is responding to what you say. An example of nonverbal feedback is a nod of the head indicating understanding.

Verbal Communication

We communicate with others by the words we speak. Although the words that you speak are important, your tone of voice also affects communication. In fact, one-third of the message is communicated through the tone and pitch of your voice. The tone and pitch of your voice can change the meaning of the communication. If the tone and pitch of your voice contradict the spoken words, the tone and pitch will overshadow the message. Be aware of the effect that the tone, pitch, and quality of your voice have on the way your message is interpreted. Choose your words carefully. Avoid using slang or words with more than one meaning. Use words that the receiver is likely to be familiar with. Speak slowly and clearly. Look at the receiver when speaking.

Paraphrasing. **Paraphrasing** is an effective method of showing that you understand what has been said. When using paraphrasing, restate your understanding of what was said. Listening to the message and paraphrasing provide feedback and show that you are sincerely interested in the conversation.

Nonverbal Communication

Attending behavior shows that you are alert and interested in what the other person is saying to you. Five components of attending behavior are:

1. Eye contact
2. Gestures
3. Posture
4. Physical distance from the other person
5. Paraphrasing

Good eye contact is important to communication. The eyes are very powerful messengers. Even if the body is still, a great deal can be learned about what a person is feeling or thinking by looking at the eyes. In fact, eye contact is often the most remembered part of making an impression. You can create a positive atmosphere by looking at the other person.

In North America, eye contact is very important to communication. This is not true in all cultures. Be sensitive to cultural differences of residents and coworkers. In North America, people who do not make eye contact may be considered dishonest or fearful. Making eye contact can open communication channels and create a bond between two people. During conversation, eye contact communicates interest, concern, warmth, trust, feelings, and credibility. Eye contact can send many different messages. Here are some common interpretations of the signals sent by the eyes:

- Avoiding eye contact may indicate that you wish to continue speaking.
- Looking directly at someone without speaking often indicates that you wish the other person to speak.
- Looking away while someone else is speaking may signal disinterest in the message.
- Glancing downward suggests modesty or insecurity.
- Glaring or staring suggests coldness, disgust, or anger.
- Wide eyes suggest excitement, wonder, amazement, disbelief, honesty, or fright.
- Raised eyebrows suggest disbelief, surprise, or curiosity.
- Excessive blinking suggests nervousness, insecurity, or dishonesty.

The best way to maintain eye contact is to look directly at the person you are speaking to for five to seven seconds. If you maintain eye contact for longer than this, the receiver of your message may think you are staring. Making eye contact is important as you finish speaking. Doing this invites the other person to speak. Learning how to use your eyes effectively in communication may take practice, but practicing this skill is a good investment of your time.

Gestures can be movements of your body or face. We gesture with our facial muscles, eyebrows, mouth, hands, and feet. We may shift restlessly about in a chair. Although we may not be aware of it, these movements send powerful messages to others.

Use gestures and facial expressions to reinforce what you say. Using positive gestures is very important to communication. Use gestures only when you speak. Avoid distracting movements, such as twisting your ring, clicking your pen, or playing with your hair. Doing these things when you are speaking suggests that you are nervous and may undermine your credibility.

When someone else is speaking, these actions suggest that you are disinterested or impatient. Smiling is a very effective way to signal your openness. If you fail to smile, people may think you are not interested, cold, or aloof. A warm smile is like hanging out a welcome sign that invites people to relate to you.

Touch is a very powerful means of communication. Touch can communicate a calm, caring attitude. All human beings need to be touched. It sends a message of compassion, caring, and acceptance. Use touch appropriate to the resident's age. For example, holding an adult resident's hand or firmly resting your hand on the forearm or shoulder communicates caring. In a child, patting or stroking the head communicates caring.

Posture is how you hold your body when you stand or sit. When you are seated, leaning forward in the chair while another person speaks shows that you are interested. Standing with the hands on your hips suggests anger, disgust, or impatience. Shaking your finger when you speak indicates anger. Communication is most effective when your body is relaxed.

Physical distance is important for effective communication. In the United States, a comfortable physical distance from others is about 18 to 36 inches. If you are closer than this, others may be uncomfortable. If you are farther away, the receiver may be offended, or the message misinterpreted because the receiver could not see or hear you correctly. The nursing assistant must realize that comfortable physical distance for communication varies with the culture of the resident and nursing assistant.

When speaking with others, always remember the impact of nonverbal communication. Your words represent only 7% of your message. The remainder of the message is interpreted through facial expressions, gestures, and overall body language. Your tone of voice represents 38% of the meaning. Gestures, facial expressions, and other body language represent 55% of your total communication.

Barriers to Communication

A **barrier** is something that interferes with communication. It can be physical, such as trying to speak with a resident whose ears are bandaged after surgery. Eliminate barriers whenever possible. If this is not possible, as in the case of the resident with bandaged ears, find other means to communicate, such as writing. Barriers can also be mental. Mental barriers occur when you have formed a negative opinion about another person or culture. Avoid forming opinions about others based on appearances. Enter each communication with an open mind.

Sometimes other barriers are present, such as with residents with mental confusion, speech and hearing disorders, or those who do not speak English. If you are not sure of the resident's ability to communicate, ask the resident's name and speak with him or her about the season or weather. Provide orienting information if necessary and evaluate the resident's response. Keep your questions simple and ask only one question at a time. If the resident does not understand, rephrase the question. Do not make fun of the resident's lack of understanding. Laugh with the resident, if appropriate. Use the information you have obtained from your evaluation of the resident's understanding to plan your care. Other barriers to communication are:

- Teasing and kidding. Although these are not always barriers, they may be offensive, so avoid them if you do not know the resident well.
- Threatening and warning. Never threaten residents that you will withhold care because of something they have said or done. Consult the nurse if a resident does not cooperate with care.
- Preaching, moralizing, or passing judgment. Do not judge the resident for what he or she has said or done. Not expressing your opinion is better. To be successful, you must try to be neutral and objective even if you disagree.
- Directing and ordering. Your tone of voice, choice of words, and body language can turn a request into an order. This can cause the resident to deliberately do the opposite of what you want. It may also frighten the resident. Select your words carefully and monitor the tone of your voice and body language to avoid sounding like you are giving the resident no choice.
- Arguing. This may make the resident defensive, angry, or upset, and the intent of the original communication will be lost.
- Pretending to be busy, or giving the resident the impression that you are rushed. This sends a message that you do not have time for the resident, or that caring for the resident is a bother.
- Using sound-alike words, such as "'haul" and "hall." This can be very confusing for elderly individuals, especially those who are confused or have difficulty hearing. Make sure the context is clear.
- Using slang or cultural terms that are not familiar to the resident, and may be misinterpreted.
- Interrupting or changing the subject. This sends a message to the resident that what he or she has to say is not worthwhile, and may inhibit the resident from future conversation.

- Giving answers such as, "Don't worry about it." This sends a message to the resident that his or her concerns are not important.
- Providing false reassurance, such as, "everything will be all right." The resident will not trust you when he or she learns you were not sincere.
- Talking to the resident about your personal problems. This is never appropriate in the long-term care setting.
- Not waiting long enough for a reply. Elderly residents may take longer to process information, especially if they have hearing problems. Allow enough time for a response.

GUIDELINES FOR COMMUNICATION

Use every contact with residents as an opportunity for communication. Show that you value the residents and respect them by calling them by their preferred names. If you do not know what they prefer to be called, use Mr. or Mrs., followed by the surname. Pet names such as "honey", "dear", and "gramps" are not appropriate. Smile and speak to residents, families, and visitors when you pass in the hallway. Speak to residents when giving care. Set aside time to talk. This shows that you like other people and are genuinely concerned for the well-being of others.

Communication should be goal-oriented. Before beginning a conversation, set a goal. Think

GUIDELINES FOR
Having a Conversation

- Knock on the door, introduce yourself by name and title, and address the resident by his or her preferred name.
- Approach the resident in a friendly, courteous manner.
- If you are in the room to perform a procedure, explain it before beginning. Allow time for the resident to ask questions and show understanding. This shows respect for the resident.
- If your time is limited, prepare the resident in advance by stating how much time you have and when you will need to leave.
- Speak in terms that are familiar to the resident.
- Make eye contact during the conversation.
- Be polite.
- Speak clearly and distinctly.
- Listen to what the resident says. Ask questions or make comments to show that you are interested.
- Use touch to communicate caring, if appropriate.

GUIDELINES TO

Use When Speaking

Techniques to use to make all types of communication more meaningful are:

- Maintain eye contact during the conversation.
- Sit at the resident's eye level, if possible (**Figure 6-2**).
- Speak clearly and distinctly.
- Use language the resident will understand. Avoid using medical terms.
- Keep your message brief and concise. This should not be difficult if you have thought about your communication and selected a goal in advance.
- Use nonverbal communication, such as touch, posture, gestures, and body language, as appropriate.
- Use open-ended questions to encourage the resident to speak.
- Be courteous and polite.
- Send positive messages by using praise, encouragement, touch, and smiles.
- Give, receive, and request feedback.

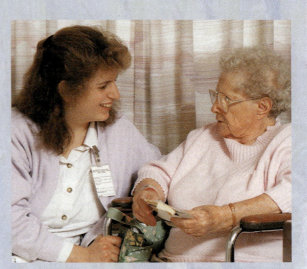

FIGURE 6-2   Sit at the resident's eye level and maintain eye contact during the conversation.

about what you want to accomplish and focus on the topic. Arrange the main points of what you would like to say in logical order. Eliminate unrelated or unnecessary information that may confuse the message.

Communication Styles

After you have set a goal for your conversation, select the style of communication that will help you meet this goal. Six types of conversations and the goal of each are listed in **Table 6-1.**

TABLE 6-1 Forms of Conversation	
Type of Conversation	**Goal**
Social conversation	To create a comfortable, relaxed atmosphere. Talk about pleasant things that the resident may be interested in. Do not discuss your problems or complaints with residents. Avoid discussing facility business or gossiping about other residents or employees.
Interviewing	To obtain information that will help you meet the resident's needs. For example, ask if the resident prefers to take a shower in the morning or evening. Interviewing helps you plan your routine and shows the resident that you are genuinely interested in his or her well-being.
Teaching	To show and tell the resident something that he or she will learn, understand, and use. All health care workers are teachers.
Reporting	To communicate accurate information. Reporting is done to the nurse. Accurate reporting involves communicating factual information.
Problem solving	To help meet the resident's needs. It is different from interviewing. In this situation, you know what the resident wants. Your objective is to find a way to do it.
Therapeutic communication	To encourage the resident to talk about feelings. This type of communication is particularly sensitive because you must be careful not to pass judgment on what the resident thinks or feels. Monitor your body language carefully.

GUIDELINES FOR
Listening

- Use open posture. Lean toward the resident. Avoid crossing your arms in front of your body or placing your hands on your hips.
- Give the resident your full attention (**Figure 6-3**).
- Maintain eye contact.
- Show interest in the resident's activities, interests, and concerns.
- Monitor the resident's body language to see if it confirms or conflicts with the verbal message the resident is sending.
- Encourage the resident to talk about feelings and concerns. Allow the resident to express anger and negative feelings without passing judgment or becoming defensive.
- Use touch to communicate caring, if appropriate.
- Use silence to allow the resident to think and continue the conversation.
- Pay attention and show interest in what the resident is saying. Ask questions if necessary. Use paraphrasing to show interest and understanding. Use noncommittal responses, such as "I understand," to show that you are listening.
- Use responses such as, "I would like to hear more about that," or "Then what happened?" to show that you are interested.
- Use responses such as, "So you felt bad about that," to show empathy.
- Wait until the resident is finished speaking before responding.
- Request help from the nurse, if needed, to solve problems.

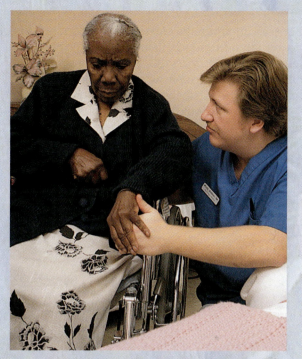

FIGURE 6-3 Pay close attention to what the resident is saying through her words and gestures.

Listening

Hearing is nothing more than being aware of sound. Listening is an active, deliberate process in which you focus and make an effort to hear and understand what the resident is saying. Listening is an important part of communication. Listening to what someone else is saying may be difficult when you have other things on your mind. Your body language may betray you by sending a message that you are not interested in what the other person is saying. Although this may not be the case, monitor your movement and expressions closely to avoid misunderstanding. Paraphrasing is a good technique to use to show that you are listening. Silence is also a good technique. Silence shows acceptance and respect. It encourages the resident to speak. You may be uncomfortable with silence. If so, work to overcome your discomfort.

GUIDELINES FOR
Ending a Conversation

- Inform the resident that you have to leave.
- Tell the resident what time you will be back, and be sure to return at this time.
- Tell the resident that you enjoyed the conversation.
- Ask if the resident needs anything before you leave.
- Before leaving the room, make sure that the resident is safe, comfortable, and has the call signal and needed personal items within reach.

COMMUNICATING WITH RESIDENTS WHO HAVE DISABILITIES AND SENSORY IMPAIRMENTS

Sensory impairments can take many forms. Some forms, such as speech, hearing, or language problems, interfere directly with communication. Other problems, such as physical impairments, may make you uncomfortable and unsure of what to say without being offensive. People with disabilities are much like you are. They have the same wants and needs. They can do many of the same things you can, but may need to adapt the environment in order to do them. Although the end result is the same, people with disabilities may perform the task differently. Their bodies work differently! As a rule, people with disabilities do not want to be treated differently from anyone else. Many are self-sufficient, have led productive lives, and are valuable and equal members of society. They may be physically challenged, but many have developed other talents and qualities using nonphysical skills.

Nursing assistants have a responsibility to emphasize the uniqueness and worth of all persons, rather than the differences between people. Your efforts will do much to encourage acceptance of people with disabilities. Treat people with disabilities the way you like to be treated. You will leave the experience feeling fulfilled and richly rewarded.

GUIDELINES FOR
Communicating with and about Residents Who Have Disabilities

- Avoid referring to the resident as a condition, such as "the paraplegic in 221." Say instead, "Mrs. Smith in 221." A person who is paralyzed has no feeling or movement. A paraplegic has no feeling or movement from the waist down. Always emphasize the person over the condition.
- Use common sense when talking to someone who has a disability. Talk to the person the same way you would anyone else. People with disabilities do not want to be treated differently.
- Do not assume that someone is not disabled or pretending because the disability is not visible. Some medical conditions are severely disabling, but the person may not appear disabled.
- Shaking hands is appropriate with people who have upper extremity disabilities. Residents with limited movement or a prosthesis are able to shake hands. A prosthesis is an artificial body part. Shake hands gently with a person who has arthritis.
- Before helping someone who has a disability, ask if you can help. It is all right to offer to help, but unless the resident is struggling, do not intervene without asking.
- It is all right to ask residents about their disabilities. Many residents are comfortable, and will talk about them, but it is also all right if they do not want to talk about it. People who are newly disabled may not have reached a point of mental acceptance and may be uncomfortable speaking about their problem.
- When caring for a resident with a disability, do not assume that the resident can or cannot do something. Assuming can be offensive. Always ask.
- Always stress the resident's ability and not the disability.
- Residents who use wheelchairs, canes, walkers, and crutches because of a disability are not always sick. Avoid making assumptions.
- Residents in wheelchairs do not like to be treated as if they are mentally impaired! Most have no mental problem. Talk to the person in the wheelchair, not to a companion.
- When talking to a resident in a wheelchair, position yourself at his or her eye level.
- Be polite. Show the same manners that you would with anyone else.
- Use good manners if you walk in front of a resident in a wheelchair by excusing yourself.
- If you are in a crowded area, such as when attending an activity, avoid standing in front of a person in a wheelchair. This blocks the resident's view.
- The wheelchair is an extension of the disabled person's body. Leaning or hanging on the chair is an invasion of the resident's personal space.
- Words such as "see," "hear," "run," and "walk" can be used when speaking with people who have disabilities.
- Choose words that are positive and nonjudgmental. Avoid using words like "cripple," "gimp," "spastic," "retard." This is demeaning and promotes negative perceptions of the physically challenged. **Table 6-2** gives examples of acceptable and unacceptable terminology to use in conversation. Remember, always emphasize the person first. Emphasizing the disease is demeaning. **Table 6-3** lists phrases to avoid when speaking about persons with disabilities.

Continues

GUIDELINES FOR

Communicating with and about Residents Who Have Disabilities, *Continued*

TABLE 6-2	Recommended Phrases for Use in Conversation
Offensive and unacceptable Do not use in conversation	**Acceptable use in conversation**
Disabled person	A person with a disability
Blind person	A person who is vision impaired
Deaf person	A person who is hearing impaired
A hunchback	A person who has curvature of the spine
The disabled	People who are disabled; the disabled community
He is a cripple (gimp)	He has a disability (or mobility problem)
Dumb (or deaf and dumb)	A person who has a speech or hearing impairment
She is nuts, crazy	She has an emotional disability or mental illness
Retard	A person with mental retardation
Birth defect	A person who is disabled from birth
Fit	Seizure
Normal person as compared with a person who has a disability	A person who is not disabled as compared with a person who is
Confined to a wheelchair	A person who uses a wheelchair
Honey, sweetie, baby, or gramps	Call the person by his or her preferred name

TABLE 6-3	Words to Avoid
Words to avoid when speaking with or about persons who are disabled	
Abnormal	Gimp
Afflicted	Invalid
Burden	Imbecile
Cerebral palsied	Maimed
Confined to a wheelchair	Moron
Courageous	Normal
	Palsied
Cripple	Poor
Crippled	Spastic
Deaf and dumb	Stricken with
Deaf mute	Sufferer
Defect	Suffers with
Defective	Suffering
Deformity	Unfortunate
Diseased	Victim
Epileptic	

- People who have disabilities like to laugh and have fun **(Figure 6-4)**. Do not leave them out!
- Canine companions, such as seeing eye dogs or hearing ear dogs, are on duty. Do not feed them or pet them without the owner's permission. This distracts them and prevents them from doing their job.

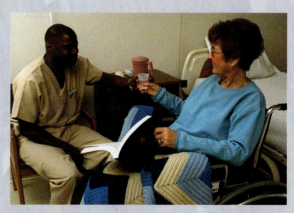

FIGURE 6-4 Residents who have disabilities like to laugh and have fun. You are privileged to share intimate moments of their lives. Enjoy the time you spend with them.

GUIDELINES FOR
Communicating with Residents Who Have Vision Loss

- Knock on the door and identify yourself by name and title before entering the room. Call the resident by the preferred name.
- Help residents clean their glasses and encourage them to wear them.
- When speaking, sit in a good light where the resident can see your face. The light source should not be behind your back, as it will shine in the resident's eyes from this position.
- Speak clearly and directly in a normal tone of voice. Blindness does not interfere with the resident's ability to hear.
- Use touch to communicate, if appropriate, but do so slowly and gently so the resident is not startled.
- When you are performing tasks in the room, tell the resident what you are doing. It is acceptable to discuss new things you see, interesting changes, and what various people are doing. This is not offensive. You are the resident's eyes!
- Always ask the resident what he or she would like to wear. Describe the color and style of the clothes.
- Tell the resident when you are finished.
- Replace everything in its original location.
- Tell the resident when you are leaving the room. Make sure the resident is comfortable and safe, with the call signal and needed personal items within reach.
- When assisting a resident who has a visual impairment to walk, have the resident hold your upper arm **(Figure 6-5)**. Walk alongside and slightly ahead of the resident. The resident can tell a great deal from feeling your body movement. Walk naturally at the resident's pace. Tell the resident when there are steps, obstacles, when to turn left or right, if you must go through a door, and so forth. Be specific when giving directions. Pause slightly before stairs, or when making a turn. Avoid revolving doors and escalators if you are in a public place. If

you are walking and are interrupted by someone, let the resident know you will be stopping.
- When using stairs, guide the resident's hand to the railing. Stop on each step before proceeding to the next step.
- When seating the resident, place the resident's hand on the back or arm of the chair.
- Do not leave a resident who is visually impaired or blind in an open area. Lead him or her to the side of a room, chair, or landmark from which he or she can obtain a direction for travel.

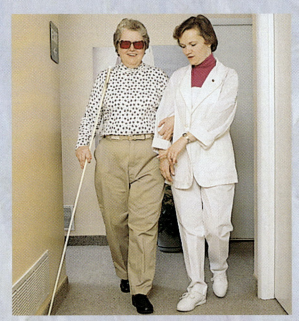

FIGURE 6-5 Have the resident hold your upper arm lightly while you walk at the resident's pace.

Communicating with Residents Who Have Vision Loss

Vision loss can range from problems that can be corrected with glasses to complete blindness. Some people are legally blind, but still have limited vision. Do not assume that residents who are wearing glasses can see. Some residents who wear glasses are severely impaired. People who are blind are like residents with other disabilities. They may have a loss in one area of their life, but they have developed other areas. Most are self-sufficient, but may need environmental adaptations. Do not rearrange furniture, equipment, supplies, or personal items in the room without the resident's approval. People with visual impairments memorize the location of items. Moving

things could result in accidents, injuries, or frustration because the resident is unable to find a needed item. When you are providing care or would like the resident to assist with a procedure, provide detailed, step-by-step directions.

Communicating with Residents Who Have Hearing Loss

Hearing loss can mean that a resident has difficulty hearing or that the resident is completely deaf. There are many causes of hearing loss. Some hearing loss can be corrected with hearing aids. Other types can be corrected with surgery. Some people have uncorrected hearing loss. People who are deaf communicate in many

GUIDELINES FOR

Communicating with Residents Who Have Hearing Loss

- Approach the resident from the front or side. Lightly touch the resident's arm or shoulder without startling the resident.
- Eliminate as much background noise and activity as possible.
- Assist the resident to use a hearing aid, if appropriate.
- Be aware that individuals with hearing loss hear and understand less well when they are ill.
- Avoid speaking from another room, when walking away, or with your back turned to the resident.
- If the resident hears better in one ear, position yourself on that side when speaking.
- Sit in a good light where the resident can see your face. The light source should not be behind your back.
- Do not chew gum, eat, or put your hands in front of your mouth when speaking.
- Be considerate and try to make the resident feel confident in you.
- Look directly at the resident when speaking.
- Speak slowly, clearly, and distinctly. Use your lips to emphasize words.
- Choose short, simple words. Use short sentences.
- Speak in a lower pitched voice than normal. You may need to raise the loudness of your voice, but do not shout. Shouting distorts the voice and makes you sound angry.

- Tell the resident what you are going to talk about.
- Use gestures, body language, and facial expressions to convey meaning.
- Write down key words, if necessary. Use communication boards or other adaptive equipment, if available.
- If the resident with hearing impairment has difficulty with letters or numbers, say, "M as in Mary, 2 as in twins, B as in boy." Say each number separately. Say "six seven" instead of "sixty-seven."
- Some residents benefit from placing a stethoscope in their ears, which amplifies the sound when you speak into the diaphragm.
- If the resident does not understand a word, use a different word instead of repeating what you said more loudly.
- Keep conversations brief and limited to a single topic.
- Do not convey impatience by your body language.
- If you do not understand what a person who is deaf or has a speech impairment says, asking him or her to repeat is acceptable.
- If an interpreter is helping you, speak to the resident, not the interpreter.
- Tell the resident when you are leaving the room. Make sure the resident is comfortable and safe, with the call signal and needed personal items within reach.

different ways. Some use sign language. This is a combination of hand signals and facial expressions. Others read lips. Some people use reading and writing as their primary form of communication. Special telephone and television communication systems and amplifiers are available for people who are deaf and hearing impaired. Residents who are hearing impaired can function independently, but as with other disabilities, may need environmental adaptations. Remember that residents with vision and hearing loss

will need help in an emergency, such as when the fire alarm sounds.

Caring for residents with hearing aids. Some residents use hearing aids to help them hear more clearly. The hearing aid amplifies the sound and improves communication. However, the resident may still be unable to hear normally, even with the hearing aid in place. Many types of hearing aids are available, but they all work on the same principle **(Figure 6-6)**. The aid contains

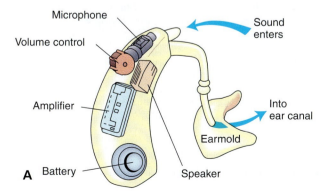

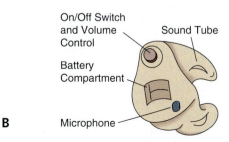

FIGURE 6-6 A. The earmold is placed in the ear canal. The rest of the hearing aid is worn outside and over the top of the ear. B. This hearing aid fits inside the outer ear canal.

GUIDELINES FOR
Caring for Hearing Aids

- The hearing aid is fragile and expensive. Avoid dropping it. Always hold the hearing aid over a soft surface or table when cleaning or caring for it.
- Keep the hearing aid clean. Remove it daily and wipe off any dust, ear wax, or body oil with a tissue. Avoid using alcohol wipes to clean the aid. Use a damp cloth.
- If the hearing aid is the cannula type, remove ear wax from the speaker opening with a pipe cleaner or special appliance cleaner. Ask the resident if he or she has a tool called a wax loop, and use this, if available. Never use a toothpick, paper clip, or other sharp object.
- When caring for a female resident, do not spray hairspray when the hearing aid is in place.
- Remove the hearing aid before using a hair dryer or blow dryer. Never apply a source of heat to the hearing aid.
- Organize your work so that male residents who shave with an electric razor can shave or be shaved before the hearing aid is applied. If this is not possible, turn the aid off or remove it before using the electric razor. The buzzing of the razor is very loud and annoying with the hearing aid in place.
- Avoid getting the hearing aid wet. If it has an outer ear mold, the ear piece may be washed with mild soap and warm water. The part of the hearing aid containing the batteries should never get wet. Allow the mold to dry thoroughly before reattaching it to the unit.

- Remove the hearing aid when bathing the resident or washing his or her hair.
- Turn the hearing aid off when it is not in the resident's ear. Opening the battery case when the aid is stored prevents unnecessary drain on the battery.
- Remove the battery at night and check it for leaks. Store the hearing aid and battery in the case. Replace worn-out or leaking batteries. Wipe the battery gently with a clean cloth before reinserting it.
- Avoid temperature extremes. Do not store the aid in a cold area, on a radiator, or in direct sunlight.
- If the hearing aid has a cord, check it for cracks or breaks.
- Insert the hearing aid properly. Sometimes the shape of the ear changes with aging and the hearing aid may need to be refitted. If the resident complains of pain or the aid is difficult to insert, this may be the problem. Advise the nurse if this occurs.
- When communicating with the resident, follow the same guidelines that you use when communicating with a resident who has a hearing impairment.
- Check the bed linen carefully before placing it in the soiled linen hamper. A hearing aid is small, expensive, and easily lost. It will not survive a trip through the washer and dryer!
- Remove the hearing aid and allow the ear to "cool" before taking a tympanic temperature.

GUIDELINES FOR
Troubleshooting Hearing Aid Problems

Never try to repair a hearing aid yourself. However, if the resident has problems with the aid, there are several things you can do that may resolve them.

- Check the hearing aid to see if it is turned on. Some models have settings marked on them. These are "M" for microphone, "T" for telephone, and "O" for off. Set the switch to the "M" setting.
- Check the volume of the hearing aid to be sure it is turned up loud enough for the resident to hear.
- Hold the hearing aid in the palm of your hand. Turn the volume up all the way. Cup the aid between your hands. You should hear a loud whistle. A weak or absent sound indicates that the battery is low.
- Before changing the battery, check the position of the old battery so you can put the new one in the same way. When inserting a new battery, place it in the unit gently. If you meet resistance, do not force it. Consult the nurse.

- Check the ear mold for wax. If wax is present, remove it.
- Ask the nurse to check the resident's ears with an otoscope for wax buildup.
- If the hearing aid is in the resident's ear and makes a loud, whistling sound, check the position. The aid should be securely in the ear. Make sure that hair, ear wax, or clothing are not interfering with the position. Check the tubing for cracks. Whistling usually indicates an air leak.
- If the hearing aid works intermittently or makes a scratchy sound, check for dirt under and around the battery. Also check the volume control and connections. If the hearing aid has a connecting wire, make sure it is plugged in tightly and is not cracked or bent.

a tiny microphone that changes sound and increases the strength of electrical signals. A tiny speaker converts the signal to a sound wave and sends the message to the resident's ear.

Communicating with Residents Who Have Problems with Language and Understanding

Some residents have illnesses or injuries that affect their ability to speak and understand what is spoken to them. They may be able to understand some things, but not others. You must assume that they understand you. Try to communicate with them as you would with other residents. Do not make the mistake of being silent when you are caring for them. Your silence may be received as a negative message by the resident. These residents may be able to speak, but what they say does not make sense. They may have certain words or phrases that have meaning to them, but not to you. Sincerely try to understand what they are saying. Be empathetic and do not show frustration. If you learn what they are saying, share this information with other members of the interdisciplinary team. This will enable all team members to help meet the resident's needs. Some residents are unable to speak correctly, but they understand what is spoken to them. Do not assume that the resident with a speech problem is mentally confused. Test the resident's ability to answer yes or no questions, or to follow

GUIDELINES FOR

Caring for Residents Who Have Problems with Language and Understanding

- Knock on the door and identify yourself by name and title before entering the room. Call the resident by the preferred name.
- Approach the resident in a friendly, courteous manner. Approach from the front to avoid startling the resident.
- Assist the resident with the use of glasses and hearing aids, if used.
- Explain what will be done.
- Use short, simple words. Pronounce them clearly and slowly.
- Focus on one topic and use short sentences.
- Use gentle touch to show that you care.
- Keep conversations short but frequent.
- Use your facial expression and gestures to convey your message.
- Allow adequate time for the resident to respond. Do not be tempted to complete a sentence for the resident.
- Listen carefully to the response. Pay close attention to what the resident is saying.
- If you think you understand what the resident is saying, use paraphrasing to give the resident feedback.
- Allow the resident time to finish speaking. Do not cut him or her off.
- Monitor your body language. Avoid communicating frustration due to your inability to understand the resident.
- Accept responsibility for being unable to understand. The resident is doing his or her best. He or she is probably more frustrated than you are. Do not discourage or blame the resident for the breakdown in communication.

- Assume that the resident understands you if you are not sure and cannot get a response.
- Encourage the resident to point to things and use gestures.
- Use adaptive devices, such as picture boards **(Figure 6-7)**, if available. The speech-language pathologist will often provide these devices and teach the resident to use them.
- Tell the resident when you are leaving the room. Make sure the resident is comfortable and safe, with the call signal and needed personal items within reach.

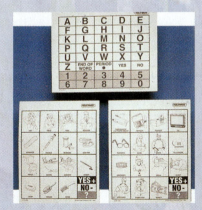

FIGURE 6-7 Picture boards are tools the resident can use to communicate wants and needs. *(Permission given for reprint/reproduction to Maddack's, Communicard Trio)*

simple directions, to determine the resident's mental status.

Communicating with Residents Who Have Problems Speaking

Some diseases and injuries leave residents unable to speak. Aphasia is a condition in which the speech center in the brain has been damaged. This commonly occurs when the resident has had a stroke. Residents with expressive aphasia have difficulty saying what they want to say. They may also have trouble with gestures and writing. Residents with receptive aphasia have trouble understanding what is spoken to them. The resident may also have trouble reading and understanding gestures. Global aphasia involves both speaking and understanding. Dysarthria is a condition in which the resident has weakness or paralysis of the lips, tongue, or throat. This is often due to a head injury or stroke. The resident may be able to make noise, but not form words. However, the resident often understands what you are saying. Do not make the mistake of thinking that a resident has a mental impairment because of the inability to speak. Over time, some residents are able to regain their speech with aggressive therapy. Some develop other methods of communication. These residents are often able to make themselves understood by gestures, writing, or with other adaptive communication devices.

Communicating with Residents Who Are Mentally Retarded

Mental retardation affects about 3% of the population in the United States. A person who is mentally retarded has experienced difficulty learning since childhood. Mental retardation is like any other disability. The condition developed because of conditions before birth or in early childhood, and was not caused by the resident. There are many levels of retardation, ranging from profound to mild. Residents with profound retardation function at the level of an infant. People with mild retardation function at the fourth-grade level. Of all people diagnosed with mental retardation, 89% are mildly retarded. People who are mentally retarded have the same needs as you, but learn more slowly and are limited in what they can learn. Most are able to live productive lives.

GUIDELINES FOR
Communicating with Residents Who Have Problems Speaking

- Knock on the door and identify yourself by name and title before entering the room. Call the resident by the preferred name.
- Approach the resident in a friendly, courteous manner.
- Assist the resident with the use of glasses and hearing aids, if used.
- Keep conversations short but frequent.
- Use questions that can be answered with yes or no answers. Tell the resident to nod his or her head in response. If the resident is unable to nod the head, tell him or her to blink the eyes once for yes and twice for no.
- Allow adequate time for the resident to respond.
- Give the resident a pen and paper to write with, if able, or use assistive communication devices such as picture or word boards.
- Listen carefully to the response.
- If you think you understand what the resident is saying, use paraphrasing to give the resident feedback.

- Do not pretend to understand the resident if you do not.
- Emphasize the positive aspects of the message, such as words and gestures that you do understand.
- Allow time to complete the conversation, to avoid sending the message that you are impatient with the resident.
- Assume that the resident understands you if you are not sure and cannot get a response.
- Use appropriate body language. Do not convey frustration at your inability to understand.
- Encourage the resident to point to things and use gestures.
- Tell the resident when you are leaving the room. Make sure the resident is comfortable and safe, with the call signal and needed personal items within reach.

GUIDELINES FOR

Communicating with Residents Who Are Mentally Retarded

- Keep your words and sentences short and simple.
- Give clear, concise instructions.
- Do not "talk down" to the resident. Treat adults as adults.
- Listen to what the resident says. Often he or she knows more than you think.
- People who are mentally retarded are very sensitive to the moods of others. If you are upset, they will be too. If you are happy and relaxed, they will be too. Ask yourself how you look to them.

- If making decisions is upsetting to the resident, limit choices to two.
- If you notice the resident becoming frustrated, slow down. Do not push.
- Praise and compliment the resident for even small accomplishments.
- Treat people who are mentally retarded with the same respect that you would give others.

Individuals who are mentally retarded need acceptance and attention. Like all other residents, they must be treated with dignity and respect. They must be able to express themselves and relieve stress. They are able to make simple choices, but may become overwhelmed if they are given too many options. If making decisions overwhelms the resident, limit choices to one of two. Residents with mental retardation respond well to consistent treatment and expectations. When caring for these residents, use of the care plan by all staff is very important because this ensures consistent care. It is important for people who are mentally retarded to feel worthwhile. They like to help and feel like they are contributing. Most are happy and loving.

People who are mentally retarded should not be pressured to learn things or perform new tasks. They can be taught, but teaching them requires great patience. They often do not function well in high-pressure situations, and may not function well in large, loud, confusing groups unless someone is there to support them. They know if others are ridiculing them, and feel hurt and rejection.

Communicating with the Resident's Family, Friends, and Visitors

You are a representative of the health care facility to visitors. Speak and smile to visitors in the hallway. If someone looks lost, ask if you can help. Maintain an open, friendly, and supportive attitude with visitors. Show them where the lounges, vending machines, cafeteria, restrooms, and smoking areas are. Answer any questions they have about your facility's policies and procedures. However, you must protect resident confidentiality, even with family members. If they ask you questions about the resident's condition, refer them to the nurse. You may tell them something about the resident's activities, such as "He ate a good lunch."

Families may react in different ways to the resident's illness. They may show anxiety or anger. Be patient and understanding. Do not argue with them. Listen carefully and be empathetic. If family members have complaints or if you notice a resident becoming upset when visitors are in the room, report this to the nurse.

Sometimes you must perform a procedure on a resident when visitors are in the room. Ask the visitors to step out until you have completed the procedure. Show them where they can wait. When you are done with the procedure, inform them that they can return to the room.

Answering the telephone. Nursing assistants are required to answer the telephone in many long-term care facilities. If this is your responsibility, answer the phone by stating the name of your facility or unit. Identify yourself by name and title. Be courteous and polite. If a physician is on the line to give orders for a resident, you must get a nurse to take the call. Unlicensed personnel cannot legally take orders from a physician. If the caller is not a physician, determine what is requested and provide the information, if possible. However, avoid giving out personal information about residents. If the caller is not a physician, obtain the information, or transfer the caller to the proper person. If the person being called cannot come to the telephone, take a clear message. Write down the date, time of the call, name of the caller, and a brief message. Sign your name and title to the message. Inform the caller that you will deliver the message. Thank the person for calling.

KEY POINTS

- Many factors influence communication.
- Health care workers communicate with many people verbally, in writing, and through gestures, touch, and body language.
- The four elements of communication are the sender, message, receiver, and feedback.
- Using goal-oriented communication involves deciding what you want to accomplish and focusing on a topic.
- People with disabilities should be treated the way you like to be treated. Some people with disabilities have special communication needs.
- Courtesy is important when answering the telephone in the health care facility.

REVIEW

A. Multiple Choice

Select the one best answer.

1. Communication may be influenced by
   a. the season.
   b. the day of the week.
   c. acute or chronic illness.
   d. the eye color of the receiver.

2. Empathy means
   a. understanding how the resident feels.
   b. feeling sorry for the resident.
   c. understanding emotional needs.
   d. solving problems for the resident.

3. The sender is the person who
   a. gets the message.
   b. initiates a communication.
   c. interprets the message.
   d. relays communication to another person.

4. Feedback is
   a. your interpretation of what the nurse said.
   b. your interpretation of what the resident said.
   c. confirmation that a message was received as intended.
   d. obtaining information to meet the resident's needs.

5. Which of the following are components of attending behavior?
   a. eye contact and gestures
   b. thinking and feeling
   c. crossing your arms and legs
   d. physical appearance and dress

6. Comfortable personal space in the United States is
   a. 8 inches to 10 inches.
   b. 18 inches to 36 inches.
   c. 28 inches.
   d. 48 inches.

7. Paraphrasing is
   a. repeating what the speaker says word for word.
   b. interpreting the message for another person.
   c. using sign language for a deaf resident.
   d. restating a message in clear, simple terms.

8. Something that interferes with communication is a
   a. gesture.
   b. barrier.
   c. suggestion.
   d. symptom.

9. Thinking about what you want to accomplish in a conversation and focusing on a topic is an example of using
   a. goal-oriented communication.
   b. paraphrasing.
   c. empathy.
   d. feedback.

10. A communication style in which you want to obtain information to meet the resident's needs is
    a. therapeutic communication.
    b. problem solving.
    c. interviewing.
    d. social conversation.

11. When communicating with a resident in a wheelchair, you should avoid using the word
    a. see.
    b. run.
    c. walk.
    d. crippled.

12. When caring for residents with vision or hearing loss, you should
    a. be as quiet as possible when you are in the room, so the resident is not disturbed.
    b. make as much noise as possible when you are in the room, so the resident knows what you are doing.
    c. announce yourself by name and title when entering the room.
    d. approach the resident from the side or rear.

13. When caring for residents who have problems with speech or understanding, you should
    a. explain the care you will be giving in medical terms.
    b. choose short, simple words and use short sentences.
    c. use sign language that the resident understands.
    d. avoid speaking whenever possible.

14. When caring for a person who is mentally retarded, you should
    a. treat the resident with courtesy and respect.
    b. not explain procedures.
    c. never smile, because this is upsetting to the resident.
    d. avoid touch as this upsets the resident.

15. You answer the telephone on your unit. The caller identifies herself as Dr. Gonzales and says that she wants to give orders for Mrs. Keene. You should
    a. ask the doctor to hold while you get the nurse.
    b. write down the orders the doctor gives you.
    c. tell the doctor to call back later.
    d. inform the doctor that the nurse is not at the desk.

B. Clinical Applications

Answer the following questions.

16. You are assigned to pass trays on Wing B. You have never passed trays on this hall before. You enter Mr. Haney's room and notice that he is standing by the dresser picking up items and feeling them. You think Mr. Haney may be visually impaired. How do you find out?

17. Mrs. Stone wears a hearing aid. You served her breakfast tray in bed. She had the hearing aid in her ear at that time. After breakfast, Mrs. Stone got out of bed and you completely changed the bed linen. Her hearing aid is missing. She says the last time she remembers using it was when she was eating breakfast. She does not know what became of it. The food trays have been returned to the kitchen. The soiled linen hamper has been taken to the laundry. What should you do?

18. Mr. White recently had a stroke and has lost the ability to speak. The speech-language pathologist is working with him. Mr. White is able to write and communicates by writing notes on a magic slate. You enter the room and ask Mr. White what time he would like his shower. He throws the magic slate against the wall and glares at you angrily. Why do you think Mr. White is behaving this way? How will you handle the situation?

19. You are assigned to care for Mrs. Chacko, a 73-year-old resident who came to the United States from India. Until recently, she lived in her daughter's home. However, the daughter was unable to care for her and admitted her to the long-term care facility. Mrs. Chacko's daughter tells you that the resident previously spoke English. However, since her stroke, she has been speaking only in her native language. You are assigned to give Mrs. Chacko a shower and walk her in the hallway. How do you explain the procedures to the resident?

20. You answer the telephone on your unit. The caller identifies himself as Mr. Peterman's brother from out of state. He says he is concerned about his brother and is requesting information about Mr. Peterman's medical condition and medications. The nurse is in a room with a resident doing a treatment and cannot come to the telephone. What should you do?

CHAPTER 7

Observations, Recording, and Reporting

OBJECTIVES

After reading this chapter, you will be able to:

- Spell and define key terms.
- Differentiate between signs and symptoms and between subjective and objective observations.
- Describe how to report and record resident information.
- List 10 guidelines for documenting in the medical record.
- Demonstrate correct use of medical terminology and abbreviations.

COMMUNICATING WITH OTHER MEMBERS OF THE HEALTH CARE TEAM

You will communicate with other members of the health care team frequently throughout your shift. Some communication is written. Some is spoken (verbal). Reporting and recording your observations and care are an important part of your job. Take this responsibility very seriously. Remember the principles of goal-oriented communication.

Report

The facility will have a procedure for report at the beginning of every shift (change-of-shift report). In most facilities, the offgoing nurse gives a verbal report to the oncoming nurse. Some facilities use a tape-recorded report. The report will provide information about the residents' conditions during the previous shift. Resident illness, pain, hospitalization, and other changes in condition will be discussed. In some facilities, all nursing staff listen to this report. In other facilities, only the nurses receive report. They in turn will have a separate report for the nursing assistants after the offgoing shift leaves. Although the procedure varies from one facility to the next, it is safe to say that you will receive some type of report at the beginning of every shift.

Having a report at the beginning of the shift helps to provide **continuity of care.** This means that all staff are working on the same goals, using the same approaches 24 hours a day to benefit the residents. The report provides information that will help you to set priorities and anticipate the care you will give the residents during your shift. It will alert you to things you should be monitoring and observing. The report is objective. Baseline information is provided, such as "Mrs. Stone's temperature was 97.8° F. She complained of feeling cold, so we gave her extra blankets." From hearing this, you know that the resident was cold, and that you should monitor her for feeling cold during your shift. The nurse may also ask you to check her temperature. If you find it is significantly different from the previous shift, this indicates a problem that must be reported immediately. Likewise, if the resident complains of feeling extremely hot for no apparent reason, this must also be reported promptly.

You will report information to the nurse throughout your shift. At the end of the shift, you will report off on all your residents. You will describe your observations, the care given, and other information. The nurse will use this as a basis for reporting off to the oncoming shift and completing her or his assessments and documentation. As you can see, your shift begins with communication. You communicate with others throughout the shift, then end the shift with more communication. Reporting and recording information on the

136

residents' records are also forms of communication. Making observations, communicating with residents and other staff, reporting, and recording are important skills to master.

Observing the Resident

The nursing assistant is responsible for making observations about the resident and reporting them to the nurse. This is an important responsibility. Because you will spend more time with the residents than other health care workers, you are in a position to notice changes immediately. You will use your senses to make observations. Many changes that you detect will be things that you can see. You may notice changes in movement, position, facial expression, or color. These changes may indicate pain or another problem.

Use your ears to observe changes you can hear. These are things such as noisy breathing or things the resident tells you. Your sense of smell is useful to detect unusual odors that may indicate a problem. You will note temperature changes or moisture on the skin with your sense of touch.

Observation of the resident is a continuous process. Important observations for which the nursing assistant is responsible are listed in **Table 7-1**.

Bath time gives you the perfect opportunity to make observations of the resident's entire body and note changes. If you see, feel, hear, or smell anything that seems abnormal, report your observations to the nurse. Even changes that seem insignificant may indicate a problem. For example, a red area on the skin may seem minor, but the area can quickly turn into a serious pres-

TABLE 7-1	Nursing Assistant Observations
Activity	**Observations**
Activities of daily living	• What the resident can do independently • The resident's need for assistance, how much assistance, type of assistance needed • The resident's ability to tolerate activity (does he become fatigued, short of breath, etc.) • The resident's motivation, preferences, abilities
Dressing and grooming	• Overall appearance—tidy, untidy, neat, clean
Walking	• Difficulty getting up and down • Need for an assistive device, such as a cane or walker • Safety awareness • Gait steady, unsteady, shuffling, rigid, etc. • Posture • Sudden onset of falls, difficulty balancing
Position, movement	• Ability to position/reposition self • Need for staff to reposition • Special positioning aids • Ability to move unassisted • Presence of contractures • Able/unable to move • Movements shaky, jerking, tremors, muscle spasms, etc. • Presence or absence of pain upon movement • Deformity, edema • Normal or abnormal range of motion • Ability to sit, stand, move, or walk
Eating	• Food likes and dislikes, refusals • Feeding ability, need for assistance, how much assistance, type of assistance needed • Percentage of meal consumed • Difficulty chewing or swallowing, coughing, choking
Drinking	• Ability to take a drink at will without assistance • Ability to drink from straw, cup, or need for special device • Need for assistance, how much assistance, type of assistance needed • Beverage preferences • Accepts or refuses water, if offered • Fluid intake • Difficulty swallowing liquids, coughing, choking

Continues

TABLE 7-1   Nursing Assistant Observations, *Continued*

Urinary elimination	• Frequency of elimination • Inability to urinate, or voiding frequently in small amounts • Will the resident use the bathroom if given the opportunity? • Is the resident incontinent? • Color, clarity, odor, amount of urine • Presence of mucus, sediment, or other abnormalities in urine • Pain, burning, frequency of urination • Does the resident have a urinary catheter; if so, is it draining properly, leaking, etc.?
Bowel elimination	• Frequency of elimination • Will the resident use the bathroom if given the opportunity? • Is the resident incontinent? • Appearance of stool, presence of blood, mucus, parasites, or foreign matter; liquid or solid stool • Abnormal color stool (black, clay color, etc.) • Small or extremely large stool • Loose, watery stool • Complaints of pain, constipation, diarrhea, bleeding • Excessive gas (flatus)
Gastrointestinal system	• Frequent belching • Fruity smell to breath • Complaints of indigestion, gas (flatus), nausea, vomiting • Choking • Abdominal pain • Abdominal distention (swelling) • Oral or rectal bleeding • Vomitus, stool, or drainage from a nasogastric tube that looks like coffee grounds • Condition of mouth and teeth; report ulcerations, pain, drainage, obvious cavities, lesions on lips or inside mouth, abscesses, cracked or broken teeth, loose teeth, abnormalities such as grinding teeth • Dentures fit properly and do not cause pain or pressure • Dentures in good repair and marked with name or initials according to facility policy • Teeth/dentures clean, breath is fresh • Moisture of lips and mucous membranes inside mouth versus dry, chapped lips or dry mucous membranes (report)
Level of consciousness	• Conscious • Unconscious • Change in consciousness, awareness, or alertness • Ability to respond verbally or nonverbally • Sleepiness for no apparent reason
Sleeping	• Ability to sleep, or can't sleep • Sleeps constantly • Awakens easily • Difficult to awaken • Moves about in sleep • Need to be awakened for toileting • Repositions self or needs to be repositioned by staff
Skin	• Skin dry, oily, normal • Redness, unusual skin color, such as blue or gray color of the skin, lips, nail beds, roof of mouth, or mucous membranes • Redness in the skin that does not go away within 30 minutes after pressure is relieved from a bony prominence or pressure area • In dark or yellow-skinned residents, spots or areas that are darker in appearance than normal skin tone • Pressure ulcers, open areas/skin breakdown, skin tears, abrasions, lacerations • Irritation, rash, bruises, skin discoloration, swelling, lumps, abnormal skin growths, change in color of a wart or mole, hives • Abnormal sweating, excessive heat or coolness to touch • Drainage • Foul odor

Continues

TABLE 7-1	Nursing Assistant Observations, *Continued*	
	• Complaints such as numbness, burning, tingling, itching • Signs of infection • Skin growths • Poor skin turgor/tenting of skin on forehead or over sternum • Edema, swelling • Moisture of lips and mucous membranes inside mouth	
Cardiovascular system	• Pulse rate, regularity, strength • Blood pressure • Presence or absence of chest pain • Color, appearance of skin, nail beds, mucous membranes	
Respiratory system	• Respiratory rate, rhythm, regularity • Respirations noisy, labored, quiet • Shortness of breath, gasping for breath, Cheyne-Stokes respirations • Wheezing • Presence or absence of coughing (dry or moist/productive) • Retractions • Skin color, color of lips, nail beds, mucous membranes	
Nervous system	• Weakness • Sensation, ability to feel touch, absence of sensation • Presence or absence of pain • Numbness, tingling • Normal, abnormal or involuntary motor function, spasticity • Ability or inability to move a body part • Coordination, lack of coordination	

sure sore. Report your observations to the nurse, who will decide on the course of action.

Reporting Your Observations

Signs are seen or observed by using your senses. The red area you noticed on the resident's skin during the bath is a sign. **Symptoms** are things residents notice about their conditions and tell you. They cannot be detected by using your senses. **Objective** observations are factual. They are made by seeing, hearing, feeling, touching, and smelling. **Subjective** observations may or may not be factual. Subjective observations are based on what you think or information the resident gives you that may or may not be true. Reporting that the resident did not eat lunch is an objective observation. Reporting that the resident ate a good breakfast and probably was not hungry at lunch is subjective. It reflects what you think. In fact, the resident may have felt nauseated, had pain, been upset, or had another reason for not eating. Information reported to the nurse should be objective.

Recording Your Observations

The resident's **chart** (**Figure 7-1**) is a notebook or binder containing the **medical record.** The

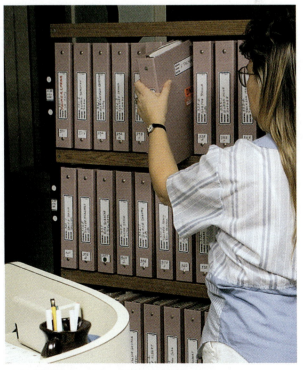

FIGURE 7-1 The resident's medical record is a confidential legal document.

medical record is a legal document. It can be subpoenaed and used in court. It is a record of the resident's true condition, progress, and care. Policies vary regarding who is responsible for recording information on the chart. You may be responsible for documenting information. A common rule in health care is, "If it is not charted, it was not done." Documentation of care given is very important and should be taken seriously. Documentation on the medical record should be objective. It should be accurate, clear, concise, and easy to read. Many facilities use flow-sheet charting **(Figure 7-2)**. This is common for vital statistics, such as vital signs, height, and weight. Routine care, such as bathing, bowel movements, and turning/repositioning, is also commonly recorded on flow sheets. Other charting is done by narrative note. Know and follow your facility policy.

Charting time. Entries in the chart are made in chronological order, by date and time. Some facilities color-code charting to identify the shift. For example, blue ink is used for the day shift, green for the second shift, and red for the night shift. A more common practice is for all shifts to document on the chart in black ink. When this is done, the time of the entry must be written using the 24-hour clock **(Table 7-2)**. When this system is used, indicating times by noting a.m. or p.m. is not necessary. The day starts at midnight, or 2400 hours. This is the same as 12:00 a.m. For the first

hour, only minutes are recorded. 12:25 a.m. is recorded as 0025. After the first hour, each hour increases by one until 24 hours are reached. 8:00 a.m. is recorded as 0800. 2:00 p.m. is recorded as 1400. 6:00 p.m. is recorded as 1800.

Confidentiality and privacy. The medical record is a private and confidential document. Protect the medical records from access by unauthorized persons. Likewise, you should not be reading resident charts out of curiosity. Medical records should be accessed only by those with a need to know the information.

In 1996, Congress passed the **Health Insurance Portability and Accountability Act (HIPAA).** This law has many provisions. One portion applies to resident privacy, confidentiality, and medical records. The HIPAA rules are:

- Increase residents' control over their medical records.
- Restrict the use and disclosure of resident information.
- Make facilities accountable for protecting resident data.
- Require the facility to implement and monitor its information release policies and procedures.

The HIPAA regulations protect all individually identifiable health information in any form. The rules apply to paper, verbal, and electronic documentation, billing records, and clinical

TABLE 7-2 The 24-Hour Clock			
Standard Clock	**24-Hour Clock**	**Standard Clock**	**24-Hour Clock**
12:00 midnight	2400 or 0000	12:00 noon	1200
1:00 a.m.	0100	1:00 p.m.	1300
2:00 a.m.	0200	2:00 p.m.	1400
3:00 a.m.	0300	3:00 p.m.	1500
4:00 a.m.	0400	4:00 p.m.	1600
5:00 a.m.	0500	5:00 p.m.	1700
6:00 a.m.	0600	6:00 p.m.	1800
7:00 a.m.	0700	7:00 p.m.	1900
8:00 a.m.	0800	8:00 p.m.	2000
9:00 a.m.	0900	9:00 p.m.	2100
10:00 a.m.	1000	10:00 p.m.	2200
11:00 a.m.	1100	11:00 p.m.	2300

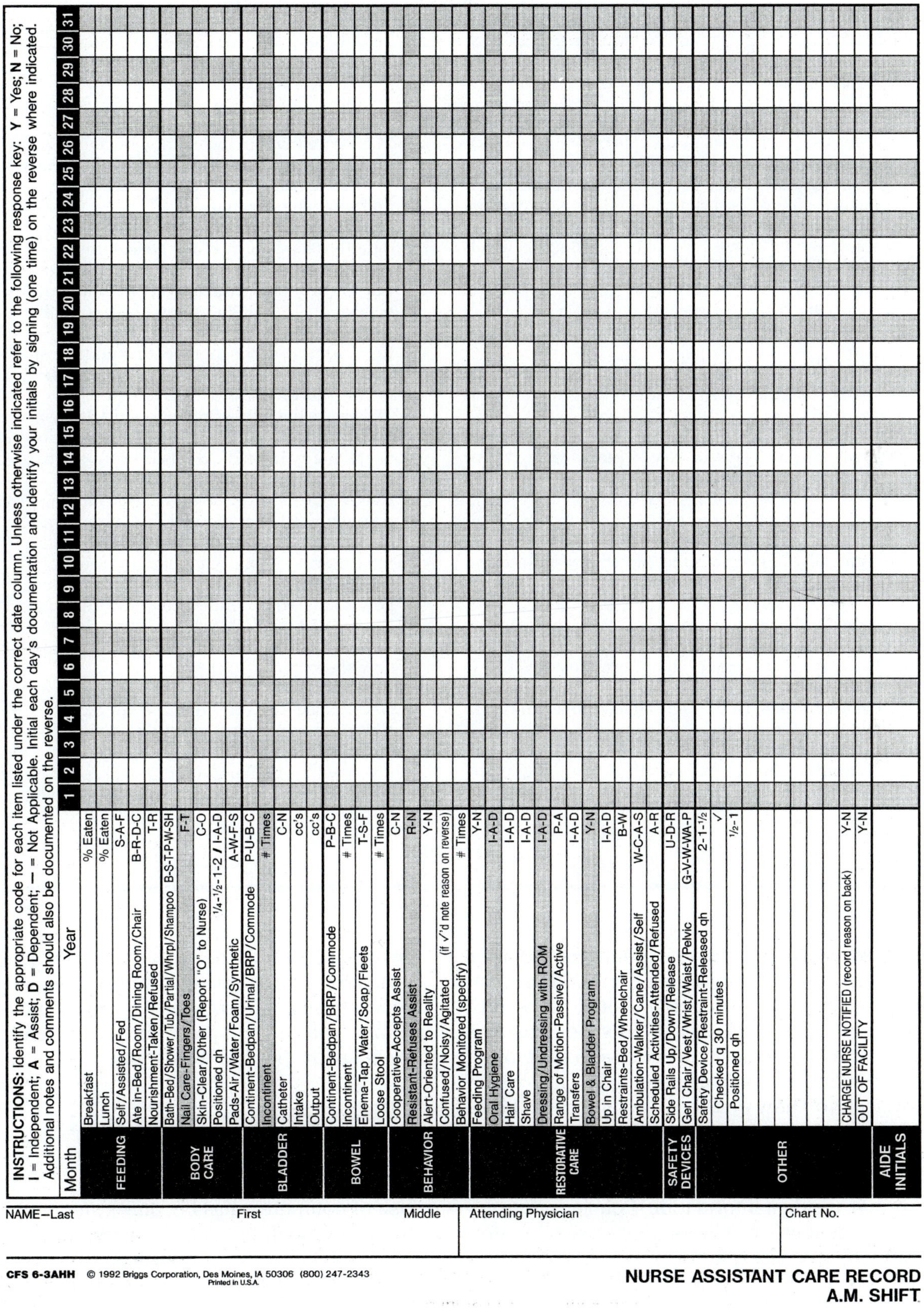

NURSE ASSISTANT CARE RECORD—A.M. SHIFT

(Reference tags: F309, F310, F312, F315-F318, F327; Cross reference tags: F221, F222, F241, F246-F247)

INSTRUCTIONS: Identify the appropriate code for each item listed under the correct date column. Unless otherwise indicated refer to the following response key: **Y** = Yes; **N** = No; **I** = Independent; **A** = Assist; **D** = Dependent; **— —** = Not Applicable. Initial each day's documentation and identify your initials by signing (one time) on the reverse where indicated. Additional notes and comments should also be documented on the reverse.

Category	Item	Code
FEEDING	Breakfast	% Eaten
	Lunch	% Eaten
	Self/Assisted/Fed	S-A-F
	Ate in-Bed/Room/Dining Room/Chair	B-R-D-C
	Nourishment-Taken/Refused	T-R
BODY CARE	Bath-Bed/Shower/Tub/Partial/Whrpl/Shampoo	B-S-T-P-W-SH
	Nail Care-Fingers/Toes	F-T
	Skin-Clear/Other (Report "O" to Nurse)	C-O
	Positioned qh	
	Pads-Air/Water/Foam/Synthetic	¼-½-1-2 / I-A-D
	Continent-Bedpan/Urinal/BRP/Commode	A-W-F-S
BLADDER	Incontinent	P-U-B-C
	Catheter	# Times
	Intake	C-N
	Output	cc's
	Continent-Bedpan/BRP/Commode	cc's
BOWEL	Incontinent	P-B-C
	Enema-Tap Water/Soap/Fleets	# Times
	Loose Stool	T-S-F
	Cooperative-Accepts Assist	# Times
BEHAVIOR	Resistant-Refuses Assist	C-N
	Alert-Oriented to Reality	R-N
	Confused/Noisy/Agitated (if ✓'d note reason on reverse)	Y-N
	Behavior Monitored (specify)	# Times
	Feeding Program	Y-N
	Oral Hygiene	I-A-D
	Hair Care	I-A-D
	Shave	I-A-D
	Dressing/Undressing with ROM	I-A-D
RESTORATIVE CARE	Range of Motion-Passive/Active	P-A
	Transfers	I-A-D
	Bowel & Bladder Program	Y-N
	Up in Chair	I-A-D
	Restraints-Bed/Wheelchair	B-W
	Ambulation-Walker/Cane/Assist/Self	W-C-A-S
	Scheduled Activities-Attended/Refused	A-R
SAFETY DEVICES	Side Rails Up/Down/Release	U-D-R
	Geri Chair/Vest/Wrist/Waist/Pelvic	G-V-W-WA-P
	Safety Device/Restraint-Released qh	2-1-½
OTHER	Checked q 30 minutes	✓
	Positioned qh	½-1
	CHARGE NURSE NOTIFIED (record reason on back)	Y-N
	OUT OF FACILITY	Y-N
AIDE INITIALS		

Days columns: 1–31

NAME—Last First Middle Attending Physician Chart No.

CFS 6-3AHH © 1992 Briggs Corporation, Des Moines, IA 50306 (800) 247-2343 Printed in U.S.A.

NURSE ASSISTANT CARE RECORD A.M. SHIFT

FIGURE 7-2 Most long-term care facilities use flow-sheet charting to record daily care. *(Compliments of Briggs Corporation (800) 247-2343.)*

GUIDELINES FOR
Charting

- Select the correct resident's chart.
- Document on the correct form.
- Charting must be accurate and legible. Follow your facility policy for printing or charting in script. Make sure the entry can be clearly read.
- Know the meaning and correct spelling of words before you write them on the chart.
- Chart in sequence.
- Chart the facts. Be specific and objective. Avoid making judgments or charting your personal opinion.
- Use the correct color pen with permanent ink. Never chart in pencil, erasable ink, or ink that runs when wet.
- Use short, concise phrases.
- Chart after an event occurs or care is given. Never chart in advance.
- Chart the exact time of the event.
- Use only facility-approved abbreviations. Never make up an abbreviation. Your facility will have a listing of abbreviations that are approved for documentation. Use abbreviations only if they are on this list.
- Leave no blank lines or spaces. Draw a single line through unused space at the end of a sentence.
- If you make a mistake, do not erase or use correction fluid. Do not mark through the entry so that it cannot be read. Draw a single line through the entry and write "error" and your initials.
- Sign your first initial, last name, and title immediately after your entry.
- Fill in all the boxes on flow-sheet charting. Blank spaces indicate that care was not given. Flow sheets are very important if the chart is involved in a lawsuit.

- Make sure that documentation of your care is complete and accurate, including turning and repositioning; feeding; food intake substitutes, snacks, and supplements; fluids given; safety measures and restraints; and range-of-motion exercises. Other data that may be carefully considered in a lawsuit are urine and bowel elimination, bathing and incontinent care, oral hygiene, ambulation, and use of special devices, such as hand rolls, restraints, and pressure-relieving mattresses.
- Read what you are documenting on flow sheets. It is easy to skip up or down a line. Be sure you are documenting on the correct line.
- Make sure the intake and output totals are accurate and recorded. If the fluid intake appears inadequate, notify the nurse. This is discussed in greater detail in Chapters 13 and 14.
- Notify the nurse if something is missing from a computerized flow sheet. The nurse will add missing information that is listed on the resident's care plan. For example, your facility routinely charts that residents are turned and repositioned every two hours. You routinely turn and reposition Mrs. Long, according to her plan of care. However, there is no place to document this important care on the flow sheet.
- Never chart for another person.
- Never chart care that you have not given.
- If you forget to chart something, follow your facility policy for making a late entry note on the chart.
- If you will be initialing a form, such as a flow sheet, make sure that you sign the initial key with your full signature and title.

records. Staff should receive only the information needed to carry out their duties. Because of this, all resident information should be used or disclosed on a need-to-know basis. For example, the dietary department would need to know if the resident was on a diabetic diet. They would not need to know that the resident has an infectious disease. The nursing assistant would need to know about both the diabetes and the infection. Facilities must monitor how and where they use resident information. Policies must protect resident charts, places where resident information is discussed, faxing resident documents, and disclosing other personal information.

The HIPAA rules ask providers to analyze how and where resident information is used, and develop procedures for protecting confidential data. This includes the areas where resident charts are stored, the places where resident information is discussed, and how residents' personal health information is distributed. The HIPAA policies and procedures for each facility are individualized to the facility.

COMPUTERS IN HEALTH CARE FACILITIES

Use of computers has become common in long-term care facilities. A large amount of information can be stored, processed, and retrieved easily. Departments can communicate with each other by computer. The information is legible and easy to read. Resident information is readily available and easy to find. Using a computer to complete the Minimum Data Set saves

GUIDELINES FOR

Documentation on the Computerized Medical Record

- Do not be afraid of computerized charting.
- When documenting on a specific resident, double-check to make sure you have entered the correct identification code.
- Do not give your identification code or password to others.
- Access only information that you are authorized to obtain.
- Document only in areas that you are authorized to use.
- Many computer programs place expert reminders or error codes on the screen. Read and follow the directions.
- Log off when leaving the computer.
- The procedure for late entry and addendum documentation will be different than in a narrative sys-

tem. Know and follow your facility policies for this type of charting.
- Keep in mind that audit trails track the machine name, user, date, time, and exactly which medical records were accessed based on the user identification.
- If you print documents from the electronic medical record, make sure they are used correctly or discarded according to facility policy. Placing them in the wastebasket is prohibited in many facilities because of privacy laws.
- Stay current. Attend continuing education programs to learn how to maximize the use of computerized charting and information systems.

a great deal of time. Statistics and data can be retrieved from the computer to spot problems and trends. Nursing units do not use the normal word processing programs for recording resident information. Special health care programs are available. These programs are usually simple to use, even for those with no computer experience. Some facilities print forms on which staff document routine care (**Figure 7-3**). Some facilities do all documentation by computer (**Figure 7-4**).

If you will be working with the computer, your facility will teach you about the programs you will be using. Do not be afraid of the computer. Becoming computer-literate may be frustrating at first, but it can make your job much easier! Look at it as an opportunity to learn something new that will benefit you and allow you to spend more time with the residents.

FAX MACHINES

Fax machines transmit printed information from one location to another over telephone lines. Long-term care facilities frequently use fax machines for laboratory and x-ray reports, physician orders, and communication with physicians and other health care agencies. You may be responsible for sending information over the fax machine. This involves placing one or more papers in the machine, dialing the telephone number of the receiving party, and pressing the start button. When sending information over the fax machine, remember that resident confidentiality laws apply. Double-check the number for accuracy before sending the documents. Your facility will teach you how to use the type of machine you will be operating.

MEDICAL TERMINOLOGY

Medicine has a language of its own. This language is used to describe the **diagnosis,** or what is wrong with the resident. Some medical terminology describes body parts, procedures, orders, measurements, treatments, activities, time, and place. Vocabulary words are listed in each chapter of your text. Learning these terms will help you master medical terminology. You will use medical terms to communicate with other members of the interdisciplinary team and to document on the resident's medical record.

Word Elements

Medical terms are a combination of word elements. You cannot expect to remember every medical term. You can, however, use your knowledge of the language of medicine to understand what unfamiliar terms mean.

The three elements of medical words are the prefix, suffix, and root. The **prefix** is the word element at the beginning of the word. A **suffix** is

```
                    Southaven Subacute Care                    Page 1
          10/03/XX Shift 2 thru 10/04/XX Shift 3

   SHIFT       SIGNATURE       TITLE   INT              57Y SEX: M
   ____  _____  _____  _____  ACCT: 0127601961  319-01  TYPE: I/P
   ____  _____  _____  _____  PHYS:                     PC:
   ____  _____  _____  _____  DOB: 01/17/32  ADM: 10/03/XX  LOS: 1
   ____  _____  _____  _____  ISO:                      SMK: NO
   ____  _____  _____  _____  ALG: paxil levaquin zithromax centr
   ____  _____  _____  _____  SGY:
   ____  _____  _____  _____  DX:  ACUTE RESP DIST COPD
   ____  _____  _____  _____               MR#: 00015435
```

DEMOGRAPHIC/PRECAUTION INFORMATION
HT: 6'0.0"/182.9cm
WT: 167lbs/75.751kg   PRECAUTIONS: FALL PROTOCOL
REL: CATHOLIC   LANG: ENGLISH

ACTIVITIES OF DAILY LIVING	0700-1500	1500-2300	2300-0700
Date Ord ADL Description			
10/03 BEDREST -A-* W/BRP ONLY			
10/03 ELIMINAT'N-E-TOILETING W/1			
10/03 HYGIENE -H-BATH-PARTIAL			
10/03 HYGIENE -H-HS CARE W/ASSIST			
10/03 I & O-Q8H			
10/03 LINEN CHG-UNOCCUPIED BED			
10/03 NUTRITION -N-FEED SELF W/TRAY SET			
10/03 POS/TURN-ASSIST ALL TRANSFERS			
10/03 SAFETY-S-* PATIENT ROUND Q2H			
10/03 SAFETY-S-LEVEL 2			
10/03 VS-ADULT-V-Q4H			

DIETARY ORDERS   Status Percent Consumption
Diet   Act   B____% L____% S____%
REGULAR (GENERAL)

CLINICAL ORDERS   Request   Stop   Freq
Dpt Description   Date/Time   Date/Time
LAB CULTURE, BLOOD, ARD   10/03/XX 1325   10/03/XX 0125P   ONCE
LAB CULTURE, BLOOD, ARD   10/03/XX 1325   10/03/XX 0125P   ONCE
EKG EKG-REVANA   10/03/XX 1330   10/03/XX 0130P   ONCE

THERAPY/MISC. ORDERS
Dpt Description   Req Date/Time
RT HAND HELD NEBULIZER   10/03/XX 2138
    : ALBUTEROL 0.5 UNIT DOSE Q4H
RT OXY 02 INCL P/H   10/03/XX 2137
    :
RT STAT BLOOD GAS   10/03/XX 1329
    :

TREATMENT ORDERS	0700-1500	1500-2300	2300-0700
10/03/XX 2142			
: IVPB MED: SOLUMEDROL 60MG Q6 X 3			
DOSES			

FIGURE 7-3 Individual care sheets are printed daily. Staff initial care when it is completed.

the word element ending the word. The **root** is the element that provides the meaning of the word. For example, the root *arth* means joint. The suffix *-algia* means pain. If you see the word arthralgia, you will know that it means pain in the joints. The letters *i* or *o* are sometimes added to the root word to make the word easier to connect and pronounce. Medical words can consist of a prefix and a suffix, a prefix and a root, a root and a suffix, or two roots.

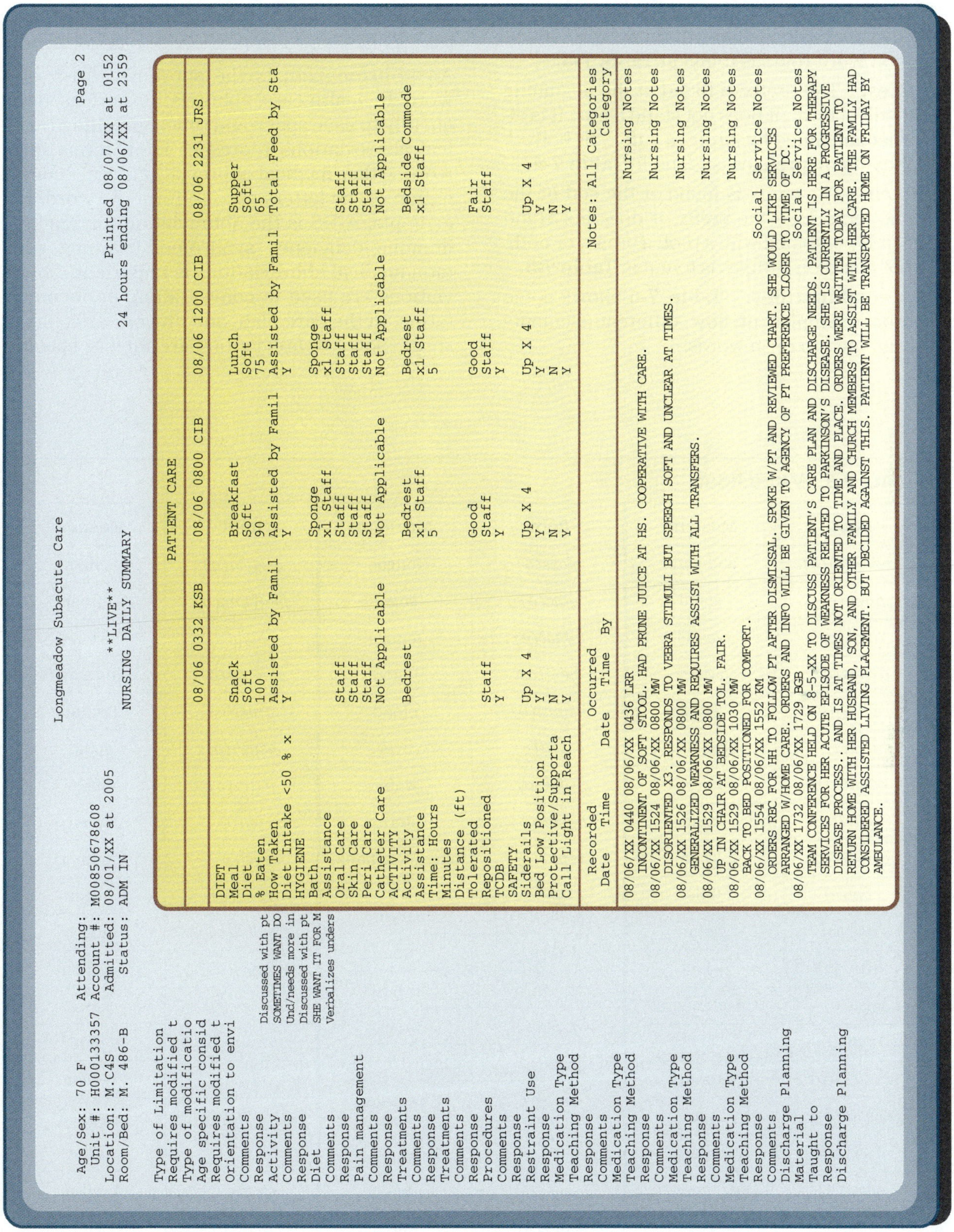

Longmeadow Subacute Care

Age/Sex: 70 F Attending: Page 2
Unit #: H000133357 Account #: M00850678608
Location: M.C4S Admitted: 08/01/XX at 2005 **LIVE** Printed 08/07/XX at 0152
Room/Bed: M. 486-B Status: ADM IN NURSING DAILY SUMMARY 24 hours ending 08/06/XX at 2359

Type of Limitation	
Requires modified t	
Type of modificatio	
Age specific consid	
Requires modified t	
Orientation to envi	
Comments	
Response	Discussed with pt
Activity	SOMETIMES WANT DO
Comments	Und/needs more in
Response	Discussed with pt
Diet	SHE WANT IT FOR M
Comments	Verbalizes unders
Response	
Pain management	
Comments	
Response	
Treatments	
Comments	
Response	
Treatments	
Comments	
Response	
Procedures	
Comments	
Response	
Restraint Use	
Response	
Medication Type	
Teaching Method	
Response	
Comments	
Medication Type	
Teaching Method	
Response	
Comments	
Medication Type	
Teaching Method	
Response	
Comments	
Medication Type	
Teaching Method	
Response	
Comments	
Discharge Planning	
Material	
Taught to	
Response	
Discharge Planning	

PATIENT CARE

	08/06 0332 KSB	08/06 0800 CIB	08/06 1200 CIB	08/06 2231 JRS
DIET				
Meal	Snack	Breakfast	Lunch	Supper
Diet	Soft	Soft	Soft	Soft
% Eaten	100	90	75	65
How Taken	Assisted by Famil	Assisted by Famil	Assisted by Famil	Total Feed by Sta
Diet Intake <50 % x	Y	Y	Y	
HYGIENE				
Bath		Sponge	Sponge	
Assistance		x1 Staff	x1 Staff	
Oral Care	Staff	Staff	Staff	Staff
Skin Care	Staff	Staff	Staff	Staff
Peri Care	Staff	Staff	Staff	Staff
Catheter Care	Not Applicable	Not Applicable	Not Applicable	Not Applicable
ACTIVITY				
Activity	Bedrest	Bedrest	Bedrest	Bedside Commode
Assistance		x1 Staff	x1 Staff	x1 Staff
Time: Hours		5	5	
Minutes				
Distance (ft)				
Tolerated		Good	Good	Fair
Repositioned	Staff	Staff	Staff	Staff
TCDB	Y	Y	Y	
SAFETY				
Siderails	Up X 4	Up X 4	Up X 4	Up X 4
Bed Low Position	Y	Y	Y	Y
Protective/Supporta	N	N	N	N
Call Light in Reach	Y	Y	Y	Y

Recorded Date Time / Occurred Date Time By / Notes: All Categories Category

08/06/XX 0440 08/06/XX 0436 LRR Nursing Notes
INCONTINENT OF SOFT STOOL. HAD PRUNE JUICE AT HS. COOPERATIVE WITH CARE.
08/06/XX 1524 08/06/XX 0800 MW Nursing Notes
DISORIENTED X3. RESPONDS TO VEBRA STIMULI BUT SPEECH SOFT AND UNCLEAR AT TIMES.
08/06/XX 1526 08/06/XX 0800 MW Nursing Notes
GENERALIZED WEAKNESS AND REQUIRES ASSIST WITH ALL TRANSFERS.
08/06/XX 1529 08/06/XX 0800 MW Nursing Notes
UP IN CHAIR AT BEDSIDE TOL. FAIR.
08/06/XX 1529 08/06/XX 1030 MW Nursing Notes
BACK TO BED POSITIONED FOR COMFORT.
08/06/XX 1554 08/06/XX 1552 KM Social Service Notes
ORDERS REC FOR HH TO FOLLOW PT AFTER DISMISSAL. SPOKE W/PT AND REVIEWED CHART. SHE WOULD LIKE SERVICES ARRANGED W/HOME CARE. ORDERS AND INFO WILL BE GIVEN TO AGENCY OF PT PREFERENCE CLOSER TO TIME OF DC.
08/06/XX 1732 08/06/XX 1729 BGB Social Service Notes
TEAM CONFERENCE HELD ON 8-5-XX TO DISCUSS PATIENT'S CARE PLAN AND DISCHARGE NEEDS. PATIENT IS HERE FOR THERAPY SERVICES FOR HER ACUTE EPISODE OF WEAKNESS RELATED TO PARKINSON'S DISEASE. SHE IS CURRENTLY IN A PROGRESSIVE DISEASE PROCESS.. AND IS AT TIMES NOT ORIENTED TO TIME AND PLACE. ORDERS WERE WRITTEN TODAY FOR PATIENT TO RETURN HOME WITH HER HUSBAND, SON, AND OTHER FAMILY AND CHURCH MEMBERS TO ASSIST WITH HER CARE. THE FAMILY HAD CONSIDERED ASSISTED LIVING PLACEMENT. BUT DECIDED AGAINST THIS. PATIENT WILL BE TRANSPORTED HOME ON FRIDAY BY AMBULANCE.

FIGURE 7-4 Nursing assistants document all daily care on the computer.

Word roots. The word root (or root word) provides the basic meaning of the word. A list of common word roots is found in **Table 7-3.**

Prefixes. The prefix is found at the beginning of a medical term. It does not stand alone. It is always accompanied by a root, a suffix, or both. A list of common prefixes is found in **Table 7-4.**

Suffixes. The suffix is found at the end of the medical term. Like the prefix, it does not stand alone. It is combined with a root, a prefix, or both. A list of common suffixes is found in **Table 7-5.**

Word combinations. Table 7-6 shows some common examples of how different elements are combined to form words.

ABBREVIATIONS

An **abbreviation** is the shortened form of a word. In health care, abbreviations are used frequently to save space and time. Sometimes medical abbreviations represent Latin terms for a word. Other medical abbreviations are a combination of the letters used to form the word. For example, AIDS is the abbreviation for acquired immune deficiency syndrome. Learning common medical abbreviations is important. Abbreviations are used in conversation, in documentation, in the care plan, and on your assignment sheet. Some abbreviations are facility specific.

TABLE 7-3 Word Roots

Root	Meaning	Root	Meaning	Root	Meaning
abdomin(o)	abdomen	gloss(o)	tongue	ped(i)(o)	child
aden(o)	gland	glyc(o)	sugar	pharyng(o)	throat
angi(o)	vessel	gynec(o)	female	phleb(o)	vein
arteri(o)	artery	hem(o)	blood	pneum(o)	lung, air
arth(o)	joint	hemat(o)	blood	proct(o)	rectum
bronch(i)(o)	bronchus	hepat(o)	liver	psych(o)	mind
cardi(o)	heart	hydr(o)	water	pulm(o)	lung
cephal(o)	head	hyster(o)	uterus	py(o)	pus
cerebr(o)	brain	lapar(o)	abdomen, flank, loin	rect(o)	rectum
chol(e)	bile			rhin(o)	nose
col(o)	colon	laryng(o)	larynx	splen(o)	spleen
crani(o)	skull	lith(o)	stone	stern(o)	sternum
cyst(o)	bladder, cyst	mamm(o)	breast	thorac(o)	chest
cyt(o)	cell	mast(o)	breast	thromb(o)	clot
dent(i)(o)	tooth	men(o)	menstruation	tox(o)	poison
dermat(o)	skin	my(o)	muscle	trache(o)	trachea
encephal(o)	brain	myel(o)	bone marrow, spinal cord	ur(o)	urine
enter(o)	small intestine	nephr(o)	kidney	urethr(o)	urethra
erythr(o)	red	neur(o)	nerve	urin(o)	urine
fibr(o)	fiber	ocul(o)	eye	uter(i)(o)	uterus
gastr(o)	stomach	ophthalm(o)	eye	ven(o)	vein
geront(o)	elderly	oste(o)	bone		

TABLE 7-4 Prefixes

Prefix	Meaning	Prefix	Meaning	Prefix	Meaning
a-, an-	without, not	hemi-	half	per-	by, through
ab-	away from	hyper-	high, above, excessive	peri-	around
ad-	toward			poly-	many
ante-	before	hypo-	low, below normal	post-	after
anti-	against	inter-	between	pre-	before
bi-	double, two	intra-	inside, within	pseud-	false
bio-	life	leuk-	white	retro-	backward
brady-	slow	micro-	small	semi-	half
circum-	around	neo-	new	septic-	infection
dys-	difficult, abnormal	non-	not	sub-	under, below
epi-	on, over	pan-	all	tachy-	fast

TABLE 7-5 Suffixes

Suffix	Meaning	Suffix	Meaning	Suffix	Meaning
-algia	pain	-meter	instrument that measures	-pnea	breathing
-alysis	analyze			-ptosis	sagging, falling
-ectomy	surgical removal	-ostomy	surgical opening	-rrhagia	excessive flow
		-otomy	surgical opening	-rrhea	discharge
-emia	blood			-scope	instrument that examines
-gram	record	-pathy	disease		
-itis	inflammation of	-penia	deficiency	-stasis	constant
-logy	study of	-phasia	speaking	-therapy	treatment
-lysis	destruction of	-plegia	paralysis	-uria	condition of urine
-megaly	enlargement				

TABLE 7-6 Combining Word Parts to Form Medical Terms

Medical Term	Prefix	Root	Suffix	Meaning
antiseptic	anti-	septic		against infection
arthritis		arthr	-itis	inflammation of joints
cardiology		cardi	-ology	study of the heart
colostomy		col	-ostomy	surgical opening into the colon
dyspnea	dys-		-pnea	difficult breathing
hemiplegia	hemi-		-plegia	paralysis in one half of the body
hypoglycemia	hypo-	glyc	-emia	low blood sugar
glycosuria		glyc	-uria	sugar in urine
leukemia	leuk-		-emia	condition of white blood cells
urinalysis	urin-		-alysis	analysis of the urine

Each facility will have a list of abbreviations approved for use in charting. Refer to this list if you do not understand the meaning of an abbreviation. Sometimes an abbreviation can mean more than one thing. For example, D/C is the abbreviation for discontinue. It can also be used to mean discharge. The context of the sentence in which it is written should give you a clue to its meaning. **Table 7-7** lists common medical abbreviations.

TABLE 7-7   Common Abbreviations

Abbreviation	Meaning	Abbreviation	Meaning
$\bar{a}$	before	B, (B), Ⓑ	bilateral, both
AAROM	active assistive (assisted) range of motion	B&B	bowel and bladder
abd	abdomen	BB	bed bath
ABT, ABX	antibiotic therapy	bid	twice a day
$\overline{ac}$	before meals	bilat	bilateral
ACT	active, actively, activities	BKA	below-the-knee amputation
AD	Activity Director	BLE	both lower extremities
ADA	American Dietetic Association, American Diabetic Association	BM	bowel movement
add.	adduction	BP, B/P	blood pressure
ad lib	as desired	BPM	beats per minute
ADLs	activities of daily living	BR	bed rest, bathroom
adm	admission	BRP	bathroom privileges
AEB	as evidenced by	BS	blood sugar
AFO	ankle/foot orthosis	BSC	bedside commode
AIDS	acquired immune deficiency syndrome	BSE	breast self-examination
aka	above-the-knee amputation, also known as	BUE	both upper extremities
alt	alternate, alternating	C	Celsius, centigrade
am	morning	$\bar{c}$	with
AMA	against medical advice	c, cm	centimeter
amb	ambulate	C1, C2, C3, etc.	first cervical vertebrae, second cervical vertebrae, third cervical vertebrae, etc.
amt	amount	CA	cancer
ant	anterior	CAD	coronary artery disease
A&P	anatomy and physiology	cal, kcal	calorie
AROM	active range of motion	cath	catheter
ASAP	as soon as possible	CBB	complete bed bath
assist	assistance	CBC	complete blood count
as tol	as tolerated	CC	chief complaint
ax	axillary (under the arm)	cc	cubic centimeter
		CHF	congestive heart failure

Continues

TABLE 7-7 Common Abbreviations, *Continued*

Abbreviation	Meaning	Abbreviation	Meaning
ck, ✓	check	*Dx*	diagnosis
ck or ✓ *freq*	check frequently	*E*	enema
cl liq	clear liquid	*ECG, EKG*	electrocardiogram
CMA	certified medication aide	*EENT*	eye, ear, nose, and throat
CNA	certified nursing assistant or certified nurse administrator	*ENT*	ear, nose, and throat
c/o	complains of	*ER, ED*	emergency room, emergency department
COLD, COPD	chronic obstructive lung (pulmonary) disease	*ESRD*	end stage renal disease
CP	care plan, clinical pathway, critical pathway	*et*	and
		ETOH	ethanol (often used to refer to alcoholic beverages)
CPM	continuous passive motion machine	*Eval*	evaluation
CPR	cardiopulmonary resuscitation	*ex.*	exercise
C & S	culture and sensitivity	*exam*	examination
cu	cubic	*ext.*	extension, extremity, external
CVA	cerebrovascular accident, stroke	*F*	Fahrenheit
CXR	chest x-ray	*FB*	foreign body
d	day	*FBS*	fasting blood sugar
D/C, DC	discontinue, discharge	*FE*	Fleet's enema
DDS	Doctor of Dental Science (dentist)	*FF*	force fluids
dep	dependent	*flex*	flexion
dept.	department	*freq*	frequently
diab	diabetes, diabetic	*FS*	frozen section, finger stick
DJD	degenerative joint disease	*FSBS*	finger stick blood sugar
DNR	do not resuscitate	*FU, F/U*	follow up
DO	Doctor of Osteopathy	*FUO*	fever of unknown origin
DOA	dead on arrival	*FWB*	full weight bearing
DOB	date of birth	*Fx*	fracture
DPM	Doctor of Podiatric Medicine	*G*	good
DR, D/R	dining room	*g/c, GC*	geriatric chair
Dr.	doctor	*GERD*	gastroesophageal reflux disease
DSD	dry sterile dressing	*GI*	gastrointestinal
DSM	Dietary Services Manager	*G/T, GT*	gastrostomy tube
DT	dietetic technician	*gtt*	drop
DVT	deep vein thrombosis (blood clot)	*GU*	genitourinary

Continues

TABLE 7-7 Common Abbreviations, *Continued*

Abbreviation	Meaning	Abbreviation	Meaning
Gyn	gynecology	*lb*	pound
h	hour	*LBP*	low back pain
H	hydrogen	*LE*	lower extremity
HAV, HBV, HCV, etc.	hepatitis A virus, hepatitis B virus, hepatitis C virus, etc.	*lg, lge*	large
		liq	liquid
hemi	half, hemiplegia	*L/min, LPM*	liters per minute
Hg	mercury	*LL*	left leg
HIV	human immunodeficiency virus	*LLE*	left lower extremity
H_2O	water	*LLQ*	left lower quadrant
H_2O_2	hydrogen peroxide	*LOC*	loss of consciousness, level of consciousness, level of care
HOB	head of bed		
HOH	hard of hearing	*LPN*	licensed practical nurse
H & P	history and physical	*lt*	left
hr	hour	*LTC*	long-term care
hs	bedtime (hour of sleep)	*LTCF*	long-term care facility
ht	height	*LTG*	long-term goal
Hx	history	*LUQ*	left upper quadrant
Ⓘ, *ind.*	independent, independently	*LVN*	licensed vocational nurse
ID	initial dose	*M*	meter
IDCP	interdisciplinary care plan	*MA*	medication aide
IDDM	insulin-dependent diabetes mellitus	*max*	maximum
IDT	interdisciplinary team	*MD*	muscular dystrophy, medical doctor
IM	intramuscular		
I & O	intake and output	*MDR*	main dining room
int.	internal	*MDS*	Minimum Data Set
IPPB	intermittent positive pressure breathing	*mech soft*	mechanical soft
		med rec	medical records
isol	isolation	*meds*	medications
IV	intravenous	*MI*	myocardial infarction (heart attack)
K, K+	potassium		
L	liter, left	*min*	minimum, minimal, minute
L1, L2, etc.	first lumbar vertebra, second lumbar vertebra, etc.	*mL or ml*	milliliter
		mm	millimeter
lab	laboratory	*mmHg*	millimeters of mercury
lat	lateral	*mod*	moderate

Continues

TABLE 7-7 Common Abbreviations, *Continued*

Abbreviation	Meaning	Abbreviation	Meaning
MRSA	methicillin-resistant Staphylococcus aureus	OT	occupational therapy
MS	multiple sclerosis	oz, ℥	ounce
mult.	multiple	℥i, ℥ii, ℥iii, etc.	1 ounce, 2 ounces, 3 ounces, etc.
NA, N/A	not applicable, nursing assistant (meaning determined by context)	$\bar{p}$	after
Na⁺	sodium	P	pulse, poor
NACEP	Nurse Aide Competency Evaluation Program	PB, PBB	partial bath, partial bed bath
NAR	no adverse reaction	$\overline{pc}$	after meals
NAS	no added salt	PCT	Patient Care Technician
NATCEP	Nurse Aide Training and Competency Evaluation Program	PE	physical examination
		peds, pedi	pediatrics
N/C, no c/o	no complaints	per	by, through
neg, −, ⊖	negative	pm	afternoon or evening
NG	nasogastric	PN	progress notes, practical nurse
NGT	nasogastric tube	po	by mouth
NIDDM	non–insulin-dependent diabetes mellitus	pos, +, ⊕	positive
NKA	no known allergies	PPE	personal protective equipment
NN	nurse's notes	PPS	post polio syndrome, prospective payment system
noc	night	preop	preoperative
NPO	nothing by mouth	prep	prepare
N/S, NSS	normal saline, normal saline solution	prn	as needed
		prog	prognosis, progress
N & V	nausea and vomiting	PROM	passive range of motion
NVD	nausea, vomiting, and diarrhea	pt or Pt	patient
NWB	nonweight-bearing	PT	physical therapy
O₂	oxygen	PUD	peptic ulcer disease
OA	osteoarthritis	PVD	peripheral vascular disease
obj	objective	PWB	partial weight bearing
OBS	organic brain syndrome	$\bar{q}$	each, every
obs	observations	$\bar{q}d$	every day
occ	occasional	$\bar{q}h$	every hour
OOB	out of bed	$\bar{q}2h$, $\bar{q}3h$, $\bar{q}4h$, etc.	every 2 hours, every 3 hours, every 4 hours, etc.
ORIF	open reduction, internal fixation	$\bar{q}hs$	every night at bedtime
os, o	mouth	qid	four times a day

Continues

TABLE 7-7 Common Abbreviations, *Continued*

Abbreviation	Meaning	Abbreviation	Meaning
$\overline{qm}$, $\overline{qam}$	every morning	SNF	skilled nursing facility
$\overline{qod}$	every other day	SNU	skilled nursing unit
$\overline{qs}$	sufficient quantity	SOB	shortness of breath
qt	quart	spec	specimen
quad	quadrant, quadriplegic	SS	social service
R	rectal, respiration, right	S/S, S & S	signs and symptoms
RA	rheumatoid arthritis, right arm	SSE	soapsuds enema
RAI	Resident Assessment Instrument	S/T	skin tear
RCP	Respiratory Care Practitioner	ST	speech therapy
RD	Registered Dietitian	stat	immediately
re:	regarding	Std prec	standard precautions
reg	regular, regulation	STG	short-term goal
rehab	rehabilitation	STNA	state tested nursing assistant
res, Res	resident	supp	suppository
resp, R	respirations	SW	social worker
RL	right leg	Sx	symptoms
RLE	right lower extremity	T, temp	temperature
RLQ	right lower quadrant	T1, T2, etc.	first thoracic vertebra, second thoracic vertebra, etc.
rm	room	TB	tuberculosis
RN	registered nurse	TF	tube feeding
RNA	restorative nursing assistant	TIAN	toilet in advance of need
R/O	rule out	TID, tid	three times a day
ROM	range of motion	TKO	to keep open
rot.	rotation	TLC	tender loving care
rt, R	right	TPN	total parenteral nutrition
RT	respiratory therapy	TPR	temperature, pulse, respiration
r/t	related to	trach	tracheostomy
RUE	right upper extremity	TT	therapeutic touch
RUQ	right upper quadrant	TTWB	toe-touch weight bearing
Rx	prescription, therapy, treatment	TWE	tap water enema
$\overline{s}$	without	Tx	traction, treatment
SBA	standby assistance	UA, U/A	urinalysis
semi	half	UE	upper extremity
sm	small		

Continues

TABLE 7-7   Common Abbreviations, *Continued*

Abbreviation	Meaning	Abbreviation	Meaning
URI	upper respiratory infection	1°	first, primary, first degree
UTI	urinary tract infection	2°	second, secondary, secondary to, second degree
vag	vaginal	3°	third, tertiary, third degree
vc, VC	verbal cues	1x, 2x, etc.	one time, one person, two times, etc.
VRE	vancomycin-resistant Enterococcus	ı̇, ı̇ı̇, ı̇ı̇ı̇, ı̇v̇, etc.	one, two, three, four, etc.
VS	vital signs	@	at
WA, W/A	while awake	//	parallel
WB	weight bearing	=	equals, equal to
WBAT	weight bearing as tolerated	>, ≥	greater than
w/c	wheelchair	<, ≤	less than
WFL	within functional limits	±, +/−	plus or minus
WNL	within normal limits	△ (triangle)	change, change to
wt	weight	°	degrees
x, X	times	Ø	zero, none, nothing
XR, X/R	x-ray	*	important
y/o	years old	♀	female
yr	year	♂	male
↑	up, increase		
↓	down, decrease		

KEY POINTS

- The nursing assistant communicates with other members of the health care team verbally and in writing.
- Observations about the resident are reported to the nurse for assessment and action.
- The nursing assistant records information about the resident in the medical record in writing or by using the computer.
- The nursing assistant will use the senses of sight, hearing, smell, and touch to make valuable observations.
- Signs can be seen or observed. Symptoms are things the resident tells you.
- Objective observations are factual. Subjective observations are based on what you think or what the resident tells you.
- The medical record is a factual, permanent record of the resident's progress and care.
- The medical record is a legal document, and entries in it must be accurate and complete.
- Understanding medical terminology and medical abbreviations is important if you are to communicate well and accurately with other members of the health care team.

REVIEW

A. Multiple Choice

Select the one best answer.

1. A sign is an observation that
   a. you detect with your senses.
   b. you think.
   c. you believe.
   d. reflects your opinion.

2. A symptom is
   a. something you know to be true.
   b. what the resident tells you.
   c. what you think.
   d. what you detect with your senses.

3. Objective means
   a. something you think and feel.
   b. a complaint of pain.
   c. something you observe.
   d. what you believe is true.

4. The medical record
   a. is a legal document.
   b. cannot be used in court.
   c. contains fictional information.
   d. can be read by any interested party.

5. When using the 24-hour clock, 5:15 p.m. is
   a. 0515 hours.
   b. 1515 hours.
   c. 1715 hours.
   d. 2015 hours.

6. The following is true about documenting in the resident's chart:
   a. Correction fluid should be used if you make a mistake.
   b. Factual information should be written on the chart.
   c. Charting is always done before care is given.
   d. Turning and repositioning need not be documented.

7. The prefix is found
   a. at the beginning of a word.
   b. at the end of a word.
   c. in the middle of a word.
   d. in the root of a word.

8. A suffix is found
   a. at the beginning of a word.
   b. at the end of a word.
   c. in the middle of a word.
   d. in the root of a word.

9. The root
   a. introduces the word.
   b. describes the suffix.
   c. provides depth.
   d. provides meaning.

10. The term *myalgia* means
    a. heart attack.
    b. infection of the bone.
    c. pain in the muscles.
    d. inflammation of the throat.

11. The term *colectomy* means
    a. removal of the colon.
    b. removal of a cyst.
    c. pain in the small intestine.
    d. irritation of the gallbladder.

12. The term *phlebitis* means
    a. infection of the lungs.
    b. inflammation of a vein.
    c. irritation of the throat.
    d. pus in a wound.

13. Hydrotherapy is
    a. a disease of the lungs.   c. water therapy.
    b. removal of the uterus.   d. oxygen therapy.

14. The nurse writes on your assignment sheet, Mr. Dominguez, room 611—"B/P at H.S." You know this means:
    a. Take the blood pressure at bedtime.
    b. Give Mr. Dominguez the bedpan at his side.
    c. The resident should have big portions for his supper.
    d. Mr. Dominguez has a blood problem with his system.

15. Mrs. Shane is to ambulate in the hallway TID. You know this means to walk the resident
    a. every other day.   c. three times a day.
    b. twice a day.   d. ten times a day.

B. Definitions

Define the meaning of the following words based on your knowledge of medical terminology.

16. tachycardia _____   22. dyspnea _____
17. bradycardia _____   23. hemolysis _____
18. gastritis _____   24. dysuria _____
19. ophthalmology _____   25. mastectomy _____
20. nephrectomy _____   26. intraabdominal _____
21. pyuria _____

C. Clinical Applications

Answer the following questions.

27. Linda Mason, CNA, is in a hurry to leave. She has an appointment as soon as she gets off work. Linda states that Mrs. Long and Mr. Thomas need to be repositioned. She completes all her other resident care, but does not get all of her charting done. She asks you to finish it for her. How should you handle this situation?

28. Your friend, John, asks if your long-term care facility has a fax machine. He asks you to fax some very important papers to another state. He said the office supply store will charge $22.00 for this and he cannot afford it. Although the fax machine is available at the nurses' station, your facility policies state that the fax is to be used for facility business only. What should you do?

CHAPTER 8

Body Mechanics, Moving and Positioning Residents

OBJECTIVES

After reading this chapter, you will be able to:

- Spell and define key terms.
- Demonstrate good body mechanics when lifting and moving residents and other heavy objects.
- Describe why positioning residents in good body alignment is important.
- Define ergonomics and describe how cumulative trauma disorders occur.
- Demonstrate proper positioning in the supine, prone, lateral, Fowler's, semisupine, and semiprone positions.
- Describe the cause of pressure ulcers and list 10 methods of preventing pressure ulcer development.
- Demonstrate procedures related to body mechanics, moving and positioning residents.

OBSERVATIONS TO MAKE AND REPORT RELATED TO BODY MECHANICS, MOVING AND POSITIONING RESIDENTS

Rash

Redness

Redness in the skin that does not go away within 30 minutes after pressure is relieved from a bony prominence or pressure area

In dark- or yellow-skinned residents, spots or areas that are darker in appearance than normal skin tone

Pressure ulcers, blisters

Abrasions, skin tears, lacerations

Irritation

Bruises

Skin discoloration

Swelling

Lumps

Abnormal skin growths

Change in color of a wart or mole

Abnormal sweating

Excessive heat or coolness to touch

Open areas/skin breakdown

Drainage

Foul odor

Complaints such as numbness, burning, tingling, itching

Signs of infection

Unusual skin color, such as blue or gray color of the skin, lips, nail beds, roof of mouth, or mucous membranes

Skin growths

Poor skin turgor/Tenting of skin on forehead or over sternum

Sunken, dark eyes

NOTE TO THE STUDENT

The direct care procedures begin in this chapter and continue through the remainder of the text. The beginning and ending steps of all procedures are the same. These steps have been printed inside the covers of your textbook for easy reference. Your text will instruct you to "Perform your beginning procedure actions." Turn to the front cover to refer to these steps. Refer to the back cover when the text instructs you to "Perform your procedure completion

TABLE 8-1 Beginning Procedure Actions

Beginning Procedure Actions	Rationale
1. Assemble equipment and take it to the resident's room.	Improves efficiency of the procedure. Ensures that you do not have to leave the room.
2. Knock on the resident's door and identify yourself by name and title.	Respects the resident's right to privacy. Notifies the resident who is giving care.
3. Identify the resident by checking the identification bracelet, or other method according to facility policy.	Ensures that you are caring for the correct resident.
4. Ask visitors to leave the room and advise them where they may wait.	Respects the resident's right to privacy. Advising visitors where to wait demonstrates hospitality.
5. Explain what you are going to do and how the resident can assist. Answer questions about the procedure.	Informs the resident of what is going to be done and what to expect. Gives the resident an opportunity to get information about the procedure and the extent of resident participation.
6. Provide privacy by closing the door, privacy curtain, and window curtains.	Respects the resident's right to privacy. All three should be closed even if the resident is alone in the room.
7. Wash your hands or use an alcohol-based hand cleaner.	Applies the principles of standard precautions. Prevents the spread of microorganisms.
8. Set up the necessary equipment at the bedside. Open trays and packages. Position items within easy reach. Avoid positioning a container for soiled items in a manner that requires crossing over clean items to access it.	Prepares for the procedure. Ensures that the equipment and supplies are conveniently positioned and readily available. Reduces the risk of cross-contamination.
9. Position the resident for the procedure. Ask an assistant to help, if necessary, or support the resident with pillows and props. Make sure the resident is comfortable and can maintain the position throughout the procedure. Drape the resident for modesty, even if you and the resident are alone in the room.	Ensures that the resident is in the correct position for the procedure. Ensures that the resident is supported and can maintain the position without discomfort. Respects the resident's modesty and dignity.
10. Raise the bed to a comfortable working height.	Prevents back strain and injury caused by bending at the waist.
11. Apply gloves if contact with blood, moist body fluids (except sweat), mucous membranes, secretions, excretions, or nonintact skin is likely.	Applies the principles of standard precautions. Protects the nursing assistant and the resident from transmission of pathogens.
12. Apply a gown if your uniform will have substantial contact with linen or other articles contaminated with blood, moist body fluids (except sweat), secretions, or excretions.	Applies the principles of standard precautions. Protects your uniform from contamination with bloodborne pathogens.
13. Apply a gown, mask, and eye protection if splashing of blood or moist body fluids is likely.	Applies the principles of standard precautions. Protects the nursing assistant's mucous membranes, uniform, and skin from accidental splashing of bloodborne pathogens.
14. Lower the side rail on the side where you are working. (Raise the rail if you must leave the bedside temporarily.)	Provides an obstacle-free area in which to work.

TABLE 8-2 Procedure Completion Actions

Procedure Completion Actions	Rationale
1. Remove gloves.	Prevents contamination of environmental surfaces from the gloves.
2. Check to make sure the resident is comfortable and in good alignment.	All body systems function better when the body is correctly aligned. The resident is more comfortable when the body is in good alignment.
3. Replace the bed covers, then remove any drapes used.	Provides warmth and security.
4. Elevate the side rails, if used, before leaving the bedside.	Prevents contamination of the side rails from gloves. Promotes resident's right to a safe environment. Prevents accidents and injuries.
5. Remove other personal protective equipment, if worn, and discard according to facility policy.	Prevents unnecessary environmental contamination from used gloves and protective equipment.
6. Wash your hands or use an alcohol-based hand cleaner.	Applies the principles of standard precautions. Prevents the spread of microorganisms.
7. Return the bed to the lowest horizontal position.	Promotes resident's right to a safe environment. Prevents accidents and injuries.
8. Open the privacy and window curtains.	Privacy is no longer necessary unless preferred by the resident.
9. Leave the resident in a safe and comfortable position, with the call signal and needed personal items within reach.	Prevents accidents and injuries. Ensures that help is available. Eliminates the need to call or stretch for needed personal items.
10. Wash your hands or use an alcohol-based hand cleaner.	Although the hands were washed previously, they have contacted the resident and other items in the room. Wash them again before leaving to prevent potential transfer of microorganisms to areas outside the resident's unit.
11. Inform visitors that they may return to the room.	Demonstrates courtesy to visitors and resident.
12. Report completion of the procedure and any abnormalities or other observations.	Informs the supervisor that your assigned task has been completed, so further care can be planned and you can be reassigned to other duties. Notifies the licensed nurse of abnormalities and changes in the resident's condition that require further assessment.
13. Document the procedure and your observations.	Ongoing progress and care given are documented. Provides a legal record. Informs other members of the interdisciplinary team of the care given.

actions." Eventually, the steps will be committed to memory and you will not have to refer to them. However, in the initial stages of your nursing assistant program, refer to them often, because they are very important. **Tables 8-1** and **8-2** summarize these important beginning and ending actions.

BODY MECHANICS

The nursing assistant routinely lifts, moves, and positions residents and other heavy objects. Good **body mechanics** involves using your body correctly. Good body mechanics should always be used when performing lifting or moving procedures, transferring residents, picking up items from the floor, and bending and lifting. Proper body mechanics means using the largest, strongest muscles to do the job. Your strongest muscles are in your legs and arms. Your weakest muscles are in your back and abdomen.

Practice the principles of good body mechanics until they become a habit. They will make your job easier and prevent fatigue by making the best use of your strength and energy. Use of proper body mechanics helps prevent injury to the nursing assistant and resident.

Posture

Good posture is the foundation on which proper body mechanics is built. Good posture is the same whether you are standing, sitting, or lying down. Keep your back straight with your feet flat on the floor and your weight distributed evenly on both feet. The feet should be at least 12 inches apart to maintain a wide base of support. Your knees should be bent slightly and your arms should be at your sides **(Figure 8-1)**.

Back Support Belts. Use a back support belt **(Figure 8-2)** if this is your preference or the

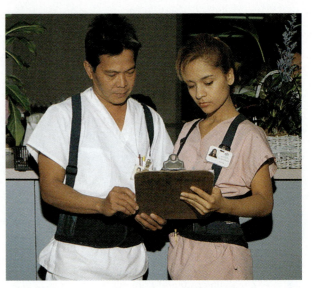

FIGURE 8-2 A back support belt reminds you to use good body mechanics. It does not make you stronger.

policy of your facility. Back injuries are very common in health care workers. Many nursing assistants feel better if they are wearing the belt for support. Several studies have shown that workers using the back support have fewer back injuries. Other studies have shown that there is no difference in the rate of injuries. The belt reminds you to keep your back straight and to use good body mechanics. Remember that wearing the back support belt does not make you stronger, and you should not lift more weight than you would if you were not wearing the belt. Using improper body mechanics when wearing the belt is difficult. For this reason alone, the belt may prove beneficial. You are less likely to become injured if you are using good body mechanics.

ERGONOMICS

Ergonomics is a method of fitting the job to the worker. When the job and the worker do not match, physical injuries can result. Ergonomic hazards are workplace conditions that place biomechanical stress on the worker. Examples of hazards are improper work methods, improper equipment, poor posture, force, repetition, and inadequate work-rest regimens.

Two types of injuries commonly affect the nursing assistant. **Instantaneous injuries** are injuries that occur suddenly and without warning, such as in an accident. An example of an instantaneous injury is a fall. **Cumulative trauma**

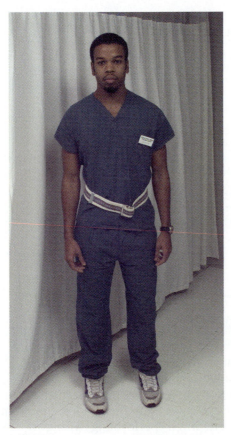

FIGURE 8-1 Good standing posture

GUIDELINES FOR

Using Good Body Mechanics

- Keep your back straight.
- Your feet should be at least 12 inches apart.
- Use the large muscles in your legs when lifting residents or heavy objects.
- Bend from the hips and knees, never from the waist.
- Face your work. Avoid twisting at the waist. If you must turn, pivot instead.
- If you must turn or change direction, take a few short steps. Turn your entire body instead of twisting your back or neck.
- Squat when lifting heavy objects from the floor.
- Keep heavy objects as close to your body as possible when lifting, moving, and carrying.
- Use both hands when lifting and moving heavy objects.
- Push, pull, or slide heavy objects instead of lifting them whenever possible. Use your body weight to help you.
- Use smooth, even movements instead of quick, jerking motions.
- Avoid unnecessary bending and reaching.

- Check the care plan before moving residents. The care plan often provides individualized instructions for moving, positioning, and transferring each resident.
- Always use a **transfer belt** for moving residents from one place to another, unless **contraindicated.** A transfer belt is a heavy canvas belt used for lifting and moving residents. The same belt is also called a **gait belt** when it is used for walking residents. Contraindicated means the belt should not be used for moving a resident because of a specific medical condition.
- Ask for help from others if you are not sure whether you can move a resident or lift an object.
- Use mechanical lifting devices for moving heavy residents.
- When giving bedside care, raise the height of the bed to a comfortable height for your body so you will not have to bend at the waist. When finished, remember to lower the bed to the lowest horizontal position.
- Avoid lifting heavy objects that are above your shoulder height.

disorders are bodily injuries to nerves, tissues, tendons, and joints that occur from repeated stress and strain over a period of months to years. Cumulative trauma disorders are caused by performing repetitious tasks, using muscular force to perform a job, doing heavy lifting without assistance, poor posture, standing in awkward positions, and inadequate rest.

Back injuries are common in workers who lift and move residents frequently. Using the principles of body mechanics will help protect you from injury. Good posture is very important as well. Use mechanical lifting devices and transfer belts for moving residents whenever possible. If the resident is not able to assist with the transfer in any way, always ask another nursing assistant to help you. Raising the height of the bed to a comfortable working height when you are performing bedside procedures is an important method of protecting your back. Avoid placing stress on your body whenever possible. Use a cart to transport heavy objects instead of carrying them. Do a job at waist height instead of bending or reaching up and down. Pivot to reach an object instead of twisting from the waist. Squat instead of bending. Always use good body mechanics when standing, lifting, moving, and turning.

PRESSURE ULCERS

The skin is the largest organ of the body, and it performs many vital functions. The skin protects the body from infection and injury. If the skin is broken, pain results, and there is an increased risk of infection. The skin also removes waste products, water, and salt through sweat. At certain places the skin joins with mucous membranes that line openings into body cavities. Some of these areas are covered with hair. The hair is a natural defense of the body to trap invading microbes and prevent them from entering. The hair and nails are considered part of the skin system.

One of the primary purposes of moving and positioning residents is to prevent **pressure ulcers.** Pressure ulcers may appear on the skin in areas where the skin is close to an underlying bone. They are the result of prolonged pressure, moisture, and other irritants. Older terms you may hear to refer to pressure ulcers are **pressure sores, bedsores, decubitus ulcers,** or **decubiti.** These areas usually develop as the result of pressure over **bony prominences,** or areas where the bone is close to the skin. **Figure 8-3** shows common sites for pressure ulcer development. Pressure ulcers can also develop in other areas if tubing or clothing is constricting, pressing, or

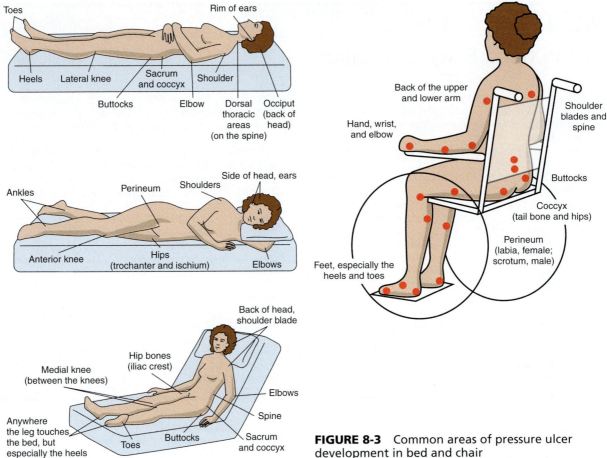

FIGURE 8-3   Common areas of pressure ulcer development in bed and chair

rubbing on the skin. Ulcers are the result of inadequate blood and oxygen flow to an area of the body. They can develop in a short time and will quickly cause tissue destruction. Residents can develop pressure ulcers while lying in bed or sitting in a chair. Pressure ulcers are painful and heal slowly. Infections and other complications may develop. They are much easier to prevent than they are to treat.

Risk Factors for Pressure Ulcers

Pressure ulcers are a very serious complication of immobility that should be prevented at all costs. Understanding the contributing causes and risk factors for pressure ulcers will help you prevent them. Many residents are identified as being at high risk of developing pressure ulcers by the minimum data set (MDS) and various assessments completed by nurses. A preventive care plan is always started when a resident is known to be at high risk. The presence of a risk factor does not make deterioration or development of a condition inevitable; rather, it is a "red flag" to staff that a serious complication or condition *may* develop. When one or more risk factors are present, staff is expected to plan and implement aggressive preventive care appropriate to the potential problem. Remember that OBRA requires facilities to maintain or improve residents' conditions whenever possible. Pressure ulcers are declines. If ulcers are present at the time of admission, the facility is expected to heal them. If the resident's skin is clear, it should remain clear. Pressure ulcers are considered unavoidable only when the resident has a medical condition that increases the risk of skin breakdown, and the:

- Resident has been accurately assessed.
- Risk of skin breakdown has been accurately assessed, and is adequately addressed in the care plan.
- Care plan is actually implemented.
- Interventions are evaluated periodically and modified according to the resident's responses to the plan of care.

When these factors are analyzed honestly, we find that most pressure ulcers are preventable.

Unfortunately, some residents slip through the cracks and their risks are not identified accurately or promptly, if at all. Serious skin breakdown can occur in a surprisingly brief period of time. Sometimes residents' conditions change quickly and breakdown occurs before the risk assessment is updated. Generally speaking, residents with low risk scores are at greater risk for developing pressure ulcers if they become ill, because no preventive plan of care is in place for them. If a resident who normally moves about independently suddenly becomes ill, he or she can develop a pressure ulcer rapidly. Thus, you must have a basic understanding of risk factors and take steps to prevent skin breakdown. Report to the nurse promptly if you feel there has been a change in a resident's condition. Tight and constricting clothing reduces oxygen and nutrients to the skin. Pressure does the same thing by reducing blood flow and nourishment. Tissues that are starved for oxygen become painful and begin to die. The full extent of the damage may not be immediately visible until the deep tissue ulcerates and sloughs off, leaving a large, deep crater in the resident's skin. An alert staff will recognize the potential danger and implement a preventive plan promptly.

Risk factors for pressure ulcer development are:

- Having a current pressure ulcer or a history of healed pressure ulcers
- Diabetes, peripheral vascular disease, edema of the feet and legs, or conditions such as stroke, in which extremities are paralyzed or sensation is impaired
- Being bedfast, chairfast, or unable to move and turn independently
- Weight loss, inadequate nutrition
- Poor fluid intake, dehydration
- Underweight (very thin) or overweight
- Skin that is dry, is thin, tears, or bleeds easily
- Confusion or coma
- Inability to communicate
- Bowel and/or bladder incontinence
- Contractures
- Restraint use

Exposure to moisture, powder, friction, shearing, chemicals, secretions, excretions, and other irritants also influences pressure ulcer development. Friction occurs when the skin rubs against another surface. Skin damage is worsened by rapid movement. Friction and shearing occur readily when residents are pulled up in a bed or chair. These minor injuries rapidly turn into pressure ulcers.

Stages of Pressure Ulcer Development

Pressure ulcers are staged according to their severity **(Figure 8-4)**. If a pressure ulcer is detected in the early stages of development, it can be prevented from worsening.

- Stage I pressure ulcers **(Figure 8-5)** begin as red areas. The redness does not go away within 30 minutes after pressure has been relieved. In a dark-skinned person, a Stage I pressure ulcer begins as a dark blue or black area on the skin. The skin is not broken in a Stage I area.
- Stage II pressure ulcers **(Figure 8-6)** are blistered or open areas. They are shallow and involve part of the top layer of skin.
- Stage III pressure ulcers **(Figure 8-7)** are areas in which the entire layer of skin is lost and the subcutaneous fat and muscle are exposed.
- Stage IV pressure ulcers **(Figure 8-8)** involve destruction of the entire top layer of skin. Damage extends through the fat into the muscle, tendon, and bone.

Prevention of Pressure Ulcers

Keeping pressure off the skin over bony prominences is the best and most important way to prevent pressure ulcers. This is done by proper positioning, padding, and moving the resident frequently. Good nutrition and hydration play important roles in keeping the body healthy and preventing skin breakdown. This will be discussed in more detail in Chapter 13. Pressure ulcers are a leading cause of lawsuits against long-term care facilities. Pressure ulcers are declines that must be prevented. Remember that the nursing assistant has an important responsibility in the prevention of pressure ulcers. Take this responsibility seriously!

Observation and Reporting

In the early stages, pressure ulcers are quite painful because the nerve endings in the skin are exposed. Early detection and treatment of pressure ulcers will prevent the areas from worsening. If the resident presently has, or has previously had, a pressure ulcer, consider this a high risk factor for further breakdown and use aggressive preventive measures. Immediately report to the nurse if you discover a red area

Stage I: Nonblanchable erythema of intact skin, the heralding lesion of skin ulceration. In individuals with darker skin, discoloration of the skin, warmth, edema, induration, or hardness may also be indicators.

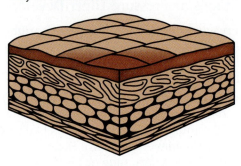

Stage II: Partial-thickness skin loss involving epidermis, dermis, or both. The ulcer is superficial and presents clinically as an abrasion, blister, or shallow crater.

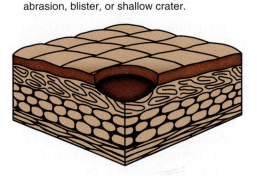

Stage III: Full-thickness skin loss involving damage to or necrosis of subcutaneous tissue that may extend down to, but not through, underlying fascia. The ulcer presents clinically as a deep crater with or without undermining of adjacent tissue.

Stage IV: Full-thickness skin loss with extensive destruction, tissue necrosis, or damage to muscle, bone, or supporting structures (e.g., tendon, joint capsule). Undermining and sinus tracts also may be associated with Stage IV pressure ulcers.

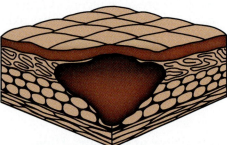

FIGURE 8-4   The pressure ulcer stages reflect the amount of tissue destruction.

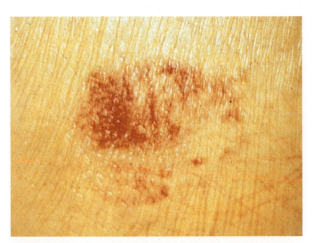

FIGURE 8-5   Stage I pressure ulcer. *(Permission to reproduce this copyrighted material has been granted by the owner, Hollister, Incorporated.)*

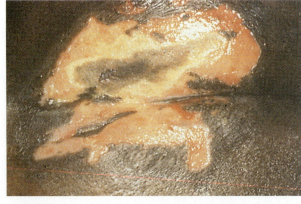

FIGURE 8-6   Stage II pressure ulcer. *(Permission to reproduce this copyrighted material has been granted by the owner, Hollister, Incorporated.)*

that does not go away after the pressure has been removed for 30 minutes. Also report blisters, **abrasions** (scrapes that rub off the skin surface), open areas, bruises, areas of pain, or areas that appear discolored.

POSITIONING RESIDENTS

The nursing assistant positions residents frequently throughout the day. You will use good posture and good body mechanics when performing these procedures. In addition, position-

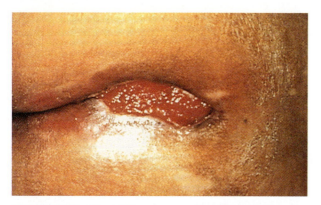

FIGURE 8-7 Stage III pressure ulcer. *(Permission to reproduce this copyrighted material has been granted by the owner, Hollister, Incorporated.)*

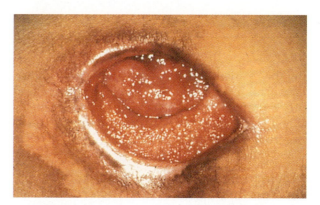

FIGURE 8-8 Stage IV pressure ulcer. *(Permission to reproduce this copyrighted material has been granted by the owner, Hollister, Incorporated.)*

GUIDELINES FOR
Prevention of Pressure Ulcers

- Turn the resident at least every two hours, and more often if necessary. Follow the care plan and the resident's individual turning schedule.
- Encourage residents who are able to move to reposition themselves frequently to relieve pressure.
- Teach residents who are seated in chairs to shift their weight every 15 minutes, if physically able, to relieve pressure.
- Residents who are sitting in chairs should also be moved and repositioned at least every two hours.
- Keep the skin clean and dry. Excessive moisture promotes skin breakdown.
- Avoid using very hot water to bathe residents.
- Use nonirritating soap to bathe residents.
- Rinse the skin well after using soap. Soap residue promotes irritation and skin breakdown.
- Avoid using powder and corn starch, which can be irritating to the skin.
- If the resident does not have control of bowel or bladder, wash the resident well with soap and water or a facility-approved cleansing agent after each episode of incontinence. Rinse the skin well. Urine and stool are very irritating to the skin.
- Use facility-approved moisturizing lotions on residents who have dry skin. Skin that is supple and well hydrated will not break as easily as dry skin.
- Keep bed linens crumb- and wrinkle-free. The pressure from wrinkles and crumbs can cause skin breakdown.
- Use lifting sheets to move residents in bed whenever possible, to avoid **friction** and **shearing.** Friction is rubbing the skin against another surface, such as bed linen. Excess friction in moving residents can cause abrasions, which can quickly worsen into pressure ulcers. Shearing **(Figure 8-9)** occurs when the skin moves in one direction while the underlying bones move in the opposite direction. The skin is stretched between the sheet (or other surface) on the outside and the bone on the inside.
- Use pressure-relieving pads in bed and chair.
- Pad areas of the resident's body where the skin or bones rub together.
- Use pillows, pads, and other props to maintain the resident's position.
- Inspect the resident's skin daily when bathing, dressing, and undressing. Report abnormal findings to the nurse.

- Check the skin folds under the breasts, abdomen, and groin for signs of redness or irritation. Dry these areas well after bathing.
- Follow the directions on the care plan for preventive skin care.
- Avoid elevating the head of the bed more than 45 degrees, to prevent shearing. If the head of the bed is elevated for any reason, help the resident change positions frequently to prevent pressure on the buttocks and hip area.
- Provide adequate nutrition to meet the resident's calorie and protein needs. Provide adequate fluids. Provide oral nourishments, supplements, and snacks as ordered.
- Wear gloves and apply the principles of standard precautions if contact with blood, moist body fluids (except sweat), secretions, excretions, mucous membranes, or nonintact skin is likely.

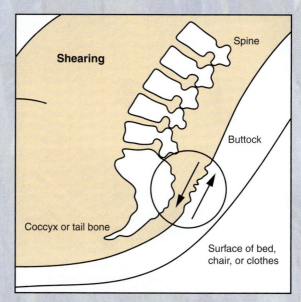

FIGURE 8-9 Shearing occurs when the skin is pulled in one direction while the underlying bone moves in the opposite direction. Many pressure ulcers develop because of shearing.

ing the resident in good alignment is very important. This means that the spine is straight and other parts of the body are in good position. When the resident is positioned correctly, function of the body systems is improved.

Moving and Positioning Devices for Comfort and Pressure Relief

Sometimes common devices are used to help you move and position residents. These devices make your job easier and the resident more comfortable. Some devices are used to help you physically turn the resident. These include the **draw sheet** and turning pads. The draw sheet is a half sheet placed horizontally across the center of the bed. Pulling the fabric on the sheet or pad is easier for you than pulling the resident. The bed positioning system **(Figure 8-10)** is similar to using a draw sheet. You pull the resident toward you, then place a long bolster to help maintain the position. Using these devices prevents accidental injury to the resident's skin and trauma to muscles, bones, and joints. The turning pad can be secured to the side rails after the move is completed to maintain the resident's position.

Foam wedges **(Figure 8-11)** are used to keep the resident in good alignment in bed. Sometimes residents will slip, move, or turn

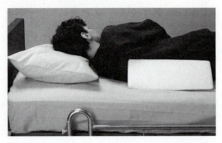

FIGURE 8-11   The foam wedge is used to support body parts and promote good alignment. *(Courtesy of Skil-Care Corporation, Yonkers, NY (800) 431-2972)*

themselves after you have positioned them. Use of the foam wedge as a prop will help maintain the resident's position. They are also useful in preventing pressure ulcers.

Pillows may also be used to position residents. They are sometimes used when the resident is in a side-lying position, to prevent rolling over to the back. Small, flat pillows or a bath blanket may also be used as pads to prevent the knees and ankles from rubbing together when the resident is lying on his or her side. Commercial devices **(Figure 8-12)** are also available for this purpose. Pillows are also used to support the forearms and may be placed under the knees when the resident is lying on his or her back. Using pillows for positioning helps the resident feel more comfortable and secure. Sheepskins **(Figure 8-13)** are synthetic devices that can be used for padding bony areas. They may also be placed on the bed to promote resident comfort and prevent friction and shearing. Heel and elbow protectors **(Figures 8-14A and 8-14B)** also increase resident comfort and prevent friction and shearing. They do not relieve pressure.

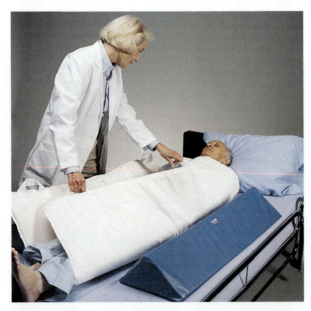

FIGURE 8-10   The bed positioning system is used for moving the resident. The positioning pad is inserted to maintain position, then Velcro fasteners are used to attach the pad to the bolster cushion. *(Courtesy of Skil-Care Corporation, Yonkers, NY (800) 431-2972)*

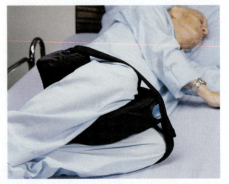

FIGURE 8-12   Keeping the legs apart will prevent pressure ulcers at the knees and ankles. The pad may also be used after some surgical procedures to position the legs. *(Courtesy of Skil-Care Corporation, Yonkers, NY (800) 431-2972)*

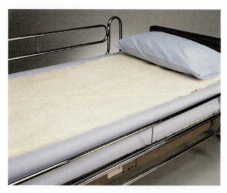

FIGURE 8-13 The sheepskin is used to prevent friction and shearing caused by skin surfaces rubbing against each other or against the sheet. It does not reduce pressure. *(Courtesy of Skil-Care Corporation, Yonkers, NY (800) 431-2972)*

A resident who is using a pressure-relieving pad or device still requires turning. Although some pressure is relieved, the devices do not remove it entirely, so further breakdown is possible. Commonly used pressure-relieving devices include:

- Foam heel elevators **(Figure 8-15)**
- Foam wedges, squares, and other foam pads
- Special foam, gel, air, and water mattresses, cushions, and overlays

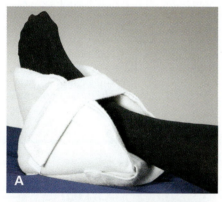

FIGURE 8-14 (A) Heel protectors and (B) elbow protectors are used to relieve pressure and prevent friction and shearing caused by rubbing against the linen. *(Courtesy of Skil-Care Corporation, Yonkers, NY (800) 431-2972)*

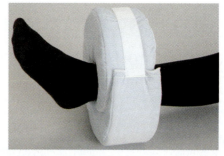

FIGURE 8-15 Foam heel elevators keep the heels off the surface of the bed, relieving all pressure. *(Courtesy of Skil-Care Corporation, Yonkers, NY (800) 431-2972)*

- Low air loss and other therapeutic beds **(Figure 8-16)**
- Other devices used by your facility.

Side rail pads **(Figure 8-17)** may be used for residents who are restless or have seizures, or diseases that cause involuntary movement of the arms and legs. The pads prevent the resident from striking or slipping through the rails, causing injury.

The **bed cradle** is used to keep the weight of the bedding off the resident's skin. This device is made of metal or plastic and fastens to the bed

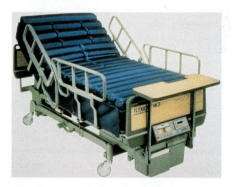

FIGURE 8-16 Low air loss and other therapeutic beds are used for residents with serious skin problems. *(Courtesy of Hill-Rom)*

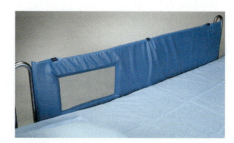

FIGURE 8-17 Side rail pads prevent serious injury. *(Courtesy of Skil-Care Corporation, Yonkers, NY (800) 431-2972)*

GUIDELINES FOR
Moving and Positioning Residents

- Evaluate the resident's ability to participate in the procedure. This involves the ability to follow directions and the ability to move, considering physical limitations.
- Ask another nursing assistant to help you if the resident is heavy, **combative** (hits or fights), unable to follow directions, unable to assist with the move, or larger than you are, or if you are unsure of your ability to move the resident alone.
- Know and follow your facility policies for positioning. In some facilities, a doctor's order is required to use certain positions.
- Consult the care plan or the nurse for specific turning and positioning instructions.
- Some facilities use "turn schedules," which specify designated positions at certain times for the resident. Follow the individual turn schedule for each resident.
- Use good body mechanics.
- Encourage residents to participate in care to the extent of their ability. Before beginning the procedure, make sure that residents understand what is expected and how to do it.
- Draw sheets, lifting sheets, and similar devices should be used whenever possible to avoid friction, shearing, and pulling on the resident's skin. Using a lift sheet to move residents helps prevent back strain for the nursing assistant as well.
- Use mechanical lifting devices, if needed.
- Use smooth, easy motions. Do not tug or jerk the resident over quickly.
- Avoid trauma and injury to the resident during the procedure.
- Use pillows, props, or other devices to maintain position, if necessary.
- Pad bony areas, such as between the knees and ankles, to prevent discomfort and skin breakdown caused by the skin surfaces rubbing together.

- Position the resident in good body alignment. The spine should be straight and supported. Sometimes residents curl up into a **fetal position** (turned on the side with the head tucked down and knees drawn up) to stay warm, or because they are in pain. If possible, identify the cause of the problem and correct it. Lying in this position for a prolonged period of time greatly increases the risk of complications. If you discover a method of positioning that reduces a resident's use of the fetal position, inform the nurse so the information can be added to the care plan.
- Support the arms, legs, or back with pillows, if needed for resident comfort. Special supportive devices may be listed on the care plan to maintain good body alignment. If so, make sure they are in place.
- Avoid tucking in the top linen too tightly. This pushes the feet downward, increasing the risk of deformities.
- If you are using a new position with a resident for the first time, check the resident frequently to be sure the position will be well tolerated.
- Monitor the location of catheters and tubing and avoid pulling them or accidentally dislodging them. After the move, position them correctly so they are not obstructed and do not put pressure on skin.
- Change the resident's position at least every two hours, and more often if indicated.
- Accurately document turning and repositioning on the flow sheet, or according to facility policy. Avoid documenting in advance. Do not document care that you did not provide. Documentation of turning and positioning residents is very important. Accurate documentation verifies that care was given as ordered, and according to the plan of care.

to provide a frame. When the resident is in bed, the sheet and blanket are placed over the top of the cradle.

A wooden or plastic **foot board** may be used at the end of the mattress. A foot board is used to prevent pressure on the heels and to keep the feet upright so deformities do not develop. When a foot board is used, the heels hang over the end of the mattress and the sole of the foot rests against the board. Other devices are available that perform the same function as the foot board. These are applied directly to the resident's foot. Supportive devices to prevent deformities are discussed in more detail in Chapter 18.

BASIC BODY POSITIONS

Four basic body positions are used for positioning residents in bed. These are the **supine** (face up), **lateral** (side-lying), **Fowler's** (semisitting), and **prone** (lying on the abdomen) positions. The semiprone and semisupine positions are variations of these positions and are excellent for relieving pressure and preventing pressure ulcers. Fowler's position also has several variations. Variations in Fowler's position are determined by the height of the head of the bed. Special positions may be used if the resident has special medical needs. The care plan and the nurse will provide specific instructions if special positioning is necessary.

PROCEDURE 12
Moving the Resident to the Side of the Bed

1. Perform your beginning procedure actions.
2. Cross the resident's arms over the chest.
3. Place your upper hand, palm side up, under the resident's shoulders.
4. Place your lower hand, palm side up, under the mid back.
5. Lift the upper part of the body toward the near side of the bed.
6. Place your hands under the resident's waist and thighs.
7. Lift the middle section of the body toward the near side of the bed.
8. Place your hands under the thighs and lower legs and lift them toward you.
9. Perform your procedure completion actions.

PROCEDURE 13
Turning the Resident on the Side Toward You

1. Perform your beginning procedure actions.
2. Move the resident to the opposite side of the bed, if necessary, following the guidelines in Procedure 12.
3. Cross the resident's arms over the chest.
4. Cross the leg farthest away from you over the near leg.
5. Place your top hand behind the resident's far shoulder. Place your bottom hand on the resident's hip **(Figure 8-18A).**
6. Instruct the resident to assist with the move by pulling on the side rail with the far hand, according to the plan of care, and as able. Keep your feet and knees separated to maintain a wide base of support. Brace your body against the side of the bed. Roll the resident toward you.
7. Raise the side rail and move to the opposite side of the bed.
8. Lower the side rail.
9. Place your hands under the resident's bottom shoulder and pull back slightly toward the center of the bed. The resident should not be lying directly on the shoulder. Repeat this action for the resident's hips **(Figure 8-18B).**
10. Roll a pillow or place a positioning device behind the resident's back to maintain the position, if necessary.
11. Raise the side rail and return to the opposite side of the bed.
12. Lower the rail.

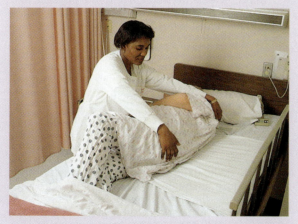

FIGURE 8-18A Place one hand on the shoulder and the other on the hip.

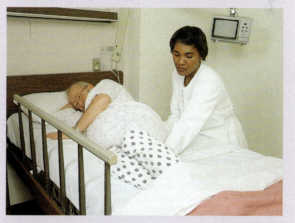

FIGURE 8-18B Pull the shoulder and hip back slightly so the resident is not lying directly on them.

Continues

13. Bend the resident's knees slightly. The upper leg should be positioned slightly ahead of the lower leg. Place a pillow or folded bath blanket from the knees to the ankles to keep the legs from rubbing together **(Figure 8-18C)**.
14. Place a pillow under the resident's upper arm, if necessary, for support.
15. Check the lower arm to be sure it is not under the resident. If the resident is not able to move the arm, place it in a position of comfort at the side of the body or bent at the elbow with the hand by the head. Make sure the resident's body is in good alignment.
16. Perform your procedure completion actions.

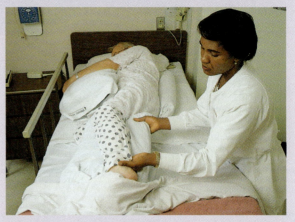

FIGURE 8-18C Place a pillow or pad between the legs for comfort and to prevent pressure.

PROCEDURE

14

Turning the Resident
on the Side Toward You
with a Lift Sheet

 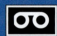

1. Arrange for another assistant to help you, as needed.
2. Perform your beginning procedure actions.
3. Make sure that a draw sheet or large pad is in place from the resident's shoulders to the knees. If not, turn the resident on the side facing you, following the guidelines in Procedure 12. Your assistant should put the draw sheet in position, then roll it in toward the resident's body.
4. Ask your assistant to turn the resident toward him or her, following the guidelines in Procedure 12. Pull the end of the lifting sheet to your side of the bed.
5. Coordinate the move with your assistant to prevent friction and shearing. Obtain additional help if necessary.
6. On a signal, use the sheet to move the resident to the far side of the bed, to provide enough space for the turn.
7. Cross the resident's arms over the chest.
8. Cross the leg farthest away from you over the near leg.
9. Roll the lifting sheet inward on the opposite side of the resident, so it is close to the body. Place your top hand on the sheet behind the resident's far shoulder. Place your bottom hand on the sheet near the resident's hip. Keep your feet and knees separated to maintain a wide base of support. Brace your body against the side of the bed.
10. Pull on the sheet to roll the resident toward you. *Note:* An alternate method is to position one hand on the resident's shoulder and the other on the

hip. On a signal, turn the resident toward you while the other nursing assistant uses the lift sheet to roll the resident.
11. Raise the side rail and move to the opposite side of the bed. (If present, the second nursing assistant performs steps 13 and 14).
12. Lower the side rail.
13. Place your hands under the resident's bottom shoulder and pull back slightly toward the center of the bed. The resident should not be lying directly on the shoulder. Repeat this action for the resident's hips.
14. Grasp the draw sheet on the opposite side of the resident at the hips and shoulders. Hold the resident on the side facing you while the second nursing assistant rolls a pillow or places a positioning device behind the resident's back (under the draw sheet) to maintain the position, if necessary. Straighten the sheet to remove wrinkles.
15. Bend the resident's knees slightly. Position the upper leg slightly ahead of the lower leg. Place a small, flat pillow or folded bath blanket from the knees to the ankles to keep the legs from rubbing together.
16. Place a pillow under the resident's upper arm, if necessary, for support.
17. Check the lower arm to be sure it is not under the resident. If the resident is not able to move the arm, place it in a position of comfort at the side of the body, or bent at the elbow with the hand by the head.
18. Perform your procedure completion actions.

PROCEDURE 15 — Turning the Resident on the Side Away from You

 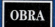

1. Perform your beginning procedure actions.
2. Move the resident to the side of the bed, if necessary, following the guidelines in Procedure 12.
3. Bend the resident's far arm at the elbow, so the hand is near the head. Cross the near arm over the chest.
4. Cross the near leg over the far leg.
5. Place your top hand on the resident's shoulder and your bottom hand on the hip. Turn the resident on the side facing away from you.
6. Roll a pillow or place a positioning device behind the resident's back to maintain the position, if necessary.
7. Raise the side rail and move to the opposite side of the bed.
8. Lower the side rail.
9. Bend the resident's knees slightly. The upper leg should be positioned slightly ahead of the lower leg. Place a pillow or folded bath blanket between the knees, calves, and ankles to keep them from rubbing together.
10. Place a pillow under the resident's upper arm, if necessary, for support.
11. Check the lower arm to be sure it is not under the resident.
12. Perform your procedure completion actions.

PROCEDURE 16 — Assisting the Resident to Move to the Head of the Bed

1. Perform your beginning procedure actions.
2. Lower the head of the bed.
3. Remove the pillow and place it against the headboard.
4. Instruct the resident to bend the knees and place the feet flat on the bed. The arms should be at the sides with elbows bent.
5. Place your top arm under the shoulders.
6. Place your bottom arm under the hips.
7. On the count of three, instruct the resident to push up with the elbows and feet while you lift.
8. Replace the pillow and straighten the bed linen.
9. Perform your procedure completion actions.

PROCEDURE 17 — Moving the Resident to the Head of the Bed with a Lifting (Draw) Sheet

1. Ask another nursing assistant to assist you.
2. Perform your beginning procedure actions.
3. Lower the head of the bed.
4. Lower the side rails.
5. Remove the pillow and place it against the headboard.
6. Roll the lift sheet inward until it touches the resident's body **(Figure 8-19).**
7. Grasp the lift sheet with your top hand at the level of the resident's shoulder and your bottom hand at the hip.
8. Face the head of the bed. On the count of three, shift your weight from the rear foot to the front foot and lift the resident toward the head of the bed.
9. Replace the pillow.
10. Straighten the lift sheet.
11. Perform your procedure completion actions.

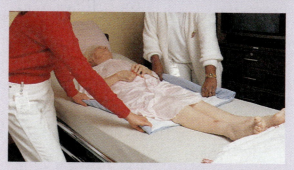

FIGURE 8-19 Roll the lift sheet inward until it touches the resident's body.

PROCEDURE 18

Moving the Resident Up in Bed with One Assistant

OBRA

1. Ask another nursing assistant to help you.
2. Perform your beginning procedure actions.
3. Lower the head of the bed.
4. Lower the side rails.
5. Remove the pillow and place it against the headboard.
6. Place your top arm under the resident's shoulders and your bottom arm under the resident's hips. Your assistant should do the same.
7. Grasp arms with your assistant.
8. Face the head of the bed. On the count of three, shift your weight from the rear foot to the front foot and lift the resident toward the head of the bed.
9. Replace the pillow.
10. Perform your procedure completion actions.

Supine Position

The resident in the supine position **(Figure 8-20)** is lying on the back. This position may be preferred for sleeping. When the body is in good alignment, the resident's head and shoulders are supported on a pillow. The spine is straight. The arms are at the sides. They may be supported on pillows for comfort. The legs are straight. A pillow may be placed behind the knees for comfort. The feet are upright. A foot board or other supportive device may be used at the end of the bed.

Semisupine Position

The **semisupine position** **(Figure 8-21)** is also called the tilt position. It should not be confused with the lateral position. The resident in this position is not lying directly on the side. When correctly used, this position relieves pressure from all bony prominences. The spine is straight and the resident is positioned so that he or she is leaning against a pillow for support. Both legs are straight. The top leg is slightly behind the bottom leg. A pillow is placed under the top leg to keep it even with the hip joint. The lower shoulder is pulled slightly forward so that pressure is distributed over the back, not the shoulder joint. The arms can be at the sides or folded across the abdomen. Support the arms on pillows for comfort.

Prone Position

The resident in the prone position **(Figure 8-22)** is lying on the abdomen. Some elderly residents cannot tolerate this position. Some facilities do not use the prone position without a physician's order. Know and follow your facility policy. When using the position for the first time, remain in the room for the first 15 minutes to make sure the resident tolerates the position without distress. After this, routinely check every 15 minutes to be sure the resident continues to tolerate the position and is not having difficulty breathing. Make sure the call signal or a manual bell is close to the resident's dominant hand.

When positioning the resident in the prone position, turn the head to one side. A small, flat pillow may be used under the head. Additional padding may be used under the shoulders if they

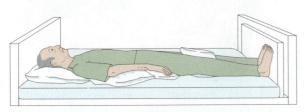

FIGURE 8-20 When the resident is in the supine position, pillows may be placed behind the knees and under the arms for comfort.

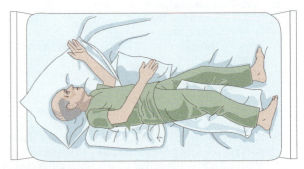

FIGURE 8-21 The semisupine position is a very comfortable position that relieves pressure from all major bony prominences.

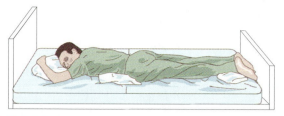

FIGURE 8-22 Check the resident frequently when using the prone position.

roll forward. The arms should be along the sides, or one arm bent so the hand is next to the head. Both arms should not be up, as this strains the shoulder muscles. Another flat pillow may be placed under the abdomen for comfort. The spine is straight. The legs are straight. The feet should be positioned so the toes are between the mattress and the end of the bed. A small pad may be used to keep pressure off the ankles.

The Semiprone Position

The **semiprone position** (Figure 8-23) is the opposite of the semisupine position. It is a very comfortable position for the resident. Like the semisupine position, it eliminates pressure on the major areas of pressure ulcer formation. To place the resident in the semiprone position, begin by placing the resident prone. Lift the resident's chest and shoulder closest to you and place a pillow under them.

If the resident has had a stroke, put the affected (paralyzed) side on top, if possible. Support the affected arm on a pillow, in a position of function with the elbow bent. Position the opposite arm behind the resident. Fold a second pillow in half and place it under the top leg. Check to make sure the legs and spine are straight, and the pelvis is not twisted. Check the hip to make sure the resident is not lying on it. Position a pillow lengthwise under the resident

from the chest to the abdomen. Support the upper leg on a pillow. Turn the resident's head to either side and place it on a small, flat pillow. Avoid a large, fluffy pillow, which may inhibit the resident's breathing.

Follow your facility policies for using the semiprone position. Like the prone position, some facilities require a doctor's order for this position. When using this position for the first time, remain in the room for the first 15 minutes to be sure the resident tolerates the position without respiratory distress. After that, check the resident at least every 15 minutes to make sure he or she is not having trouble breathing. Position the call signal close to the resident's unaffected (good) hand.

Lateral Position

A resident in the lateral position **(Figure 8-24)** is lying on either side. The spine is straight. The bottom shoulder and hip are pulled slightly forward so that there is no pressure directly on the joint. A pillow may be rolled behind the back to hold the resident in this position. The arms can be positioned where they are most comfortable for the resident. Usually, the elbow of the bottom arm is flexed and the hand placed near the head. The upper arm is folded across the abdomen and supported on a pillow. The upper leg is flexed and pulled slightly ahead of the bottom leg. A pillow is used to support the upper leg and keep the knees from rubbing together.

Fowler's Position

A resident in Fowler's position is lying on the back with the head elevated. This position is used for residents who are receiving tube feedings, or having difficulty breathing. The knee of the bed may also be elevated slightly for

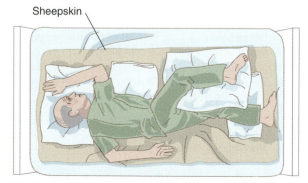

FIGURE 8-23 The semiprone position is very comfortable for the resident.

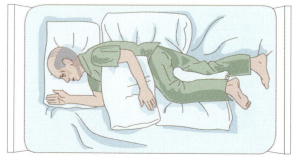

FIGURE 8-24 Use pillows to support the resident in the lateral position.

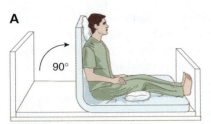
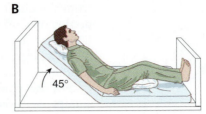
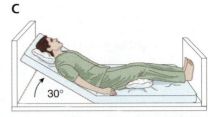

FIGURE 8-25 (A) High Fowler's position is used for meals and for residents who have difficulty breathing. (B) Fowler's position. (C) Semi-Fowler's position.

comfort. This position places extra pressure on the resident's buttocks and spine and increases the risk of pressure ulcer formation, so careful attention must be paid to skin care. You may be directed to position residents in three different Fowler's positions **(Figure 8-25):**

- High Fowler's position—the head of the bed is elevated 90 degrees
- Fowler's position—the head of the bed is elevated 45 degrees
- Low Fowler's position—the head of the bed is elevated 30 degrees

KEY POINTS

- Good body mechanics are used when lifting and moving residents and other heavy objects.
- Ergonomics is a method of fitting the job to the worker to prevent injuries.
- Residents must always be positioned in good body alignment.
- The primary cause of pressure ulcers is lack of oxygen and circulation to the skin, caused by pressure.
- Pressure ulcers are easier to prevent than to treat.
- Wearing a back support belt does not make you stronger; avoid lifting more weight than you would if you were not wearing the belt.
- Pressure ulcers are declines; most pressure ulcers are preventable.
- Residents with current pressure ulcers or a history of healed pressure ulcers are at high risk for additional skin breakdown.
- Documentation of turning and positioning residents is very important; accurate documentation verifies that care was given as ordered, and according to the plan of care.
- Lying in the fetal position for a long time greatly increases the risk of complications.
- Positioning residents in the semiprone and semisupine positions relieves pressure from all major bony prominences.

REVIEW

A. Multiple Choice

Select the one best answer.

1. Using your body correctly to do the job is good body
   a. maintenance.
   b. mechanisms.
   c. muscles.
   d. mechanics.

2. Your strongest muscles are in the
   a. back.
   b. abdomen.
   c. legs.
   d. shoulders.

3. Using your body correctly involves
   a. keeping your feet eight inches apart.
   b. using the strong muscles in your legs when lifting.
   c. lifting heavy objects instead of pushing them.
   d. bending from the waist and knees.

4. Which of the following is true about pressure ulcers?
   a. They are the result of inadequate blood and oxygen to the skin.
   b. Pressure ulcers take a long time to develop.
   c. Infections are not a consideration in preventing pressure ulcers.
   d. Pressure ulcers usually heal quickly.

5. A Stage II pressure ulcer may
   a. be a large, red area with intact skin.
   b. look like a blister or abrasion.
   c. involve the subcutaneous fat.
   d. involve muscle, tendon, and bone.

6. A Stage IV pressure ulcer
   a. is a large, red area with intact skin.
   b. looks like a blister or abrasion.
   c. involves only the top layer of skin.
   d. involves muscle, tendon, and bone.

7. A pressure ulcer in the early stages of development on a person with dark skin may appear
   a. black.
   b. pink.
   c. red.
   d. gray.

8. Which of the following measures prevents pressure ulcers?
   a. Turning the resident every four hours.
   b. Padding areas where bones and skin rub together.
   c. Using the Fowler's position.
   d. Positioning the resident on bony prominces.

9. When moving and positioning residents, the nursing assistant should *always*
   a. use the mechanical lift.
   b. use a gait belt.
   c. avoid friction and shearing.
   d. elevate the head of the bed.

10. Residents should be repositioned every
    a. two hours.
    b. three hours.
    c. four hours.
    d. shift.

11. Millie Davis is an obese, dependent resident. You are assigned to move her up in bed. Mrs. Davis has a pressure ulcer on her left hip. The best way to move her is to
    a. lift the resident by yourself.
    b. lift her on a draw sheet with one or more helpers.
    c. ask another assistant to lift the hips while you lift the feet.
    d. use a mechanical lift.

12. A resident in the supine position is lying
    a. face up.
    b. face down.
    c. on the abdomen.
    d. on the side.

13. A resident in the prone position is lying on the
    a. back.
    b. abdomen.
    c. left side.
    d. right side.

14. The nurse asks you to place Mr. Kay in Fowler's position while his tube feeding is running. You know the head of the bed should be elevated
    a. 15 degrees.
    b. 30 degrees.
    c. 45 degrees.
    d. 90 degrees.

15. The resident in the lateral position is lying
    a. face up.
    b. face down.
    c. with the head elevated.
    d. on the side.

B. Short-Answer

Answer the following questions.

16–20. List five methods the nursing assistant can use to prevent pressure ulcers.

16. _____   19. _____

17. _____   20. _____

18. _____

21–30. List 10 rules of good body mechanics.

21. _____   26. _____

22. _____   27. _____

23. _____   28. _____

24. _____   29. _____

25. _____   30. _____

C. Clinical Applications

Answer the following questions.

31. Martha Harris is an underweight, dependent resident. The care plan states that she is at high risk for skin breakdown and must be turned and repositioned every hour. It is very difficult to maintain Martha's position because she turns herself over onto her back as soon as you leave the room. You changed Martha's position at 9 a.m. When you left the room, she was on her right side. You got busy and forgot to return exactly at 10 a.m. When you returned at 10:30, Martha was lying on her back. When you turned her onto her left side, you noticed a very red area on her coccyx. What action should you take?

32. You must turn and reposition Mr. Taylor in bed. Mr. Taylor is very heavy and is more than six feet tall. He is unable to assist in the move. The care plan states to use a draw sheet to turn the resident, then place pillows behind his back for support. Mr. Taylor has slipped down in bed and needs to be moved up to the head of the bed before he is turned. What should you do?

33. You are assigned to position Mrs. Strong in the prone position. This position has never been used for the resident before. After you position the resident on her abdomen, what should you do next? How often should you check on her?

34. It is almost time to leave for the day when you discover that one of your assigned residents is wet and soiled. You change and clean the resident and discover a new open area that looks like a Stage II pressure ulcer. You did not notice the open area this morning. After cleaning the resident, you plan to report your observation to the nurse. The nurses are in report. Your ride is waiting outside. What action will you take?

35. You are assigned to give Mr. Walecki a shower. He has a loose dressing covering a pressure ulcer on his hip. The tape has fallen off two sides of the dressing. What action will you take?

CHAPTER 9

Assisting Residents with Mobility

OBJECTIVES

After reading this chapter, you will be able to:

- Demonstrate how to lift and move residents from one location to another using the rules of good body mechanics.
- Describe how to check the wheelchair to ensure it fits the resident properly.
- List at least eight guidelines for positioning residents in a chair or wheelchair.
- Describe how to prevent pressure ulcers in residents who are chairfast.
- List at least twelve guidelines for safe use of a wheelchair.
- Discuss how to transport a resident by wheelchair and by stretcher.
- Demonstrate how to assist residents with ambulation.
- Demonstrate procedures related to assisting residents with mobility.

OBSERVATIONS TO MAKE AND REPORT RELATED TO ASSISTING RESIDENTS WITH MOBILITY

Pain
Deformity
Edema
Immobility
Inability to move arms and legs
Inability to move one or more joints
Limited/abnormal range of motion
Shortening and external rotation of one leg in a
    resident with a history of fall

Sudden onset of falls, difficulty balancing
Jerking, tremors, shaky movements, muscle
    spasms
Weakness
Sensory changes, dizziness
Changes in ability to sit, stand, move, or walk
Pain upon movement
Changes in ability to assist with procedure

ASSISTING RESIDENTS WITH MOBILITY

The nursing assistant frequently helps **transfer** residents. A transfer is done to move a resident from one location to another. The procedures in this section involve helping residents to get out of bed. Make sure that your uniform fits loosely enough to allow you to lift and move residents without tearing or binding. As with the other procedures, use of good body mechanics and helping residents maintain proper body alignment in both bed and chair are very important.

Assisting Residents to Sit on the Side of the Bed

Sitting on the side of the bed with the legs over the edge of the mattress is called **dangling.** This is the first step to getting out of bed. Sitting on

PROCEDURE 19

Assisting the Resident to Sit Up on the Side of the Bed

1. Perform your beginning procedure actions.
2. Place the bed in the lowest horizontal position.
3. Elevate the head of the bed.
4. Assist the resident to move to the side of the bed closest to you.
5. Place your arm closest to the head under the resident's shoulders, palm side up.
6. Place your other arm under the resident's knees, palm side up.
7. Lift the back and knees up and pivot the resident so the legs are hanging over the side of the bed and the back is straight.
8. Help the resident maintain balance, if necessary.
9. If the resident will be getting out of bed, assist him or her to put on a robe and footwear appropriate to the floor surface.
10. Stay with the resident and observe for changes in color and moisture of the skin.
11. To return the resident to bed, reverse the procedure and pivot the resident back to the supine position.
12. Perform your procedure completion actions.

the side of the bed helps residents who have been lying down to balance before getting up. The resident may become dizzy after lying down for a long time. Dangling helps to equalize the system before the resident is transferred to the chair or begins to walk. The resident should sit in this position for a few minutes before getting up. This helps prevent fainting and loss of balance. Stay with the resident while dangling.

Monitor the skin for perspiration or pale color. If these changes occur, return the resident to the supine position and notify the nurse.

Assisting Residents Out of Bed

If the resident tolerates dangling without difficulty, the next step is to assist the resident out of bed. The nursing assistant should evaluate the

GUIDELINES FOR
Assisting Residents with Mobility

- Wear a back support belt if this is your preference or facility policy.
- Refer to the care plan or nurse for specific instructions.
- Explain the procedure to the resident. Before beginning the move, make sure the resident understands what is to be done and what is expected.
- Always use a transfer belt (unless contraindicated) to prevent injury to yourself and the resident.
- Adjust the bed to the lowest horizontal position. Elevate the head of the bed 90 degrees to make it easier for the resident to get up.
- Lock the brakes on beds, wheelchairs, lifts, stretchers, or other equipment before beginning the move.
- Use lifting devices, if needed.
- Make sure that mechanical lifts and other moving devices are in good working condition.
- When transferring a resident with a weak or paralyzed side, move toward the stronger side.
- Support the resident's weaker side during transfers.
- Be alert to catheters and other tubes so they are not accidentally pulled or removed.

- Have the resident wear footwear appropriate to the floor surface if standing during the transfer.
- Apply artificial limbs and braces correctly before transferring the resident.
- Make sure the resident's feet are firmly on the floor before standing.
- Avoid lifting the resident under the arms. This can cause pain, dislocation, and other injuries.
- The resident should never place hands or arms around your neck during the transfer.
- When ambulating residents, look for hazards on the floor and approach corners slowly, watching for approaching traffic.
- Check the tips of canes, crutches, and walkers. If they are worn through, do not use them.
- If you will be transferring the resident into a wheelchair, check the position of the small front wheels. The large part of the small wheels should be facing forward before you begin the transfer.

resident and check the care plan before moving the resident. Follow the directions for transfer on the care plan. If the resident is larger than you are, cannot follow directions, or is otherwise unable to help you with the transfer, ask another nursing assistant to help you.

Before beginning, explain the procedure to the resident. Tell him or her what is expected. Get feedback to make sure the resident understands. Use simple commands or counts to time your movements. For example, tell the resident, "We will move when I count to three," or, "We will move when I say lift." Moving simultaneously with the resident is important. This helps prevent injury to you and the resident.

Transferring the Resident into a Wheelchair

If you will be transferring the resident into a wheelchair, you must position the chair and lock the brakes before beginning the transfer. The footrests should be removed or pushed up and out of the way during the transfer. (If you remove the leg rests, make sure to replace them immediately upon completion of the procedure.) Before beginning the transfer, position the wheelchair at a 45° to 60° angle to the surface from which you are transferring. If the resident has a strong side, position the chair so the strongest leg moves toward the chair. Pay close attention to the small, front caster wheels of the wheelchair. These wheels provide the ability to move in all directions. The large part of the wheel faces back when the chair is moving. During transfers, position the large part of the small front wheels to face forward **(Figure 9-1)**. This changes the center of gravity of the chair and reduces the risk of tipping. To reposition the wheels, back the chair up, then move forward until the wheels are in good alignment, then lock the brakes.

The resident must be able to move to the side of the bed or front edge of the chair before standing, and for most transfers. Sitting in this position moves the resident's center of gravity over the base of support in the feet, making standing easier and safer. Several methods can be used for moving the resident forward. If he or she cannot scoot forward independently, the care plan will list the method to use.

The Transfer Belt

The transfer belt is a heavy canvas belt. In some facilities, each resident is given a belt

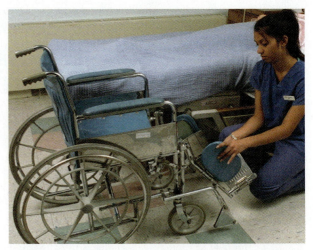

FIGURE 9-1 Prepare for the transfer by positioning the chair correctly at a 45° to 60° angle. Position the large part of the small front wheels facing forward. Lock the brakes. Move the footrests back or up and out of the way.

that is used only for that resident. Other facilities require the nursing assistant to wear the belt and use it to transfer all residents. Use of the transfer belt is safer for both you and the resident. It prevents pulling and tugging on the resident's skin. The belt makes it easier for you to move the resident and gives you control if the resident starts to slip or fall. The belt should be used for most routine transfers. Never use the belt on a pair of pants in place of a transfer belt.

Contraindications for use of the transfer belt. The transfer belt may be contraindicated in residents with some conditions. Facilities have different policies for use of the transfer belt. Know and follow your facility policy. Check with the nurse or the resident's care plan for specific instructions. In general, contraindications to use of the transfer belt are:

- A **colostomy,** a surgical procedure in which the colon is attached to the outside of the body and waste is eliminated into a plastic bag attached to the skin
- A **gastrostomy** tube, or feeding tube that is surgically inserted into the resident's stomach with the end extending through the side of the abdomen
- Recent abdominal surgery or a fresh surgical **incision** (cut in the skin made with a knife)
- Severe cardiac and respiratory disease
- Fractured ribs or vertebrae
- Pregnancy

GUIDELINES FOR
Using the Transfer (Gait) Belt

- The resident should be dressed before the belt is applied. Do not apply it over bare skin.
- Make sure the resident is wearing footwear appropriate to the surface of the floor. If you are unsure, check with the care plan or nurse. As a rule, nonslip soles are used in facilities with tile floors. Leather or plastic soles may be used on carpeting. The physical therapist will evaluate the resident to determine what type of sole is safest for the resident.
- The belt is placed around the waist and buckled in front.
- For a female resident, be sure the breasts are not under the belt.
- Thread the belt through the teeth side, then back through the opening on the other side so that it is double-locked **(Figure 9-2)**.
- Check the fit of the belt by placing three fingers under it. The belt should be snug, but there should be enough space for your fingers to fit comfortably.
- Before attempting to move the resident, be sure his or her feet are flat on the floor. If they are not, use the belt to assist the resident to the edge of the bed until the feet are resting firmly on the floor.
- If you are transferring a resident into or out of a wheelchair, the footrests should be out of the way during the transfer. After the resident is seated, the legs should not dangle. The feet are supported on the floor or on the wheelchair footrests.
- Teach the resident to assist by pushing off the bed with the hands when you count to three.

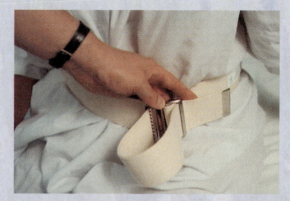

FIGURE 9-2 Threading the transfer belt through the teeth ensures that the belt will not slip during the transfer.

- Always hold the belt with an underhand grasp. For transfers, one hand should be on each side of the buckle in front.
- When the resident is standing, pivot to transfer.
- The chair should be close enough so the resident can feel the back of the chair with the hands after you pivot.
- The belt is removed after the resident is seated.
- Keep your belt clean. Wash it at least weekly, and whenever it becomes soiled.

- An abdominal **pacemaker.** This is a surgically implanted device that regulates the rate of the heartbeat. Most commonly, the pacemaker is implanted in the chest, but occasionally it is placed in the abdomen. You will see the shape of the device beneath the skin surface.
- Implanted medication pumps. Some residents have implanted medication pumps under the skin of the abdomen. These are not always visible, although an incision will be present over the implant. The care plan, nurse, or resident will inform you if such a device is present. If the surgical site is well healed, it is probably safe to use the gait belt. However, you should always follow the care plan or check with the nurse before using a gait belt to move a resident with any type of implanted device.
- Abdominal **aneurysm.** An aneurysm is a ballooning of the wall of an artery due to a struc-

tural weakness. If the aneurysm ruptures, the resident will die.

Moving the Resident with a Mechanical Lift

Several types of mechanical lifts are available. Some are hydraulic. Others are electric. The most commonly used lift is the hydraulic lift. It is used when a resident is heavy, unable to assist, or unbalanced, or has an amputation or other condition that makes transfer with a belt difficult or impossible. For safety reasons, the hydraulic lift should be operated by two or more nursing assistants. Never attempt to operate it alone. Some electric and battery-operated lifts can safely be used by one person. Know and follow your facility policy for use of the mechanical lift.

PROCEDURE 20

Assisting the Resident to Transfer to Chair or Wheelchair, One Person, with Transfer Belt

1. Perform your beginning procedure actions.
2. Assist the resident to dress and put on footwear appropriate to the floor.
3. Apply the transfer belt snugly around the resident's waist and check it with three fingers for tightness.
4. Stand in front of the resident. Keep your feet apart, knees bent, and back straight. Place one hand under each side of the transfer belt, using an underhand grasp **(Figure 9-3A).**
5. Move the resident so the feet are touching the floor. The resident's knees should be separated to provide a wide base of support.
6. Instruct the resident on the count of three to lean forward and push up from the bed with the hands

while you lift up on the belt. Support the resident's knees and feet by placing your knees and feet firmly against them **(Figure 9-3B).**
7. Assist the resident to pivot until the knees touch the back of the chair and the resident can reach the armrests with his or her hands.
8. Bend your knees and assist the resident to lower himself or herself into the chair.
9. Remove the transfer belt.
10. Adjust the wheelchair legs and footrests.
11. Perform your procedure completion actions.
12. Reverse the procedure to return the resident to bed.

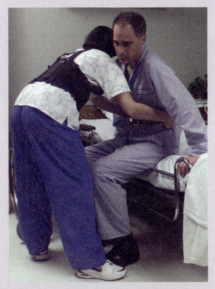

FIGURE 9-3A   Always use an underhand grasp for transferring and ambulating residents.

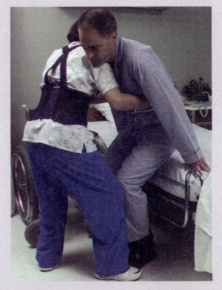

FIGURE 9-3B   Supporting the resident with your knees and feet reduces the risk of slipping.

Because the mechanical lift is a hydraulic unit, check the floor by the lift each time you use it. If you see an oily substance on the floor, do not use the lift until it has been checked and repaired. The fluid may be hydraulic fluid. If hydraulic fluid is leaking, the lift may slip, causing injury to both the resident and the nursing assistant. Check the sling, release mechanisms, attachment straps, and chains for safety before using the lift. If anything is in need of repair, do not use the lift. Follow your facility policy for tagging the lift out of service. Obtain safe equipment before attempting to move the resident.

Assisting the Resident to Transfer to Chair or Wheelchair, Two Persons, with Transfer Belt

OBRA

1. Perform your beginning procedure actions.
2. Assist the resident to dress and put on footwear appropriate to the floor.
3. Apply the transfer belt snugly around the resident's waist and check it with three fingers for tightness.
4. Stand in front of the resident. Keep your feet apart, knees bent, and back straight. Each nursing assistant places one hand under the front of the belt and one hand under the back of the belt, using an underhand grasp **(Figure 9-4)**.
5. Move the resident so the feet are touching the floor. The resident's knees should be separated to provide a wide base of support.
6. On the count of three, both nursing assistants move the resident at the same time. Coordination of movement is important.
7. The nursing assistant on the side closest to the chair stands in a position so that he or she can pivot and move away, allowing the resident unobstructed access to the chair. This nursing assistant should stand with one leg behind the other, so that he or she can step back quickly.

8. The other nursing assistant uses one knee to support the resident's weak leg. This nursing assistant's other leg is positioned further back.
9. Instruct the resident to lean forward and push off the bed, using the palms of the hands, on the count of three.
10. The resident's knees should be spread apart. Instruct the resident to put both feet down with the stronger foot behind the weaker foot.
11. Both nursing assistants bend their knees, squat slightly, and spread their feet to provide a wide base of support.
12. On the count of three, the resident is lifted to a standing position. The nursing assistants pivot slowly and smoothly by moving their feet, legs, and hips to the left side until the resident can feel the back of the wheelchair with his or her legs.
13. Instruct the resident to place his or her hands on the armrests of the chair and lean forward slightly.
14. Both nursing assistants bend their knees and lower the resident into the chair **(Figure 9-5)**.
15. Remove the transfer belt.
16. Adjust the wheelchair legs and footrests.
17. Perform your procedure completion actions.
18. Reverse the procedure to return the resident to bed.

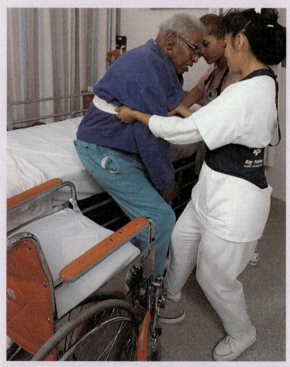

FIGURE 9-4 During a two-person transfer, each assistant places a hand on the front and back of the belt.

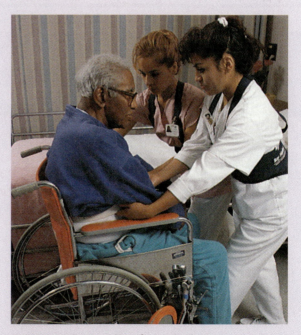

FIGURE 9-5 Bending from the knees and using good body mechanics, lower the resident into the chair.

PROCEDURE 22

Assisting the Resident to Transfer from Bed to Chair or Wheelchair, One Assistant

OBRA

1. Perform your beginning procedure actions.
2. Assist the resident to dress and put on footwear appropriate to the floor.
3. Bring the resident to the edge of the bed so the feet touch the floor. The resident's knees should be separated to provide a wide base of support.
4. Place your hands under the resident's arms and around the back of the shoulders (**Figure 9-6**).
5. Brace the resident's knees and feet with your knees and feet.
6. On the count of three, pull the resident to a standing position. Avoid pulling upward under the arms.
7. Pivot the resident until the knees touch the back of the chair and the resident can reach the armrests with his or her hands.
8. Bend your knees and assist the resident to lower himself or herself into the chair.
9. Adjust the wheelchair legs and footrests.
10. Perform your procedure completion actions.
11. Reverse the procedure to return the resident to bed.
    Note: For the safety of both the nursing assistant and the resident, use this procedure only if use of the transfer belt is contraindicated.

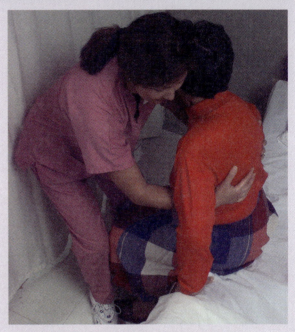

FIGURE 9-6 Place your arms around the resident to the back of the shoulders. Avoid pulling under the arms.

PROCEDURE 23

Transferring the Resident Using a Mechanical Lift

OBRA

1. Perform your beginning procedure actions.
2. Place the chair at right angles to the foot of the bed, facing the head.
3. Lower the side rail on the side nearest you.
4. Roll the resident on the side.
5. Position the sling under the resident's body so that it supports the shoulders, buttocks, and thighs. Straighten the sling.
6. Roll the resident onto the sling and properly position it on the other side (**Figure 9-7A**).
7. Position the lift over the bed (**Figure 9-7B**). Spread the legs of the lift to the widest open position to maintain a broad base of support.
8. Attach the suspension straps or chains to the sling. The "S" hook should face away from the resident to prevent injury (**Figure 9-7C**).
9. Position the resident's arms comfortably inside the sling.
10. Attach the straps or chains to the lift frame.

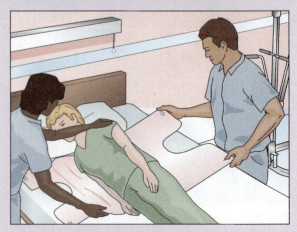

FIGURE 9-7A Position the sling between the shoulder blades and thighs.

Continues

Transferring the Resident Using a Mechanical Lift, *Continued*

OBRA

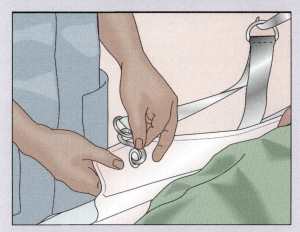

FIGURE 9-7B Center the lift over the resident.

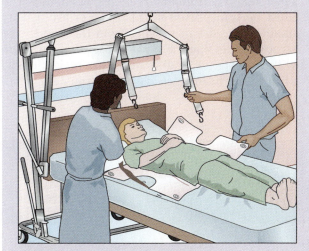

FIGURE 9-7C Fasten the straps with the "S" hooks facing outward, to prevent injury to the resident.

11. Reassure the resident, lock the hydraulic mechanism, and slowly raise the boom of the lift until the resident is suspended over the bed.
12. Slowly guide the lift away from the bed.
13. Position the lift above the chair.
14. The nursing assistant helping you holds the sling back and helps lower the resident slowly into the chair, keeping the hips back while you slowly release the hydraulic and lower the lift.
15. When lowering the lift, monitor the location of the resident's feet and arms to prevent injury **(Figure 9-7D).**
16. Unhook the straps or chains and remove the lift. The lift seat remains under the resident.
17. Position the footrests to support the feet.
18. Perform your procedure completion actions.
19. Reverse the procedure to return the resident to bed. When raising the resident from the chair, monitor the position of the "S" hooks, which sometimes catch under the arms of the chair.

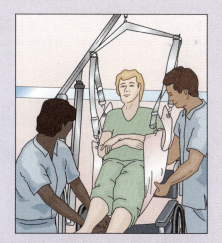

FIGURE 9-7D Slowly lower the lift while monitoring the resident's legs and arms and guiding the hips back into the chair.

SLIDING BOARD TRANSFERS

A sliding board **(Figure 9-8)** transfer is used for residents who have good upper body strength and sitting balance. This type of transfer is commonly used for residents with paraplegia. The procedure is performed by doing a series of pushups. The resident locks the elbows and pushes with the hands. To transfer, the resident must be able to lift the buttocks off the bed.

After lifting the buttocks, he or she lowers onto the sliding board, then lifts and slides until the transfer is complete.

The wheelchair must have removable armrests when a sliding board is used. The resident must have clothing on the lower half of the body. Blue jeans do not slide well on the board. Cotton or synthetic slacks are best. If the resident has difficulty sliding on the board, draping a pillowcase across the board may be helpful. (Do not

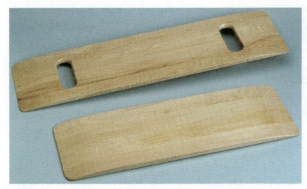

FIGURE 9-8 The sliding board is used when the wheelchair has removable arms and swing-away leg rests. Make sure the resident is wearing pants that will slide easily across the surface. *(Photo courtesy of Briggs Corporation)*

encase the board in the pillowcase as you would a pillow.) The board can also be waxed to maintain a slippery surface. Some residents perform this transfer independently, whereas others need help. If you will be assisting, always use a transfer belt.

Two assistants can move dependent residents by using a sliding board. One assistant stands in front and the other behind the resident. At the count of three, both assistants hold the belt and slide the resident across the board.

Toilet Transfers

A survey of long-term care facility workers revealed that toilet transfers were the most difficult. This is because the bathrooms in most facilities are small. Many meet the OSHA definition of "confined spaces." Working in a confined space increases the risk of injury. The wheelchair takes up a great deal of space. The toilet is close to the wall. There is little room for the assistant to move during the transfer. Follow all safety precautions carefully to prevent injury to the resident and yourself.

TRANSPORTING A RESIDENT BY STRETCHER

Most long-term care facility residents are ambulatory or can be safely transported by wheelchair. Residents who are comatose or bedfast may need to be transported on a stretcher. A stretcher may also be needed for transporting residents in certain emergencies. Residents who must be transported in this manner are usually unable to assist in moving from the bed to the stretcher and back. Four or more staff members will be needed to safely move the resident. The **sliding technique** is used for transfers when

---

PROCEDURE 24

Sliding Board Transfer from Bed to Wheelchair

1. Perform your beginning procedure actions.
2. Remove the arm of the wheelchair closest to the bed. Remove the legs or fold them back.
3. Position the wheelchair parallel to the bed, or at a slight (about 35°) angle. Lock the brakes.
4. Apply a transfer belt. Check the fit with three fingers.
5. Assist the resident to move close to the edge of the bed.
6. Tell the resident to lean away from the wheelchair. Place the sliding board well under the buttocks, with the beveled side of the board facing up. Avoid pinching the resident's skin between the board and the bed.
7. Place the opposite end of the board well onto the seat of the wheelchair.
8. Instruct the resident to push up with the hands, lock the elbows, and move across the board. Repeat until the resident is seated in the chair with one buttock on the board.

Note: The resident may push on the opposite armrest of the wheelchair with one hand. This will help achieve greater height in the pushups. The resident may also push on the board. Caution the resident to avoid placing the fingers under the edges of the board.

9. Be prepared to assist by lifting the resident's buttocks during the sitting pushup. If the resident is having trouble balancing, place your hands on the shoulders for support.
10. Support and move the resident's legs with your hands, if necessary.
11. Instruct the resident to lean away from the bed. Remove the board.
12. Remove the transfer belt.
13. Position the legs on the leg rests, or as instructed. Replace the arm on the chair.
14. Perform your procedure completion actions.
15. Reverse the procedure to return the resident to bed.

PROCEDURE 25

Transferring the Resident from Wheelchair to Toilet

1. Perform your beginning procedure actions.
2. Position the wheelchair at a right angle to the toilet, if possible. Position the chair so that the toilet is on the resident's strong side, if possible.
3. Lock the brakes.
4. Remove the wheelchair legs or fold them back.
5. Apply the transfer belt.
6. Assist the resident to unfasten clothing.
7. Instruct the resident to place the hands on the wheelchair armrests and slide forward in the chair.
8. Tell the resident to pull the feet back under the body, placing them firmly on the floor.
9. Have the resident lean forward and push up, turning to the strong side **(Figure 9-9)** until he or she feels the toilet seat on the legs. Hold the transfer belt, but assist only to the degree necessary.
10. Instruct the resident to hold the grab rail and use the other hand to undress. Assist as needed.
11. Tell the resident to hold the rail and slowly lower his or her body to the toilet seat.
12. Remove the transfer belt, or leave it on according to resident preference and facility policy.
13. Provide privacy. Instruct the resident to call for assistance when done.
14. Perform your procedure completion actions.
    Note: Reverse this procedure to return the resident to the chair. If possible, position the wheelchair on the resident's strong side. To rise from the toilet, the resident holds the rail. Tell the resident to slide forward slightly. Then remind the resident to pull the feet back and lean forward. He or she pushes up with the hands on the rails, or pulls up using the rail on the wall. Remind the resident to face forward, keeping the head over the feet. After the resident is seated in the chair, assist him or her to the sink. Provide supplies or assist with handwashing.

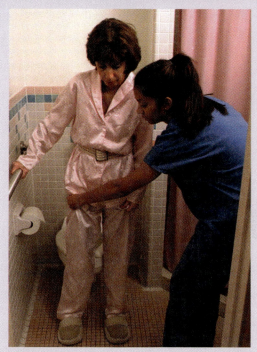

FIGURE 9-9 Assist the resident to pivot or back up until his legs touch the toilet. Hold the belt for support, if necessary, when adjusting the resident's clothes.

the resident cannot bear weight. Use this technique for moving residents on a sheet, such as from bed to stretcher. Use your body weight to hold the two surfaces together during the transfer. This keeps them from separating. One or more caregivers stand on each side of the resident. The sheet is rolled close to the resident's body. On the count of three, lift the sheet, pulling and sliding the resident over to the stretcher.

WHEELCHAIRS

The wheelchair is an important piece of equipment in the long-term care facility. Many residents use wheelchairs for mobility. Some will progress to ambulation. Others will always use the wheelchair to move about. Whenever possible, the facility should restore the resident's ability to ambulate. If the resident is unable to ambulate, it may be best to use the wheelchair to move from one location to another, then transfer into a regular chair. For example, the resident propels the wheelchair to the dining room. For pressure relief and mealtime positioning, transferring her into the dining room chair may be best. Follow your facility policies and the residents' care plans.

Because residents spend so much time in wheelchairs, careful attention to fitting the chair

PROCEDURE 26 — Transferring the Resident from Bed to Stretcher

1. Perform your beginning procedure actions.
2. Gather your supplies:
   • Stretcher
   • Bath blanket
3. Ensure that three to four other staff members are available to assist in moving the resident.
4. Raise the bed to a horizontal position equal to the height of the stretcher. Lock the wheels. Lower the side rail on the side where you are working.
5. Cover the resident with the bath blanket.
6. Remove the linen by pulling it down from underneath the blanket. Avoid exposing the resident. Fanfold the linen at the foot of the bed or dispose of it according to facility policy.
7. Roll the turning sheet up against the resident's body on both sides. The turning sheet should be long enough to support the resident's torso from the knees to the shoulders. If no turning sheet is available, use the bottom bed sheet.
8. Move the stretcher in next to the bed. Lock the brakes.
9. Two or three people stand on the open side of the stretcher. One or two more go to the other side of the bed and lower the rail. The staff on this side should be prepared to get on their knees in the bed during the transfer, if necessary, to avoid back injury from lifting and reaching. If another assistant is available, he or she should stand at the head of the bed to support the resident's head.
10. All staff grasp the sheet using an overhand grasp.
    • The assistant(s) at the end of the bed grasps the lifting sheet by placing one hand on the lower leg area and one at the hip area.
    • The middle assistant(s) grasps the lifting sheet by placing one hand at the hip and one at the shoulder.
    • The assistant at the head (if present) grasps the sheet on either side of the resident's head.
11. On the count of three, all staff lift, push, and pull the sheet from the bed to the stretcher **(Figure 9-10)**.

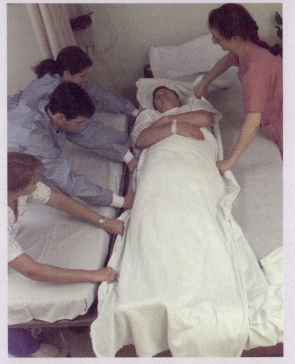

FIGURE 9-10 On signal, all staff move the sheet from the bed to the stretcher.

12. Center and position the resident in good body alignment, with a pillow for comfort.
13. Secure the safety straps.
14. Raise the side rails on the stretcher.
15. Transport the resident as directed. When complete, return to the unit to straighten the bed and prepare for the resident's return.
16. Perform your procedure completion actions.

to the resident is very important for comfort and pressure ulcer prevention. Sometimes wheelchairs are ordered or modified to meet special resident needs. For example, some residents with hemiplegia can propel the wheelchair independently. They use the strong arm on the wheel and push the strong leg on the floor. The leg rest is removed on this side.

Wheelchair Size

For safety, the wheelchair must be used correctly and must fit the resident properly. There is no "one size fits all" wheelchair. Residents may not be able to propel a wheelchair that does not fit correctly. Fewer positioning aids are necessary if the chair fits the resident. A wheelchair that is the wrong size causes discomfort, contributes to skin breakdown, and increases the need for restraints. Positioning residents upright, in good body alignment, is difficult and further increases the risk of complications. As you can see, attention to chair size is very important.

The therapist or restorative nurse will evaluate the chair to determine whether it fits the resident. The type of chair selected is determined by:

- An assessment of the resident's physical condition
- The resident's special needs
- The needs of caregivers
- The environment in which the chair will be used

Brakes

The brakes are an important safety feature of the wheelchair. Several types of brakes are available. The most common type uses a lever system to lock the chair. The brakes must be secure during transfers. Set them when the wheelchair is parked. If the chair slips even slightly, the brakes are not working properly. Notify the nurse or the appropriate person in your facility if you believe the brakes are not working correctly. Do not transfer the resident into or out of the chair until the brakes have been repaired. If a transfer is essential, have another assistant immobilize the chair while you transfer the resident.

Some residents do not lock the brakes on the wheelchair because they cannot reach them. For example, a resident with hemiparesis may not be able to reach the brake on the affected side. Extensions are available to lengthen the brake handle **(Figure 9-11).** Some facilities create brake extensions by attaching PVC pipe.

Caster Wheels

The small, front caster wheels of the chair provide the ability to move in all directions. The

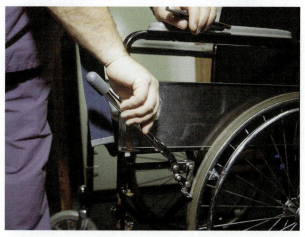

FIGURE 9-11 The brake extension is attached so the resident can reach it with the opposite arm, if necessary.

large part of the wheel faces back when the chair is moving. Before beginning a transfer, and when parking the chair, position the large part of the front wheel facing forward. This will stabilize the chair by changing its center of gravity. Back the chair up, then move it forward until the wheels are properly positioned.

Drive Wheels

The large, rear wheels are the drive wheels. The most common type of wheel is made from solid rubber.

The outer rim of the drive wheels is used for pushing the chair. Propelling the wheelchair independently is better for the residents. It provides exercise, and permits them to move about the facility at will. This is much more satisfying than having to wait for someone to transport them.

Seat Depth

The depth of the seat is very important. The seat must be deep enough to support the pelvis and thighs correctly. A short seat can be very uncomfortable for residents with long legs. If the seat is too long, the resident's weight is shifted toward the sacrum. This causes discomfort and increases the risk of skin breakdown. A long seat also makes it more difficult for the resident to propel the chair. Some residents slide to the front edge of the wheelchair. A seat that is too long is often the problem. Facilities often look for restraints and alternatives to keep residents from sliding when a different wheelchair may be all that is necessary! Staff members may not recognize this problem. When the resident is seated properly in the chair, the hips should be near the back. The front edge of the seat should end two or three inches before the back of the knees.

Seat Width

Proper seat width is also important for comfort. It affects ease in moving the drive wheels and resting the arms on the armrests. A wheelchair that is too wide is difficult for residents to move. The resident may lean to one side. A seat that is too narrow increases pressure on the thighs, buttocks, and hips. If the seat width fits the resident correctly, there should be enough space to slide your hand in on either side between the resident's hips and the side of the wheelchair.

Back Height

The height of the chair back is determined by the resident's need for back support. The back should be supported from the hips to the bottom of the shoulder blades. If the resident uses a foam cushion in the wheelchair, the back must be the proper height with the cushion in place. Some wheelchairs have an extension piece that is elevated to provide head support, if needed.

Armrests

Armrests can be removable or nonremovable. Removable armrests are necessary for use of sliding boards, and for some other transfers. Armrest height is important for comfort and good sitting posture. If the armrests are too high, shorter residents will have problems propelling the chair.

Armrests are available in two lengths. The desk-length armrest is lower in the front than in the back. This enables the resident to get close to tables. The chair works well for residents who sit in wheelchairs at mealtime. The full-length armrest is most common and is comfortable when the resident is seated. However, getting close to tables may be a problem. Elevating the table height does not solve the problem. Raising the table allows the resident to move closer. However, most residents are too short to benefit from the increased table height. They may end up eating with their elbows in the air because the table is too high. This is very uncomfortable and causes shoulder strain. It may cause some residents to have problems eating. Attaching a lap tray to the armrests corrects the problem.

Leg Rests and Footrests

Many wheelchairs have removable leg rests. Remove the leg rests or fold the footrests up during transfers. If they fall down, notify the nurse. The footrest is easily tightened. If you remove the leg rests, make sure to replace them when you finish. Facilities have many different types of wheelchairs. If the parts become separated from the chair, matching them up may be difficult.

Some wheelchairs have swing-away or pivoting legs. A lever on the side releases the leg. These leg rests can be folded to the sides during transfers. When using wheelchairs with fixed legs, raise the footrests during transfers.

Some residents with edema or fractures need chairs with elevating legs. This type of leg rest may also be used for residents with contrac-

tures, or those who cannot flex the knees. A lock on the side holds the leg rest in place. For safety, support the leg with one hand while operating the lock with the other. Support the calf with a pad when the leg rests are elevated.

Residents' feet must be supported when the chair is being moved. Their feet should never dangle in the air or drag on the floor. The length of the chair legs can be adjusted to provide proper support. If the leg rest cannot be adjusted, a footrest elevator (**Figure 9-12**) may be used. Your maintenance department may make footrest elevators out of wood. When the wheelchair is parked, the resident's legs should be supported on the footrests or the floor. Allowing the legs to dangle is uncomfortable and increases the risk of blood clots. Advise residents to avoid

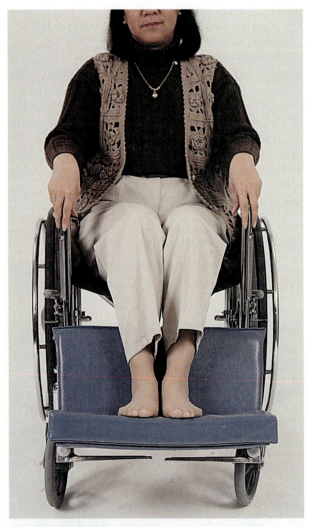

FIGURE 9-12 The feet must always be supported when the resident is seated. The foam footrest elevator may be used if the feet do not reach the footrests. *(Courtesy of Skil-Care Corporation, Yonkers, NY, (800) 431-2972)*

leaning forward or picking up items from the floor. If the feet are on the footrests, the chair will tip. There should be at least two inches of clearance from the bottom of the footrest to the floor.

Reclining Chairs

Reclining-back wheelchairs **(Figure 9-13A)** and geriatric chairs **(Figure 9-13B)** should be used only for residents who cannot sit upright. The chair back supports the head and neck. Adjust the back for comfort and maximum functional ability. When adjusting the back, support the resident. Suddenly releasing the lock will cause him or her to fall back quickly, frightening the resident and causing pain and potential injury.

Avoid placing residents in reclining chairs unless such a chair is medically necessary. At first glance, using a recliner looks like a good way to position the resident comfortably in a chair without using restraints. However, placing a resident in a reclining chair unnecessarily can cause serious physical and mental declines. If a recliner must be used, avoid reclining the back farther than necessary. This often causes loss of orienta-

tion. The resident looks at the ceiling all day and cannot see people or activity in the room. He or she becomes more dependent because the resident cannot perform activities, such as feeding, in this position. Use of reclining chairs is discussed in greater detail in Chapter 15.

Preventing Skin Tears

Torn armrests and seats on wheelchairs are a common cause of skin tears and resident injury. Surveyors will write up deficiencies if they observe worn wheelchairs. The armrests and seats should be replaced if they become cracked or torn. Notify your supervisor if you observe a chair in disrepair.

POSITIONING THE RESIDENT IN A CHAIR OR WHEELCHAIR

Proper positioning is as important for residents who are sitting in chairs as it is for residents who are in bed. Use foam or padding on the chair seat if the resident will be sitting for long periods. Assist the resident to stand or shift weight periodically. Before leaving a resident seated in a

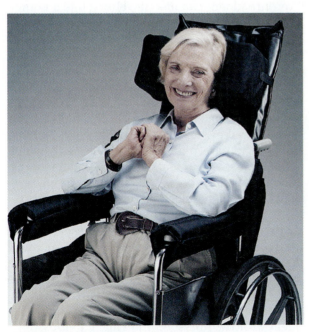

FIGURE 9-13A   The reclining wheelchair may be used for residents who do not have trunk, head, or neck control. Keep the back as upright as possible to maintain orientation to the environment. *(Courtesy of Skil-Care Corporation, Yonkers, NY, (800) 431-2972)*

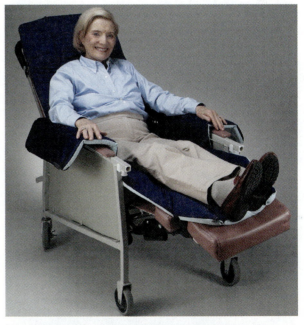

FIGURE 9-13B   The reclining geriatric chair is a restraint if the resident cannot get out of it at will. Keep the chair as upright as possible so the resident can interact with the environment. *(Courtesy of Skil-Care Corporation, Yonkers, NY, (800) 431-2972)*

Positioning the Resident in a Chair or Wheelchair

1. Perform your beginning procedure actions.
2. Make sure the brakes are locked and that the small, front caster wheels on the wheelchair are properly positioned before beginning.
3. Seat the resident upright so the head is erect and centered over the spine.
4. Position the resident's arms for comfort.
5. The back of the wheelchair should be at the lower level of the resident's shoulder blades.

6. The hips and back are positioned at a 90° angle.
7. The edge of the seat should be two to three inches from the back of the resident's knees. Position the legs at a 90° angle. If the knees touch the seat, place a cushion behind the back to move the resident forward.
8. Position the feet and ankles at 90° angles on the footrests or floor.
9. Perform your procedure completion actions.

---

chair, make sure that he or she is in good alignment **(Figure 9-14).** Good sitting posture begins with positioning the pelvis correctly. Position the resident upright in the center of the chair seat, with the hips to the back. The resident's hips and knees are positioned at a 90° angle. Make sure the weight is evenly distributed on the buttocks. You should be able to place a flat hand between the armrests and the resident's hips. If the resident leans to the side, use props to bring him or her to an upright position. Position the arms on the armrests. Check to

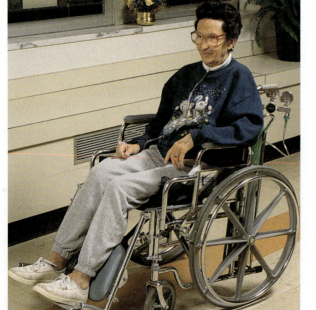

FIGURE 9-14   This resident is sitting in good body alignment and the chair fits her properly. These two factors improve her body function and ability to propel the chair.

make sure the shoulders are not pushed up. Check behind the knees. There should be three or four finger widths between the knees and the seat. Adjust the feet and legs so they are in line with the pelvis. Support the feet on the footrests so the legs do not dangle.

PRESSURE RELIEF IN THE CHAIR

Years ago, pressure ulcers were called decubitus ulcers. The term *decubitus* means lying down. Pressure ulcers can also develop while a person is sitting in a chair, so the name was changed to more accurately describe the cause of the problem. Residents who sit in chairs for long periods can develop skin breakdown. Anticipate this risk. If the resident is wearing a gown, cover the seat of the chair with a sheet or bath blanket. If a resident will be sitting in a chair for a prolonged period, make sure the seat is well padded. Follow the care plan for guidance as to which device to use. However, even with padding, pressure relief must be provided by assisting residents to move regularly to relieve pressure.

You will work with many residents who are **chairfast,** or confined to chairs. Assist and remind the residents to perform pressure-relieving activities. When the resident is learning pressure-relieving techniques, stay with him or her to give directions and encouragement. The therapist or restorative nurse will recommend a frequency for the pressure-relieving activities.

Wheelchair pushups

Wheelchair pushups are the best method of relieving pressure when the resident is seated. The resident places the palms on the armrests of the

PROCEDURE 28

Assisting with Wheelchair Pushups

OBRA

1. Perform your beginning procedure actions.
2. Position the small front wheels of the wheelchair facing forward. Lock the brakes.
3. Remove the leg rests or fold them back. Place the resident's feet on the floor.
4. Position yourself in front of the resident.
5. Instruct the resident to place both hands on the armrests, push the body up, lock the elbows, and lift the hips off the seat **(Figure 9-15)**.
6. If the resident can use one or both legs, instruct him or her to push on the floor with the feet while pushing up with the hands.
7. Instruct the resident to unlock the elbows, slowly flex the knees, and lower gradually to the seat.
8. Repeat as instructed by the restorative nurse or therapist.
9. If the resident can perform the procedure independently, remind him or her to practice.
10. Assist the resident to return the leg rests and legs to a position of comfort.
11. Perform your procedure completion actions.

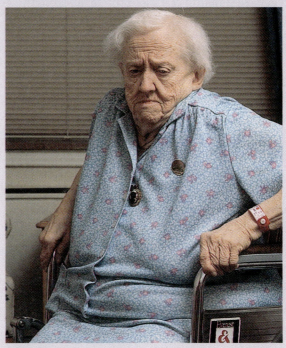

FIGURE 9-15 To perform wheelchair pushups, position the small front wheels facing forward. Elevate the footrests and place the resident's feet on the floor. Lock the brakes. Teach the resident to push on the armrests with the hands and raise the body off the seat.

PROCEDURE 29

Leaning to the Side for Pressure Relief

OBRA

1. Perform your beginning procedure actions.
2. Position the small front wheels of the wheelchair facing forward. Lock the brakes. For extra security, back the wheelchair against a wall.
3. Remove the leg rests or fold them back. Place the resident's feet on the floor.
4. Position yourself in front of the resident.
5. Instruct the resident to lean forward slightly, then lean back.
6. Have the resident lean from side to side. Advise him or her to lift as much weight off the buttocks as possible. Repeat five times, or as stated in the care plan.
7. Assist the resident to return the leg rests and legs to a position of comfort.
8. Perform your procedure completion actions.

wheelchair. The feet are flat on the floor. Caution the resident against performing pushups with the feet on the footrests. Instruct the resident to push down with the hands, extend the elbows, and lift the buttocks from the chair. This should

be done at least five times, or the frequency specified by the care plan.

Wheelchair pushups relieve pressure on the hips, buttocks, and coccyx. They are helpful to the resident who sits in a chair for long periods of time. Wheelchair pushups increase upper body strength. This helps prepare the resident for transfer procedures. The care plan will list directions.

Leaning to the Side for Pressure Relief. Some residents do not have the arm strength or trunk control to perform pushups. These residents can lean to the sides and front of the chair to relieve pressure. For more dependent residents, have the resident grab your hands. Instruct the resident to pull on your hands to shift the weight off the buttocks.

WHEELCHAIR MOBILITY

The wheelchair is a mobility device, not a transportation device. Propelling the wheelchair independently is good exercise. It promotes communication, independence, confidence, and self-esteem. Wheelchair mobility provides opportunities for residents to make choices and decisions. They can decide where they will go and what activities to attend. A facility emphasis on efficiency may create problems with wheelchair mobility. Pushing the chairs is faster for staff, but it deprives residents of much-needed exercise and independence. Some residents do not propel their wheelchairs because of physical problems. However, adaptations may allow them to move independently. Some do not propel the chair because it does not fit correctly. Fitting wheelchairs and teaching residents to use them is best. The therapy and restorative nursing departments will work with the residents to teach them to move their wheelchairs independently. For example, a resident may propel the chair by pushing with the foot on one side. Assist and encourage residents with independence whenever possible.

ASSISTING RESIDENTS WITH AMBULATION

Walking, or **ambulation,** is an excellent form of exercise. The body functions more efficiently in an upright position. Residents may have difficulty walking because of illness, injury, surgery, or weakness. In the initial stages of ambulation, the nursing assistant will assist residents until

GUIDELINES FOR
Wheelchair Safety

- Make sure the wheelchair fits the resident correctly and has all necessary parts, such as leg rests and brakes.
- Position the small front wheels in the forward position when transferring the resident into and out of the chair, and when the chair is parked.
- Keep the brakes locked during transfers and when the chair is parked.
- Position the resident in good body alignment; reposition as often as necessary.
- Support paralyzed body parts so they do not slip over the chair arm, drag the floor, or become entangled in the wheels.
- Cover the resident's lap with a lap blanket or bath blanket, as needed for modesty and warmth. This is especially important for a female resident who is wearing a skirt or dress. Make sure the blanket and the resident's clothing do not drag on the floor or become entangled in the wheels.
- Remind residents about wheelchair safety, including:
  - locking the brakes when the chair is parked.
  - parking the chair with the large part of the small front wheels facing forward.
  - holding the armrests and feeling the chair with the back of the legs before sitting.

- not reaching down between the knees or bending over to pick up items from the floor.
- Push the wheelchair from behind by guiding it with the handgrips. Avoid walking too fast. Slow down and look before turning corners.
- Approach swinging doors with caution. Prop the door open before entering, if possible. If not, back the wheelchair through the doorway.
- Always back over the thresholds of doorways.
- Lock the elevator, turn the wheelchair around, and back in. When the elevator stops at your destination, lock it again, turn the chair around, and back out. (Remember to go back and unlock the elevator.)
- To transport a wheelchair up a ramp, instruct the resident to lean forward slightly. Push the resident up, from behind the chair.
- To move a wheelchair down a ramp, turn the chair around. Position yourself behind the chair and walk backward. Guide the chair by using the handgrips. Periodically look over your shoulder to make sure the path is clear. Walk slowly, using your body to guard the chair. Avoid very steep ramps, if possible.

GUIDELINES FOR

Transporting a Resident by Stretcher

- Make sure the side rails are up and all safety belts are fastened.
- Push the stretcher by standing at the resident's head.
- Approach corners slowly and look before you go around them.
- Slow down and look for oncoming traffic when approaching a swinging door. Prop the door open to propel the stretcher through the door. If this is not possible, back through swinging doors.
- When entering an elevator, push the stop button to lock the doors open. Back the stretcher into the elevator by walking backward and pulling the head end.
- Stand by the resident's head while an elevator is in motion. When the elevator stops, push the stop button to lock the door open. Push the stretcher out so the feet exit the elevator first. (Remember to go back and unlock the elevator.)

  If the elevator threshold is uneven, go to the foot end of the stretcher and pull it out of the elevator. After the stretcher is safely out of the elevator, unlock the door mechanism.
- When transporting a stretcher down a ramp or incline, walk backward, slowly guiding the stretcher from the head end. Periodically look over your shoulder to make sure the path is clear.
- When parking a stretcher, avoid blocking a doorway.
- Never leave a resident unattended and unsupervised on a stretcher.

---

they regain strength and become more independent. Some residents may never become independent. However, walking them is important so that they do not lose the use of their legs. You will be assigned to walk residents a specified distance each day to help them maintain the ability to walk. If the resident is in a physical therapy or restorative nursing program, the care plan will contain specific instructions for you to follow during ambulation.

Make sure the resident's shoes are appropriate for the floor surface. Residents should not ambulate with bare feet or stocking feet. Ambulate residents on a tile floor whenever possible. Uneven surfaces make walking more difficult. They may also cause fatigue and loss of balance. Use good judgment when ambulating residents. Safety is always a primary concern. Check for hazards on the floor, such as spills, or objects that could cause the residents to fall.

Goal–Oriented Ambulation

The therapist or restorative nurse develops assessment-based ambulation goals for each resident **(Figure 9-16).** They try to consider goals that will be useful or purposeful for the resident. For example, going to the dining room is a functional skill. In this case, the care plan will state to ambulate the resident to and from the dining room for meals. Instead of ambulating in the hallway, walking to and from the dining room gives the activity a useful purpose. Other purposeful goals are ambulating residents:

- To and from activities programs
- To and from the bathroom
- To the nurses' station for medications

If the ambulation care plan involves walking back and forth in the hallway, residents may not see the functional purpose of the ambulation. Because of this, they view the activity as exercise, and will depend on their wheelchairs for

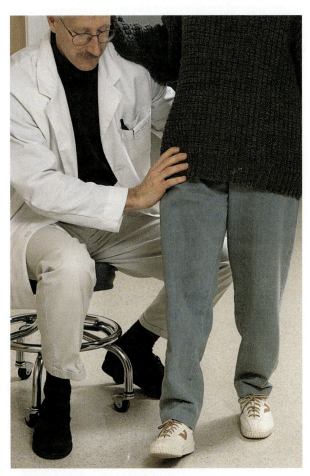

FIGURE 9-16 The physical therapist evaluates the resident's gait.

mobility instead. The overall goals of ambulation are to:

- Maintain or improve the resident's ability to ambulate
- Ensure that the resident can ambulate safely
- Prevent the loss of independence
- Prevent **atrophy,** or muscular wasting from lack of use
- Provide a safe, consistent, purposeful ambulation activity for residents who otherwise would be unable or unwilling to ambulate regularly
- Increase residents' endurance for ambulation outside their rooms
- Increase residents' confidence and sense of well-being

Gait

The way a person walks is called the **gait.** Residents with certain musculoskeletal and neurologic problems have a gait that is peculiar to the illness. For example, residents with Parkinson's disease walk with a shuffling gait. This is because of muscle rigidity. Residents with some neurological problems walk with an **ataxic** gait. The residents appear uncoordinated. They keep their legs farther apart. This makes the residents more stable. Residents with an ataxic gait need a very wide base of support to prevent falls. Their movement is somewhat irregular. They may walk with jerking movements. Residents having pain may walk slowly. The resident's body language and facial expression may appear strained. The resident may move the painful area differently or abnormally.

Normal Gait.   The normal gait pattern consists of two steps. The resident begins with the feet flat on the floor. He or she raises a leg, dorsiflexes the foot, and begins walking. The heel strikes the floor first. The resident rolls forward on the sole of the foot, and moves ahead. The arms swing back and forth, in the same direction as the opposite leg **(Figure 9-17).** The care plan will list special approaches to use for a resident with an abnormal gait, and special risk and safety factors.

Some residents may require more than one assistant for safe ambulation. The physical therapist or restorative nurse will determine if this is necessary. The therapist or restorative nurse will also decide whether the resident would benefit from use of an assistive device.

When developing ambulation goals, the interdisciplinary team determines the distance that

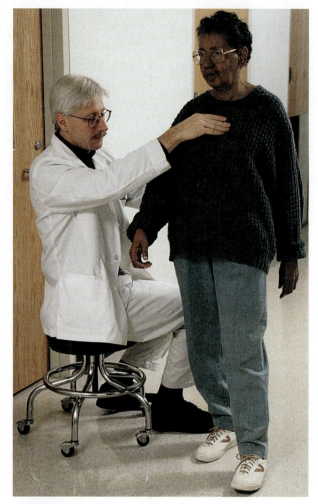

FIGURE 9-17   The arms swing in the same direction as the opposite leg.

the resident can ambulate safely. Preventing increased pain, edema, shortness of breath, or weakness is important. If you observe these problems when you are walking a resident, stop the activity. Notify the nurse promptly

Assisting the Resident to Walk with a Cane, Walker, or Crutches

Canes, crutches, and walkers are used to provide support during ambulation. They redistribute the balance of the resident's weight, shifting the center of gravity over a wider area. The device helps prevent loss of balance. Usually, the physical therapist will provide the device and teach the resident how to use it correctly. Use of these devices enables residents who are weak or unsteady to be independent with ambulation. Check the rubber tips before the resident ambulates. If the rubber is worn through, the tip must be replaced before the resident gets up. If the

GUIDELINES FOR

Assisting Residents with Ambulation

- Check the resident's shoes to make sure they are appropriate for the floor surface. Never ambulate a resident who has bare feet or is wearing only socks.
- Dress the resident in street clothes. If this is not possible, make sure the resident's body is covered. Avoid long pants, long robes, and slippers that could cause the resident to trip.
- Assist the resident to dangle, then stand at the bedside to balance before ambulating. If the resident feels weak, dizzy, or faint, return him or her to bed. Notify the nurse.
- Always use a gait belt, even if the resident is steady on his or her feet.
- If an assistive device is ordered, have the resident practice using it. The therapist or restorative nurse will determine the gait pattern to use. Ambulate the resident with the device for the distance and time ordered.
- If the care plan or your assignment is not specific, ask for clarification.
- Practice good body mechanics for both yourself and the resident.
- Teach and remind the resident to practice safety.
- Position your body so it moves with the resident's body. You should not interfere with the resident's movement. Match the resident's stride.
- Support the resident's weak side (if any). Stay close, slightly behind and to the resident's side. Hold the center back of the gait belt with an underhand grasp **(Figure 9-18)**.
- Encourage the resident to stand upright and erect when walking. The head, shoulders, hips, knees, and feet should be aligned.
- Encourage the resident to take moderate, even steps. Make sure he or she maintains a wide base of support. The distance between the feet should be about equal to the resident's shoulder width.
- Allow adequate time for ambulation. Avoid making the resident feel rushed.
- Allow the resident time to rest, if necessary.
- Provide only the amount of assistance necessary.

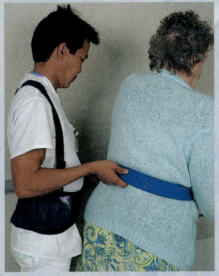

FIGURE 9-18 Stand behind and to the side of the resident, grasping the center of the belt with an underhand grasp.

- If the resident is not motivated, place a chair ahead of him or her. Tell the resident the goal is to walk to the chair.
- Have another assistant follow behind you with a wheelchair, if the resident's endurance is in doubt.
- Inform the nurse if you believe the resident is unsafe.
- Stop ambulation immediately if the resident shows signs of illness, pain, extreme fatigue, shortness of breath, dizziness, sweating, or anxiety. Notify the nurse.
- Never leave the resident standing unattended. When you are through, leave the resident safely sitting in a chair.

PROCEDURE
30

Ambulating the Resident with a Gait Belt

1. Perform your beginning procedure actions.
2. Lower the bed to the lowest horizontal position.
3. Assist the resident to dangle.
4. Assist the resident to dress and put on footwear appropriate to the floor.
5. If the resident is not familiar with the gait belt, explain how and why it will be used.
6. Check the fit of the belt with three fingers.
7. Using an underhand grasp, place your hands under the belt on each side and bring the resident to a standing position.
8. Walk behind and slightly to one side of the resident. Maintain a firm, underhand grasp at the center back of the gait belt.

Continues

Ambulating the Resident with a Gait Belt, *Continued*

9. Encourage the resident to use the handrails in the hallway.
10. Walk the distance specified by the care plan, physical therapist, or nurse's instructions.
11. Monitor the resident for signs of fatigue. If fatigue occurs, assist the resident to sit in a chair.
12. If the resident starts to fall, pull him or her close to your body. Protect the resident's head. Using good body mechanics, hold the belt securely and ease the resident down your leg to the floor **(Figure 9-19)**. Bend your knees as you lower the resident. Do not attempt to hold the resident up. This could cause injuries to the resident and nursing assistant. Use of the belt gives you control of the fall and helps prevent head injuries.
13. After the ambulation, return to the resident's room.
14. Assist the resident to sit in the chair or return to bed.
15. Remove the gait belt.
16. Perform your procedure completion actions.
17. Upon completion of this procedure, you may be asked to record the distance the resident walked and the resident's vital signs.

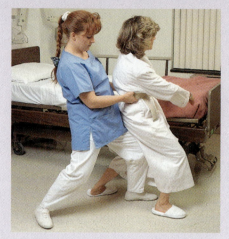

FIGURE 9-19 Keep your back straight and bend from the hips and knees. Guide the resident down your leg to the floor.

ambulation device has nuts, bolts, or pushbutton locks, make sure they are securely fastened before ambulating the resident. Each leg of the walker has a pushbutton lock. All four legs must be the same height before the resident uses the device. If you feel that a resident is not using the assistive devices correctly, notify the nurse, who will contact the therapy department.

Canes. Canes are ordered for residents who have balance problems, pain, or weakness in the legs. One or two canes may be used. They are most commonly used when only one side of the body is weak. Many types of canes are available **(Figure 9-20)**. The standard cane is shaped like an upside-down letter J. The **quad cane** has four feet. Of the canes available, it is the most stable. The resident can release the hand grip and it will not fall to the floor. The base of the quad cane comes in two sizes, small and large. The large base provides the greatest stability. However, its size may make maneuvering in tight spaces difficult. Canes are available with many different types of hand grips. Some have an offset shaft, which changes the center of gravity. This shifts the weight over the tip of the J cane or the center of the base of the quad cane.

For safety, the cane must fit the resident. The hand grip of the cane should be at the panty-line level. If the cane is the correct height, the resident's shoulders will be even and not raised. Wooden canes can be adjusted only by cutting them. Metal canes are adjusted by releasing the pushbutton lock and moving the telescoping shaft.

The physical therapist will select the gait pattern to use, depending on the resident's problem. The most common gait pattern involves holding the cane in the hand opposite the weak leg. The cane and the weak leg move forward at the same time. This provides extra support and balance on the weak side.

Walkers. Walkers are commonly used for elderly residents. Indications for using a walker are:

- Debilitating conditions
- Generalized weakness in one or both legs
- Need to reduce weight bearing on one leg
- Poor coordination
- Injury to one leg
- Inability to use crutches
- Difficulty balancing without support

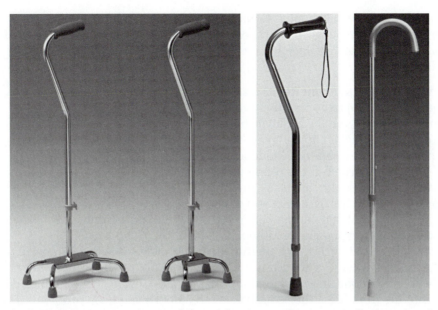

FIGURE 9-20 Various types of canes. *(Courtesy of Lumex Medical Products)*

The walker provides a sturdy base of support. The resident propels the walker by using elbow extension and shoulder depression. Residents who are recovering from hip fractures often begin ambulation using a walker. Several different types of walkers are available **(Figure 9-21)**. The therapist will select the type that meets the resident's needs. The walker is adjusted so that the handgrip is at panty-line height. If the shoulders are raised during ambulation, the walker is too high. Platforms may be attached to the walker to support the arms.

The therapist will measure the walker height to fit the resident. The walker is adjusted by turning the device upside down. Each leg has a pushbutton lock. Depress the lock and push or pull the telescoping leg to adjust the height. All four legs should be the same height before the resident uses the device.

The most common types of walkers are pictured in Figure 9-21. The aluminum walker with rubber tips on all four legs is used most often. Walkers are also available with two and four wheels. These are used for residents who cannot

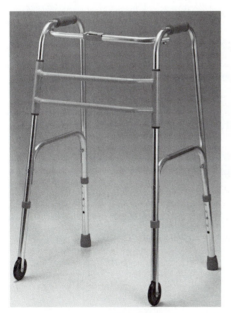
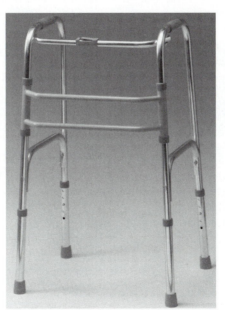
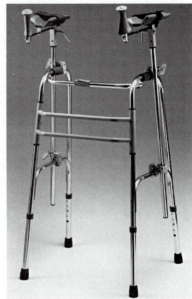

FIGURE 9-21 Various types of walkers. *(Courtesy of Lumex Medical Products)*

lift a walker, or who have weak hands. Some walkers have brakes on the wheels. The brakes lock automatically when weight is placed downward on the walker.

Safety Precautions for Ambulating Residents with a Walker. The therapist or restorative nurse will recommend a gait for the resident to use. The standard walker is picked up and placed a comfortable distance ahead of the resident. Comfortable distance is important. If the resident must lean forward to reach the handles, the walker is too far away. If you are assisting, stand on the resident's weak side, holding the gait belt in the center back with an underhand grasp. All four legs of the walker should strike the floor at the same time. Some residents have a tendency to touch the back legs on the floor first, rocking the walker forward onto the front legs. This is an unsafe practice that causes falls. When all four legs are securely on the floor, the resident steps forward. He or she steps into the walker with the weak leg, then the strong leg. If the resident has visual or cognitive deficits, assist with steering. Place one hand on the gait belt and one hand on the walker, guiding the resident.

Some residents pick up the walkers and carry them. This also increases the risk of injury. If the resident can carry the walker, he or she probably does not need the device, or may do better with a different type of device. Consult the nurse.

Many residents want to use the walker as a transfer device. They may try to hold the walker while they get into or out of the chair. This is an unsafe practice, as the walker is not stable and may tip, resulting in a fall. The resident should be taught to push against the arms of the chair when sitting and rising.

Crutches. Crutches are used by residents who have only one leg, or have an injury to one leg. The correct height of the crutch is three finger-widths below the armpit. Several different gaits are used in crutch walking, depending on the resident's medical problem. The therapist will teach the resident the correct gait for his or her condition.

Crutches are not commonly used by elderly residents. Most do not have sufficient arm strength to lift the body. Balance and coordination may also be a problem.

KEY POINTS

- A transfer involves moving a resident from one location to another.
- Sitting on the side of the bed is called dangling; this is the first step in the transfer procedure if the resident has been bedfast.
- A transfer belt should always be used when moving residents, unless contraindicated.
- Lock the brakes on the bed and wheelchair before transferring the resident.
- Move the footrests out of the way if the resident is transferring into a wheelchair.
- A key to maintaining stability of a wheelchair is positioning the large part of the front caster wheels facing forward.
- Always lock the brakes during transfers into and out of a wheelchair, and when the chair is parked.
- Position the resident in the wheelchair in good body alignment.
- The resident's legs must be supported on the footrests or the floor when the resident is seated in a wheelchair.
- The mechanical lift is a two-person device.
- A resident with good upper body strength can use a sliding board to transfer from the bed to a wheelchair and back.
- The wheelchair must fit the resident properly for comfort, safety, and to reduce the use of restraints.
- Pressure ulcers can develop when a resident is seated in the wheelchair; pressure relief must be provided.
- The wheelchair is a mobility device, not a transportation device. The resident should propel the chair independently whenever possible.
- The care plan will list purposeful activities for maintaining residents' ambulation ability.
- Residents may need canes, walkers, or crutches for balance, stability, and support during ambulation.

REVIEW

A. Multiple Choice

Select the one best answer.

1. Sitting a resident on the side of the bed is called
   a. proning.
   b. supining.
   c. semisitting.
   d. dangling.

2. When transferring residents from one place to another, you should
   a. lock the brakes of the bed, wheelchair, or stretcher.
   b. adjust the bed to the highest horizontal height.
   c. use a transfer belt only if the resident has had a stroke.
   d. advise the resident not to help, for safety.

3. Contraindications for using the transfer belt include residents who have
   a. had a stroke.
   b. head injuries.
   c. a gastrostomy.
   d. confusion.

4. When moving a resident (by yourself) with a transfer belt,
   a. use an underhand grasp.
   b. use an overhand grasp.
   c. stand behind the resident.
   d. lift from the side.

5. When using the mechanical (hydraulic) lift,
   a. ask another nursing assistant to help you.
   b. apply a transfer belt to the resident.
   c. fasten the "S" hooks facing inward.
   d. unlock the brakes so the wheelchair can be moved.

6. You are assigned to ambulate Mr. Wells using a gait belt. You are in the middle of the hallway, and the resident starts to fall. You should
   a. let go of the belt.
   b. hold Mr. Wells up and call for help.
   c. ease the resident down your leg.
   d. tell the resident to grab the handrail.

7. The correct height for the hands on a walker or cane is at the
   a. waist level.
   b. panty-line level.
   c. mid-thigh level.
   d. wrist level.

8. When transferring the resident from the bed to the wheelchair, position the wheelchair
   a. facing the door.
   b. at a 90° angle.
   c. at a 45° to 60° angle.
   d. on the resident's weak side.

9. When a resident transfers using the sliding board, he or she should wear
   a. cotton pants.
   b. a hospital gown.
   c. blue jeans.
   d. underwear only.

10. When transferring a resident from the bed to a stretcher,
    a. lower the bed to the lowest horizontal height.
    b. ensure that three or four people are available to help.
    c. logroll the resident onto the stretcher.
    d. lift the resident from the head and feet.

11. For wheelchair safety, all of the following are correct *except*
    a. lock the brakes during transfers and when the chair is parked.
    b. the small part of the front wheel faces sideways during transfers.
    c. the resident's feet should be supported when seated in the chair.
    d. the wheelchair must fit the resident properly.

12. Pressure ulcers
    a. can develop in chairfast residents.
    b. are not a concern in elderly persons.
    c. develop only when the resident is in bed.
    d. occur if the resident is not moved every four hours.

13. When pushing a wheelchair or stretcher, you should
    a. always avoid ramps and inclines.
    b. make sure the resident faces forward to enter an elevator.
    c. not use belts or rails, to avoid restraining the resident.
    d. back over thresholds and uneven surfaces.

14. If the resident's hips slide forward in a wheelchair, you should
    a. apply a restraint.
    b. check the chair depth.
    c. get a larger chair.
    d. shorten the leg rests.

15. Ideally, the resident who is chairfast should
    a. relieve pressure every 15 minutes.
    b. be moved by staff every four hours.
    c. use a five-inch foam or eggcrate cushion.
    d. stand up at least once each hour.

B. Short Answer

Answer the following questions.

16–20. List at least five contraindications for using the gait (transfer) belt.

16. _____   19. _____

17. _____   20. _____

18. _____

21–30. List at least 10 guidelines for proper chair positioning.

21. _____

22. _____

23. _____

24. _____

25. _____

26. _____

27. _____

28. _____

29. _____

30. _____

C. Clinical Applications

Answer the following questions.

31. You must transfer Mr. Hall from the chair to his bed. The care plan states that a transfer belt should be used for moving Mr. Hall. You cannot find a transfer belt. Mr. Hall has a belt on the trousers he is wearing. What should you do?

32. You have never transferred Mrs. Livingston before. The resident is smaller than you are. The care plan states that she uses a one-person transfer, but the resident is confused, agitated, and seems fearful. She is not following your directions. What will you do?

33. Mrs. Tsai asks you to take her to the bathroom. Because of the design of the room, the toilet is on her paralyzed side. How will you safely transfer this resident to the toilet?

34. You enter Mr. Secrest's room to walk him to the dining room for lunch, as listed on the care plan. The resident tells you he has a headache and feels weak. What action will you take?

35. After getting Miss Hegle up in the wheelchair, you discover that one leg rest is missing. The resident is confused. You were instructed to transport her to the activities room for a church service. What will you do?

CHAPTER 10

Care of the Environment

OBJECTIVES

After reading this chapter, you will be able to:

- Spell and define key terms.
- Describe the furniture found in a typical resident unit.
- Describe how to maintain separation of clean and soiled items in the resident's unit.
- List the nursing assistant's responsibilities in keeping the unit safe and clean.
- Demonstrate procedures related to care of the environment.

OBSERVATIONS TO MAKE AND REPORT RELATED TO CARE OF THE ENVIRONMENT

Residents have a call signal within reach at all times

Call signals are answered promptly

Doors to rooms are closed when care is being provided

Privacy curtain and window curtains are closed when care is being provided

Residents are covered completely in bed, chair, or hallways so they are not exposed

Staff knock on the door before entering a room and wait for a response

If the resident's door is open, staff knock on the door frame or other surface, and wait for permission to enter

Residents have fresh water at least once a shift and as requested

Water pitchers are always covered with lids

Water pitchers are washed regularly

Water pitchers are identified by resident name, bed number, or other method

Staff pours water for residents; offers to assist, assists dependent residents

Staff offers fluids each time they enter the room, or according to facility policy

Bedpans and urinals are marked with residents' names and properly stored

Bedpans and urinals are covered during transport

Gloves are not worn in public areas

One-glove technique or other method is used to prevent contamination of environment

Personal care items, such as combs, toothbrushes, and hygienic supplies, are properly stored and labeled with residents' names

Clean and soiled items are separated in bedside stands

Clean and soiled equipment are separated by at least one room's width in the hallway

Housekeeping carts and soiled linen hampers are removed from the hallway when meals are being served, or stored according to facility policy

Items in the refrigerator are covered, labeled, and dated

Refrigerator thermometer is present, temperature is below 45°F

Food and beverages are not stored in the same refrigerator with medications or laboratory specimens

Food and beverages are covered when carried in a hallway

PPE is readily available in areas of use

OBSERVATIONS TO MAKE AND REPORT RELATED TO CARE OF THE ENVIRONMENT, *CONTINUED*

Gloves and PPE are available in a variety of sizes; nonlatex and powder-free products are available upon request

Standard precautions are consistently used in the care of the environment and cleaning procedures

Staff avoid environmental contamination with soiled gloves

Gloves and other PPE are discarded in covered containers, or according to facility policy

Sharps containers are available in areas of use

Fire exists are marked; evacuation plan is posted

Only clean items are stored in clean utility room

Chemicals are properly labeled and stored in locked areas

Soiled utility room is used for soiled items only

Staff carry clean and soiled items away from uniforms

Clean linen is at least 18 inches from ceiling in clean linen storage room

Clean linen carts are covered when not in use

Only needed linen is taken into resident rooms

Linen hampers and barrels are not overflowing; lids fit tightly

Soiled linen is never placed on the floor

Facility policies describe routine cleaning tasks, dating and labeling of clean items

Tubs, shower chairs, and permanent equipment items are disinfected before and after each use

Medication room is not accessible to unauthorized persons

Charts and medical records are not accessible to unauthorized persons

RESIDENT'S UNIT

The resident's **unit** is the area for the resident's personal use **(Figure 10-1)**. The unit is the resident's personal space, consisting of a bed, chair, overbed table, bedside stand, wastebasket, dresser, and closet. Most of the personal care you deliver is done here. Caring for the resident includes caring for the unit. Some health care facilities also provide a telephone, television set, or radio as part of the unit. In others, residents who use these items provide their own.

The resident has a right to be treated with respect and dignity. You protect this right by knocking on closed doors and providing privacy when visitors are present. When providing personal care in the room, you must close the door, pull the privacy curtain, and close the drapes on the window, even if no one else is present.

Safety and Infection Control

Think *safety* when you enter and leave the room. The nursing assistant is responsible for keeping the unit safe.

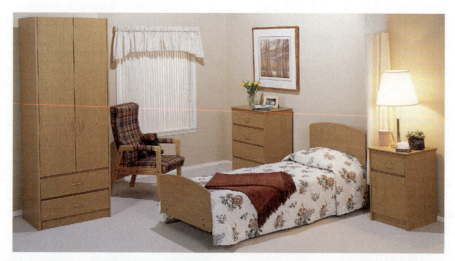

FIGURE 10-1 The resident's unit should be neat and tidy when the resident is admitted. Encourage residents to bring in personal items to create a comfortable, homelike environment. *(Courtesy of Medline Industries, Inc. 1-800-MEDLINE)*

GUIDELINES FOR
Caring for the Resident's Unit

- Check the call signal daily. The call signal should be within the resident's reach at all times, even if the resident is mentally confused.
- When the resident is in bed or in a chair, place the call signal, water, tissues, and other needed personal items within reach. This reduces the risk that the resident will reach for an item and fall.
- Cleaning the unit is usually the job of other departments. The nursing assistant is responsible for caring for the resident's personal items. You are expected to wipe tabletops after care, if food is spilled, or if soiling occurs.
- Controlling odors is very important. The best way to do this is to eliminate the source of the odor.
- Follow all infection control guidelines for separation of clean and soiled items in the resident's unit. Know which surfaces can be used to hold clean and soiled items.
- Follow your facility policy for disposing of gloves. Many facilities require that gloves be discarded in a closed container, and not in the open wastebasket in the unit.
- Always respect the resident's choices about arrangement of personal items. Avoid moving the resident's personal belongings without permission. This shows you care about the resident as a person.

- Know and follow your facility policy for storage of food, hygienic products, chemicals, and over-the-counter medications in the unit.
- Some long-term care facilities allow residents to self-administer medication. The medication may be kept in the unit. If this is the case, it must be stored in a secure location.
- Respect the resident's right to privacy when you are performing a procedure that involves exposing the body. Even if all the curtains and doors are closed, use of a **bath blanket** is necessary to preserve the resident's dignity. A bath blanket is a soft cotton or flannel blanket used to protect resident privacy and provide warmth during procedures in which the body is exposed.
- Check the floor for items and equipment that could cause the resident to fall.
- Clean spills on the floor immediately, and place a "wet floor" sign until the floor dries. Follow your facility policies for cleaning and disinfecting blood and body fluid spills.
- If you feel that an electrical or mechanical safety hazard exists, follow your facility policy for having the equipment locked and tagged out until it can be removed and repaired.
- If the resident uses the bathroom at night, leave a night light on.

Bedside Stand

The **bedside stand** is an important piece of furniture that is used to store personal items and articles used to deliver care. Bedside stands vary in design. Most have at least one drawer. The lower part of the stand may have a cupboard-type door or several drawers. Clean and soiled items must be kept separate in the cupboard and drawers. For example, the drawer in the top of the bedside stand is often used to store personal hygiene items, such as a toothbrush, brush, and comb. These items should not come into contact with each other. The lower part of the bedside stand usually stores the washbasin, bedpan and urinal. The washbasin is considered a "clean" item. It should not be stored next to the bedpan or urinal, which are considered "soiled." The inside of the cupboard-type bedside stand is divided by two shelves. Most facilities store the washbasin on the top shelf and the bedpan and urinal on the bottom shelf. In bedside stands with drawers, store these items in separate drawers **(Figure 10-2)**.

Overbed Table

The **overbed table** is a narrow table on wheels that is used to hold only clean items. The height of the table can be adjusted to a high or low position. It is also used for meal trays, if the resident eats meals in bed. The resident's drinking water may also be placed here. Wipe the top of the overbed table as often as necessary to keep it clean at all times.

THE HOSPITAL BED

The hospital bed is the most important piece of furniture in the resident's unit. As a nursing assistant, you must learn to meet all basic personal care needs for bedfast residents. This may mean adapting some normal procedures, such as bathing. For the bedfast resident, the hospital bed becomes the focal point for care. The bed will have some type of a privacy barrier, such as a curtain or screen. This curtain must be closed

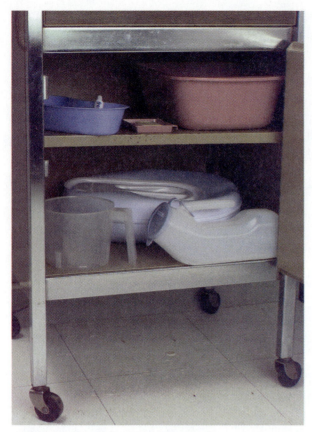

FIGURE 10-2 Clean and soiled items must be separated in the bedside stand.

when personal care is being provided, even if you are alone in the room with the resident.

The hospital bed may be electric or manual. Specialty (therapeutic) beds may be used for medical treatments, such as pressure ulcer management and care of the resident with pneumonia. You must learn the purposes of any specialty beds used in your facility and how to operate them when you are caring for the residents.

The head and knee areas can be raised or lowered in all regular hospital beds. Changing the angle of the head or knee of the bed is done for resident comfort, and to meet medical needs. Most beds also have a high-low function that raises and lowers the height of the bed. This feature has no therapeutic benefit for the residents. Always keep the height of the bed in the lowest horizontal position for resident use. Using the high-low feature makes your job easier and reduces the risk of injury to your back when you are working at the bedside. The bed is raised only when you are providing care, or performing a procedure such as making the bed. It is lowered when you are finished, before you leave the

room. You must become familiar with the operation of the hospital beds used in your facility:

- The **gatch handles** are used to change the height of manually operated beds. The gatch handles are at the foot of the bed **(Figure 10-3A)**. They are turned clockwise to raise the bed and counterclockwise to lower the bed. The handle on the left raises and lowers the head of the bed. The handle on the right raises and lowers the foot of the bed. The center handle is used to control the horizontal height of the bed. Use this handle to adjust bed height so the bed is in a comfortable working position for you. To prevent injuries to residents and staff, always fold the gatch handles under the bed when not in use **(Figure 10-3B)**.
- Wheels on the hospital bed enable you to move the bed, if necessary. All four wheels should be locked in place, except when the bed is being moved.
- Hospital beds are designed to be used with side rails. Some beds have a full-length rail on either side of the bed. Others have two small half rails on each side, one at the head and one at the foot. You must elevate the rails when you are caring for the resident with the bed in the highest horizontal position. Lower the rail only when you are at the bedside providing care. Raise it if you must step away, even for a moment. Keep the rail up on the opposite side of the bed. Some residents use the bed rails to pull on when positioning and turning in bed. Aside from these two situations, side rails may not be used for some residents. Check the care plan for instructions for each of your assigned residents. The use of side rails is discussed further in Chapter 15.
- Many facilities use electric beds. Switches are used to change the position of the head, knee, and horizontal bed height. In some beds, these

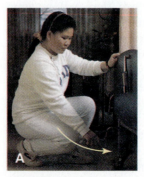
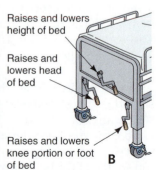

Raises and lowers height of bed

Raises and lowers head of bed

Raises and lowers knee portion or foot of bed

FIGURE 10-3 (A) For safety, fold the gatch handles under the bed when not in use. (B) Gatch handles

controls are permanently mounted on the bed rail.

- Always check the bed carefully for lost items before removing the linen. Items such as dentures, glasses, and hearing aids are commonly left on the bed. These items are very expensive and will not survive a trip through the washer and dryer.

Low Beds

Low beds **(Figure 10-4)** are commonly used in health care facilities for residents at risk of falls, for whom use of side rails is not desirable. The bed frame is four to six inches from the floor to the top of the frame deck. These beds reduce the risk of injury if the resident falls from the bed. Some facilities place pads on the floor next to the bed to further reduce the risk of injury.

Low beds are wonderful tools for reducing resident injuries, but the nursing assistant must use good body mechanics and common sense to prevent back injuries when lifting, moving, and caring for residents, and when making beds. Some low beds have high-low features, but many are stationary, which increases the risk of back injury. If the bed you are using has a high-low feature, use it whenever caring for the bedfast resident, transferring the resident, and making the bed. A mat on the floor reduces the risk of injury when a resident falls, but it can also be a trip hazard. Move slowly and carefully when working near a floor mat. Avoid entering the room in the dark. Leave a nightlight on, or turn the light on when entering. Squat or kneel on the floor mat when caring for the resident, to reduce back

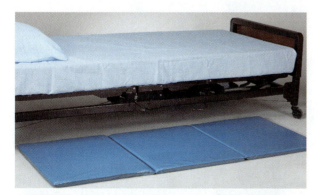

FIGURE 10-4 Low beds may be used for residents who are at risk for falls. Organize the bedmaking procedure carefully to avoid injury to your back. *(Courtesy of Skil-Care Corporation, Yonkers, NY, (800) 431-2972)*

strain caused by bending at the waist. Use good body mechanics, a transfer belt, or a mechanical lift when assisting residents into and out of low beds, to prevent back injuries. The care plan will provide resident-specific instructions. Avoid bending at the waist when moving the resident.

The bedmaking procedure is the same as it is for hospital beds. To make this task easier:

- Mentally plan and prepare yourself for the procedure.
- Organize your work well to reduce the total number of motions required to complete the task.
- Make sure you have everything you need before entering the room.
- Elevate the bed, if possible.
- Place linen and needed items on the resident's chair or within close reach.
- Maintain a neutral posture and bend from the legs, not the waist. Avoid twisting.
- Slowly remove the bed linen several pieces at a time. Avoid trying to remove all the linen in one bundle. The weight of the linen and your posture increase the risk of back injury.
- Make one side of the bed at a time. This is faster, more efficient, and conserves energy.
- Use a fitted bottom sheet to reduce the number of movements necessary for making the bed, thereby lowering the risk of back strain.

MAKING THE BED

The nursing assistant is responsible for making the bed each day. A clean, wrinkle-free bed promotes resident comfort and prevents skin breakdown. If the resident is out of bed, the unoccupied bedmaking procedure is used. A wide variety of linen is available for bedmaking. Flat sheets may be used on both the top and bottom. Many facilities use fitted sheets on the bottom. Most facilities place draw sheets (lift sheets) under residents who must be turned by the staff. Disposable or reusable underpads are placed under the buttocks if the resident is incontinent or uses the bedpan or urinal in bed. A plastic or rubber draw sheet covered with a cotton sheet may also be used, but many facilities have eliminated these in favor of large underpads. Thermal blankets are usually used for warmth. Many different types of bedspreads are available.

You may be instructed to make the bed in several different ways. **Table 10-1** describes different bedmaking methods.

TABLE 10-1 Bedmaking Methods

Method of Bedmaking	Procedure Variations	Rationale
Unoccupied bed	Most common type of bedmaking procedure; used for making all types of beds.	Making the unoccupied bed is easier and faster for the nursing assistant. It is more comfortable for the resident.
Occupied bed	Used when the resident is confined to bed.	Changes wet or soiled linen for resident comfort and prevention of skin breakdown; provides fresh, clean linen for feeling of comfort and security.
Closed bed	The bed is made with the top sheet, blanket, and spread pulled all the way to the top. The pillow may be covered or placed on top of the spread, depending on facility policy. The open end of the pillow case faces away from the door.	Used when the resident is expected to be out of bed all day or when making a bed after the resident has been discharged; presents a neat, tidy appearance.
Open bed	The bed is made in the normal manner. The top sheet and spread are fan-folded to the foot of the bed.	This procedure is used when the resident is temporarily out of bed. The resident can be covered easily and quickly upon return to bed.

Planning Your Work

Plan your work before making the bed. Bring all necessary linen into the room and stack it in the order of use. Before making the bed, adjust the height so that it is comfortable for you. Lower the head and knee so the bed is flat. Avoid walking around the bed many times. Make one side of the bed at a time, then go to the other side to complete the bedmaking procedure. It may take (text continues on page 208)

GUIDELINES FOR
Handling Clean and Soiled Linen

- Wash your hands before handling clean linen.
- Carry all linen (clean or soiled) away from your uniform.
- Bring only the necessary amount of linen to the room. Extra linen cannot be removed and used for other residents until it has been washed.
- Do not shake linen. Unfold clean linen.
- Check the bed linen for lost articles before removing it from the bed.
- Roll soiled linen with the soiled side in.
- Wash your hands immediately after handling used linen, even if it is not visibly soiled.
- Follow your facility policy for placement of clean and soiled linen in the resident's room.
- Soiled linen is never placed on the floor. Some facilities allow the soiled linen hamper in the room and some do not. If you cannot bring the hamper into the room, you may be able to place soiled linen in a plastic bag or pillowcase draped over the back of the chair. Follow your facility policy.
- If you are handling linen contaminated with blood, body fluids, secretions, or excretions, you must wear gloves (Figure 10-5). Wear a gown if your uniform will have substantial contact with soiled linen.

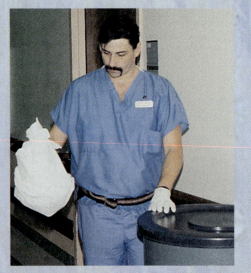

FIGURE 10-5 Wear gloves when handling linen soiled with blood, body fluids, secretions, or excretions. Hold soiled linen away from your uniform.

GUIDELINES FOR

Handling Clean and Soiled Linen, *Continued*

- Linen contaminated with blood or body fluids may be placed in plastic bags that are tied or secured at the top. If the outside of the bag accidentally becomes contaminated during the bagging process, the first bag should be placed in a clean outer bag. If the outside is not contaminated or torn, double bagging is not necessary.
- Some facilities use water-soluble bags for wet linen contaminated with blood or body fluids. These bags dissolve in the washer. Water-soluble bags must always be double-bagged inside a regular plastic bag. The wet linen may cause the water-soluble bag to dissolve before it reaches the laundry.
- After you have discarded the soiled linen, remove your PPE and wash your hands. Doing this will prevent contamination of clean linen and other envi-

ronmental surfaces. Gloves are not necessary for handling clean linen.
- Keep the lids on soiled linen hampers. Soiled linen should not overflow under the lid. Most facilities require that hampers be taken to the laundry when they are three-quarters full, to avoid overflowing.
- Clean and soiled linen should never touch each other.
- Follow your facility policy for separation of clean linen carts and soiled linen hampers in the hallways. Most facilities require a one room-width separation of clean and soiled equipment.
- Follow your facility policy for removal of linen hampers from the hallways when food carts are on the unit.

PROCEDURE

31 Making the Unoccupied Bed

1. Perform your beginning procedure actions.
2. Gather needed supplies: disposable gloves, mattress pad (if used), two large sheets (or one flat and one fitted sheet), a linen draw sheet (if used), underpad (if used), pillowcase, laundry bag or hamper, and blanket or bedspread (if needed). Stack the linen in the order of use.
3. Carry clean linen away from your uniform **(Figure 10-6)**.
4. Stack the linens on a clean area near the bed in the order of use, with bottom linen on top.
5. Lower the head so the bed is flat.
6. Remove and fold the bedspread if you are reusing it.
7. Apply gloves if linen is wet or soiled.
8. Check the linen for lost items. Remove the soiled linen from the bed by rolling it in a ball, soiled side facing in. Follow your facility policy for wiping the mattress. If the mattress is soiled with excretions or secretions, it should be wiped with disinfectant.
9. Place soiled linens in the hamper or laundry bag. Avoid contaminating environmental surfaces with your gloves during this procedure.
10. Remove gloves and discard them according to facility policy.
11. Wash your hands.
12. Straighten the mattress pad (if used). Center the lengthwise middle fold of the bottom sheet in the middle of the bed.

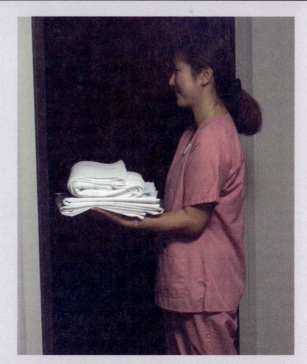

FIGURE 10-6 Carry clean linen away from your uniform.

Continues

13. Open the sheet.
14. Place the end with the small hem even with the foot of the mattress **(Figure 10-7)**.
15. Tuck the top of the sheet under the mattress.
16. **Miter** the corner **(Figure 10-8)** by folding it at a 45° angle perpendicular to the mattress, or tuck the corners of the fitted sheet over the edge of the mattress.
17. Beginning at the head of the bed, tuck in the sheet, working from head to foot.
18. Place the draw sheet across the center of the bed.
19. Tuck the edge of the sheet under the mattress.
20. Center the lengthwise middle fold of the top sheet in the center of the bed.
21. Open the sheet and position it so the top edge is even with the top of the mattress.
22. Place the blanket or bedspread on the bed.
23. Miter linens at the foot of the bed by tucking the sheet in at a 45° angle perpendicular to the mattress.
24. Move to the other side of the bed.
25. Pull and straighten the bottom sheet.
26. Pull the sheet tightly, and tuck the bottom sheet under the mattress at the head of the bed.
27. Miter the corner of the sheet at the head of the bed or tuck in the corners of the fitted sheet **(Figure 10-9)**.

28. Pull the bottom sheet tightly and tuck it under the mattress.
29. Pull the linen draw sheet tightly and tuck it under the mattress. Tuck the center of the sheet first, then the edges.
30. Check to be sure the bed is smooth and wrinkle-free.
31. Straighten the top sheet.
32. Straighten the blanket or spread.
33. Tuck the sheet and blanket or spread under the foot of the mattress.
34. Miter the top linens at the foot of the bed.
35. Fold the spread back about 30 inches at the top edge.
36. Fold the top sheet back about 4 inches at the top edge of the sheet.
37. Place the pillow on the bed.
38. Grab the center end of the pillowcase with your dominant hand. Fold it up over your arm **(Figure 10-10A)**. Grab the pillow with this hand **(Figure 10-10B)**. Unfold the pillowcase over the pillow **(Figure 10-10C)**.
39. Straighten the pillowcase.
40. Place the pillow at the head of the bed with the open end facing away from the door.
41. Cover the pillow with the bedspread.
42. Perform your procedure completion actions.

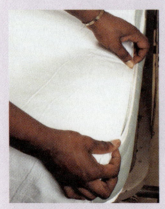

FIGURE 10-7 Place the rough edge down, even with the end of the mattress.

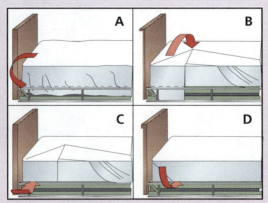

FIGURE 10-8 Making a mitered corner. (A) The sheet is hanging loose at the side of the bed. (B) Pick up the sheet about 12 inches from the head of the bed to form a triangle. (C) Tuck in the sheet at the head of the bed. Pick up triangle and place your other hand at the edge of the bed, near the head, to hold the edge of the sheet in place. Bring triangle over the edge of the mattress and tuck smoothly under the mattress. (D) Tuck in the rest of the sheet along the side of the mattress. Make sure the sheet is wrinkle-free.

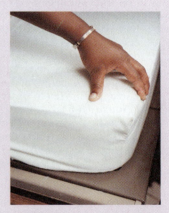

FIGURE 10-9 Tuck the fitted sheet securely under the mattress.

PROCEDURE

31

Making the Unoccupied Bed, *Continued*

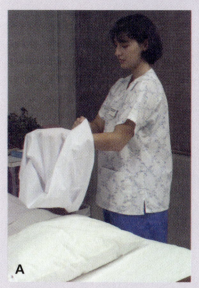 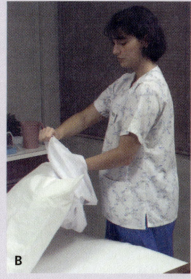 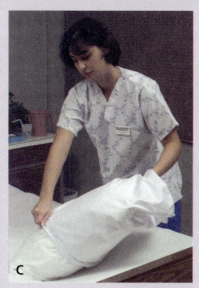

FIGURE 10-10 (A) Grasp the pillowcase at the seam and fold it back and over your wrist, inside out. (B) Grab the end of the pillow in the center with your pillowcase-covered hand. If the pillow has a tag, grasp the end with the tag on it. (C) Unfold and smooth the pillowcase over the pillow.

PROCEDURE

32

Making the Occupied Bed

1. Perform your beginning procedure actions.
2. Gather supplies needed: disposable gloves, two large sheets (or one flat and one fitted sheet), a linen draw sheet (if used), underpad (if used), pillowcase, laundry bag or hamper, and blanket or bedspread (if needed). Stack the linen in the order of use.
3. Carry clean linen away from your uniform.
4. Stack the linens on a clean area near the bed in the order of use, from bottom to top.
5. Lower the head so the bed is flat. Check with the nurse for directions on residents with tube feeding, using oxygen, or those with respiratory distress.
6. Remove the bedspread and blanket. Fold them and place them on the chair.
7. Apply gloves if linen is wet or soiled.
8. Cover the top sheet with a bath blanket. Remove the sheet by sliding it out underneath without exposing the resident. Place the used sheet in the soiled linen container.
9. Turn the resident on the side away from you, following the guidelines in Procedure 16.
10. Loosen the bottom sheet.
11. Check the bed for lost items. Roll the soiled bottom sheet(s) inward and tuck them along the resident's back.
12. Center the lengthwise middle fold of the bottom sheet in the middle of the bed.
13. Open one half of the sheet lengthwise.
14. Place the end with the small hem even with the foot of the mattress, or fit the corner of the fitted sheet.
15. Tuck the top of the sheet under the head of the mattress on the side where you are working.
16. Miter the corner.
17. Beginning at the head of the bed, tuck in the sheet, working from head to foot.
18. Place the draw sheet across the center of the bed.
19. Tuck the edge of the draw sheet under the mattress.
20. Roll the remaining half of the sheets and tuck them under the soiled sheet.
21. If an underpad or lift sheet is used, place it on top of the draw sheet and roll it inside.
22. Help the resident roll over the linen on the side facing you.

Continues

23. Raise the side rail.
24. Go to the other side of the bed.
25. Lower the side rail.
26. Remove the soiled linens.
27. Dispose of linens according to facility policy. *Do not put soiled linen on the floor.* Raise the side rail if leaving the bedside. Avoid contaminating environmental surfaces with your gloves during this procedure.
28. Remove gloves and discard according to facility policy.
29. Wash your hands.
30. Return to the bedside and lower the side rail.
31. Pull the bottom sheet over the mattress.
32. Tuck the bottom sheet tightly under the head of the mattress.
33. Miter the corner of the sheet at the head, or fit the corner of the fitted sheet.
34. Pull the bottom sheet tightly and tuck it under the mattress.
35. Pull the draw sheet tight, and tuck it in. If an underpad is used, smooth and straighten it.
36. Help the resident roll on his or her back. Keep the resident covered with the bath blanket.
37. Place the top sheet over the bath blanket, centering the center fold.
38. Pull the bath blanket out from under the clean sheet without exposing the resident.
39. Place the blanket and bedspread over the sheet.
40. Fold the top sheet over the edge of the blanket.
41. Tuck the top linens under the foot of the mattress, allowing room for the resident's toes. Make a **toe pleat** by folding the top linen over two to three inches at the end of the bed **(Figure 10-11)**. The toe pleat provides extra space and keeps the linen from pulling the feet downward. This is more comfortable for the resident and reduces the risk of contractures, such as foot drop (see Chapter 18).

42. Miter the corner of top linens at the foot of the bed.
43. Raise the side rail.
44. Go to the other side of the bed.
45. Lower the side rail.
46. Miter the corner of the top linens at the foot of the bed.
47. Remove the pillow and soiled pillowcase.
48. Place a clean pillowcase on the pillow.
49. Fold and store the bath blanket or place in the soiled linen hamper, according to facility policy.
50. Perform your procedure completion actions.

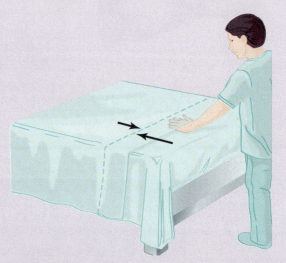

FIGURE 10-11 The toe pleat provides space for movement of the feet. The resident will be more comfortable, and the risk of contractures is reduced.

a little practice to learn to make the bed this way, but it saves your strength and energy and reduces fatigue and injury to your back.

Making the Occupied Bed

Sometimes residents have conditions that require them to stay in bed all the time. When residents are confined to bed, you must make the bed using the **occupied bedmaking** procedure. Sometimes only part of the linen is changed while the resident is in bed. If the resident is bedfast, you will have to check the bed linen and straighten it as often as necessary during your shift. Keeping the linen clean, dry, and wrinkle-

free enhances resident comfort and reduces the risk of skin breakdown.

Always apply the principles of standard precautions when changing the bed. Wear gloves if contact with blood, body fluids (except sweat), secretions, or excretions is likely. Wear a gown if your uniform will have substantial contact with linen contaminated by these substances.

OTHER IMPORTANT AREAS

The residents' rooms are part of a larger nursing unit. The area may be called a nursing station, section, hall, floor, or unit. Other important resident care and service areas on the larger nursing unit are:

- Nurses' station—This is a work area for nursing personnel. Reports and assignments are usually given at the nurses' station. Medical records are stored here, and documentation is completed in this area **(Figure 10-12)**. Remember that resident records and documents are confidential. These things should be protected from access by unauthorized persons. Lists of resident names, such as the nourishment list, restraint list, bowel and bladder records, and assignment sheets, should not be placed where they can be viewed by the public.
- Medication room—This is a smaller, locked area in the nurses' station. Access is limited to nurses, certified medication aides (if permitted by state law), and other licensed personnel. Other employees (such as the housekeeper) can enter this room only under the direct supervision of a licensed nurse. This room is used for storage and preparation of medications. The door is kept locked when not in use.
- Clean utility room—This area is used only for storage of clean and sterile supplies. New personal care items, such as lotions, toothpaste, and denture cups, may be stored here. Soiled items should never enter this room.
- Soiled utility room—The soiled utility room is used for cleaning soiled supplies. Clean items are removed as soon as they are washed, disinfected, and dried. Clean supplies must never be brought into this room. Personal protective equipment (PPE) should be available for use during cleaning procedures. Apply the principles of standard precautions and select the PPE appropriate to the procedure. A hopper

or utensil washer may be available for washing bedpans and urinals. Disinfectants and other chemicals will be stored here. These should be kept in locked cupboards when not in use. (Some facilities keep the door to the soiled utility room locked as well.) Make sure chemicals are stored in the original, labeled containers. Use them only according to manufacturers' directions. Some facilities use this area as a holding room for soiled linen until it is transported to the laundry.
- Linen room—This room is used for clean linen storage. Linen should not be stored on the top shelf closer than 18 inches to the ceiling. If linen is closer than this, the sprinkler system will not be effective in a fire. Most facilities have a central linen storage area. Smaller amounts of linen are removed and placed on wheeled carts that are pushed into the hallways **(Figure 10-13)**. The door to the linen room should be kept closed. The smaller linen carts should be covered except when linen is being added or removed.
- Dining room—Most residents eat their meals in a community dining area. Some facilities have a dining room on each nursing unit, whereas other facilities have a larger dining room that is used by residents from all nursing units. The unit dining room may also be used

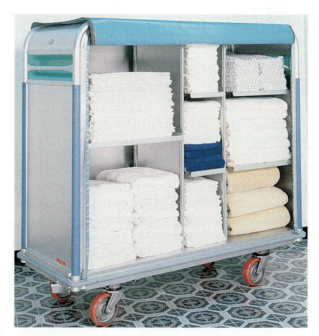

FIGURE 10-13 The clean linen room holds the primary linen supply. Linen is loaded onto smaller carts for use in the hallways. Keep the door closed when not in use. Always keep the carts covered in the hallway, except when removing clean items. *(Courtesy of Medline, Inc. 1-800-MEDLINE)*

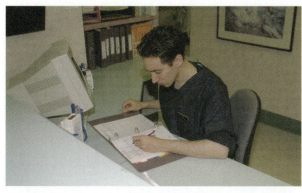

FIGURE 10-12 The nurse's station is a work area for personnel. Medical records are stored behind the station where they are not accessible to the public.

as a day room, television lounge, and activity room. Eating is a social occasion. Most people do not like to eat alone. Residents' appetites are usually better if they eat their meals with others in a pleasant community area.

- Tub/Shower room—Residents are bathed in community tub and shower areas in some facilities. Shower curtains, privacy curtains, or doors are used to separate residents who are using the room at the same time. Take care to avoid exposing residents in this community area. These are clean areas, and soiled linen should not be placed on the floor.
- Pantry—Some facilities also have a pantry area on each unit in which resident snacks are stored. In many facilities, the ice machine or clean ice chest is stored in the pantry. The refrigerator in the pantry will have a thermometer. Refrigerator temperatures must be checked daily. Temperature should not exceed 45°F. This is a clean area and soiled items should not be stored here. The refrigerator is for food items only. Laboratory specimens and medications are not stored in this refrigerator. Food items should be covered, wrapped, and sealed. Open items should be dated and discarded according to facility policy.

CLEANING ASSIGNMENTS

Nursing assistants are usually given a cleaning assignment that is completed during or at the

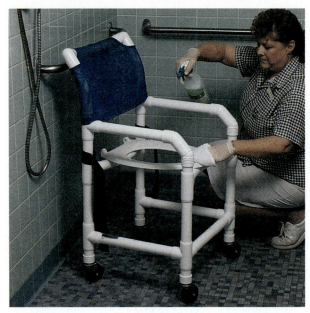

FIGURE 10-14 All staff must complete a cleaning assignment during their shift.

end of the shift. You may be responsible for tidying the service areas listed here (**Figure 10-14**). In some facilities, items such as bedpans, urinals, and wheelchairs are cleaned on a regular schedule. Your assignment may include these responsibilities during your shift. All nursing personnel are responsible for maintaining a clean, homelike, sanitary environment on the nursing unit.

KEY POINTS IN CHAPTER

- The resident's unit is an area for personal use.
- Respect the resident's rights when giving care and handling personal belongings.
- Think safety when you enter and leave each resident's room.
- Follow your facility infection-control policies for separation of clean and soiled items.
- Follow your facility policies for handling soiled linen.
- Practice the principles of standard precautions when making the bed if contact with blood, moist body fluids (except sweat), secretions, or excretions is likely.
- Personal protective equipment is removed after soiled linen is discarded. The hands are washed before handling clean linen and touching other environmental surfaces.
- The nursing assistant is responsible for keeping resident rooms tidy. You may also be responsible for routine cleaning assignments that must be completed during or at the end of the shift.

REVIEW

A. Multiple Choice

Select the one best answer.

1. When giving personal care to the resident,
   a. close the door only; there is no need to close the privacy curtain unless someone else is in the room.
   b. always drape the resident with a bath blanket even if no one else is present in the room.
   c. you may leave the door open after visiting hours, but close the privacy and window curtains.
   d. close the door and privacy curtain; closing the window curtain is not necessary during daylight hours.

2. The following is true about the use of side rails:
   a. Side rails should be kept up for all residents.
   b. Side rails should be kept down for all residents.
   c. Consult the care plan to see if side rails are indicated.
   d. The resident always determines if side rails are used.

3. The overbed table is used for
   a. clean items, food, and water.
   b. holding soiled linen and toilet articles.
   c. storing the bedpan and urinal.
   d. medical procedures only.

4. When caring for a resident in a bed with gatch handles, which handle always elevates the head of the bed?
   a. Right.
   b. Left.
   c. Center.
   d. It varies with the bed.

5. Which of the following is true about storing items in the bedside stand?
   a. The hairbrush and urinal are stored on the top shelf.
   b. The washbasin and bedpan are stored on the bottom shelf.
   c. The washbasin and urinal are stored on the top shelf.
   d. The bedpan and urinal are stored on the bottom shelf.

6. Which of the following is true about handling linen?
   a. Clean and soiled linen are always carried away from your uniform.
   b. Extra linen in a room can be removed and used for another resident.
   c. Soiled linen may be placed on the floor.
   d. Gloves are used for handling both clean and soiled linen.

7. You are assigned to make an unoccupied bed in room 931. The linen is saturated with fresh blood. Select the correct personal protective equipment to wear:
   a. Mask, gown, gloves.
   b. Gown, gloves.
   c. Gloves, mask, face shield.
   d. Mask, face shield.

8. When making the unoccupied bed,
   a. raise the bed to a comfortable working height.
   b. raise the side rail on the side opposite from where you are working.
   c. elevate the head of the bed at least 30 degrees when you are done.
   d. roll the resident from side to side so you can tighten the bottom sheet.

9. Clean linen should be
   a. stored at least 8 to 12 inches from the ceiling.
   b. covered when being transported on carts in the hallway.
   c. placed next to the soiled linen hamper in the hallway for convenience.
   d. carried from one resident's room to the next in a stack.

10. A toe pleat
    a. makes the finished bed look neater.
    b. is used only in the unoccupied bedmaking procedure.
    c. reduces resident discomfort and complications.
    d. is an older method that is no longer used.

11. The temperature of the pantry refrigerator should be
    a. 45°F or below.
    b. at least 50°F.
    c. appropriate for laboratory specimens.
    d. 36°F or below.

12. Soiled linen
    a. should be placed on the floor when making an occupied bed.
    b. is put on the overbed table until it can be removed.
    c. is not the nursing assistant's responsibility.
    d. should be placed in a plastic bag or covered hamper.

B. True/False

Answer each statement true (T) or false (F).

13. _____ Shake soiled linen before placing it in the hamper to check for lost items.

14. _____ The call signal is placed close to alert residents only, because residents who are mentally confused don't know how to use it.

15. _____ A bath blanket is used to drape the resident when providing personal care.

16. _____ Only authorized personnel can access the medication room unless directly supervised.

17. _____ Instruments used in resident care are brought to the clean utility room for cleaning.

18. _____ Chemicals in the soiled utility room must be stored in locked cabinets.

19. _____ Licensed nurses are responsible for the personal care of residents using specialized (therapeutic) beds.

20. _____ The nursing assistant should check the bed for lost items before removing soiled linen.

C. Clinical Applications

Answer the following questions.

21. Beverly Fry's room is very cluttered. She has food, newspaper, trash, and numerous personal items in disarray all over the room. The nurse states that the room is a health hazard and assigns you to clean it. When you enter the room, Beverly starts yelling at you and tells you to get out. She says she will sue you if you throw anything away. What should you do?

22. You are making an occupied bed. The bed linen is soiled and must be changed. The resident is lying on his side. You remove the soiled linen behind his back. No one else is in the room to assist you. There is no soiled linen hamper in the room. What do you do with the soiled linen until you can take it to the hallway and discard it in the hamper?

CHAPTER 11

Personal Care Skills

OBJECTIVES

After reading this chapter, you will be able to:

- Spell and define key terms.
- Describe how personal care affects self-esteem.
- List four daily care routines and describe the type of care given in each.
- Demonstrate routine oral hygiene, special oral hygiene, and care of dentures.
- List the general guidelines for assisting residents with bathing and perineal care.
- Demonstrate the back rub procedure.
- List the guidelines for assisting residents with personal grooming.
- Demonstrate hand, foot, and nail care.
- Demonstrate correct application of antiembolism stockings.
- Describe measures to protect the resident's arms and legs from injury.
- Demonstrate dressing and undressing a dependent resident.
- Demonstrate procedures related to personal care skills.

OBSERVATIONS TO MAKE AND REPORT RELATED TO PERSONAL CARE SKILLS

Rash

Redness

Redness of the skin that does not go away within 30 minutes after pressure is relieved from a bony prominence or pressure area

In dark- or yellow-skinned residents, spots or areas that are darker than normal skin tone

Pressure ulcers, blisters

Abrasions, skin tears, lacerations

Irritation

Bruises

Skin discoloration

Swelling

Lumps

Abnormal skin growths

Change in color of a wart or mole

Abnormal sweating

Excessive heat or coolness to touch

Open areas/skin breakdown

Drainage

Foul odor

Complaints such as numbness, burning, tingling, itching

Signs of infection

Unusual skin color, such as blue or gray color of the skin, lips, nail beds, roof of mouth, or mucous membranes

Skin growths

Poor skin turgor, tenting of skin on forehead or over sternum

Sunken, dark eyes

PERSONAL CARE OF THE RESIDENT

Good personal **hygiene** (cleanliness) is essential to maintaining or restoring health. Good hygiene prevents infection, eliminates odors, promotes relaxation, stimulates circulation, and enhances self-esteem. Hygienic habits and practices are developed over a person's lifetime. They may be influenced by culture or religion. Some adaptations of routines and customary practices may be necessary in the long-term care facility. Even minor changes can be upsetting to the resident. Personal care and hygiene is a very private matter for most people.

Providing personal care is a major responsibility of the nursing assistant. It is also an area in which you must be sensitive to the needs, feelings, emotions, and cultural practices of others. Most personal care involves exposing and touching the resident's body. Often, you are bathing and caring for private areas. Think of how you would feel if someone else had to do these things for you. Remember, the resident feels this way, too. The resident may feel embarrassed or ashamed because he or she is unable to care for himself or herself. Be kind, compassionate, and sensitive to the resident's feelings and do not show disgust if you must care for a resident who has lost control of bowel or bladder. If you react in a negative way, this will further lower the resident's self-esteem. Always provide privacy. Use proper terms when referring to elimination. Avoid slang, which may be degrading to the resident.

Activities of Daily Living

Activities of daily living, or ADLs, are personal care activities that people do every day to meet their human needs. Examples of ADLs are bathing; shaving; caring for the hair, mouth, and nails; and applying makeup. Dressing, eating, and toileting are also activities of daily living. These activities fall at the lower levels of Maslow's hierarchy of needs, so they are the most basic. If the resident cannot meet these needs independently, the nursing assistant must assist or provide care that meets them. Personal care of the resident includes care of the mouth, teeth, skin, hair, nails, and feet. It may involve cleaning body excretions if a resident is **incontinent.** Incontinence is the inability to control the bowel, bladder, or both, and is often the result of a medical problem over which the resident has

no control. It may be temporary. A resident who becomes incontinent may feel guilty and embarrassed. You must be sensitive to the resident's feelings. Personal care also involves bathing, dressing, and grooming the resident. Good personal hygiene prevents skin breakdown; gives the resident a secure, comfortable feeling; and enhances self-esteem.

The resident has carried out ADLs throughout his or her life. Sometimes the resident is able to continue to do all or part of these skills. If so, he or she should be encouraged to continue. You must provide the supplies needed and arrange them conveniently so the resident can use them. It may take longer, but you will reinforce the resident's feelings of self-worth by allowing him or her to do these things. Organize your work so that you can do something else while the resident is performing self-care skills. This makes good use of your time. If the resident is unable to complete a task, you will finish it for him or her. This is part of providing restorative nursing care.

Daily Care Routines

Personal care is given as often as necessary to maintain comfort and keep residents clean. Residents who can be out of bed may be able to continue with their regular routines, but you must assist residents who are weak, mentally confused, or bedfast.

Routine care is given at certain times. The names for the procedures may differ slightly in your facility, but the care given at certain times of day is an important part of the daily routine for all residents. You may be assigned to give AM care, morning care, afternoon care, or HS care. Staff on duty in the early morning are responsible for providing **AM care.** Residents are prepared for breakfast early in the morning. Routine bathing and skin care measures are usually done during **morning care.** Many residents like to have **afternoon care** before visitors arrive. **HS care** may also be called evening care or bedtime care. This care makes the resident comfortable and improves the ability to rest and relax. A summary of the routine hygienic measures performed is found in **Table 11-1.**

Changing the Resident's Gown. Most residents are up and dressed during the day. Some bedfast residents wear hospital gowns. The gown may have to be changed frequently if it becomes wet or soiled. Avoid exposing the resident during this procedure.

TABLE 11-1 Routine care tasks

Type of Care	Responsibilities
AM care (may also be called early AM care)	1. Assisting with using the bathroom, bedpan, or urinal. 2. Cleansing incontinent residents and changing wet or soiled linen. 3. Assisting the resident to wash face and hands for breakfast. 4. Providing oral care, or assisting the resident to brush teeth. 5. Straightening the bed. 6. Assisting the resident to dress, or put on robe and slippers if getting out of bed for breakfast. 7. Transferring the resident to the chair, or assisting the resident to a comfortable position for eating in bed, if necessary. 8. Tidying the unit and removing unnecessary articles before breakfast. 9. Passing fresh drinking water and assisting the resident to drink, if necessary. 10. Clearing and wiping the overbed table in preparation to receive the breakfast tray, or assisting the resident to go to the dining area.
Morning care (may also be called AM care)	1. Assisting with using the bathroom, bedpan, or urinal. 2. Cleansing incontinent residents and changing wet or soiled linen. 3. Assisting the resident to wash face and hands immediately after breakfast. 4. Providing oral care, or assisting the resident to brush teeth after breakfast. 5. Providing bed baths, partial baths, perineal care, whirlpool baths, tub baths, and showers. 6. Shaving male residents. 7. Assisting female residents to put on makeup. 8. Performing range-of-motion exercises (Chapter 18), if indicated on the care plan. 9. Assisting residents to change pajamas or dress in street clothes, according to preference and facility policy. 10. Brushing and caring for the hair and nails. 11. Assisting residents with walking and other activity. 12. Transporting residents to other areas for treatments and activities. 13. Changing the bed linen, or making the bed, according to facility policy. 14. Tidying the unit.
Afternoon care (may also be called PM care)	1. Assisting with using the bathroom, bedpan, or urinal. 2. Cleansing incontinent residents and changing wet or soiled linen. 3. Assisting the resident to wash face and hands after lunch. 4. Providing oral care, or assisting the resident to brush teeth after lunch. 5. Changing the resident's clothing, if necessary. 6. Assisting residents to return to bed for a nap. 7. Assisting residents out of bed after they have rested. 8. Assisting residents to brush hair or freshen makeup, if desired. 9. Assisting residents with ambulation. 10. Performing range-of-motion exercises (Chapter 18), if indicated on the care plan. 11. Straightening the bed linen. 12. Passing fresh drinking water and assisting the resident to drink, if necessary.
HS care (may also be called evening care)	1. Assisting with using the bathroom, bedpan, or urinal. 2. Cleansing incontinent residents and changing wet or soiled linen. 3. Assisting with a bedtime snack, supplement, or nourishment. 4. Assisting the resident to wash face and hands before bedtime. 5. Providing oral care, or assisting the resident to brush teeth at bedtime. 6. Assisting residents with a partial bath before bedtime. 7. Assisting residents into gowns or pajamas for bed (or change, if necessary or desired). 8. Giving back rubs. 9. Straightening the bed linen. 10. Tidying the unit. 11. Passing fresh drinking water and assisting the resident to drink, if necessary.

PROCEDURE 33

Changing the Resident's Gown

1. Perform your beginning procedure actions.
2. Reach behind the resident and untie the gown strings.
3. Remove and loosen the gown under the resident's body.
4. Unfold the clean gown and drape it across the resident's chest, on top of the bath blanket or top sheet.
5. Remove the resident's arms from the sleeves of the gown, but keep the chest covered. If the resident cannot pull the arms from the sleeves, insert your hand into the sleeve to support the resident's hand, and pull the sleeve down and off.
6. Assist the resident to insert the arms into the sleeves of the clean gown. If the resident has a paralyzed arm, place that arm in the sleeve first. If the resident cannot place the arms in the sleeves, put your hand in the sleeve on the outside of the gown. Grab the resident's hand. Slide the gown off your hand, then up over the resident's hand and arm.
7. After both arms are in the sleeves, remove the soiled gown by pulling it under the clean gown, without exposing the resident.
8. Tie the strings and straighten the clean gown under the bedding.
9. Perform your procedure completion actions.

ORAL HYGIENE

Oral hygiene involves cleaning the mouth, teeth, gums, and tongue. One of your responsibilities is to provide good mouth care for the resident. Residents need mouth care even if they have no teeth and no dentures. When a person is ill, there may be a bad taste in the mouth caused by the illness or medication. The tongue may be coated with a substance that spoils the appetite. One purpose of oral hygiene is to remove food particles and make the mouth feel fresh and clean. Having a clean mouth helps the resident's appetite, prevents bad breath and mouth odor, and reduces the incidence of pneumonia and some other medical conditions to which elderly persons are susceptible.

Good oral hygiene also reduces the buildup of **plaque,** an acidic, decay-causing substance.

GUIDELINES FOR

Giving Oral Hygiene

- Encourage the resident to do as much self-care as possible.
- Allow the resident to brush his or her own teeth. Take the resident to the bathroom sink, if possible.
- Always wear gloves when performing oral hygiene. Avoid contaminating environmental surfaces and clean supplies with your gloves.
- Observe and report any signs of irritation, sores, loose teeth, pain, swelling, or other abnormalities to the nurse.

Everyone has bacteria in the mouth. Many foods cause the bacteria to produce acids. Sugars and starches are the worst culprits, but other foods in combination with bacteria produce plaque as well. Plaque also irritates the gums, making them red, tender, or bleed easily. The gums may pull away from the teeth. Pockets form and fill with pus and more bacteria. Untreated, the condition worsens until the bone around the teeth is destroyed. The teeth may become loose or have to be removed. Gum disease is a leading cause of tooth loss in adults.

Many elderly persons have reduced saliva, which causes the mouth to be dry and uncomfortable. Residents who breathe mainly through the mouth also have dry mucous membranes. Providing mouth care is partly a comfort measure that creates a feeling of well-being. It is also an opportunity for observation. While assisting with oral care, you have an opportunity to observe the resident's mouth and inspect it for abnormalities and pocketed food.

Special Oral Hygiene

You will recall from Chapter 7 that NPO is the abbreviation for "nothing by mouth." Residents who are NPO, unconscious, receiving tube feeding, or using oxygen require more frequent mouth care. The mucous membranes of the mouth dry out quickly and become coated with mucus. Sometimes they crack and bleed. The purpose of providing special oral hygiene is to keep the mucous membranes and lips moist. This procedure may also be used for residents who have no teeth.

PROCEDURE

34

Brushing and Flossing the Resident's Teeth

1. Perform your beginning procedure actions.
2. Gather supplies needed: disposable gloves, fresh water, disposable drinking cup, straw, soft-bristle toothbrush, toothpaste, mouthwash, **emesis basin,** and towel. (An emesis basin is a kidney-shaped basin used for oral care procedures.)
3. Sit the resident upright, or elevate the head of the bed as much as possible. Drape the towel across the resident's chest.
4. Mix equal parts of water and mouthwash in the cup.
5. Let the resident rinse his or her mouth with mouthwash.
6. Hold the emesis basin under the chin so the resident can spit out the mouthwash.
7. Wet the toothbrush and apply toothpaste.
8. Gently insert the toothbrush in the mouth with the bristles pointing down. Then rotate the toothbrush so the bristles face the teeth. Brush all surfaces of the teeth. The bristles must reach into the space between the teeth and the gums. Hold the brush at a 45° angle against the teeth, then scrub *gently*, using a short back-and-forth motion, or small circular motion. Scrubbing too hard will damage the gums—be gentle!
9. Brush all surfaces of the teeth **(Figure 11-1).** Do the outside, insides, bottom, and top. Clean all areas where food can get stuck. To reach the upper front teeth, use the "toe" end of the brush. Rotate the brush vertically, then use the bristles near the end. Move the brush gently up and down.

10. Brush the tongue gently, avoiding the back of the tongue. Contact with the back of the tongue or throat may cause the resident to gag.
11. Hold the emesis basin under the chin and allow the resident to spit out the toothpaste.
12. Break off about 18 inches of dental floss. Wind most of it around the middle finger of one gloved hand. Wind the remaining floss around the middle finger of the other hand. Use this finger to take up the used floss as it becomes dirty. Hold the floss tightly between your thumbs and forefingers.
13. Keep your fingers close to the resident's teeth for good control. Gently guide the floss between the resident's teeth, using a gentle rubbing motion. Avoid snapping the floss into the gums. When you reach the gum line, curve the floss into a C-shape against one tooth. Slide it gently into the space between the tooth and the gum.
14. Hold the floss tightly against the tooth. Gently rub the side of the tooth, using an up-and-down motion as you move the floss away from the gum. Continue until you have flossed all teeth.
15. Let the resident rinse his or her mouth with the mouthwash solution.
16. Hold the emesis basin under the chin and allow the resident to spit out the mouthwash.
17. Wipe the mouth with a towel.
18. Perform your procedure completion actions.

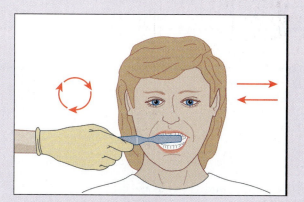

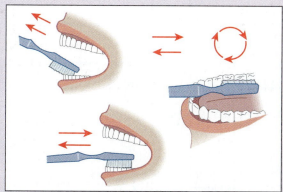

FIGURE 11-1 Gently brush all surfaces of the teeth and gums.

Care of Dentures

Dentures are artificial teeth made of a hard plastic material. Most are removable. Some are permanently attached inside the mouth. They are necessary for eating, retaining the shape of the face and jaw, and giving the resident a sense of well-being. Many people are sensitive about wearing dentures and will not allow others to see them without their teeth. Always provide privacy when caring for dentures. Dentures are very expensive and break easily if dropped, so handle them carefully.

| PROCEDURE 35 | Special Oral Hygiene | |

1. Perform your beginning procedure actions.
2. Gather supplies needed: disposable gloves, emesis basin, two towels, commercially prepared swabs, lubricant for lips, plastic bag. If commercial swabs are not available, obtain tongue depressors, gauze sponges, a disposable cup, mouthwash, and water.
3. Cover the pillow with a towel. Use the second towel to cover the resident's chest.
4. Turn the resident's head to the side. Tip the head forward slightly so that fluid and secretions will not run down the throat.
5. Place the emesis basin against the resident's chin.
6. Gently open the mouth.
7. Dip the prepared sponge applicators into water, mouthwash, or solution used by the facility. Press against the side of the cup to remove extra fluid. Limit the amount of fluid used if the resident is unable to spit or swallow.
8. If prepared applicators are not available, wrap a gauze sponge around the tongue depressor. Dip the depressor into a cup containing a solution of half water and half mouthwash. Press the applicator against the side of the cup to remove extra solution.
9. Wipe the gums, teeth, tongue, and inside of the mouth with applicators.
10. Discard the used applicators in the plastic bag.
11. Apply lubricant or lip balm to the lips.
12. Perform your procedure completion actions.

GUIDELINES FOR
Giving Special Oral Hygiene

- This procedure is done for bedfast residents who are unresponsive or poorly responsive.
- Always wear gloves when performing this procedure.
- Explain the procedure to the resident even if he or she is confused or unresponsive.
- Turn the resident's head to the side when cleaning the mouth, to avoid getting liquids into the lungs.
- Moisten the lips with lip balm or other lubricant according to facility policy. If oxygen is in use, use a water-soluble lubricant.

GUIDELINES FOR
Denture Care

- Always wear gloves when performing this procedure. Avoid contaminating environmental surfaces and clean supplies with your gloves.
- Handle dentures carefully.
- Let the resident remove the dentures from the mouth, if able.
- Dentures must be brushed daily. Soaking dentures in solution does not eliminate the need for daily brushing.
- Rinse dentures well before brushing under running water. Do not rinse them in standing water in the sink.
- If you must place items such as the toothbrush, toothpaste, or dentures on the counter, put them on a clean paper towel. Never place them in the sink or on an unprotected countertop.
- Check the dentures for cracks, chips, or loose teeth.
- Store dentures in a marked denture cup. Some dentures are stored dry, but most are stored in water. Follow the directions for the type of dentures you are caring for. If in doubt, store the dentures in clean, cool water. Avoid hot water, which will cause them to warp. Consult the nurse if necessary.
- Change the soaking solution and wash the denture cup with soap and water daily. Rinse well.
- The tissues and gums in the mouth must be brushed daily, even if the resident has no teeth. Use a soft-bristle brush to clean the mouth. This improves circulation and removes oral debris.

PROCEDURE 36

Denture Care

1. Perform your beginning procedure actions.
2. Gather supplies needed: disposable gloves, emesis basin, denture cup, denture brush or soft-bristle toothbrush, denture paste or powder, towel, tissues, a disposable cup, paper towels, mouthwash, and water. If you will be removing the dentures, obtain a gauze sponge to place under your gloved hand. The gauze gives you a firm grip on the dentures to avoid slipping. Obtain a small plastic bag to dispose of the gauze sponge and gloves.
3. Drape the towel across the resident's chest.
4. Line the emesis basin with paper towels. A washcloth or hand towel may also be used.
5. Ask the resident to remove the dentures, if able, and place them in the emesis basin.
6. Offer the resident a tissue to wipe the mouth after removing the dentures.
7. If the resident is unable to remove the dentures, apply gloves. Cover your fingers with a gauze sponge and grasp the center of the upper denture with the thumb and index finger of your hand. An alternative is to place your index fingers on both sides at the back of the denture plate. Gently move the denture up and down to break the seal. Pull the denture out of the mouth and place it in the emesis basin.
8. To remove the lower denture, cover your gloved fingers with a gauze sponge and gently grasp it with your thumb and index finger. Turn it to the side slightly and lift it from the mouth. Place it in the emesis basin. Discard the gauze sponge in the plastic bag.
9. Raise the side rail.
10. Line the bottom of the sink with paper towels, a washcloth, or a hand towel. Fill the sink half-full of cool water so the dentures do not break if they drop **(Figure 11-2).** You may also place the dentures in an emasis basin under running water.
11. Rinse the dentures well under cool running water to remove food particles and other debris.
12. Wet the toothbrush and apply the denture paste or powder. If you have not yet applied gloves, do so at this time.
13. Hold the dentures securely and brush all surfaces.
14. Rinse the dentures well under cool running water. Place them in the denture cup.
15. Return to the bedside and lower the side rail.
16. Let the resident brush his or her gums and tongue, then clean and rinse the resident's mouth with a solution of equal parts water and mouthwash before replacing the dentures.
17. Hold the emesis basin under the chin and allow the resident to spit out the solution.
18. Hand the resident the denture cup and ask him or her to insert the dentures, if able. Some residents

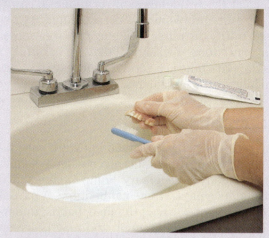

FIGURE 11-2   Line the sink with a paper towel and fill it half-full with water to avoid breakage if the dentures accidentally drop.

may ask for denture paste or powder to hold the dentures in place. Apply it according to the directions on the package. For a paste, a dot on each back corner and a dot in the front center are usually enough.
19. If the resident is unable to insert the dentures, grasp the middle front of the upper denture firmly with your thumb and index finger. Raise the upper lip with your other hand and slide the denture into the mouth. Place both index fingers in the mouth on each side of the upper denture and press firmly to ensure that the denture is in place.
20. Grasp the middle front of the lower denture securely with your thumb and index finger. With your other hand, pull the lower lip down and slide the denture into the mouth. Place both index fingers in the mouth on each side of the denture and press firmly to ensure it is in place.
21. Raise the side rail.
22. Remove the towel and discard according to facility policy.
23. Rinse and dry the denture cup and return it, with your other supplies, to the top drawer of the bedside stand. If the resident does not want the dentures in his or her mouth, store them in the cup in the bedside stand. Some dentures are stored dry, but most should be kept moist. Ask the resident how the dentures should be stored. If in doubt, fill the cup with clean, cool water, and place the dentures in it. Cover the cup and place it in the bedside stand.
24. Perform your procedure completion actions.

BATHING THE RESIDENT

Bathing is done to eliminate odor, stimulate circulation, provide mild exercise, and refresh and relax the resident. Bath time is an excellent time to inspect the resident's skin for redness, irritation, or other problems. If skin problems are observed, notify the nurse. Washing removes secretions, excretions, dirt, and oil that are harmful to the skin. Bath time is a good time for you to communicate with the resident.

Types of Baths

Many types of baths are given in health care facilities. A **complete bath** is given when washing the entire body is necessary. Some facilities give all residents a **partial bath** at bedtime. A partial bath consists of washing the face, hands, underarms, back, and genital area, and may be given as often as necessary to meet the resident's needs. Follow your facility policy for washing the hair. Some facilities do not consider a shampoo part of the bathing procedure, and may require a doctor's order to wash the hair. Some female residents have their hair done at the beauty parlor each week. If this is the case, get permission from the nurse before washing their hair. Doing so will remove the curl and style the beautician has created.

Most residents can take a tub, shower, or whirlpool bath. Some facilities require a doctor's

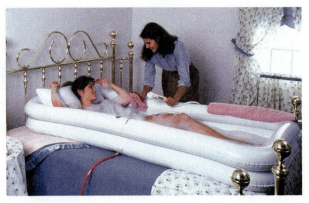

FIGURE 11-3 Special tubs may be used to bathe bedfast residents. *(Courtesy of Medline Industries, Inc. 1-800-MEDLINE)*

order for certain types of baths, so follow your facility policy. Special shower chairs are available for residents to sit in while taking a shower. Tub baths and showers are given two or more times a week, according to your facility policy and individual resident needs. Some facilities have special tubs that may be used to immerse bedfast residents in water for bathing **(Figure 11-3).** These are very comforting and appreciated by the residents. Refer to the care plan for information about the type of bath and other special hygiene and grooming needs.

Residents who must stay in bed or are either too weak or ill to receive a tub bath or shower

GUIDELINES FOR
Bathing Residents with the Waterless Bathing System

- Commercially prepared waterless bathing products are designed to be used for one bath. A full-size kit contains eight cloths. Smaller kits containing four cloths are also available for partial baths and perineal care. The package may be resealed if you do not use all the cloths.
- The washcloths may be used at room temperature, but many facilities microwave them for comfort. Monitor the temperature carefully to prevent overheating and intermittent hot spots that could injure the resident.
- Peel the label back or open the package before heating to avoid bursting in the microwave.
- Follow manufacturers' directions for heating the package. One minute is usually sufficient to warm the contents to a comfortable temperature.
- The cloths in the package are for a single use only.

- The procedure is similar to a bed bath, with cleansing done in the same order:
  1. Face and neck
  2. Far arm and hand
  3. Chest and abdomen
  4. Near arm and hand
  5. Far leg and foot
  6. Near leg and foot
  7. Back and buttocks
  8. Perineum
- Discard used cloths properly, according to facility policy. Avoid flushing them down the toilet. A plastic bag at the bedside works well for cloth disposal.
- If you have extra cloths at the end of the procedure, reseal and date the package. Discard unused cloths within 72 hours of opening, or immediately if they are dry.

are given a **bed bath.** The nursing assistant cleans the resident's entire body, one part at a time, while the resident remains in bed. The resident who receives a complete bed bath probably will be unable to assist you.

Waterless Bathing

When residents are bathed in bed, a basin of water and soap are traditionally used. Over the past few years, a newer system of bathing, developed by a nurse, has become popular. This system is

---

GUIDELINES FOR
Assisting with Bathing and Personal Care

- Consult the care plan for information about the type of bath to be given, special information, resident's self-care ability, routines, use of adaptive devices or other equipment, resident needs, goals related to bathing and grooming, and general care. Your care should be consistent with the care plan goals.
- Gloves are worn for part of the bathing procedure. You will have to change your gloves and wash your hands several times during a complete bath to apply the principles of standard precautions.
- If you have open cuts or sores on your hands, you will have to wear gloves for the entire bathing procedure. To apply the principles of standard precautions, you must remove your gloves, wash your hands, and reapply clean gloves immediately before contacting mucous membranes or nonintact skin.
- Moving the resident to the side of the bed near you may be helpful, if you are bathing the resident in bed. Follow the guidelines in Procedure 12.
- Provide privacy by closing the door, window curtains, and privacy curtain.
- Many personal care procedures involve exposing the resident, so be sure the room is warm and comfortable.
- Before beginning a procedure, organize your work. Anticipate what you will need and gather it in advance.
- Keep the resident's body covered with a bath blanket for modesty and warmth and expose only the part of the body on which you are working.
- Bathe only one part of the body at a time, keeping the rest of the resident covered.
- Offer the resident choices. Personal care should be given according to the resident's preference, considering medical needs. Also consider culture, religion, social, and familial practices, as well as individual preference.
- If you find a technique that improves resident self-esteem or independence, share this information with other members of the interdisciplinary team.
- Change the water if it cools off or becomes soapy or dirty.
- Soap can be irritating and drying to the skin. Be sure it is rinsed off.
- When not using the soap, keep it in the soap dish and not in the wash basin.
- If you will be using liquid soap from a dispenser mounted on the wall, avoid putting the soap directly into the bath water. Dispense some soap into a small cup and carry it to the bedside. Pour the liquid soap onto the washcloth as needed.
- In some facilities, bar soap is not permitted. If refillable liquid soap bottles are used, each resident should have a bottle labeled with his or her name. The soap from that bottle is used for that resident only.
- The shower bath is commonly given in the long-term care facility. Keep the spray of warm water on the resident's body during the entire procedure to prevent chilling.
- If you wash the resident's hair in the shower, placing cotton in the ears will prevent problems if the spray is misdirected. Bring an extra towel and wrap the resident's head after rinsing out the shampoo.
- A bottle of lotion can be placed in the bath water at the beginning of the bath to warm it. After the bath it can be used on the resident's hands, arms, and back.
- When applying lotion to resident's arms and legs, rub or pat it on lightly. Avoid vigorous up-and-down massage, as this may cause circulatory complications.
- After the bath, dry the skin well. Pay special attention to skin folds, creases, and the area between the toes. Drying helps prevent infection and skin breakdown.
- Follow your facility policy for use of powders. If permitted, use sparingly. Too much powder is not good for the skin. Powder can cause respiratory problems if inhaled.
- Apply deodorant after the bath, unless the resident objects.
- Upon completion of the bathing procedure, dress the resident in appropriate clothing. If the resident must wear a hospital gown or other nightwear, cover the body as much as possible.
- Clothing should be appropriate for the resident's age and gender. Consider the season and color-coordinate clothing as much as possible. Let the resident select the clothing, if possible.
- Assist the resident to put on proper undergarments. Avoid using a hospital gown under clothing in place of undergarments.
- If the resident will be getting out of bed, put socks and footwear appropriate to the floor surface on the feet.

called **waterless bathing.** It may also be called basinless bathing or bag bath. The waterless bathing system is prepackaged **(Figure 11-4A).** A package of moistened washcloths is used in place of the water basin and soap. The package may be used at room temperature, or heated in a microwave or commercial warmer **(Figure 11-4B),** according to facility policy and resident preference. Advantages to the waterless bathing system include:

- Faster and more economical for the facility; each bath takes approximately 8 to 10 minutes
- Less fatiguing for the resident
- Conserves moisture, reduces drying, and is gentler to skin than soaps

- Less friction, because the cloths are softer than regular washcloths and towels, and drying is eliminated

Perineal Care

The **perineum** is the area between the anus and vagina in the female; the area between the anus and scrotum in the male. **Perineal care** is also called **peri-care.** This procedure involves washing the genital area. Peri-care must be given frequently when residents are incontinent. Urine and stool are very irritating and will promote skin breakdown.

SAFETY GUIDELINES FOR
Personal Care Procedures

- Test the temperature of the bath water with a thermometer. As a rule, water that is 105°F is comfortable for bathing. Use common sense with water temperature. Ask the resident if the temperature is comfortable for him or her. Check the temperature with your elbow or wrist to make sure it is not too hot.
- If you will be transporting the resident in the hallway to a tub or shower room, be sure that the resident's body is covered.
- Use the transfer belt over the clothing to move the resident.

- Use safety belts on tub lifts and shower chairs.
- Make certain that bath mats are secure.
- Help residents in and out of the tub and shower.
- *Never leave the resident unattended in the bathtub, whirlpool, or shower.*
- If the resident becomes weak or dizzy in the tub or shower, stay in the room and pull the emergency call signal. Begin to drain the water from the tub. Cover the resident with a bath blanket for warmth.

INFECTION CONTROL GUIDELINES FOR
Personal Care Procedures

- Apply the principles of standard precautions and wear gloves and other personal protective equipment when indicated.
- Use of gloves is not necessary or desirable for the entire bathing procedure. Use them only when contact with blood, body fluids (except sweat), secretions, excretions, mucous membranes, or nonintact skin is likely. Change gloves as often as necessary to comply with standard precautions.
- If you are wearing gloves, remove them, wash your hands, and reapply new gloves *immediately before* contact with mucous membranes or nonintact skin. Mucous membranes are found in the eyes, nose, mouth, and **genital area.** The genital area is the part of the body where the external reproductive organs are located.
- Avoid contaminating equipment or items in the

room and environment with gloves used for resident care.
- Dispose of gloves according to facility policy.
- Wash from the cleanest area to the least clean.
- Change water, washcloth, and gloves after washing a contaminated or "dirty" area.
- Once a towel has been used below the waist, avoid using it above the waist.
- The handheld shower spray should be placed on the hook when not in use. Do not let it hang down or touch the floor, which is always considered dirty.
- Disinfect the tub, shower chair, or whirlpool according to facility policy before and after each use.
- Follow your facility infection-control policies for handling clean and soiled linen. Soiled linen or towels should not be left on the tub or shower room floor.

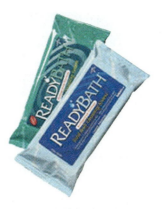

FIGURE 11-4A A waterless bath or "bag bath" is a popular, comfortable, time-saving alternative to the traditional bed bath. *(Courtesy of Medline Industries, Inc. 1-800-MEDLINE)*

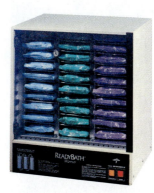

FIGURE 11-4B Warmed bag bath is very comfortable and soothing for the resident. The commercial warmer reduces the risk of hot spots and overheating in the microwave. *(Courtesy of Medline Industries, Inc. 1-800-MEDLINE)*

| PROCEDURE **37** | Giving a Bed Bath | |

1. Perform your beginning procedure actions.
2. Gather supplies needed: basin, bath thermometer, soap, washcloth, two towels, clean gown or clothing, bath blanket, lotion, comb or brush, disposable gloves, and plastic laundry bag or hamper.
3. Place clean equipment on the resident's overbed table. Follow your facility policy for covering the overbed table with a barrier.
4. Check the temperature of the room. Make sure it is not too cold.
5. Offer the resident the bedpan or urinal before beginning the procedure. If you will be assisting, apply the principles of standard precautions.
6. Remove the bedspread and blanket. Fold and place them on the chair.
7. Place the bath blanket over the top sheet. Ask the resident to hold the blanket in place. Remove the sheet by pulling it down from underneath the blanket. Avoid exposing the resident. Place the soiled sheet in the hamper or dispose of it according to facility policy.
8. Remove the gown and dispose of it according to facility policy. Keep the resident covered with the bath blanket. Expose only the part on which you are working.
9. Raise the side rail.
10. Fill the basin with warm (105°F) water. Check the temperature with a thermometer.
11. Return to the bedside and lower the side rail.
12. Place a towel across the resident's chest.
13. Allow the resident to wash his or her own face, if possible. If the resident is unable, you will wash the face. Check for the resident's preference regarding soap. Some people do not use soap on the face.
14. Apply disposable gloves to wash the eyes.
15. Make a mitten by folding the washcloth around your hand **(Figure 11-5)**.

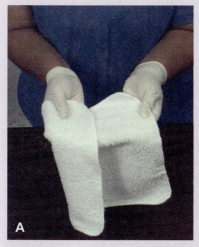 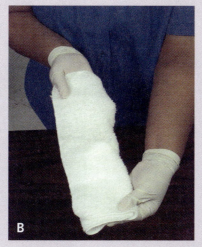 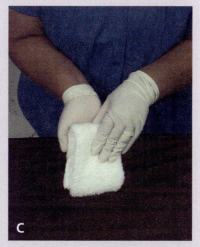

FIGURE 11-5 Make a washcloth mitt. Wear gloves if there is potential for contact with blood, body fluids, secretions, excretions, mucous membranes, or nonintact skin.

Continues

16. Wash the eyelids from the inner corner to the outer corner, using plain water without soap. Use a separate part of the washcloth for each eye.
17. Dry the washed area.
18. Rinse the washcloth.
19. Remove the gloves and discard according to facility policy.
20. Wash and dry the remainder of the face, neck, and ears.
21. Place a towel lengthwise under the resident's arm farthest from you.
22. Hold the arm up. Wash the arm from the shoulder to the wrist and fingertips, using long, firm, circular strokes.
23. Rinse and dry the arm.
24. Wash, rinse, and dry the armpit, or **axilla.**
25. Repeat for the other arm.
26. If possible, place the resident's hands in water. Wash, rinse, and dry hands, fingers, and nails. Clean under the nails with an orange stick, if soiled.
27. Place the towel across the chest **(Figure 11-6).** Pull the bath blanket down to the abdomen.
28. Fold the towel to expose half the chest.
29. Wash, rinse, and dry the chest. In the female resident, dry under the breast well. Repeat for the other side of the chest.
30. Cover the chest with the towel.
31. Pull the bath blanket down to expose the abdomen.
32. Wash, rinse, and dry the abdomen.
33. Cover the resident with the bath blanket.

34. Remove the towel from under the blanket.
35. Uncover the leg farthest from you. Place the towel lengthwise under the leg. Bend the knee and place the foot on the bed, if the resident is able.
36. Wash, rinse, and dry the leg from the groin area to the toes.
37. Repeat for the other leg.
38. If the resident is able, place the basin on the towel and place the feet in the basin one at a time **(Figure 11-7).**
39. Wash, rinse, and dry the feet. Wash, rinse, and dry well between the toes. Check the appearance of the toes and skin between the toes for redness, cracking, or irritation.
40. Cover the legs with the bath blanket.
41. Raise the side rail.
42. Empty the basin, rinse, and refill with clean (105°F) water.
43. Return to the bedside and lower the side rail.
44. Assist the resident to turn so that his or her back is toward you.
45. Place the towel lengthwise on the sheet against the resident's back.
46. Wash, rinse, and dry the back and outer buttocks. Observe for signs of redness, irritation, or skin breakdown.
47. Put lotion on the resident's back, following the guidelines in Procedure 43.
48. Remove the towel and assist the resident to turn on his or her back.
49. Ask the resident if he or she would like to wash the genital area. If the resident is unable, apply disposable gloves.

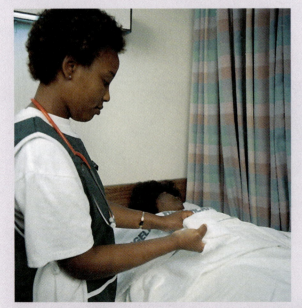

FIGURE 11-6 Respect the resident's modesty by covering her body with a towel and draping with the bath blanket.

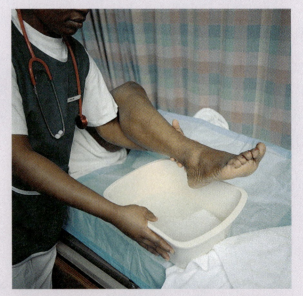

FIGURE 11-7 If the resident is able, soak the feet in a basin, one at a time.

Continues

| PROCEDURE **37** | Giving a Bed Bath, *Continued* | 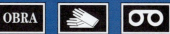 |

50. Wash, rinse, and dry the genital area from the front to the rectal area, following the guidelines in Procedure 41 (42 for male residents).
51. Place the soiled linen in the hamper or plastic bag, according to facility policy.
52. Remove gloves and dispose of them according to facility policy.
53. Apply deodorant and put a clean gown on or dress the resident.
54. Raise the side rail.
55. Wash your hands.
56. Return to the bedside and put the side rail down.
57. Comb the hair and assist with other grooming requests (Procedure 45).
58. Replace bed linens, if indicated, or straighten the bed.
59. Perform your procedure completion actions.

| PROCEDURE **38** | Giving a Partial Bath |  |

1. Perform your beginning procedure actions.
2. Gather supplies needed: basin, soap, washcloth, two towels, clean gown or clothing, bath blanket, lotion, comb or brush, hamper or plastic laundry bag for soiled linen, and disposable gloves.
3. Place the equipment on the overbed table. Follow your facility policy for covering the overbed table with a barrier.
4. Offer the resident the bedpan or urinal. Apply the principles of standard precautions if you will be assisting with this procedure.
5. Remove the bedspread and blanket. Fold and place them on the chair.
6. Place the bath blanket over the top sheet. Ask the resident to hold the blanket in place. Remove the sheet by pulling it down from underneath the blanket. Avoid exposing the resident. Place the soiled sheet in the hamper or dispose of it according to facility policy.
7. Fill the basin with warm (105°F) water. Check the temperature with a thermometer.
8. Remove the gown and dispose of it according to facility policy
9. Place a towel across the resident's chest.
10. Allow the resident to wash his or her own face, if possible. If the resident is unable, you will wash the face. Check for the resident's preference regarding soap.
11. Apply disposable gloves to wash the eyes, because of the potential for mucous membrane contact.
12. Make a mitten by folding the washcloth around your hand.
13. Wash the eyelids from the inner corner to the outer corner, using plain water without soap. Use a clean area of the washcloth for each eye.
14. Dry the washed area.
15. Rinse the washcloth.
16. Remove the gloves and discard according to facility policy.
17. Wash the remainder of the face, neck, and ears.
18. Place the towel under the hand farthest from you.
19. Wash, rinse, and dry the hand.
20. Repeat for the other hand.
21. Place the towel under the axilla.
22. Wash, rinse, and dry the axilla.
23. Repeat on the opposite side.
24. Assist the resident to turn so that his or her back is toward you.
25. Place the towel lengthwise on the sheet against the resident's back.
26. Wash, rinse, and dry the back and outer buttocks. Observe for signs of redness, irritation, or skin breakdown.
27. Put lotion on the resident's back, following the guidelines in Procedure 43.
28. Remove the towel and assist the resident to turn on his or her back.
29. Use gloves to wash the genital area. Wash from the front of the genital area to the rectal area, following the guidelines in Procedure 41 (42 for male residents).
30. Place the soiled linen in the hamper or plastic bag, according to facility policy.
31. Remove gloves and dispose of them according to facility policy.
32. Apply deodorant, if desired, and put a clean gown on the resident.
33. Raise the side rail.
34. Wash your hands.
35. Return to the bedside and put the side rail down.
36. Comb the hair and assist with other grooming requests.
37. Replace bed linens, if indicated, or straighten the bed.
38. Perform your procedure completion actions.

PROCEDURE 39

Waterless Bed Bath

 OBRA

1. Perform your beginning procedure actions.
2. Gather supplies needed: disposable gloves, bed linen; bath blanket; hospital gown/resident's nightclothes; bath towel; lotion for back rub; waterless bathing product (heated according to facility policy or resident wishes); basin of warm water for soaking hands (optional); comb; brush; supplies for oral hygiene, as needed; supplies for nail care, as needed; deodorant; small plastic bag to discard used bathing cloths; large plastic bag or hamper for soiled linen.
3. Place clean supplies on overbed table.
4. Offer the bedpan or urinal. Put on gloves if you will be assisting with this procedure.
5. Lower the head of the bed and the side rail on the side where you will be working.
6. Loosen the top bedclothes. Remove and fold the blanket and spread and place them over the back of the chair.
7. Place the bath blanket over the top sheet and remove the sheet by sliding it out from under the bath blanket. Place the sheet in the laundry hamper.
8. Leave one pillow under the resident's head. Place any extra pillows on the chair.
9. Remove the resident's gown and place it in the laundry hamper.
10. Assist the resident to move to the side of the bed near you.
11. Open the package of bathing cloths. (If a microwave was used to heat the package, check cloths for hot spots.) Remove one cloth and cleanse the resident's face and neck. (Solution can safely be used around the eyes.)
12. Place a towel over the resident's chest. Fold the blanket down to the waist and cleanse the chest. Be sure that the area under the breasts is carefully cleaned.
13. Fold the bath blanket down to the pubic area and wash the abdomen. Replace the bath blanket over the abdomen and chest. Remove the towel by sliding it out from under the bath blanket. Discard the used cloth in a plastic bag.
14. Uncover the far arm. Remove another cloth from the package and wash the arm and hand **(Figure 11-8).** Soaking the opposite hand in a basin of warm water, while you wash one arm, is a nice touch. This is refreshing to the resident if he or she cannot be out of bed to bathe. Wash the axilla. Apply deodorant. Discard the used cloth in a plastic bag. Cover the arm with the bath blanket.
15. Uncover the near arm. Remove a new cloth from the package. Wash the arm, hand, and axilla. Apply deodorant. Discard the used cloth in a plastic bag. Cover the resident with the bath blanket.
16. Provide nail care as needed.
17. Ask the resident to flex the far leg, if possible. Fold the bath blanket up to expose the thigh, leg, and foot. Remove a new cloth from the package. Cleanse the thigh, leg, and foot. Be sure the area between the toes is left dry. Discard the used cloth in a plastic bag. Cover the leg and foot with the bath blanket.
18. Repeat step 17 with the near thigh, leg, and foot.
19. Make sure the side rail on the opposite side of the bed is up. Help the resident turn on the side away from you. Place a bath towel lengthwise next to the resident's back.
20. Remove a new washcloth from the package. Draw the bath blanket back to expose the back. Wash the back and outer buttocks. Discard the used cloth in a plastic bag. A back rub (Procedure 43) may be given at this time. Cover the resident with the bath blanket.
21. Assist the resident to turn on the back. Position a towel under the buttocks by asking the resident to lift the hips, if possible. Remove a new cloth from the package. Hand the resident the cloth and instruct him or her to wash the perineum. Assist if necessary. (Wear gloves if you will be assisting.) Follow the guidelines in Procedure 41 (42 for male resident). Discard your used gloves and the cloth in a plastic bag. Remove the towel.
22. Wash your hands.
23. Assist the resident to put on a clean gown (Procedure 33).
24. Cover the pillow with a towel. Comb or brush the hair (Procedure 45). Assist with oral hygiene (Procedure 34 or 35), if needed.
25. Change the bed linen, following the occupied bedmaking procedure. Put soiled linen in a plastic bag or the linen hamper.
26. Perform your procedure completion actions.

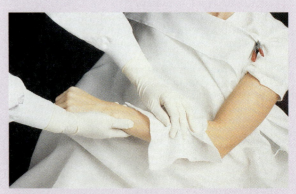

FIGURE 11-8 Wash the far arm and hand. The waterless bath product is kind to the skin and dries quickly. *(Courtesy of Sage Products, Inc.)*

PROCEDURE 40

Assisting The Resident with a Tub or Shower Bath

1. Perform your beginning procedure actions.
2. Check to see if the tub or shower room is available. Disinfect the tub or shower chair according to facility policy. Adjust the temperature in the room, if necessary. Place a bath mat on the floor of the tub or shower, and a disposable or cloth bath mat in front of the tub.
3. Gather supplies needed: disposable gloves, plastic laundry bag or hamper, washcloth, two or three towels, bath blanket, bath thermometer, soap, lotion, and personal grooming supplies.
4. Go to the resident's room and assist with toileting, if necessary. Apply the principles of standard precautions if you will be assisting with this procedure.
5. Assist the resident to the tub or shower room.
6. Regulate the water temperature. Always turn the cold water on first and off last. Check the water temperature with a thermometer. It should be comfortably warm, or 105°F. Double-check the temperature by allowing the water to run over your inner forearm or wrist.
7. If the resident is taking a tub bath, fill the tub half-full of water.
8. Assist the resident to undress, if necessary. Give the resident a towel to place in front of the waist and lower abdomen.
9. Assist the resident to transfer to the tub or shower chair. If the resident is being transferred to a chair with a footrest, push the footrest back during the transfer, then pull it out to support the resident's feet.
10. Push the shower chair into the shower and position it so you can support the resident from the front if he or she starts to fall. In the tub, position the resident so that he or she faces the controls.
11. Lock the wheels to the shower chair in position so the chair will not move.
12. Wash the back.
13. Allow the resident to complete the bath. If unable, you will wash and rinse the resident. Apply the principles of standard precautions if contact with blood, body fluids, secretions, excretions, mucous membranes, or nonintact skin is likely. You may

have to change your gloves several times during this procedure to avoid cross-contamination.
14. Assist the resident in washing the lower legs and feet, if necessary. Make sure to wash and rinse well between the toes. Discard the washcloth in the hamper.
15. Assist with washing the hair, if needed. If you will be doing this procedure, bring an extra washcloth, towel, and two cotton balls into the shower room. Place the cotton balls in the resident's ears before beginning, and remove them when finished. Give the resident a clean, dry washcloth to cover the face. Wrap the resident's head with the towel after rinsing to prevent chilling.
16. Assist with perineal care, if necessary. Apply gloves. Wash the genitalia from the front of the chair. Then squat down and wash the remainder of the perineum by reaching underneath the chair. Wash the rectal area from the back of the chair, following the guidelines in Procedure 41 or Procedure 42. Always wash from front to back (most clean to least clean). Turn the cloth frequently. Rinse well.
17. Upon completion of the bathing procedure, assist the resident out of the tub or shower. Wrap with a bath blanket for modesty and warmth.
18. Pat the resident dry, or allow the resident to dry independently. Make sure to dry the perineal area and the areas between the resident's toes well.
19. Apply lotion to the back, and to other areas if the resident desires. Avoid the area between the toes. Applying lotion to this area promotes fungal growth.
20. Return to the resident's room and assist with dressing and other personal care needs. Keep the resident's body completely covered in the hallways. You may dress the resident in the shower room as facility environment and procedures permit.
21. Perform your procedure completion actions.
22. After the resident is safe and comfortable, return to the tub or shower room. Discard the linen according to facility policy. Wear gloves when removing wet linen. Clean and disinfect the tub, shower chair, and handrails.

GUIDELINES FOR

Giving a Whirlpool Bath

- Check with the nurse before giving a whirlpool bath to a resident with an infection, surgical incision, or pressure ulcer.
- If the resident is combative or disoriented, check with the nurse before giving the resident a whirlpool

bath. The noise from the whirlpool may worsen agitation in some residents.
- Disinfect the whirlpool tub immediately before and after each use.

Continues

GUIDELINES FOR
Giving a Whirlpool Bath, *Continued*

- The water temperature in the whirlpool tub is usually set at 97°F to 100°F because the temperature in the tub remains constant. (Use common sense; if the tub is steaming, the water is probably too hot. Use a thermometer to check the water temperature.) The constant movement of warm water stimulates the resident's circulation.
- Never leave the resident alone in the whirlpool tub, even for a minute **(Figure 11-9).**
- Always fasten the safety belt when moving a resident into or out of a whirlpool tub with a hydraulic lift seat. The safety belt should remain fastened throughout the procedure.
- The resident may be frightened when using the hydraulic lift for the first time. Explain the procedure and reassure the resident.
- Drape the resident's genital area with a bath towel for modesty during the whirlpool bath.
- Use low-suds or no-suds products that are designed specifically for whirlpool use.
- Never pour liquid soap or shampoo into the whirlpool tub. Even a tiny bit of liquid soap will result in an abundance of suds. If the resident accidentally creates a suds problem, rub a bar of soap against the walls of the tub to reduce the bubbles.
- The whirlpool activity provides a cleansing action. However, if you will be assisting the resident with bathing, apply the principles of standard precautions.
- Wrap the resident with a bath blanket for warmth and modesty immediately after removing him or her from the whirlpool tub.

- The jets in some whirlpool tubs have the potential to harbor dangerous pathogens. Follow facility policies for carefully cleaning the tub with the proper disinfectant solution. Make sure that you follow directions correctly and run the disinfectant through the tub for the correct length of time.
- When the bath is completed, raise the lift seat out of the soapy water and rinse with the hose, using comfortably warm water.

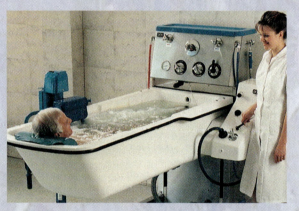

FIGURE 11-9   Never leave the resident alone in the whirlpool. Keep the safety belt fastened on the lift chair. If the resident becomes ill, use the call signal to get help. Drain the tub.

GUIDELINES FOR
Giving Peri-Care

- Always wear gloves during this procedure. Be careful not to contaminate clean supplies and environmental surfaces with your gloves.
- Be kind and sensitive. Most people are very uncomfortable about having someone else clean their genital area.
- Protect the resident's modesty and privacy by exposing only the part of the body on which you are working.
- If the perineum is soiled with excretions, remove them with tissues or disposable wipes. Place them in the bedpan for removal. Change the underpad if it is wet or soiled. If the resident is wet, place on a dry underpad before beginning. After the heavy soiling is removed, discard your gloves. Wash your hands and reapply clean gloves before continuing the procedure.

- Use warm, soapy water. Wash the cleanest area first. In the female, this means you will wash from front to back. In the male, begin at the end of the penis and move down toward the body, under the scrotum, then back to the rectum. Turn the washcloth so you are using a clean section each time you move to a new area. Use a second washcloth if necessary. Avoid rubbing back and forth. Rinse the soap off well and dry thoroughly. Some facilities use special products for peri-care. Follow your facility policy.
- If the resident has a catheter, wash it gently to remove urine, stool, mucus, or dried secretions. Catheter care is described in Chapter 14.
- When washing the catheter, begin at the urinary meatus and wash downward three to four inches on the catheter. Do not rub back and forth.

Continues

GUIDELINES FOR
Giving Peri-Care, *Continued*

- In the female resident, keep the labia separated as much as possible during the procedure. Avoid placing your fingers on an area after washing it. You may need several washcloths to perform the procedure without contamination. (Some states require a second, clean washcloth for rinsing; the used cloth is not put back into the water basin.)
- If using a mitt is difficult for you, an alternate method is to fold the washcloth in fourths. One edge will have corners that can be folded down separately. Wet the washcloth and squeeze out excess water. Place a drop of liquid soap on each corner of the edge. Fold these corners back, one at a time, to expose a clean area of the cloth with each

stroke. Turn the cloth around and use the other area of the washcloth to cleanse the perineum.
- Usually, the nursing assistant is expected to give perineal care to residents of both sexes.
- Many facilities apply barrier products to protect the skin after performing perineal care. Know and follow your facility policy. Some barrier products contain alcohol. Avoid applying these products to red or broken skin. If you are applying barrier cream after perineal care, remove your gloves, wash your hands, and apply new gloves. Your gloves become contaminated during the peri-care procedure, and you must use new (clean) gloves to apply barrier cream.

PROCEDURE
41
Female Perineal Care

Note: The guidelines and sequence for this procedure vary slightly from state to state. Your instructor will inform you if the sequence in your state differs from the procedure listed here. Know and follow the required sequence for your state.

1. Perform your beginning procedure actions.
2. Gather supplies needed: basin, soap, washcloth, towels, clean gown or clothing, bath blanket, bed protector, hamper or plastic laundry bag, and disposable gloves.
3. Place the equipment on the overbed table. Follow your facility policy for covering the overbed table with a barrier.
4. Offer the resident the bedpan or urinal. Apply the principles of standard precautions if you will be assisting with this procedure.
5. Remove the bedspread and blanket. Fold and place them on the chair.
6. Place the bath blanket over the top sheet. Ask the resident to hold the blanket in place. Remove the sheet by pulling it down from underneath the blanket. Avoid exposing the resident. Place the soiled sheet in the hamper or dispose of it according to facility policy.
7. Remove the gown and dispose of it according to facility policy.
8. If the linen is wet or soiled, remove and dispose of it according to facility policy. Be sure the resident is lying on a clean, dry surface.
9. Assist the resident to raise her hips. Place a bed protector under the buttocks. Remove the soiled bed protector, if present. Wear gloves if you will be handling a wet or soiled bed protector.
10. Raise the side rail.

11. Fill the basin with warm (105°F) water. Check the temperature with a thermometer.
12. Return to the bedside and lower the side rail.
13. Position the bath blanket so the area between the legs is exposed.
14. Assist the resident to separate and bend the knees, placing the feet on the bed, if able.
15. Put on disposable gloves.
16. Make a mitten by folding the washcloth around your hand.
17. Wet the washcloth and apply soap. Avoid using too much soap, which can be irritating to the skin.
18. Separate the labia with one hand. If a urinary catheter is present, hold the tubing securely to one side and support against the leg to avoid unnecessary movement or traction on the catheter. Keep the tubing and drainage bag below the level of the bladder.
19. With the other hand, wash the center of the labia, using a single downward stroke from top to bottom **(Figure 11-10)**. Stop at the base of the labia.
20. Turn the washcloth to a clean area.
21. Wash the far side of the labia, using a single downward stroke from top to bottom.
22. Turn the washcloth to a clean area.
23. Wash the near side of the labia, using a single downward stroke from top to bottom.
24. Continue to alternate from side to side, working outward to the thighs, using the same technique. Turn the washcloth or use a new washcloth, if necessary, so a fresh section is used to cleanse each area.
25. If a urinary catheter is present, wash, rinse, and dry the perineal area surrounding the urinary

Continues

Female Perineal Care, *Continued*

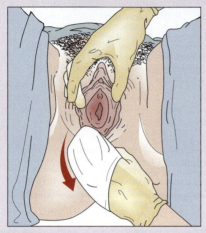

FIGURE 11-10 Wash from top to bottom with a single stroke. Avoid rubbing back and forth. Use a clean section of the washcloth for each downward stroke.

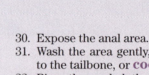

FIGURE 11-11 Turn the resident on the side and wipe from the rectal area to the coccyx.

meatus and catheter. Change the washcloth. Wash the catheter beginning at the urinary meatus, down the catheter approximately three to four inches. Use a single downward stroke. Do not rub back and forth. Rinse and dry in the same direction. Hold the catheter firmly to avoid pulling and traction. After washing the catheter, continue with perineal care.

26. Rinse the area from top to bottom with the washcloth. Rinse in the same sequence, beginning in the center and moving outward from side to side. Turn the washcloth so a clean surface is used for each downward stroke. Avoid rubbing back and forth.

27. Gently pat the area dry with a towel. Dry in the same sequence, beginning in the center and moving outward from side to side. Position the towel so a clean surface is used for each downward stroke. Avoid rubbing back and forth.

28. Assist the resident to turn on the side away from you. Flex the upper leg forward, if possible.

29. Wet the washcloth and make a mitt. Apply soap.

30. Expose the anal area.

31. Wash the area gently, wiping from the perineum to the tailbone, or **coccyx** (**Figure 11-11**).

32. Rinse the washcloth, then rinse the area well.

33. Gently pat dry with a towel. Avoid rubbing back and forth.

34. Assist the resident to return to her back.

35. Remove and dispose of the bed protector according to facility policy.

36. Place the soiled linen in the hamper or plastic bag, according to facility policy.

37. Remove one glove and raise the side rail with the ungloved hand. Dispose of both gloves according to facility policy.

38. Wash your hands.

39. Return to the bedside and lower the side rail.

40. Replace the top covers and remove the bath blanket.

41. Help the resident into a clean gown or other clothing of choice.

42. Perform your procedure completion actions.

Male Perineal Care

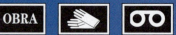

Note: The guidelines and sequence for this procedure vary slightly from state to state. Your instructor will inform you if the sequence in your state differs from the procedure listed here. Know and follow the required sequence for your state.

1. Perform your beginning procedure actions.

2. Gather supplies needed: basin, soap, washcloth, towels, clean gown or clothing, bath blanket, bed protector, hamper or plastic laundry bag, and disposable gloves.

Continues

Male Perineal Care,
Continued

3. Place the equipment on the overbed table. Follow your facility policy for covering the overbed table with a barrier.
4. Offer the resident the bedpan or urinal. Apply the principles of standard precautions if you will be assisting with this procedure.
5. Remove the bedspread and blanket. Fold and place them on the chair.
6. Place the bath blanket over the top sheet. Ask the resident to hold the blanket in place. Remove the sheet by pulling it down from underneath the blanket. Avoid exposing the resident. Place the soiled sheet in the hamper or dispose of it according to facility policy.
7. Remove the gown and dispose of it according to facility policy.
8. If the linen is wet or soiled, remove and dispose of it according to facility policy. Be sure the resident is lying on a clean, dry surface.
9. Assist the resident to raise his hips. Place a bed protector under the buttocks. Remove the soiled bed protector, if present. Wear gloves if you will be handling a wet or soiled bed protector.
10. Raise the side rail.
11. Fill the basin with warm (105°F) water. Check the temperature with a thermometer.
12. Return to the bedside and lower the side rail.
13. Position the bath blanket so the area between the legs is exposed.
14. Assist the resident to separate and bend the knees, placing the feet on the bed, if able.
15. Put on disposable gloves.
16. Make a mitten by folding the washcloth around your hand.
17. Wet the washcloth and apply soap. Avoid using too much soap, which can be irritating to the skin.
18. With one hand, grasp the penis gently and wash. Wash the urinary meatus in a circular motion.
19. Continue to wash down the penis and the rest of the perineal area, including the scrotum, using downward strokes and working outward to the thighs **(Figure 11-12).** Lift the scrotum and wash the perineum.
20. If the resident is not circumcised, gently pull the foreskin back and wash it **(Figure 11-13).** Rinse the penis, dry gently, and replace the retracted foreskin.
21. If a urinary catheter is present, wash, rinse, and dry the area surrounding the urinary meatus and catheter. Wash the catheter beginning at the urinary meatus, down the catheter approximately three to four inches. Use a single downward stroke. Do not rub back and forth. Rinse and dry in the same direction. Avoid pulling on the catheter.
22. Wash the scrotum, then gently lift it and wash the perineum.

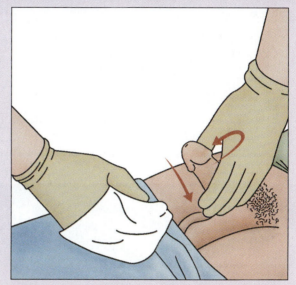

FIGURE 11-12 Wash the meatus area in a circular motion. Wash the shaft using downward strokes.

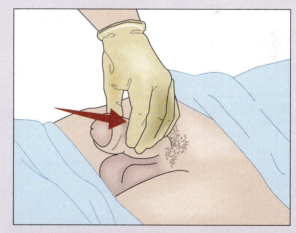

FIGURE 11-13 Gently push the foreskin back to wash the head of the penis.

23. Rinse the washcloth.
24. Make a mitten. Gently rinse the urethra, shaft of penis, scrotum, and perineal area well, working in the same direction until the entire area is clean and soap-free.
25. Gently dry the area with a towel.
26. Assist the resident to turn on the side away from you. Flex the upper leg forward, if possible.
27. Wet the washcloth and make a mitt. Apply soap.

Continues

PROCEDURE

42

Male Perineal Care, *Continued*

28. Expose the anal area.
29. Wash the area, stroking from the perineum to the coccyx.
30. Rinse the washcloth, then rinse the area well.
31. Gently pat the area dry with a towel.
32. Assist the resident to return to his back.
33. Remove and dispose of the bed protector according to facility policy.
34. Place the soiled linen in the hamper or plastic bag, according to facility policy.

35. Remove one glove and raise the side rail with the ungloved hand. Dispose of both gloves according to facility policy.
36. Wash your hands.
37. Return to the bedside and lower the side rail.
38. Replace the top covers and remove the bath blanket.
39. Help the resident into a clean gown or other clothing of choice.
40. Perform your procedure completion actions.

PROCEDURE

43

Giving a Back Rub

1. Perform your beginning procedure actions.
2. Gather supplies needed: basin of water (105°F), soap, washcloth, towel, hamper or plastic laundry bag for soiled linen, and disposable gloves if contact with nonintact skin or any moist body fluid is likely.
3. Place the equipment on the overbed table. Follow your facility policy for covering the overbed table with a barrier.
4. Assist the resident to turn on the side away from you. Expose the back and upper buttocks.
5. Place the bottle of lotion in the basin of water to warm it **(Figure 11-14)**.
6. Wash, rinse, and dry the back.
7. Apply a small amount of lotion to one hand.
8. Warm the lotion by rubbing it between your hands, if necessary.
9. Apply lotion to the back.
10. Rub the back with both hands, using gentle, firm strokes in a circular motion. Massage from buttocks to shoulders:

a. Begin at the base of the spine and rub up the center of the back with long, soothing strokes.
b. Move your hands in a circular motion as you massage down from the shoulders to the buttocks.
c. Repeat this procedure for three to five minutes **(Figure 11-15)**.
11. Wipe off excess lotion.
12. Close and retie the gown, or change the gown if necessary.
13. Straighten and tighten the bottom sheet and draw sheet.
14. Assist the resident to a comfortable position.
15. Perform your procedure completion actions.

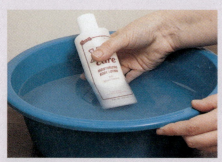

FIGURE 11-14 Warming the lotion in the bath water for a few minutes makes it much more comfortable for the resident.

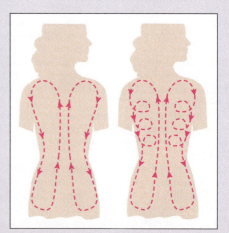

FIGURE 11-15 The back rub is very soothing to the resident. It stimulates circulation and prevents skin breakdown. Avoid rubbing red or open areas.

Shampooing the Resident's Hair

Follow your facility policy for washing the resident's hair. Some facilities require a doctor's order for this procedure. If permitted, the hair can be washed in the tub or shower. Offer the resident a washcloth or towel to hold over the face when washing and rinsing hair. For residents on complete bed rest, this procedure must be done in bed. Some facilities use dry chemical shampoos that are brushed out. No-rinse shampoos are also available for bedfast residents.

Shampoo caps **(Figure 11-16)** are a popular alternative for bathing bedfast residents. These are most comfortable for residents if they are warmed in a microwave for 30 seconds or less, or in the product warmer. The cap is placed on the resident's head, then rubbed gently for one to two minutes for short hair and four to five minutes for long hair. After this time, the cap is removed and the hair towel-dried and combed. Shampoo caps reduce tangling and do not leave residue like some dry chemical products.

Care of African American Residents' Hair

African American residents have special hair care needs. Hair texture of these residents can vary from soft and silky to coarse and thick. Residents with coarse hair need special care to prevent damage, tangling, and breaking. Asking the resident or family how to care for the hair is not offensive. In fact, it shows that you care about meeting the resident's needs. They have been caring for the hair for years, and are experts at it. They also know what products work and which do not.

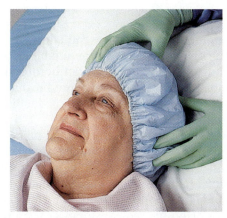

FIGURE 11-16 Shampoo caps simplify the hairwashing procedure for bedfast residents. The products leave the hair feeling clean and tangles are reduced. *(Courtesy of Medline Industries, Inc. 1-800-MEDLINE)*

In general, avoid using hair products designed for Caucasian persons. Most of these are designed to eliminate oil. Eliminating the oil from the hair is one of the worst things to do when caring for a person of color. Use a shampoo marketed specifically for "black hair." In most cases, the resident or family will provide a product that works. Wash the hair once every week or two, as specified on the care plan. Washing more often than this dries the hair and causes breakage. If a special shampoo is not available, baby shampoo works best. Wash the hair using the guidelines in Procedure 44. Use a detangling conditioner according to product directions. After washing the hair, gently towel-dry. Cover the shoulders with a dry towel. Use a wide-toothed comb or pick to comb through the damp hair. Be gentle and patient. It may take time to work through the tangles.

Persons of color need additional oil on the hair at all times. Some residents use products they refer to as hair "grease." If the resident does not have a product preference, apply baby oil *to the scalp, not the hair*. Then, using a soft brush, brush from the scalp to the ends of the hair until all the hairs are covered with oil. You may need to apply this heavily. If it is too oily, wipe the excess with a towel. If you use enough, the hair will appear shiny.

The resident's hair can be braided while damp. Run the wide-toothed comb through the hair to remove tangles, following the guidelines in Procedure 45. Gently twist the hair and apply a hair tie. Avoid using rubber bands, if possible. These cause breakage and damage hair. If a rubber band must be used, apply hair grease or baby oil liberally to your fingers. Roll the rubber band around in the hair grease until it is well coated, then apply it to the hair. Style the hair in a pony tail, then section and braid it. When you get to the end, apply more grease. Wrap the ends around a barrette and snap it shut, or use a hair tie or grease-coated rubber band.

APPLYING LOTION TO THE RESIDENT'S SKIN

Massaging the resident's skin is comforting and refreshing. Massage can stimulate circulation and helps prevent skin breakdown. Refer to the care plan to see if massage is indicated. Each facility has a house lotion used for massaging residents' skin. Applying moisturizing lotion immediately after the bath helps to seal moisture in the skin, preventing dryness. Always massage the skin in smooth, light strokes. Do not massage

PROCEDURE

44

PROCEDURE 44 — Shampooing the Hair

OBRA

1. Perform your beginning procedure actions.
2. Gather supplies needed: shampoo, conditioner, cotton balls, washcloth, two towels, pitcher if needed for rinsing, comb or pick, hair dryer (optional). Additional supplies for bed shampoo include shampoo tray, waterproof bed protector, pitcher of warm (105°F) water.
3. Place cotton balls in the resident's ears. Remove the resident's hearing aid(s) and glasses, if worn.
4. Have the resident cover the face with the washcloth.
5. Tip the resident's head back, if possible.
6. Use the shower head or pitcher of water to wet the resident's scalp and hair well **(Figure 11-17A)**.
7. Apply shampoo to the palm of your hand. Rub your hands together. Apply the shampoo to the resident's scalp, rubbing with your fingertips (not fingernails) to work up a lather **(Figure 11-17B)**. Wash all areas of the scalp well, using gentle, massaging motions.
8. Have the resident tip the head back. Rinse with warm water from the shower head or water pitcher.
9. Continue rinsing until all soap is removed.
10. Apply conditioner, if the resident desires, or as needed to remove tangles. Follow directions for the product used. Rinse or leave in according to product instructions. (An alternate to reduce tangling is to use a solution of one part white vinegar to five parts warm water. Apply to hair and rub in well. Rinse with warm water. Avoid vinegar if the resident has a fresh permanent; it may remove the curl.)
11. Towel-dry the hair.
12. Wrap the hair with a dry towel.

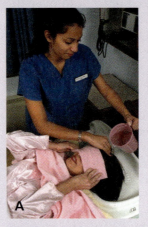
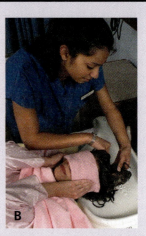

FIGURE 11-17 (A) Cover the eyes with a washcloth and pour water over the hair to wet it thoroughly. (B) Use your fingertips to work up a lather. Wash all areas of the scalp.

13. Remove the towel and comb or pick hair following the guidelines in Procedure 45. Avoid brushing wet hair.
14. Dry with a hair dryer if permitted. Hold the dryer 8 to 10 inches from the head. Follow all safety precautions and facility policies for use of the hair dryer. Direct the heat to the hair, not the scalp. Keep the dryer moving. Use the dryer only on the low heat setting. Never use a handheld hair dryer in a wet area. Avoid placing the hair dryer on the resident's lap.
15. Finish styling the resident's hair when it is dry.
16. Perform your procedure completion actions.

---

red areas that may be Stage I pressure ulcers. Massaging these areas causes tissue destruction. Avoid massaging the legs. Massaging the legs can cause complications related to blood clots. If the resident uses lotion on the legs, pat it on.

GROOMING THE RESIDENT

Proper grooming is important for the resident's self-esteem. Grooming includes combing hair, shaving, nail care, and applying makeup.

Shaving Residents

Most men shave daily as part of the morning routine. If the resident can shave himself, provide the equipment and supplies and allow him to do it. If the resident is weak or unable, you will shave him. Check the care plan before shaving residents. Some residents may not be shaved because of their medical condition or medications they are taking.

Elderly women may grow facial hair as a result of hormonal changes in aging. Coarse hair is common on the chin. Most women prefer to have facial hair removed. Many women also prefer to have hair removed from their legs and underarms. Honor the resident's preferences. Know your facility policy for removing facial hair from female residents. Some facilities use depilatories. Some facilities shave women in the same manner in which men are shaved.

GUIDELINES FOR
Assisting Residents with Grooming

- Allow the resident to determine the routine. Respect the resident's preferences and choices.
- Encourage self-care. Assist by setting up supplies and providing equipment.
- Provide privacy.
- Dress and groom the resident appropriately for age, gender, and season, within the limitations of the resident's condition.

- Keep clean grooming items separate from soiled supplies.
- Clean all grooming items after using them.
- Discard disposable razors in the puncture-resistant sharps container.

PROCEDURE 45

Combing the Hair

1. Perform your beginning procedure actions.
2. Gather supplies needed: towel, comb, and brush.
3. Cover the pillow with a towel, or place the towel over the shoulders if the resident is sitting in a chair.
4. Section the hair with one hand. Begin at the scalp and work toward the end of the hair **(Figure 11-18)**.

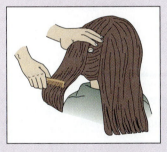

FIGURE 11-18
Beginning at the scalp, comb each section downward.

5. Brush the hair well.
6. If the resident is in bed, assist him or her to turn away from you so that you can brush the back of the hair.
7. If the hair is tangled, separate it with the comb. Start with a small section of hair. Beginning at the end, comb downward. Hold the hair above where you are combing with your other hand so you do not pull on the resident's scalp. Continue working upward until you reach the scalp.
8. Style the hair attractively. If the resident has long hair, consider braiding it or putting it up. Coarse, tightly curled hair may require special treatment.
9. Remove the towel and discard according to facility policy.
10. Perform your procedure completion actions.

PROCEDURE 46

Shaving the Male Resident

1. Perform your beginning procedure actions.
2. Gather supplies needed: disposable gloves, washcloth, towel, electric or safety razor, shaving cream or preshave lotion, basin of water (105°F), mirror, and aftershave lotion.

3. Place the equipment on the overbed table. Follow your facility policy for covering the overbed table with a barrier.
4. Provide privacy.

Continues

> **PROCEDURE**
> ## 46
> **Shaving the Male Resident,**
> *Continued*

  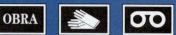

5. Drape a towel across the resident's chest.
6. Fill the washbasin with warm (105°F) water and place it on the table.
7. Soften the beard by placing a warm, moist washcloth over it for two to three minutes. Apply pre-shave lotion if using an electric razor.
8. Moisten the face with water and apply shaving cream.
9. Put on disposable gloves.
10. Hold the skin taut in front of the ear (**Figure 11-19**).
11. Starting at the sideburns, move the razor down over the cheeks to the chin, using short, even strokes. Continue until the entire cheek is shaved. Rinse the razor between strokes.
12. Repeat with the other cheek.
13. Ask the resident to tighten the upper lip. Shave from the nose to the upper lip in short, downward strokes.
14. Ask the resident to tighten the chin. Shave the chin in downward strokes.
15. Assist the resident to tip his head back.
16. Apply shaving cream to the neck.
17. Hold the skin taut under the chin, and shave the neck area in short, smooth, upward strokes.
18. Wash and dry the face and neck.
19. Apply aftershave lotion if the resident desires.
20. Remove the basin, empty and dry it, and return it to its storage place.
21. If you accidentally nick the resident, apply a small piece of tissue over the cut to stop the bleeding. Report the cut to the nurse.
22. Perform your procedure completion actions.

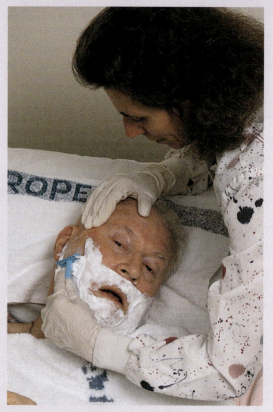

FIGURE 11-19 Hold the skin taut with one hand while shaving in a downward motion with the other.

GUIDELINES FOR
Providing Hand, Foot, and Nail Care

- Know and follow your facility policy for who is allowed to clip and clean nails.
- Cleaning and trimming nails is easier immediately after they are soaked or bathed.
- Avoid the use of nail files and other sharp objects for cleaning nails. An orange stick is a disposable, pointed, wooden stick that can be used safely.
- If your facility allows you to clip fingernails, use clippers, not scissors.
- When trimming nails, be very careful not to accidentally clip or damage the skin surrounding the nail.
- If you observe any abnormalities, such as redness, cracking, or signs of infection by the finger or toenails, report this finding to the nurse.

- Fingernails are clipped straight across, then rounded at the edges with an emery board (**Figure 11-20A**).
- Push the cuticles back with a washcloth or the dull end of the orange stick (**Figure 11-20B**).
- After washing the feet, dry well between each toe and inspect for red or cracked areas. Moisture promotes fungal growth and skin breakdown, which can lead to more serious complications.
- Lotion may be applied to the hands or feet if the skin is dry. Do not apply lotion between the toes, as this promotes fungal growth.

GUIDELINES FOR

GUIDELINES FOR
Providing Hand, Foot, and Nail Care, *Continued*

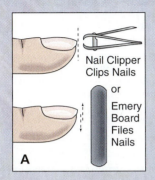
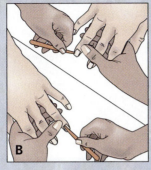

Nail Clipper
Clips Nails

or

Emery
Board
Files
Nails

A

B

FIGURE 11-20 (A) Clip the nails straight across, then use an emery board to round the edges. (B) Gently push the cuticles back.

Shaving may be done with an electric razor or a disposable razor. Electric razors are usually the residents' personal property. They are used for one resident only and cleaned according to manufacturer's directions after each use. This usually involves brushing the heads with a small brush designed for this purpose. All hair should be removed from the head of the razor. Some electric razors must be recharged periodically. Electric razors are expensive. Handle the razor carefully and avoid dropping it. If the electrical cord is frayed or worn, report to the nurse and remove the razor from use. If an electric razor is not available, a disposable safety razor is used. If you are using a disposable razor, always wear gloves because of the high probability of contact with blood during this procedure. Do not recap the razor. Discard the used razor in the sharps container.

Caring for the Resident's Hands, Feet, and Nails

Nails and feet require special attention to prevent injury and infection. In many agencies, only licensed personnel are allowed to cut fingernails, although the nursing assistant is expected to clean them. As a rule, the nursing assistant is not allowed to cut toenails, but is responsible for keeping the feet clean and dry.

The resident's feet require special care. Poor blood circulation to the feet is common, particularly in the elderly and people with diabetes. Ingrown toenails cause pain and breaks in the skin, which can lead to infection. The skin on the feet heals slowly if injured. Protecting the feet from injury is important. Know and follow your facility policy for foot and toenail care. Report to the nurse if the nails need to be cut or if other abnormalities are noted.

PROCEDURE

47

Hand and Fingernail Care

1. Perform your beginning procedure actions.
2. Gather supplies needed: disposable gloves if contact with moist body fluid or nonintact skin is likely, soap, towel, disposable bed protector, basin of warm water (105°F), lotion, nail clippers, orange stick, and emery board.
3. Cover the overbed table with a bed protector. Place the equipment on the overbed table.
4. Position the overbed table in front of the resident and adjust the height.

5. Fill the washbasin with warm (105°F) water and place it on the table.
6. Instruct the resident to place his or her hands in the water. A soft brush can be used to clean under the nails when the hands are soaking.
7. Soak the hands for 10 minutes. Placing a towel over the resident's hands and the basin will keep the water warm. Add more warm water if necessary. (Remove the resident's hands when adding water.)

Continues

PROCEDURE 47
Hand and Fingernail Care, *Continued*

8. Ask the resident to wash his or her hands. Gently push the cuticles back.
9. Lift the hands out of the water and dry them with the towel.
10. Clip the nails if permitted by facility policy. The nail clippings will fall on the bed protector to be discarded later.
11. Round the edges of the nails with the emery board. Apply fingernail polish if requested by a female resident.

12. Rub the hands with lotion.
13. Remove the basin, empty and dry it, and return it to its storage place.
14. Remove the bed protector containing the nail clippings and discard according to facility policy.
15. Perform your procedure completion actions.

SUPPORT HOSIERY

Support hosiery is used for residents who have circulation problems. It is also used during and after surgery to prevent blood clots and other complications. Support hose may also be used to prevent edema. The hose apply pressure to the legs, increasing the blood flow. The stockings are made of stretchable elastic and fit tightly. Support stockings may be knee length or cover the entire leg. They are called **antiembolism stockings,** or often referred to by the brand name, such as TED Hose.

PROTECTING THE ARMS AND LEGS

Some residents have very fragile, paper-thin skin. The skin bruises easily and commonly tears if it is bumped even slightly, such as on the side rail. Skin tears are unsightly and painful for the

PROCEDURE 48
Foot and Toenail Care

1. Perform your beginning procedure actions.
2. Gather supplies needed: disposable gloves if contact with moist body fluid or nonintact skin is likely, soap, towel, bed protector, basin of warm water (105°F), lotion, orange stick or soft brush.
3. Place the equipment on the overbed table. Follow your facility policy for covering the overbed table with a barrier.
4. Transfer the resident to a chair at the bedside. Remove the resident's shoes and socks.
5. Place a bed protector on the floor under the resident's feet.
6. Fill the washbasin with warm (105°F) water and place it on the bed protector.
7. Assist the resident to place his or her feet in the water.
8. Soak the feet for 10 minutes. Placing a towel over the resident's feet and the basin will keep the water warm. Add more warm water if necessary. Check the temperature of the water you add. It should be no more than 105°F. Remove the resi-

dent's feet from the water temporarily while you add more water, to avoid accidental burns.
9. Wash the resident's feet. Gently clean under the toenails with the orange stick or a soft brush.
10. Wash the feet with soap, and rinse well.
11. Lift the feet out of the water and dry them with the towel. Dry well between the toes.
12. Inspect the feet for red, dry, cracked, or open areas. Check for bruises, corns, or other abnormalities.
13. Rub the feet gently with lotion. Avoid vigorous massage. Avoid applying lotion between the toes.
14. Apply nail polish if requested by a female resident.
15. Remove the basin, empty and dry it, and return it to its storage place.
16. Assist the resident to put on socks and shoes.
17. Remove the bed protector and discard according to facility policy.
18. Perform your procedure completion actions.

GUIDELINES FOR
Applying Antiembolism Stockings

- The care plan will specify the wearing schedule for the stockings, according to physician orders and facility policies. For most residents, the hosiery is applied during the day and removed at bedtime. The care plan will specify when the stockings should be put on and removed.
- It is best to apply the stockings before the resident gets out of bed in the morning. Elevating the legs for 20 to 30 minutes before applying the hosiery will reduce swelling and make stockings easier to apply.
- Antiembolism stockings come in several sizes. The resident is measured with a tape measure to find the correct size. The hose must fit well to be effective.
- To preserve the life of the stockings, avoid contact with lotions, ointments, or oils containing lanolin or petroleum products. These products deteriorate the elastic.
- Do not apply the hosiery over open areas, fractures, or deformities. If the resident has an open or abnormal skin area, fracture, or deformity on the legs or feet, inform the nurse.

- The stockings must be applied smoothly with no wrinkles.
- A light application of powder or cornstarch on the feet and legs will make the hosiery easier to apply.
- Placing a plastic sandwich bag over the foot allows the hosiery to slide on easily. After the hose are applied, remove the bag through the opening in the toe area.
- Check the stockings periodically to be sure the tops have not rolled or turned down. Keep the fabric straight.
- Most elastic stockings have a hole in the toe end to allow access for circulation checks. In some stockings, the hole is on the top of the foot, and in others it is on the bottom. As long as the heel is centered, the hole will be in the correct place.
- Monitor circulation in the resident's toes every four hours, or as specified on the care plan. Note color, sensation, swelling, temperature, and ability to move. Report abnormalities to the nurse.
- Follow your facility policy for washing antiembolism stockings. These must be hand-washed and drip-dried. The hose are damaged by the commercial washers and dryers used in the health care facility.

PROCEDURE 49
Applying Antiembolism Stockings

1. Perform your beginning procedure actions.
2. Obtain hosiery in the correct size.
3. Expose one leg.
4. Insert one hand into the stocking as far as the heel pocket. Holding the heel pocket, turn the stocking inside out.
5. Carefully position the stocking over the foot and heel.
6. Place the index and middle fingers of both hands into the stocking foot.
7. Face the resident and ease the stocking up over the foot, stretching sideways as you go. Center the heel pocket. An acceptable alternative is to face the foot, then pull the stocking up, similar to the manner in which you apply your own socks.
8. Continue pulling the stocking up over the ankle and calf, smoothing and stretching the elastic. The top of a knee-high stocking should be one to two inches below the knee. The top of a thigh-high stocking should be one to three inches below the groin.
9. Check the fit to be sure the stocking is even and that there are no wrinkles. Pull up slightly on the toes to ensure that the stocking is not too tight (Figure 11-21).

10. Expose the other leg.
11. Repeat the procedure.
12. Perform your procedure completion actions.

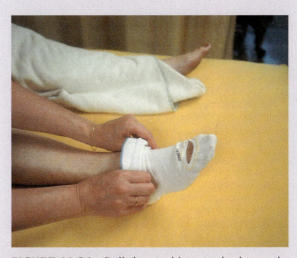

FIGURE 11-21 Roll the stocking up the leg and smooth any wrinkles.

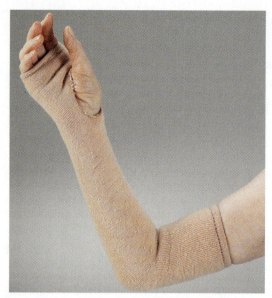

FIGURE 11-22 Skin sleeves offer excellent skin protection against skin tears and bruises. Leg protectors are also available. *(Courtesy of Skil-Care Corporation, Yonkers, NY (800) 431-2972)*

sible. The sleeve covers the hand and arm, leaving the fingers free. It may also be used as a restraint alternative, to prevent the resident from pulling out an IV or other medical device. To apply a skin sleeve:

- Grasp the sleeve near the upper arm opening.
- Roll and gather the sleeve until you reach the thumb opening.
- Slip the resident's hand into the sleeve, fitting the fingers into the large opening, and the thumb into the smaller opening for the hand.
- Unroll the sleeve up over the arm. Smooth the fabric so it is wrinkle-free.

The care plan will specify when the sleeve is to be worn. Monitor the resident's skin under the sleeve when it is removed. Report skin tears, bruises, or other injuries to the nurse. The skin sleeves should be hand-washed or machine-washed on a gentle cycle. Hang them to dry.

resident. They can occur when the resident is transferred into and out of the wheelchair. Keeping the skin moisturized and well lubricated will reduce the risk of injury slightly, but some residents need additional protection. The care plan will specify measures to use, such as wearing long sleeves or keeping the arms and legs covered. Many residents use skin sleeves **(Figure 11-22)**. The skin sleeve protects fragile skin. Some skin sleeves have additional padding. They are available in light and dark flesh tones to match the resident's skin color as closely as pos-

PROSTHESIS CARE

Some residents use a prosthesis to replace a body part. Many types of prostheses are used. A resident may have an artificial eye or breast. Others have artificial arms, hands, legs, or feet. The prosthesis helps the resident function as normally as possible. Remember, the prosthesis is part of the resident's body and should be treated with care. You will be responsible for keeping the prosthesis clean. This usually involves washing with mild soap, rinsing, and drying. Follow the instructions on the care plan or check with the nurse.

GUIDELINES FOR
Caring for a Resident Who Has a Prosthesis

- Always check the care plan for special instructions regarding applying, removing, and caring for the prosthesis.
- The prosthesis and the skin under the prosthesis must be kept clean and dry.
- Check the skin under the prosthesis. Notify the nurse of any redness, irritation, dark spots, open areas, or blisters.
- Follow the directions on the care plan for covering the extremity under the prosthesis. A **stump sock** is a garment used to protect the extremity from irritation caused by rubbing against the prosthesis and is usually worn under artificial limbs.
- For residents with lower extremity amputation, position the remaining joints in extension (as straight

as possible). Residents with leg amputation are at risk for contracture development. Follow the positioning instructions on the care plan. Avoid elevating the stump on pillows.
- Report to the nurse if you feel that the prosthesis needs repair. Do not attempt to fix it yourself.
- An artificial eye is usually cared for by the nurse or resident. If you will be caring for residents with artificial eyes, make sure you are properly trained. Follow facility policy. Handle the eye carefully. The eye socket and the artificial eye must be cleaned as indicated on the care plan. Apply the principles of standard precautions when inserting, removing, and cleaning the eye.

GUIDELINES FOR

Dressing and Undressing Residents

- Provide privacy and avoid exposing the resident.
- Wear gloves and apply the principles of standard precautions if you anticipate contact with blood, body fluids (except sweat), secretions, excretions, mucous membranes, or nonintact skin.
- Check the care plan for special instructions and use of adaptive equipment.
- Encourage the resident to do as much self-care as possible.
- Allow the resident a choice of clothing. The clothing should be appropriate for age and season, and color-coordinated. Follow your facility policy for having torn items replaced or repaired. Do not put torn clothing on a resident.
- If the resident has one paralyzed or weak side, remove the clothing from the strong side first. Put

clothing on the weak side first. Always support the weak or paralyzed extremity.
- It is easier to dress residents who can assist if they are standing or sitting.
- It is easier to dress a dependent resident in bed.
- Residents who are dressed in street clothes should wear proper undergarments. Apply underwear and socks first.
- When dressing residents who use catheters or tubes, treat the tubes as part of the person's body. Avoid pulling on them or obstructing them. Do not disconnect them. Avoid elevating a urinary catheter above the level of the bladder during the dressing procedure. Consult the nurse for assistance.
- Gather the pant legs and sleeves before putting them on the resident.

DRESSING AND UNDRESSING THE RESIDENT

Most residents in the long-term care facility can be up and dressed each day. Self-esteem is improved when the resident is dressed and well-groomed. It also affects other people's perception about the resident's health. All people dress and undress several times a day. In the morning,

we remove night clothing and dress in day wear. At bedtime, we remove clothing and put on night wear. Sometimes in health care, more frequent changes of clothing are necessary due to tests, procedures, medical treatments, and accidental soiling of clothes. Some residents cannot dress and undress themselves. Others may need limited assistance. Residents with paralysis have special dressing needs.

PROCEDURE

50

Assisting the Resident with Dressing

1. Perform your beginning procedure actions.
2. Gather needed supplies: bath blanket, clothing, deodorant, and disposable gloves.
3. If the resident has a weak or paralyzed arm, work from the strong side.
4. Cover the resident with the bath blanket and remove the upper linens without exposing the resident.
5. For pants:
   a. Put one foot at a time into underwear. Slide them up over the feet and ankles.
   b. Gather the leg of the pants on the weak side. Slide the pant leg over the foot and ankle. Repeat with the strong leg.
   c. Slide the pants and underwear up the resident's legs.
   d. Ask the resident to raise the hips and buttocks while you pull underwear and pants into position.

   e. If the resident is unable to assist, roll him or her onto the strong side. Pull the underwear and pants up on the weak side (**Figure 11-23**). Turn the resident to the weak side and finish pulling the clothing up. Fasten at the waist, if necessary.
6. Apply deodorant before putting on a shirt or sweater.
7. To put on garments that go over the arms or head:
   a. Stretch the garment neck as wide as possible and pull it over the resident's head (**Figure 11-24**).
   b. Put your hand into the sleeve of the garment on the resident's weaker side. Grasp the resident's weak hand. Slide the sleeve off your wrist and pull the resident's hand and wrist through the sleeve.
   c. Pull the sleeve up and adjust it at the shoulder.

Continues

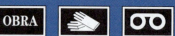

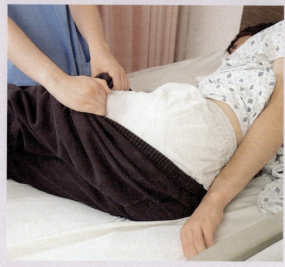

FIGURE 11-23 Pull the pants up on the weak side first.

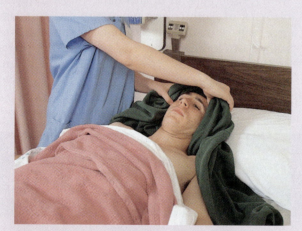

FIGURE 11-24 Stretch the neck and pull the garment over the resident's head.

d. Lift the resident's arms and shoulders. Adjust the garment in the back.

e. Ask the resident to put the strong arm into the other sleeve. If unable, repeat step 7b.

f. Lift the resident's arms and shoulders, or roll the resident to the side. Pull down the garment and adjust it in back.

8. To put on a shirt or blouse that opens in front:

a. Put your hand into the sleeve of the garment on the resident's weaker side. Roll the sleeve over your wrist. Grasp the resident's weak hand. Slide the sleeve off your wrist and over the resident's hand and wrist.

b. Pull the garment up the arm and adjust it at the shoulder.

c. Lift the resident's head and shoulders and pull the garment around the back. If you cannot lift the resident, roll him or her toward you and tuck the garment under him or her. Turn the resident away from you and pull the garment out. Then return the resident to the supine position.

d. Ask the resident to put his or her strong arm into the other sleeve. If unable, repeat step 8a.

e. Pull the garment up the arm and adjust it at the shoulder.

f. Fasten the garment in the front.

9. Gather the sock back from the opening to just below the heel. Support the foot and slip the sock over the toes. Pull it up and over the heel. Straighten and smooth the top over the calf. Repeat with other sock. (You may find it easier to apply the socks first, when you apply the undergarments. This is an acceptable alternative.)

10. Loosen shoe laces and pull the tongue up in shoes. Slip the resident's foot into the shoe and adjust for comfort. Repeat with the other shoe. If possible, have the resident stand before adjusting laces and tying shoes. If the resident is unable to stand, tie the shoe immediately after putting it on.

11. Perform your procedure completion actions.

12. Reverse the procedure for undressing the resident. Remember to remove clothes from the strong side first.

KEY POINTS

- Good personal hygiene is essential to proper health.
- Activities of daily living are things people do every day to meet their health and hygiene needs.
- The nursing assistant assists residents to meet health and hygiene needs when they are unable to take care of these needs independently.
- Oral hygiene is the cleaning of the resident's mouth, teeth, gums, and tongue.
- Special oral hygiene is given frequently to residents who are unconscious, NPO, receiving tube feedings, or receiving oxygen.

- Dentures are artificial teeth that require special care and handling.
- Bathing is done to cleanse the skin, stimulate circulation, provide exercise, and refresh and relax the resident.
- Bath time is an excellent time to make observations of the resident's skin and body.
- Bath water temperature is checked with a thermometer. A comfortable temperature for bathing is 105°F.
- When bathing residents, wash from clean to dirty areas.
- The bed bath is given to residents who are on complete bed rest. The resident's entire body is cleaned.
- The partial bath involves washing the resident's face, hands, underarms, back, and genital area.
- When giving perineal care to a female, wash from front to back. Avoid rubbing back and forth.
- When giving perineal care to a male, wash from the tip of the penis to the rectum.
- Massaging the resident's back is comforting, refreshing, and stimulating to circulation. Giving a back rub helps prevent skin breakdown.
- In most agencies, the nursing assistant does not cut fingernails and toenails.
- Antiembolism hose increase blood flow to the legs and prevent blood clots, edema, and other complications.
- A prosthesis is used to replace a missing body part.
- The resident's self-esteem is enhanced when he or she is dressed and well-groomed.

REVIEW

A. Multiple Choice

Select the one best answer.

1. Hygienic habits
   a. are easily changed.
   b. are not influenced by culture and religion.
   c. are a private matter for most people.
   d. are determined by the nursing assistant.

2. ADLs are
   a. all daily learning.
   b. activities of daily living.
   c. all done lovingly.
   d. activities during life.

3. Incontinence is
   a. loss of bowel or bladder control.
   b. difficulty breathing.
   c. inability to move or feel a body part.
   d. not a medical condition.

4. Always brush the resident's teeth with
   a. a stiff-bristle toothbrush.
   b. an abrasive cleanser.
   c. a soft-bristle toothbrush.
   d. the brush vertical to the teeth.

5. You are assigned to give Mr. Lee a partial bath. You know this means to wash the
   a. face, abdomen, legs, underarms, and feet.
   b. face, hands, underarms, back, and perineum.
   c. face, arms, hands, perineum, and legs.
   d. face, underarms, perineum, and feet.

6. When bathing residents, always wash
   a. vigorously in a circular motion.
   b. from the dirtiest area to the cleanest.
   c. from clean to dirty.
   d. the weakest side first.

7. The temperature of bath water should be
   a. 85°F.
   b. 95°F.
   c. 105°F.
   d. 115°F.

8. Which of the following is *not* true about wearing gloves during the bathing procedure?
   a. Gloves are worn for the entire procedure.
   b. Gloves are changed immediately before contact with nonintact skin.
   c. Gloves are changed immediately before performing perineal care.
   d. Gloves should be changed if they become heavily soiled.

9. When assisting the female resident with perineal care, wash
   a. from back to front.
   b. in a back-and-forth motion.
   c. in a circular motion.
   d. from front to back.

10. You are assigned to bathe Mrs. Lloyd. You notice that her toenails are long and dirty. You should
   a. clean and cut the nails.
   b. clean the nails and consult the nurse.
   c. do nothing, as you are not allowed to care for nails.
   d. clean the nails and file them with an emery board.

B. True/False

Answer each statement true (T) or false (F).

11. _____ Massage stage I pressure sores well with lotion.

12. _____ Shave a man's face using downward strokes.

13. _____ Assist the resident to sit up in a chair before applying antiembolism stockings.

14. _____ Always dress and undress the paralyzed arm first.

15. _____ A prosthesis is an artificial body part.

16. _____ HS care is given to prepare the resident for bed at night.

17. _____ Always wear gloves when giving oral care.

18. _____ It is not necessary to wear gloves when shaving residents with a disposable razor.

19. _____ Always brush dentures while they are in the resident's mouth.

20. _____ Wear gloves when washing the resident's eyes.

C. Clinical Applications

Answer the following questions.

21. You are assigned to give Mrs. Green a tub bath. After you transfer Mrs. Green into the bathtub, she tells you that she wants privacy and asks that you leave her alone in the tub. Your facility policy is that residents are not to be unattended in the bathtub. What should you do?

22. Mr. Hill is a mentally confused resident with very poor personal hygiene. He does not like to bathe. If his soiled clothes are not removed from the room when he goes to bed at night, he will put them on again the next morning. Today is Mr. Hill's shower day. He tells you he does not want to take a shower. What should you do?

23. Helen Spencer is at high risk of skin breakdown. She is frequently incontinent of bowel and bladder. Helen will not tell anyone when she is wet or soiled. Her skin becomes red and breaks down quickly. What can a CNA do?

24. Carmen Hernandez has arteriosclerotic heart disease. She has a history of blood clots. Carmen has very dry skin. She asks you to massage lotion on her legs to relieve the dryness. What actions should you take?

25. When you arrive on duty at 7 a.m., Mrs. Street is sitting up in the chair in her room. After breakfast, you give her a shower. After the shower, you are dressing the resident and discover that her feet and lower legs are very edematous. The care plan states that Mrs. Street must wear antiembolism stockings when she is out of bed. What should you do?

CHAPTER 12

Comfort, Pain, Rest, and Sleep

OBJECTIVES

After reading this chapter, you will be able to:

- Spell and define key terms.
- Explain why nursing comfort measures are important to residents' well-being.
- List six observations to make and report for residents who have pain.
- Describe nursing assistant measures to increase comfort and relieve pain.
- List nursing comfort measures that promote rest.
- Describe the phases of the sleep cycle and the importance of each.
- List nursing measures to promote sleep.
- Define religion and spirituality and explain how they are different.
- Describe methods of supporting residents' spirituality.

OBSERVATIONS TO MAKE AND REPORT RELATED TO COMFORT, PAIN, REST, AND SLEEP

Chest pain
Pain that radiates
Pain upon movement
Pain during urination
Pain when having a bowel movement
Splinting an area upon movement
Grimacing, or facial expressions suggesting pain
Body language suggesting pain
Moaning or sighing

Pattern of behavior suggesting pain, such as screaming upon movement
Acute headache
Complaints of binding pain or sensation around forehead
"Splitting" headache
Unrelieved pain after pain medication has been given
Pain is *never* normal; *all* complaints of pain should be reported to the nurse promptly

RESIDENT COMFORT

All humans need comfort, rest, and sleep for physical and emotional well-being, health, and wellness. **Comfort** is a state of physical and emotional well-being. The resident is calm and relaxed, and is not in pain or upset. Assisting residents with their comfort needs is a major nursing assistant responsibility. In fact, assisting residents with physical or emotional comfort needs is at the very heart of nursing care. Many factors affect residents' comfort. Environmental factors that in-terfere with comfort are unfamiliar environment, lack of privacy, noise, odor, temperature, lighting, and ventilation. Personal and uncontrollable factors that increase or contribute to discomfort include age, activity, injury, illness, surgery, stress, and pain. As a rule, residents are uncomfortable when their physical or emotional needs are not met. Unmet needs cause tension and anxiety, and interfere with comfort and rest **(Figure 12-1).** Using basic nursing measures to meet residents' needs promotes comfort and relaxation, and provides a sense of well-being.

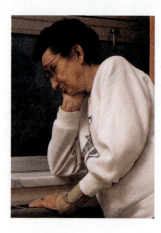

FIGURE 12-1 This resident's body language betrays the emotional distress she is feeling.

PAIN

Pain (Figure 12-2) is a state of discomfort that is unpleasant for the resident. Pain is always a warning that something is wrong. It interferes with the resident's optimal level of function and self-care. Residents may limit movement when they are having pain. Unrelieved pain contributes to complications of immobility, increasing the risk of pneumonia, skin breakdown, and other problems. Pain decreases quality of life, and may cause hopelessness, anxiety, depression, and a feeling of helplessness. Pain may cause acting out, crying, and other strange, belligerent, or combative behavior. It is a major preventable public health problem that slows recovery in individuals with acute illness, complicates chronic illness, and increases health care costs. Relieving pain has always been an important nursing responsibility. Nursing staff must identify residents who are having pain, and those who are at risk for pain, then take the appropriate action to make the residents as comfortable as possible.

Residents' Responses to Pain

Residents' responses to pain vary widely. Some individuals do not feel pain as acutely as others.

Some try to ignore the pain. Other residents may try to deny pain because they are afraid of what it means. Ignoring or denying pain increases the risk of injury, because the normal warning that pain gives goes unrecognized or unheeded. Confused residents may display behavior problems when they are having pain. Some moan, sigh, or yell during movement. Never ignore body language or other signs of pain in residents. Always report signs and symptoms of pain to the nurse. Your observations are a valuable contribution to the nursing assessment and residents' comfort.

Residents' responses to pain may be related to culture. People from some cultures are very emotional when they are in pain. Others are very stoic. Some think that showing pain is a sign of weakness, whereas others believe that pain is a punishment from a higher power. Pain causes stress and anxiety, interfering with comfort, rest, and sleep (Figure 12-3). Rest and sleep are necessary for the body to restore strength and energy, and to repair itself. Inability to sleep, restlessness, and disturbed sleep may be caused by pain.

Identifying Residents in Pain

Pain is a serious condition that affects well-being and quality of life. Residents have the right to timely pain assessment and management. Many factors affect residents' reactions to pain. The reactions may be different from one moment to the next, and one resident to the next. Four types of pain are listed in **Table 12-1**. Monitor the residents' body language for signs of pain. Regularly ask residents if they are in pain. Some will not volunteer this information if not asked directly. Some residents will yell or cry out during transfers or movement. This may be interpreted as confusion instead of pain.

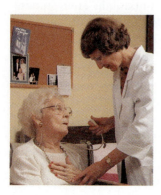

FIGURE 12-2 This resident is having severe pain.

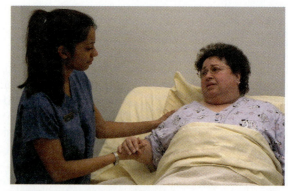

FIGURE 12-3 This resident's pain is interfering with her ability to sleep.

TABLE 12-1	Types of pain
Type of Pain	**Description**
Acute pain	Occurs suddenly and without warning. Acute pain is usually the result of tissue damage, caused by conditions such as injury or surgery. Typically, acute pain decreases over time, as healing takes place.
Persistent (chronic) pain	Persistent pain lasts longer than six months. (Another, older term for this type of pain is *chronic pain*). It may be intermittent or constant. Persistent pain may be caused by multiple medical conditions.
Phantom pain	Phantom pain occurs as a result of an amputation. The resident has had a body part, such as a leg, removed, but complains of pain in the missing toes. The pain is real, not imaginary.
Radiating pain	Radiating pain moves from the site of origin to other areas. For example, when a resident is having a heart attack, the pain may radiate from the chest to the jaw or arm.

Body language is often the first clue that a resident is having pain. This may be the only clue in some cognitively impaired residents, those from other cultures, and residents who are comatose. Look for pain upon movement, facial expressions, crying, moaning, rigid posture, and guarded positioning. The resident may withdraw when he or she is touched or repositioned. Watch for restlessness, irregular or erratic respirations, periodic breath-holding, dilated pupils, and sweating. The resident may favor one extremity. He or she may become irritable, fatigued, or withdrawn. The resident may refuse to eat for no apparent reason. The resident may act opposite of normal. For example:

- A cognitively impaired resident who is normally very quiet becomes noisy
- A resident with garbled speech accurately describes his or her pain
- The agitated and combative resident becomes quiet and nonverbal
- A friendly and outgoing resident cries easily and withdraws
- The resident who is normally active becomes still and quiet

Always suspect pain if the resident's behavior changes. Although the resident may not display an outward appearance of pain, asking if he or she is having pain is the best way to find out. Report your observations to the nurse compared with the normal behavior for the resident. If the behavior changes back to normal after the nurse administers an **analgesic** (pain-relieving) medication, this confirms that the change in body language or behavior was caused by pain. The nurse will inform the interdisciplinary team that further evaluation is necessary to determine the best ways of managing the pain.

The resident's self-report of pain is the most accurate indicator of the existence and intensity of pain, and should be respected and believed. Avoid making assumptions about a resident's pain. Although many residents with pain display outward signs through their body language and behavior, avoid making assumptions about the presence or absence of pain if the resident is laughing, talking, or sleeping. For example, some health care workers assume that residents who are smiling or laughing cannot be in pain. Vital signs may be normal. These workers believe that residents who are having pain should be grimacing, frowning, or crying. This is untrue. Some residents may appear comfortable while having severe pain. Once again, avoid judging the resident. His or her self-report of pain is the most accurate and reliable indicator of pain. Notify the nurse without passing judgment.

When asking about pain, make sure the resident can see and hear you. Allow enough time for the resident to process your questions and respond. Be patient. Use language that is appropriate for the resident's age and mental status. Remember that residents may use different words for pain, such as "hurt," "sore," or "tender." Residents who are mentally confused may surprise you. Some can describe their pain accurately. Some residents will admit to having pain only if you ask them directly, so do not omit this important step. Always ask residents who are crying, those whose body language suggests pain, and those with behavior suggesting pain.

Observing and Reporting Signs and Symptoms of Pain

Pain always requires further intervention. It should never be ignored. Always report verbal complaints of pain, describing the pain in the resident's exact words. Be aware of signs and symptoms of pain in residents who have difficulty communicating, such as residents who cannot speak and residents who are cognitively impaired. Facial expressions and grimacing; moaning; refusing to move; stiff, rigid, or limited movements; and crying, yelling, or screaming may be clues that the resident is having pain. Inform the nurse promptly. Pain is always an observation that must be reported immediately. A nursing assessment of pain involves many different factors. Your observations contribute to this assessment and the resident's well-being.

Using a Pain Rating Scale. Your facility will have policies and procedures for pain management. Most facilities have adopted several different pain rating scales to evaluate the level of residents' pain. In fact, many facilities now consider pain the "fifth vital sign." In these facilities, pain is regularly and frequently evaluated.

Because pain is personal and subjective, consistent pain evaluation among health care workers is a concern. Using a pain rating (assessment) scale helps nurses assess the resident and keeps caregivers from forming their own opinions about the level of the resident's pain. Using a pain scale prevents subjective opinions, provides consistency, eliminates some barriers to pain management, and gives the resident a means of describing the pain accurately. Pain scales are important tools for communication. The resident selects the scale that helps *best describe* his or her pain. Pain rating scales can be used to evaluate pain in residents of all ages and cultures.

Although you will not be directly assessing the residents' pain, you must understand the purpose of the scales used in your facility and how they are interpreted. Many facilities use a 0 to 10 scale, with 0 meaning no pain and 10 meaning intolerable pain. If the resident tells you that she is having pain at "level 5," for example, you must know what this means and report the problem to the nurse. Likewise, if the resident complains of pain at "level 9" an hour after receiving pain medication, this suggests a potentially serious problem and must be reported immediately.

Many different pain scales are used in health care **(Figure 12-4).** These scales are only examples. Your facility may use similar or different tools for evaluating pain. Pain scales use pictures, words, or numbers to help the resident describe pain intensity. Most scales range from no pain to very severe pain. Picture scales use smiling faces, neutral faces, frowns, and tears.

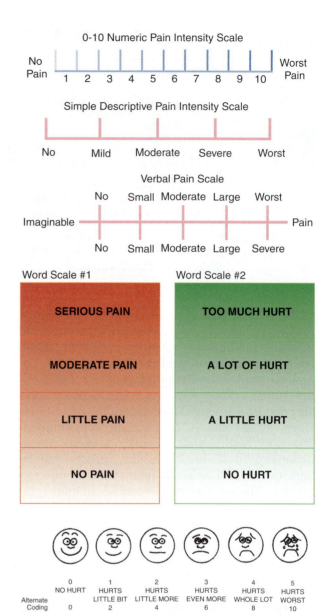

FIGURE 12-4 The resident will select the pain scale that best helps him or her communicate the level and intensity of his or her pain. *(FACES scale from Wong D. L. et al. Wong's Essentials of Pediatric Nursing, ed. 6, St. Louis: Mosby, 2001, p. 1301. Reprinted with permission.)*

Managing Pain

Unrelieved pain has a negative effect on the resident's health and functional status. Notify the nurse as soon as the resident complains, before pain becomes severe or out of control. Report your observations objectively. Observe the resident carefully after pain medications have been given, and report your observations to the nurse.

Sometimes the physician orders several different medications for each resident's pain. The nurse will select which drug to use based on an assessment of the resident. Your observations, the resident's self-report of pain intensity, and physical assessment findings are all considered when determining which medication to administer, when more than one is ordered. If the first drug does not relieve the pain, the nurse may have the option of administering another, so always report unrelieved pain. The quality of pain control is influenced by the education, experience, and attitude of the health care providers caring for the resident.

Pain management is an important part of resident care. Take complaints of pain very seriously. Respect and support the residents' right to pain assessment and management without judgment or disbelief. You are responsible for promptly reporting the information to the nurse, who will assess the resident and take the appropriate action. Avoid passing judgment on residents who take narcotic medications to control their pain. Many health care workers try to discourage residents from taking these drugs because of the potential for addiction. Studies have shown that very few residents with severe pain become addicted to the drugs.

Although the nursing assistant is not directly responsible for pain management, your observations and nursing care are very important, because you work so closely and intimately with the residents. Understanding the responsibilities that health care providers have for pain relief will help you provide nursing comfort measures, monitor for signs and symptoms of pain, and report your observations to the nurse.

Nursing Assistant Comfort Measures. As a nursing assistant, you can provide many basic nursing measures to make the resident more comfortable. Relieving discomfort helps reduce pain and anxiety. These include:

- Telling residents what you plan to do and how you will do it
- Providing privacy
- Assisting the resident to get into a comfortable position **(Figure 12-5)**
- Repositioning the resident to relieve pain and muscle spasms
- Changing the angle of the bed to relieve tension on surgical sites or injured areas
- Avoiding sudden, jerking movements when moving or positioning the resident
- Performing passive range-of-motion exercises to reduce stiffness and maintain mobility
- Using pillows to support the affected body part(s) **(Figure 12-6)**

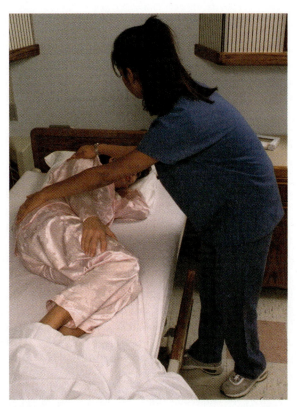

FIGURE 12-5 Help the resident find a comfortable position.

- Providing extra pillows and blankets for comfort and support
- Straightening the bed and linen
- Giving a back rub
- Washing the resident's face and hands
- Providing a cool, damp washcloth on the resident's forehead
- Providing oral hygiene

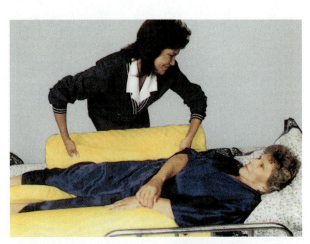

FIGURE 12-6 Use pillows, props, and supports to position body parts for comfort. *(Courtesy of Briggs Corporation, Des Moines, IA (800) 247-2343)*

- Providing fresh water, food, or beverages as permitted
- Playing soft music to distract the resident
- Listening to resident's concerns
- Providing emotional support
- Touching the resident, if appropriate
- Maintaining a comfortable environmental temperature
- Providing a quiet, dark environment
- Eliminating unpleasant sights, sounds, and odors from the environment
- Waiting at least 30 minutes after the nurse administers pain medication before moving the resident or performing procedures or activities
- Timing resident care to coincide with pain medication

Regularly incorporate these steps into your resident care. Follow the individual directions on the care plan. The nurse may also direct you to apply warm or cold applications (Chapter 4) to make the resident more comfortable.

REST

Rest is a state of mental and physical comfort, calmness, and relaxation. The resident's basic needs of hunger, thirst, elimination, and pain must be met before effective rest is possible. He or she should be dressed comfortably and feel fresh and clean. The resident may sit or lie down, or may do things that are pleasant and relaxing. Some residents have rituals, such as reading the Bible **(Figure 12-7)** or saying the rosary. The

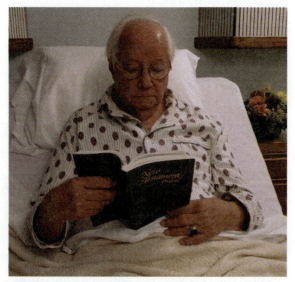

FIGURE 12-7   Reading the Bible is a pleasurable activity that helps this resident rest.

environment should be calm and quiet to promote rest. If basic care is tiring for the resident, allow him or her to rest before continuing. Some residents feel refreshed after 15 minutes of rest. Others need more time. Some residents must rest frequently throughout the day. Plan your schedule and activities to allow for rest periods. Providing a back rub, nursing comfort measures, or other relaxation activities may assist the resident to rest. Follow the care plan and the nurse's instructions.

SLEEP

Sleep is a period of continuous or intermittent unconsciousness in which physical movements are decreased, allowing the mind and body to rest. Sleep is a basic need of all humans. Adequate sleep is necessary for the body and mind to function properly. Sleep occurs in a cycle that lasts for several hours at a time.

The body repairs itself during sleep. Because movement and activity are limited, the body's metabolic needs are reduced. The resident may need a blanket because he or she is not moving, and may become cold. It is common for vital signs to decrease during sleep. The need for sleep decreases as a person ages. Infants and children require more sleep than adults. Elderly residents require less sleep than younger adults or middle-aged residents. Children require more sleep than adults. In fact, newborns may sleep as much as 20 hours a day. Sleep needs by age group are listed in **Table 12-2.** Weight loss may decrease the need for sleep, whereas weight gain often increases the need for sleep.

Many factors affect sleep. Sleep problems often result from a combination of many factors. Obvious problems that may interfere with the quality and quantity of sleep are:

- Pain
- Hunger
- Thirst
- Need to eliminate
- Illness
- Exercise
- Noise
- Temperature
- Ventilation
- Light intensity
- Physical discomfort
- Some medications
- Caffeine intake
- Alcohol, drugs
- Some foods and beverages

TABLE 12-2	Sleep needs throughout the life cycle

- Newborn infants sleep in 3- to 4-hour intervals for a total of 16 to 20 hours of sleep a day
- Infants require 12 to 16 hours of sleep a day
- Toddlers require 12 to 14 hours of sleep a day, usually broken into 10 to 12 hours of sleep at night, with one or more daytime naps
- Preschool children require 10 to 12 hours per day
- Elementary school children require 10 to 12 hours a day
- Adolescents require 8 to 10 hours per day
- Young adults aged 18 to 40 require about 7 to 8 hours a day
- Middle-aged adults aged 40 to 65 require about 7 hours a day
- Elderly adults over the age of 65 require about 5 to 7 hours per day

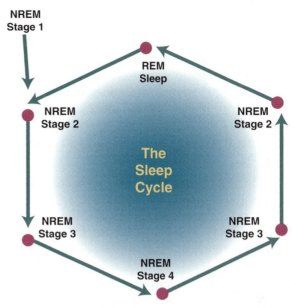

FIGURE 12-8 The sleep cycle

- Lifestyle changes
- Anxiety, stress, fear, emotional problems
- Changes in the environment, unfamiliar environment
- Treatments and therapies
- Staff providing routine care

Worry is another factor that interferes with comfort, rest, and sleep. Residents worry about many things, such as:

- What the future will bring
- How much the stay in the facility will cost
- Who is taking care of their responsibilities
- Whether they are dying

You will not have the answers to all these pressing concerns. You can listen, however. Share these concerns with the nurse. This is not gossiping. The nurse and the other members of the staff may be able to help the resident solve the problems. With worries reduced, the resident will rest easier.

The Sleep Cycle

Each person has a sleep–wake cycle. An internal biological clock tells the person when it is time to sleep and wake up. The sleep cycle includes two types of sleep **(Figure 12-8)**.

- **Nonrapid eye movement (NREM) sleep** has four phases, progressing from light to very deep. This part of the sleep cycle begins when the resident first falls asleep. In the first two phases, the resident is easily aroused. As he or she progresses through the cycle, arousal becomes more difficult and sleep becomes deeper.

- **Rapid eye movement (REM) sleep** restores mental function. If you look closely, you will see the resident's eyes moving behind closed lids during this phase. Avoid awakening a resident who is in REM sleep, whenever possible. This is the part of the cycle in which dreams occur. The resident passes into REM sleep within approximately 60 to 90 minutes after falling asleep. Hospitalized residents may not experience prolonged periods of sleep time, so total REM time is less than normal. They awaken feeling less rested and may be more tired during the day.

Sleep is important to prevent feelings of fatigue, and for healing of medical and surgical problems. Getting enough sleep and rest allows residents to function at their highest level. Moving through the stages of the sleep cycle uninterrupted is important. Some residents become irritable if they do not have enough sleep. Elderly residents who do not sleep well may become disoriented. This correctable problem may be mistaken for confusion! It is easily solved by allowing uninterrupted sleep. Other signs and symptoms of inadequate sleep are:

- Slow mental and physical responses
- Decreased attention span
- Forgetfulness, difficulty remembering things
- Reduced reasoning and judgment
- Puffy, red, swollen eyes
- Dark circles under the eyes
- Disorientation
- Mood swings, moodiness
- Lethargy, sleepiness, fatigue

- Agitation, restlessness
- Clumsiness, incoordination
- Difficulty finding the right word(s) to say
- Slurred speech
- Hallucinations in severe **sleep deprivation,** or prolonged sleep loss (inadequate quality or quantity of REM or NREM sleep).

Nursing Assistant Measures to Promote Comfort, Rest, and Sleep

Basic nursing comfort measures, such as those used to relieve pain, are also effective in helping residents to rest and sleep. Specific measures for each resident will be listed in the care plan. Measures that promote comfort, rest, and sleep are:

- Helping the resident into loose-fitting, comfortable clothing or nightwear
- Assisting with toileting, cleanliness, oral care, and personal hygiene needs
- Providing a warm bath or shower, if permitted
- Avoiding serving beverages containing caffeine after the evening meal
- Providing a snack, if desired; snacks with protein and/or calcium, such as meat, cheese, milk, nuts, and peanut butter, promote sleep (peanut butter is not permitted in some facilities and states)
- Straightening the bed
- Assisting the resident into a comfortable position, providing pillows and props as needed for comfort
- Giving a back rub **(Figure 12-9)**
- Providing a comfortable environmental temperature and ventilation
- Providing an extra blanket, if desired
- Eliminating unpleasant odors
- Eliminating noise
- Adjusting the lighting to a comfortable level, darkening the room as much as possible for sleep or providing a nightlight, if desired

- Reporting pain to the nurse
- If the resident is having pain, waiting for at least 30 minutes after pain medication before performing procedures
- If the resident is anxious, listening to what he or she says and eliminating the cause of the anxiety, if possible
- Not startling the resident
- Handling the resident gently during care
- Organizing routine care to allow the resident uninterrupted sleep or rest
- Avoiding physical activity or other activities that are upsetting to the resident before bedtime
- Assisting with personal bedtime rituals, if any
- Allowing the resident to select his or her own bedtime
- Allowing the resident to read, watch television, or listen to the radio, if desired
- Reading to the resident from a favorite book
- Assisting with relaxation exercises and activities, as directed **(Figure 12-10)**
- If the resident receives a sleeping medication, making sure the resident is ready for sleep before the nurse administers the medication
- Closing the door to the resident's room

SPIRITUALITY

Spirituality and religion can provide great comfort and support to residents, particularly during times of illness and emotional distress. Many people believe that spirituality and religion are the same thing, but they are not. *Spirituality* is a broader term that includes:

- Our perceptions of our place in the universe **(Figure 12-11)**
- Belief in a higher power (if any)
- Our ideas about responsibilities to others
- Our fears and beliefs about living and dying

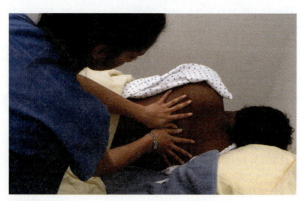

FIGURE 12-9   A back rub is relaxing and relieves muscle tension.

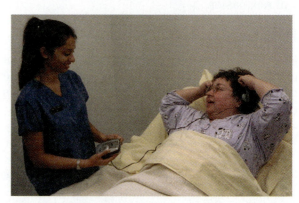

FIGURE 12-10   This resident uses music as a form of relaxation.

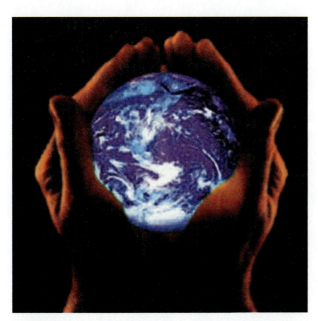

FIGURE 12-11 Spirituality involves our perceptions of our place in the universe.

The need for spirituality may be fueled by experiences, relationships, and opportunities that provide the motivation for deeper healing and growth throughout life. Illness can be a powerful motivator for eliminating emotional, mental, and physical patterns that limit and restrict spiritual growth. A key to caring for residents' spiritual needs is respecting each resident as an individual, and remembering that no two people are alike.

When residents use spirituality for healing, they allow the power of the spirit to work more fully in their lives, leading to greater harmony and balance. It is usually a quiet time for introspection and questioning. Healing may require making changes. It involves blending of the physical, mental, emotional, and spiritual aspects of self. When a person experiences deep physical or emotional healing, all parts of the self are changed. Physical problems often involve thoughts and emotions. Residents sometimes have surprises during periods of intense spirituality. They may release a great emotional burden instead of experiencing a physical recovery. The lifting of the emotional burden often brings a great sense of inner peace.

Nursing Assistant Actions

The nursing assistant must recognize that all humans are spiritual beings, although we all choose different paths. Be sensitive to the residents' paths and choices. Avoid passing judgment about residents' religious, spiritual, ethnic, and cultural practices and choices in health care treatment. Although spiritual beliefs are usually considered a private concern, the need for spiritual caring is fundamental when serious health problems occur. The resident may question the meaning and purpose of life, the sense of hope, belief in self, belief in caregivers' ability, belief in the physician's ability, and belief in a higher power. Health care personnel are privileged to have a presence and role in these very personal times of significant stress and turmoil in residents' lives. Pay attention to what the resident is saying. Your role is to listen, to reflect, and to clarify information. Never try to interpret or define spiritual meaning or truth to the resident. Avoid imposing your beliefs on the resident. Avoid pat, uncaring answers to questions. Never give residents false hope. Never use problem-solving techniques to analyze spiritual truths for residents. Admitting that you do not know an answer is all right.

Remember that caring for residents during very private moments is a privilege. Do not be so distracted with your workload or the environment that you fail to show sensitivity when residents express spiritual concerns. Provide privacy and support while they work through challenges to their health and well-being. Inform the nurse or social worker of the resident's concerns. They may be able to provide assistance, intervention, or referrals to other sources of help.

KEY POINTS

- All humans need comfort, rest, and sleep for physical and emotional well-being, health, and wellness.
- Comfort is a state of physical and emotional well-being.
- Pain is a state of discomfort that is unpleasant for the resident; it is always a warning that something is wrong.
- Residents' responses to pain may be related to culture.
- Body language may be the first (and only) clue that a resident is having pain.
- Relieving pain is an important nursing responsibility.

- The resident's self-report of pain is the most accurate indicator of the existence and intensity of pain, and should be respected and believed.
- Residents may have pain when they are laughing, talking, or sleeping; vital signs may be normal.
- Pain rating scales are important tools for communication. They prevent subjective opinions, provide consistency, eliminate some barriers to pain management, and give the resident a means of describing the pain accurately.
- The incidence of drug addiction is very low in individuals with persistent pain who take narcotic analgesics.
- Rest is a state of mental and physical comfort, calmness, and relaxation. The basic needs of hunger, thirst, elimination, and pain must be met before effective rest is possible.
- Sleep is a period of continuous or intermittent unconsciousness in which physical movements are decreased and the mind and body rest.
- Sleep is a basic need. Adequate sleep is necessary for the body and mind to function properly.
- Less sleep is required as people age.
- Rapid eye movement sleep restores mental function.
- Spirituality and religion can provide great comfort and support during times of illness and emotional distress.
- Spirituality and religion are not the same thing.
- Spirituality includes our perceptions of our place in the universe, belief in a higher power (if any), ideas about our responsibilities to others, and our fears and beliefs about living and dying.
- Caring for residents during very private moments is a privilege. The nursing assistant should show sensitivity when residents express spiritual concerns.

REVIEW

A. Multiple Choice

Select the one best answer.

1. Pain is
   a. not the nursing assistant's responsibility.
   b. a sign of something wrong.
   c. always a sign of acute illness.
   d. a normal condition in the elderly.

2. Pain
   a. never interferes with rest and sleep.
   b. is not stressful or worrisome.
   c. negatively affects well-being.
   d. can usually be ignored.

3. If a resident expresses her problems and worries, the nursing assistant should
   a. stay out of the resident's business.
   b. avoid sharing the information with the nurse.
   c. allow her to talk about it; be a good listener.
   d. provide answers to the problems.

4. Pain assessment is considered to be the
   a. primary vital sign.
   b. frequency at which pain is evaluated.
   c. fifth vital sign.
   d. effectiveness of pain medication.

5. The resident who is having pain
   a. may be laughing or sleeping.
   b. will have abnormal vital signs.
   c. will always limit movement.
   d. always displays painful body language.

6. A state of mental calmness, comfort, and relaxation is
   a. security.
   b. sleep.
   c. leisure.
   d. rest.

7. A period of continuous or intermittent unconsciousness in which physical movements are decreased is
   a. relaxation.
   b. comfort.
   c. sleep.
   d. diversion.

8. When a resident is sleeping,
   a. vital signs may be lower than usual.
   b. temperature increases.
   c. movement increases.
   d. the pulse decreases and respirations increase.

9. During the REM sleep cycle, the resident
   a. dreams.
   b. awakens readily.
   c. progresses through four sleep phases.
   d. may feel hot to the touch.

10. Sleep deprivation is
    a. getting too much sleep.
    b. not getting enough sleep.
    c. a condition caused by snoring.
    d. a sign of mental confusion.

11. Spirituality
    a. is the same as religion.
    b. includes perceptions about one's place in the universe.
    c. is a very private matter between the resident and God.
    d. should be managed only by a qualified social worker.

B. True/False

Answer each question true (T) or false (F).

12. _____ The nurse selects the pain scale for the resident to use.

13. _____ Lack of privacy can affect a resident's comfort.

14. _____ Unrelieved pain can lead to complications of immobility.

15. _____ Persistent pain never lasts longer than one month.

16. _____ Acute pain results from tissue damage.

17. _____ Phantom pain is imaginary pain.

18. _____ Radiating pain always encircles the area in which the pain originates.

19. _____ Assume that the resident is not in pain if he or she does not complain.

20. _____ Rest and sleep are necessary for the body to restore strength and energy, and to repair itself.

21. _____ Pain always indicates something wrong.

22. _____ Culture has no effect on residents' responses to pain.

23. _____ The resident's self-report of pain is the most accurate indicator of the existence and intensity of pain.

C. Matching

Choose the correct term from Column II to match the phrases in Column I. Write the letter of that term in the blank.

	Column I	Column II
24. _____	state of physical and emotional well-being	a. sleep deprivation
25. _____	period of unconsciousness in which movements are decreased	b. analgesic c. REM sleep d. rest
26. _____	progresses from light to very deep	e. pain f. comfort
27. _____	restores mental function	g. NREM sleep h. sleep
28. _____	pain-relieving medication	
29. _____	mental and physical comfort, calmness, and relaxation	
30. _____	inadequate sleep	
31. _____	state of discomfort	

D. Fill in the Blank

32-39. *Complete the statements by writing in the correct word from the following list:*

acute	comfort	pain
amputation	NREM	phantom
persistent	REM	radiating

32. Full-color dreaming occurs during the _____ phase of the sleep cycle.

33. _____ is a state of well-being.

34. _____ sleep restores mental function.

35. _____ is an unpleasant state of discomfort that indicates something is wrong.

36. _____ pain occurs as a result of the removal of an extremity, or _____.

37. Pain that lasts longer than six months is _____ or chronic pain.

38. _____ pain moves from the site of origin to other areas.

39. _____ pain is usually the result of tissue damage; it occurs suddenly and without warning.

E. Clinical Application

Mr. Wong is grimacing and supporting his right side with his hands when you enter the room. He smiles and nods at you. Answer questions 40-44 regarding this resident.

40. Can Mr. Wong smile if he is having pain?

41. If Mr. Wong's right side hurts, how can you position him for comfort and support?

42. Should Mr. Wong's body language be reported to the nurse?

43. Should you ask Mr. Wong if he is having pain?

44. List six nursing assistant measures you can take to make Mr. Wong more comfortable.

Mrs. Lee is a mentally confused resident. She often cries during your shift, but despite your best efforts, you are unable to comfort her. Mrs. Lee goes to therapy several times a week for a warm paraffin wax treatment on her hands. The nurse tells you the resident has arthritis. When the resident leaves the therapy department, she is often smiling. Answer questions 45-47 regarding this resident.

45. Can pain cause crying in a cognitively impaired resident?

46. List four observations you will make of this resident's crying behavior to report to the nurse.

47. List one nursing assistant approach to use for this resident when she is crying.

CHAPTER 13

Nutrition and Hydration

OBJECTIVES

After reading this chapter, you will be able to:

- Spell and define key terms.
- Describe how proper nutrition influences health.
- List the six categories in the food pyramid and give the recommended number of daily servings from each.
- List five common categories of diets served in health care facilities.
- Describe how the nursing assistant assists residents to meet their nutritional needs.
- Describe general care and list the risks for the resident with dysphagia and swallowing problems.
- Identify residents who are at risk of malnutrition and list measures to promote adequate food intake.
- State the purpose of calorie counts and food intake studies.
- List three alternative methods of feeding.
- Explain why elderly individuals are at risk of dehydration and list nursing assistant actions to prevent dehydration.
- Identify the normal daily fluid requirement for adults.
- Demonstrate accurate measurement of oral fluid intake.
- List the general rules for passing fresh drinking water.
- Demonstrate the procedure related to nutrition and hydration.

OBSERVATIONS TO MAKE AND REPORT RELATED TO NUTRITION AND HYDRATION

Sores or ulcers inside the mouth
Difficulty chewing or swallowing food
Unusual or abnormal appearance of feces
Blood, mucus, parasites, or other unusual substances in stool
Unusual color of feces
Hard stool, difficulty passing stool
Extremely small or extremely large stool
Loose, watery stool
Complaints of pain, constipation, diarrhea, bleeding
Frequent belching
Changes in appetite
Excessive thirst
Fruity smell to breath
Complaints of indigestion

Excessive gas (flatus)
Nausea, vomiting
Choking
Abdominal pain
Abdominal distention (swelling)
Oral or rectal bleeding
Vomitus, stool, or drainage from a nasogastric tube that looks like coffee grounds
Increase or decrease in food (caloric) intake
Increase or decrease of body weight
Diabetic residents who do not eat all their food, or who eat more than allowed on diet
Residents on restricted diets who do not adhere to their diet
Refusal to accept meal, supplement, snack

Refusal to accept food substitute for meat or vegetable

Meal intake of less than 50% (or 75%, according to facility policy)

Drinking less than six cups of liquid a day

Dry mouth

Cracked lips

Sunken eyes

Dark urine

Urine output less than usual for resident

Urine dark and concentrated in appearance

New onset of difficulty swallowing food or liquids

Diarrhea, vomiting, or fever

New onset of mental confusion or worsening mental confusion

Weak or tired

Lethargy, difficulty staying awake

(Additional signs and symptoms of dehydration and fluid balance problems are listed in Chapter 14)

Important Observations of Diabetic Residents

Inadequate food intake

Eating food not allowed on diet

Refusal of meals, supplements, or snacks

Nausea, vomiting, or diarrhea

Inadequate fluid intake

Excessive activity

Complaints of dizziness, shakiness, racing heart

Signs and Symptoms of Abnormally High Blood Sugar (Hyperglycemia, Diabetic Coma)

Nausea, vomiting

Weakness

Headache

Full, bounding pulse

Fruity smell to breath

Hot, dry, flushed skin

Labored respirations

Drowsiness

Mental confusion

Unconsciousness

Sugar in the urine

Signs and Symptoms of Abnormally Low Blood Sugar (Hypoglycemia, Insulin Shock)

Complaints of hunger, weakness, dizziness, shakiness

Feeling faint or lightheaded

Skin cold, moist, clammy, pale

Rapid, shallow respirations

Nervousness and excitement

Rapid pulse

Unconsciousness

No sugar in the urine

NUTRITION

Good nutrition is essential for good health. The nursing assistant must maintain good health to be effective in the job. Residents need good nutrition to restore their health and promote healing. The body will not heal if it is not adequately nourished. **Nutrients** are chemical substances in food that are necessary for life. Six nutrients are essential for good health. These are:

1. Water
2. Vitamins
3. Minerals
4. Carbohydrates
5. Proteins
6. Fats

Vitamins are organic compounds found in foods. They perform vital functions and regulate processes in the body. Each vitamin has a specific function. Absence of vitamins causes disease. **Minerals** are essential parts of all cells and contribute to the formation of the bones, teeth, and nails. They also help rebuild body tissues. **Carbohydrates** are food products that provide fuel and energy for the body. Sources of carbohydrates are fruits, vegetables, and grain products. **Proteins** are the fundamental structural element of all cells. They are sometimes called "nature's building blocks," and are essential for growth, healing, and good health. Sources of protein are meat, fish, eggs, and milk products. **Fats** are food products such as butter and oil, which are used as a source of energy and heat.

FOOD GUIDE PYRAMID

The United States Department of Agriculture (USDA) is a governmental agency that studies nutrition and makes recommendations. The USDA has grouped foods into six categories. The **food pyramid** (**Figure 13-1**) was developed to provide an easy-to-understand picture of daily nutritional requirements. Although the pyramid has six levels, the items in the small triangle do not fit in any of the major food cate-

gories. The sixth level at the top of the food pyramid is not considered a food group. The food guide pyramid recommends eating foods from the five major food groups shown in the three lower sections of the pyramid. Each of these food groups provides some, but not all, of the nutrients you need each day. Foods in one group cannot replace those in another. No one food group is more important than another. For good health, you need them all. The categories and USDA recommended servings are:

- Bread, rice, cereal, and pasta group—six to eleven servings a day.
- Fruit group—two to four servings a day.
- Vegetable group—three to five servings a day.
- Milk, yogurt, and cheese group—two to three servings a day.
- Meat, poultry, fish, dry beans, eggs, and nut group—two to three servings a day.
- Fats, oils, and sweets—use sparingly.

Eating according to the recommendations on the food pyramid will provide a well-balanced diet. **Table 13-1** lists the recommended portion sizes from each category.

70+ Food Guide Pyramid

In 1999, researchers at the USDA's Human Nutrition Research Center on Aging at Tufts

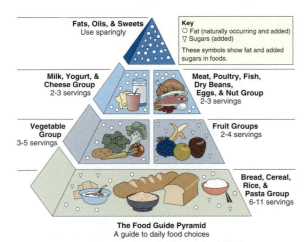

FIGURE 13-1 The USDA Food Guide Pyramid. *(Courtesy of the U.S. Department of Agriculture)*

TABLE 13-1 Portion sizes for the food guide pyramid food groups			
Food Group	**One Serving from this Group is:**	**Food Group**	**One Serving from this Group is:**
Bread, cereal, rice, and pasta	1 slice of bread 1 tortilla ½ cup cooked rice, pasta, or cereal 1 ounce ready-to-eat cereal ½ hamburger bun, bagel, or English muffin 3-4 plain crackers 1 pancake (4-inch diameter) ½ large croissant ½ medium doughnut or danish $\frac{1}{16}$ cake (average-size cake) 2 medium cookies $\frac{1}{12}$ of an 8-inch pie	Fruit group	1 piece fruit or melon wedge ¾ cup fruit juice ½ cup chopped, cooked, or canned fruit ¼ cup dried fruit
		Milk, yogurt, and cheese group	1 cup milk or yogurt 1½ ounces cheese (natural) 2 ounces cheese (processed) 1½ cups ice cream or ice milk 1 cup frozen yogurt
Vegetable group	½ cup chopped raw or cooked vegetables 1 cup raw, leafy vegetables ¾ cup vegetable juice ½ cup scalloped potatoes ½ cup potato salad 10 french fries	Meat, poultry, dry beans, eggs, and nuts group	2½ to 3 ounces cooked lean beef, pork, lamb, veal, poultry, or fish (a portion the size of a deck of cards)
			½ cup cooked beans, 1 egg, or 2 tablespoons peanut butter, or ⅓ cup of nuts equal 1 ounce of meat
		Fats, oils, sweets	Use sparingly

TABLE 13-2 Food guide pyramid comparison

USDA Food Guide Pyramid	70+ Food Guide Pyramid
	Adds a small supplement flag to the top, suggesting that supplements for three nutrients—vitamin D, calcium, and vitamin B12—may be appropriate for some, but not all, individuals.
Fats, oils, and sugars used sparingly	Fats, oils, and sugars used sparingly.
2 to 3 servings of milk	3 or more servings of milk; lowfat products recommended.
2 to 3 servings of meat	2 or more servings of meat.
3 to 5 servings of vegetables, 2 to 4 servings of fruits	3 or more servings of vegetables, 2 or more servings of fruit. Fiber-rich, whole fruits and vegetables are recommended instead of juices. Deeply colored yellow, green, orange, and red fruits and vegetables are recommended, as well as vegetables like cabbage, cauliflower, and broccoli.
6 to 11 servings of grain-based food	6 or more servings, emphasizing increased fiber and nutrient density.
	8 eight-ounce glasses of liquid form the base of the pyramid. This includes any nonalcoholic, caffeine-free beverage.
	A fiber icon (f+) has been added for good sources of fiber. Fiber is important for elderly individuals.

University, Boston, proposed changes to the food guide pyramid for adults aged 70 and older **(Figure 13-2)**. These changes make the food guide pyramid a more appropriate tool for elderly individuals, and are designed to help them optimize their food intake. Some dietitians use this food pyramid when planning meals for long-term care facility residents. **Table 13-2** compares the two food pyramids.

HEALTH CARE FACILITY DIETS

Physicians write diet orders for residents based on the residents' individual medical and nutritional needs. Food served in the health care facility is prepared by the dietary department. A licensed dietitian writes the menus to be sure that diets are well-balanced. The dietitian writes special menus for people with certain diseases to ensure that the nutrients provided meet their needs.

Many types of diets are served in long-term care facilities. Each facility has a listing of the types of diets served. Facilities post the menu each day. Some facilities have a selective menu. This menu allows each resident to select what he or she wants to eat. The common categories for diets served in long-term care facilities are:

- Regular, or general diets
- Liquid diets
- Soft or bland diets
- Mechanically altered diets
- Therapeutic diets

The Food Guide Pyramid for Older Adults

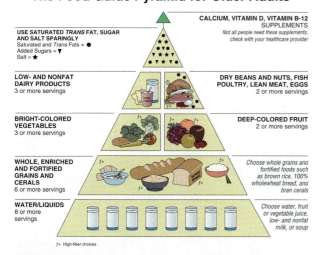

FIGURE 13-2 The Tufts University 70+ food pyramid. The liquid at the base of the pyramid is an important part of its structure. The liquids include water and any nonalcoholic, caffeine-free beverage. The fiber symbols throughout the pyramid remind the user to select foods that are high in fiber. *(Courtesy of Tufts University)*

Regular Diets

The **regular diet** is a normal, unrestricted diet. This diet is served to residents with no dietary restrictions. The diet is well balanced and has a variety of foods from the food pyramid.

Liquid Diets

Liquid diets are served to residents after surgery, and before some tests. They are also used for residents who have nausea, vomiting, or diarrhea. They are not nutritionally complete and should only be used for a short time. The two main types of liquid diets are:

- **Clear-liquid diet.** This diet is high in water and carbohydrates and consists of liquids that you can see through **(Figure 13-3).** It includes broth, tea, soup, gelatin, popsicles, and strained fruit juices. Clear soda pop and ginger ale are also served with this diet.
- **Full-liquid diet.** This diet consists of all clear liquids plus milk-based liquids. It includes cream soups, milk, ice cream, eggnog, and yogurt.

Soft Diets

Soft or **bland diets** are served to residents who have conditions of the digestive system or those who cannot eat spiced or seasoned food. A soft diet limits seasoning and is low in residue. Food served on this diet includes soups, white meat and fish, cream cheese and cottage cheese, breads, crackers, and milk products.

Mechanically Altered Diets

Mechanically altered diets are served to residents who have chewing, swallowing, or digestive disorders. Any kind of diet can be blender-

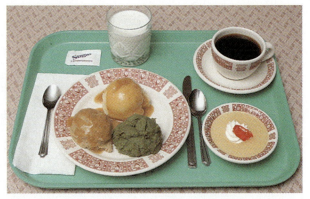

FIGURE 13-4   The pureed diet should have a firm consistency. Liquid should not run from the food.

ized to alter the mechanical consistency of the food. The two main types of mechanically altered diets are:

- **Pureed diet.** This diet is blended with liquid so the food is smooth without large particles **(Figure 13-4).** It is the consistency of baby food, but should not appear runny or watery. If the diet is blended properly, a plastic spoon will stand upright in the food without falling over.
- **Mechanical soft diet.** This diet is usually served to residents with chewing problems **(Figure 13-5).** It includes some foods, such as bread, that are not blended. Hard-to-chew items, such as meats, are ground until they are finely chopped. The food is not reduced to liquid in this diet.

Therapeutic Diets

Therapeutic diets are served to treat certain medical diseases or conditions. The licensed dietitian plans these diets very carefully to meet the resident's treatment needs. Regular food is used, but preparation of the food may be different from

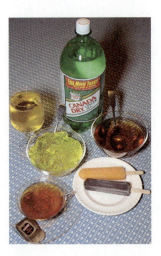

FIGURE 13-3   Items on a clear liquid diet include only liquids that you can see through.

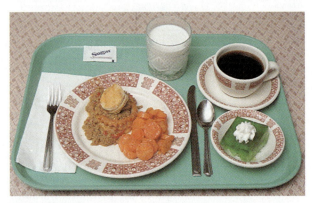

FIGURE 13-5   The mechanical soft diet includes ground meat. Foods that can be easily chewed are not blended.

that of a regular diet. For example, certain foods on a regular diet are prepared with salt. A resident on a salt-restricted diet would have the same food item prepared without salt. Each therapeutic diet has special requirements, and some foods may be restricted on certain diets. There are four common types of therapeutic diets.

Diabetic Diet. The **diabetic diet** serves normal foods, but the diet is prepared without sources of free sugar. This type of diet is served to residents with diabetes mellitus. Some diabetic diets count calories. Other diabetics are served a **no concentrated sweets diet,** which restricts forms of concentrated sweets, such as sugar packets, fruits canned in sugar, cakes, pies, and sweetened desserts. The recommended distribution of calories in a diabetic diet is 60 percent carbohydrate, 20 to 30 percent protein, and 20 to 30 percent fat.

Meal intake is very important for the diabetic resident. Meals and snacks must be served in a timely manner to maintain the resident's blood sugar. Diabetics receive medication to control their diabetes based on their food intake. If intake is inadequate, or meals are missed or delayed, serious complications may result. If a diabetic resident does not eat, report this information to the nurse. You will usually be instructed to offer the resident another food of similar nutritive value, to replace the uneaten items.

Calorie-Controlled Diets. **Calorie-controlled diets** usually are served to residents who are overweight. These diets are nutritionally complete, but the portions are usually smaller than those of a regular diet. Like the diabetic diet, sugar and forms of concentrated sweets are avoided on this type of diet.

Sodium-Restricted Diets. The **sodium-restricted diet** is served to residents with heart or kidney disease. Sodium-restricted diets are some of the most difficult diets to follow. The average American consumes 2 to 6 grams of sodium in food each day. Table salt is a major source of sodium in the diet. The doctor may order a diet prepared completely without sodium (salt), or the resident may be allowed sodium in a limited amount. In this diet, salt packets are not served on trays. Some facilities use salt substitutes if the doctor agrees. Foods that are usually low in sodium are fresh fruits, vegetables, and some cereals. Some foods have a high sodium content and should be avoided. Some examples are:

- Potato chips and similar snacks
- Lunch meats and processed meats, ham, and bacon
- Certain soft drinks
- Pickles and olives
- Many canned foods

Lowfat/Low-Cholesterol Diets. **Lowfat** and **low-cholesterol diets** are served to residents with heart, blood vessel, liver, and gallbladder disease. Sources of fat are limited or avoided in food preparation, and fats such as butter, margarine, and oil are limited or restricted. This diet includes lean meats that are baked or broiled, fruits and vegetables, and lowfat dairy products.

Other Types of Diets. Residents have many unique needs, and sometimes other types of diets are necessary. Some diets restrict sources of fiber. Others may serve a high or low amount of protein. Some are high in calories. High-calorie diets are commonly served to residents with burns, or those who need extra nutrition for healing. Some residents are on special diets because of religious prohibitions of certain foods. Special dietary requirements of cultural and religious groups in the United States are listed in **Table 13-3.**

Supplemental Feedings

Supplemental feedings are served to many residents. Supplements are served to meet special nutritional needs. Many residents have poor appetites and are underweight. Supplements are served to assist residents to maintain their weight, and gain if possible. Serving supplements and assisting residents to consume them is a very important nursing assistant responsibility. Sometimes common foods or beverages, such as milkshakes, ice cream, or juices, are served as supplements. Some facilities offer canned beverages, such as Ensure **(Figure 13-6).** Ensure and other

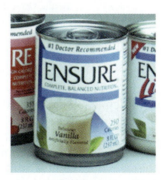

FIGURE 13-6 Oral supplements are an important part of the diet for underweight residents and those who need extra protein and calories for healing. Supplements require a physician order. Documentation should support supplement intake and the percentage of supplement consumed by the resident. *(Used with permission of Ross Products Division, Abbott Laboratories, Columbus, Ohio)*

TABLE 13-3	Dietary considerations for cultural and religious groups in the United States
Religion/Group	**Food Requirements and Prohibitions**
Adventist, Seventh Day	Alcohol, coffee, and tea are prohibited. A vegetarian diet is encouraged.
American Indian	In some tribes, sharing food is customary. Explain to visitors that they should not share the resident's food in the health care facility. After prayer and certain ceremonies, berries, corn, and dried meat are consumed. These foods may be provided by family members or other members of the tribe.
Buddhist	Buddhists do not eat meat.
Catholic	Some residents do not eat meat on Fridays and other holy days. Avoid food for one hour before Communion.
Chinese Americans	Believe in the balance of heat and cold in the body and use food to maintain this balance, as well as to treat disease. Rice and noodles are staples in the diet. Very little meat is eaten. Meat is usually mixed with cooked vegetables. Family members may bring in special foods to treat certain illnesses. Also use herbs and herb preparations to treat illnesses.
Christian Scientist	Alcohol prohibited. Some abstain from coffee and tea.
Church of Jesus Christ of Latter Day Saints (LDS or Mormon)	Alcohol, coffee, and tea not allowed.
Hindu	Most Hindus are vegetarians. A light meal is eaten for breakfast, a heavy meal for lunch, and a light meal for supper. Dietary customs state that the right hand is used for eating and the left hand for toileting and personal hygiene.
Islam	Alcohol, pork, and some shellfish are not allowed.
Jewish	Milk and meat are not eaten together. Predatory fowl, shellfish, and pork are not allowed. Fish with fins and scales are permitted. Other types of fish are not allowed. Some Jewish residents request kosher food, which requires very special preparation.
Mexican American	Prefer fresh, natural ingredients in food preparation. Beans, corn tortillas, and rice are staples of the Mexican American diet. Tomatoes are used extensively in preparation of sauces. Food is highly spiced with onions, cilantro, and chilies. Mexican Americans believe that the properties of some diseases are hot or cold. Foods are served to complement the hot or cold disease state. The terms do not refer to food temperature, but rather to the effect the food has on the body.
Puerto Rican	Some observe traditional coffee time at 10 a.m. and 3 p.m. Coffee is traditionally prepared with boiled milk and sugar. Rice, beans, and plantains are served with most meals. Do not eat red meat or chicken during certain religious events.

canned supplements require a physician's order for administration. The percentage of supplement the resident consumes is documented on a flow sheet. In some facilities, the nursing assistant is responsible for documenting this. In others, licensed nurses document this information. Know and follow your facility policy. Supplemental feedings are always served between meals. If they are served too close to mealtime, the resident may not be hungry and will not eat. Diabetic residents are often given medication to control their diabetes. If supplements are served to a diabetic, the total calorie value of the supple-

ment is included in the diet. The diabetic medication given is calculated based on the calorie count. Supplements must be given as ordered to maintain a proper balance between the food and medication.

Bedtime Snacks. Most facilities offer residents a light bedtime snack, such as milk, juice, graham crackers, cookies, or fruit. This is an important part of the residents' diet, and should be offered to all residents before they go to sleep. Most facilities document that the resident accepted or refused the bedtime snack.

Some facilities document snack consumption according to the percentage of the snack consumed. Know and follow your facility policy.

ASSISTING RESIDENTS WITH NUTRITION

Illness and certain medications can affect the resident's appetite. When preparing residents for meals, it is important to make the environment and the food as pleasant and appealing as possible. Washing residents' hands before meals is also important.

Preparing Residents for Meals

Before mealtime, prepare residents for meals so that when meals arrive they can be served quickly. This maintains proper temperature. Food can be a source of infection if the temperature is not maintained. Hot foods should be served hot, and cold foods served cold.

Follow your facility policy for preparing the nursing unit for meals. Some facilities require removal of laundry hampers and housekeeping carts from hallways before tray carts arrive. Bring a clothing protector **(Figure 13-7)** to the room if needed by the resident. Do not call a clothing protector a bib. "Bib" is a demeaning term to most adults.

When assisting residents to be seated at dining tables, or using an overbed table, proper positioning is very important. The resident should sit upright with feet supported on footrests or the floor. Monitor the resident's distance from the table. The resident should not have to stretch and reach to eat. Monitor the height of the table.

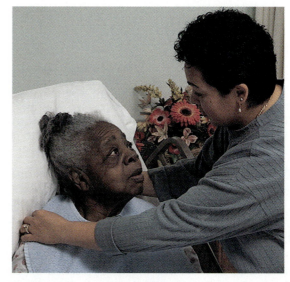

FIGURE 13-7   An adult clothing protector. Avoid referring to this garment as a bib.

Some short residents may be sitting too low. They should not have to eat with their elbows in the air to reach the food. The elbows should be below the level of the hands when eating. Some adjustments in the type of table used, table height, or type of chair may be necessary to make eating easier. If the resident has to work to eat, he or she may not eat as well. It is usually easier to seat the resident in a straight-backed chair than it is to use a wheelchair. A straight-backed chair usually has lower armrests (or no armrests), making it easier to get close to the table. Wheelchair arms may not fit under the table and increase the distance that the resident has to stretch. Chairs that are used in health care facility dining rooms are usually the correct height for the tables. If an overbed table is used

GUIDELINES FOR
Preparing Residents for Meals

- Make the environment as pleasant as possible. Remove bedpans, urinals, and other objectionable items. Eliminate odors.
- Assist the resident with toileting and elimination needs before mealtime. Provide incontinent care, if necessary. Apply the principles of standard precautions if you are assisting with this procedure.
- Assist the resident to wash his or her hands.
- Be sure the resident has dentures, glasses, and hearing aid, if used.

- If the resident will be eating in bed, elevate the head to the high Fowler's position. Assist the resident to sit in a chair, if allowed.
- Monitor the resident's position and distance from the food and make necessary adjustments.
- Clear the top of the overbed table to receive the tray. Wipe the top of the table with a damp paper towel or according to facility policy.
- Apply a clothing protector, if used by the resident.

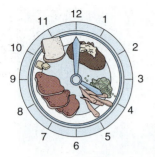

FIGURE 13-8 When serving a tray to a resident with visual impairment, describe the arrangement of the food compared with the face of a clock.

to serve meals, adjust the height and distance from the arms when you serve the tray.

Many residents use adaptive devices to help them eat independently. These are special cups, dishes, utensils, or placemats that enable them to feed themselves with dignity. Special adaptive devices used at mealtime are usually listed on the diet card and provided by the dietary department. Use of adaptive devices is discussed in Chapter 18.

When serving a meal tray to a resident who is visually impaired or blind, describe the location of food items compared with a clock **(Figure 13-8)**. Say, "The meat is at eight o'clock, the bread is at eleven o'clock, and the potato is at one o'clock."

Socialization is a very important part of meal service in the long-term care facility. Residents should be seated with others with whom they can socialize at tables. Residents should face each other and should not be positioned so that they are looking out a window or at a wall during meal service.

Most residents in long-term care facilities eat in community dining rooms. They look forward to mealtime. Help to make mealtime special. Make the atmosphere as pleasant as possible. If residents are satisfied with the quality of food and food service in the facility, they tend to look at the entire facility in a positive light. Many resident complaints to surveyors are about food and meal service. Make sure that residents have condiments and other seasonings of choice. Honor resident requests for substitutes and extra portions, if allowed on the diet. Facilities are required to prepare a substitute for the meat and vegetable at each meal. If the resident eats less than 50 to 75 percent of these foods, a substitute is automatically offered. There is no requirement to substitute desserts, breads, and beverages. If these foods are requested by the resident, follow your facility policy for serving them. Use common sense, and do your best to make mealtime satisfying. Know and follow your facility policy for substitutes. Many facilities provide a glass of ice water on food trays. Many confused residents will drink whatever liquids are placed in front of them. Offer residents a second cup of coffee when they are finished with the meal. When dining in a restaurant, a glass of water and additional coffee are always provided. Long-term care residents will appreciate this gesture and benefit from the fluid intake. Making mealtime special will pay off in resident satisfaction.

Serving Meals. In most health care facilities, food is served on trays. The trays will be delivered to the dining room and nursing units in carts. Each tray is labeled with the resident's name, room number, and type of diet. After all trays are passed, check on residents while they are eating. If food is not being eaten, offer a substitute. Offer to replace or reheat food that has become cold.

Food Thickeners. Residents with certain diseases and disorders may have trouble swallowing

GUIDELINES FOR
Serving Meals

- Plan and organize your time so you are available to pass trays as soon as the cart is delivered. Food must be served promptly to maintain temperature.
- Wash your hands.
- Check the tray card for the resident's name and room number.
- Check the food on the tray to see if it should be served on the resident's diet. If you think a food item is not appropriate, consult the nurse.
- Keep food covered during transportation to maintain temperature and prevent contamination.
- Leave trays on the food cart until you are ready to feed residents. Do not put a tray in front of a resi-

dent who must be spoon-fed until you are available to assist with the meal.
- Take the tray to the room, identify the resident, and place the tray on the overbed table.
- Prepare the tray, if necessary, by opening milk cartons, cutting meat, buttering bread, and putting condiments on food.
- Provide adaptive eating devices, if used.
- Feed the resident, if necessary.
- Serve all uneaten trays before returning used trays to the food cart. Do not return used trays if uneaten food remains on the cart.

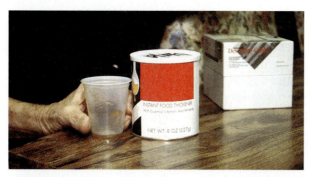

FIGURE 13-9 The speech-language pathologist will order the type of thickener and consistency to use.

beverages, soup, and thin liquids. Residents who have had a stroke, or have Parkinson's disease or multiple sclerosis, are at high risk of choking on liquids.

Food thickeners **(Figure 13-9)** are nonprescription, powdered products that are mixed into beverages and some foods to make swallowing easier and prevent aspiration. The consistency of the liquid depends on the amount of powder added. It is important to add exactly the amount that has been ordered. Thickeners do not change the flavor of food or liquids, but they may change the intensity, making it taste stronger. Prethickened liquids are also available.

The care plan will specify the type and amount of thickener to use to achieve the necessary texture. For example, the therapist may recommend that liquids be mixed to the consistency of peach juice, nectar, honey, or pudding. Milk products may take longer to thicken than other liquids, and coffee and hot beverages must be stirred very well, because the thickener has a tendency to lump. Add the thickener immediately before serving the product. Follow the therapist's directions exactly. When adding thickeners:

- Use the correct product
- Use the correct amount of thickener in the correct amount of liquid
- Follow manufacturers' directions
- Stir the thickener well (make sure the container is large enough to permit stirring)
- Stir again if product settling occurs
- Allow the beverage to stand for the recommended time to thicken
- Follow the speech therapist's instructions and plan of care for positioning and feeding

Feeding the Resident. Some residents are not able to eat by themselves and must be fed. The resident may feel embarrassed and childish. Be sensitive to the resident's feelings.

After Meals. After meals, pick up trays and return them to the tray cart. Wipe spilled food off the overbed table, if necessary. Facilities record how much residents have eaten in different ways. Some write "good," "fair," or "poor." Other facilities use fractions or record the percentage of the diet consumed **(Figure 13-10)**. Know and follow your facility policy. Notify the nurse if the resident eats less than 75% of the meal. Follow the nurses' instructions. Record the amount of liquid taken if the resident is on intake and output. Before leaving the room, return the bed to a position of comfort and assist the resident to use the toilet, wash face and hands, and meet other hygienic needs. Make sure that there is no food on the face, hands, or clothing. Change the resident's clothing if soiled. Wait until all uneaten trays have been passed before returning used food trays to the cart.

GUIDELINES FOR
Feeding Residents

- Sit at or below the resident's eye level, if possible. This is less intimidating than standing over the resident. It also prevents the resident from choking, which could be caused by bending the head back and looking up at you.
- Check the food temperature before feeding. Place a drop of hot food on your wrist to be sure it is not too hot.
- Tell the resident what is on the tray. Ask what the resident would like to eat first.
- Sometimes residents cannot handle utensils, but are able to eat their own finger foods, such as bread, crackers, or cookies. Encourage them to do this, if able.

- Offer liquids at intervals. Using a straw will make it easier for residents to drink. For some residents, sipping from a small, flexible cup works best. The care plan will list the approach to use.
- Make pleasant conversation while feeding. Avoid making conversation if the resident has difficulty swallowing. Responding to conversation may cause accidental choking.
- Avoid rushing the resident.
- Be emotionally sensitive to the residents' needs. Focus on residents when feeding. Avoid having conversations with others in the room.

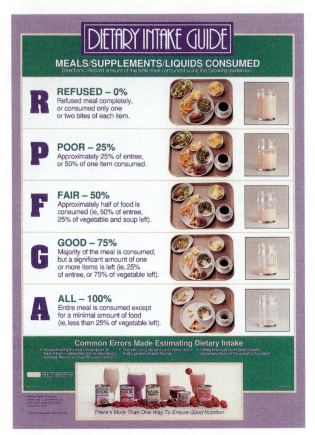

FIGURE 13-10 Accurate documentation of meal intake is an important nursing assistant responsibility. *(Used with permission of Ross Products Division, Abbott Laboratories, Columbus, Ohio)*

DYSPHAGIA

Some residents have **dysphagia,** or difficulty swallowing food and liquids. This condition may occur in residents who have:

- Had a stroke
- Neurological diseases
- Cancer of the head, neck, or esophagus
- Undergone radiation therapy to the head or neck
- Dementia

People who take medications that cause sedation or reduce saliva production are also at risk of dysphagia. Signs and symptoms of dysphagia are:

- Taking a long time before beginning to swallow
- Swallowing three or four times with each bite of food
- Frequent throat clearing or coughing
- Lack of a gag reflex or weak cough
- Difficulty controlling liquids and secretions in the mouth
- Wet, gurgling voice

- Refusing to eat, spitting food out, or pocketing food in cheeks
- Unintentional weight loss
- Tightness in the throat or chest
- Feeling as if food is sticking in the esophagus or sternal area

If you observe any of these signs or symptoms, inform the nurse. Residents with dysphagia are at high risk of developing malnutrition and dehydration. Consultation with a speech-language pathologist and diagnostic tests for dysphagia may be necessary.

Dysphagia is treated with swallowing exercises, practicing proper swallowing techniques, and altering the consistency of food and beverages. The dietitian will work closely with the speech-language pathologist to ensure that the food is the proper consistency to meet the resident's needs and reduce the risk of aspiration. The goal is to keep the look, taste, and food consistency as close to normal as possible, while considering the resident's safety needs. Extra gravies or sauces may be added to some foods. Adults may be resistant to eating pureed food because it resembles baby food. Molds and special methods of preparation are used to enhance the appearance of pureed foods, making them more acceptable to the resident. You may be instructed to monitor the resident's food and fluid intake accurately. Inform the nurse if the resident has special dietary requests. The physician may order frequent weight monitoring.

Residents with dysphagia will have special approaches for eating and drinking to prevent aspiration and ensure proper intake. The speech therapist works closely with these residents. Liquids are usually the most difficult to swallow. The speech professional may recommend using food thickeners to slow the movement of fluid through the esophagus.

Assisting with Meals for Residents Who Have Swallowing Problems

Residents who have difficulty swallowing may require one-to-one assistance, prompting, or supervision at meals. The speech therapist recommends special techniques and positions for improving swallowing and preventing aspiration. These will be listed on the care plan. The therapist may work closely with each staff member who feeds the resident. In general:

- Before serving food or beverages, make sure the resident is fully awake and alert
- Position the resident in an upright position, as upright as possible

- The head should face forward, with the neck flexed forward slightly
- During the meal, reduce distractions
- Limit conversation. The resident with dysphagia should not try to carry on a conversation while eating. Focus the resident on eating
- Direct the food to the unaffected side of the mouth
- Prompt or feed the resident slowly, offering small bites. Remind him or her to chew and swallow the food well. Check the mouth to make sure the resident has swallowed the food

The speech-language pathologist may order other special positions and exercises, depending on the resident's medical condition and needs. The care plan will provide additional directions, such as reminding the resident to tuck the chin in when swallowing. In some types of dysphagia, this changes the position of the airway, further reducing the risk of aspiration. In other types, this technique increases the risk. Because dysphagia care is highly individualized, many staff members must work as a team to ensure that the resident's nutritional needs are safely met.

MALNUTRITION

Malnutrition is inadequate nutrition due to poor diet or inability to absorb nutrients. This is a serious condition that causes serious complications. It can and does occur in long-term care facility residents, despite their being served a balanced diet and having nutritional supplements available.

Nursing Assistant Actions

Mealtime is very busy in the long-term care facility, especially on the day shift, when two meals are served. Do not get so busy that you overlook residents who are having difficulty or who are not eating. Residents who are at greatest risk of malnutrition and unintentional weight loss are those who:

- Forget what they ate, or if they ate, or forget to eat altogether
- Lose interest or become distracted before the meal is consumed, or during the meal
- No longer know the purpose of food
- Do not know what utensils are used for
- Cannot recognize or identify feelings of hunger or thirst
- Need help eating and drinking
- Eat less than half their meals and/or planned snacks
- Have mouth pain

- Have no dentures, or have dentures that do not fit correctly
- Have difficulty chewing or swallowing or need to be prompted to chew and swallow
- Have difficulty getting utensils or glasses to their mouth
- Cough or choke while eating
- Are sad, have crying spells, or withdraw from others
- Are confused, wander, pace, or have increased calorie needs because of activity
- Have diabetes, lung disease, cancer, HIV, or other chronic diseases

To increase food intake and prevent weight loss and malnutrition, create a pleasant, positive dining atmosphere for the residents. Be aware of each resident's self-feeding ability and changes in eating patterns. Report your observations and changes in residents' conditions and appetite to the nurse. You should also:

- Provide oral care before meals
- Position residents correctly for feeding
- Honor food preferences, likes, and dislikes
- Prompt and cue the resident, if necessary
- Before feeding the resident, use hand-over-hand technique (see Chapter 18)
- Offer substitutes according to facility policy
- Serve meals promptly so that foods are at the proper temperature; check foods by dropping a small amount on your wrist
- Assist residents in using condiments, as allowed on diet
- Offer a variety of foods and beverages
- Help residents who are having trouble feeding themselves
- Provide adaptive utensils and dishes, as ordered
- Notify nursing staff if a resident has difficulty feeding himself or herself, eating, or using utensils
- Encourage residents to eat
- Allow enough time for residents to finish eating; avoid rushing
- Reheat cold food items if necessary
- Ask what's wrong if a resident's appetite decreases, or he or she seems sad
- Accurately record the resident's intake at each meal
- Assist and prompt residents to consume planned, ordered snacks and supplements

Calorie Counts and Food Intake Studies

The physician or dietitian may order special food intake studies for residents who are at risk

Diet _____

CALORIE/PROTEIN SUMMARY

RESIDENT _____   ROOM # _____

DAY 1					DAY 2					DAY 3				
DATE ___ / ___ / ___					DATE ___ / ___ / ___					DATE ___ / ___ / ___				
	% 0–25	% 25–50	% 50–75	% 75–100		% 0–25	% 25–50	% 50–75	% 75–100		% 0–25	% 25–50	% 50–75	% 75–100
Breakfast					**Breakfast**					**Breakfast**				
Meat					Meat					Meat				
Milk					Milk					Milk				
Fruit					Fruit					Fruit				
Starch					Starch					Starch				
Fat					Fat					Fat				
Other					Other					Other				
AM Supp.					AM Supp.					AM Supp.				
Noon Meal					**Noon Meal**					**Noon Meal**				
Meat					Meat					Meat				
Milk					Milk					Milk				
Juice					Juice					Juice				
Starch					Starch					Starch				
Vegetable					Vegetable					Vegetable				
Bread					Bread					Bread				
Fat					Fat					Fat				
Dessert					Dessert					Dessert				
Other					Other					Other				
PM Supp.					PM Supp.					PM Supp.				
Evening Meal					**Evening Meal**					**Evening Meal**				
Meat					Meat					Meat				
Milk					Milk					Milk				
Juice					Juice					Juice				
Starch					Starch					Starch				
Vegetable					Vegetable					Vegetable				
Bread					Bread					Bread				
Fat					Fat					Fat				
Dessert					Dessert					Dessert				
Other					Other					Other				
PM Supp.					PM Supp.					PM Supp.				
Total Kcal					**Total Kcal**					**Total Kcal**				
Total Pro					**Total Pro**					**Total Pro**				
Avg. for 3 days Kcal:					**Avg. Protein for 3 days:**									

PLEASE RETURN COMPLETED FORM TO NUTRITION CARE MANAGER

FIGURE 13-11 The calorie count provides an accurate picture of the resident's calorie and nutrient intake over a three-day period. The information is used to adjust the resident's diet and nutritional plan of care.

of malnutrition, and those with special nutritional needs. The resident's food intake is carefully recorded for a period of time, usually three days. The food intake is analyzed for nutritional adequacy and number of calories consumed. The dietitian uses this information to plan a diet to meet the resident's special medical needs.

If the physician orders a food intake study, a special food documentation form **(Figure 13-11)** is prepared and placed on the medical record or other designated location. The food intake study usually begins with the breakfast meal on the day after the physician writes the order. In some facilities, each food item is weighed or measured. At the end of each meal, you will accurately record the resident's food intake on the form. Facility policies vary on how food intake is documented, but this is usually done by recording an accurate percentage of each individual meal item. You will also accurately document intake of all snacks, liquid nutritional beverages, and food items brought from home by visitors.

At the end of the study period, the form is returned to the dietitian. He or she will use the information to calculate the amount of protein, carbohydrates, fat, and calories the resident consumed each day. In some facilities, nutrient, vitamin, and mineral intake are also calculated. The dietitian will use this information to adjust the resident's diet and nutritional plan of care. The results of the study and the dietitian's recommendations are communicated to the physician, who may order extra vitamin or mineral supplements necessary for the resident's medical condition. Completing a food intake or calorie count study requires a team effort, good communication, and very accurate documentation.

ALTERNATIVE METHODS OF FEEDING

Sometimes residents cannot eat solid food and are fed by other methods. The nursing assistant does not administer these feedings, but must have a basic understanding of how to care for residents who are being fed by alternative methods.

Tube Feeding

Feeding tubes **(Figure 13-12)** are used for residents who have certain medical problems or are unable to swallow. A **nasogastric tube** is inserted through the nose and threaded through the esophagus to the stomach. This tube is for short-term use, usually six weeks or less. A **gastrostomy tube (Figure 13-13)** is surgically inserted through the abdominal wall into the stomach. This tube is inserted when long-term feeding-tube use is necessary. It is often, but not always, permanent. The tube can be removed if the resident regains his or her ability to eat. The resident is fed liquid formula through the tube. Feedings are commonly administered through a pump **(Figure 13-14),** which delivers the solution at a slow rate over a long period of time. Several other methods of tube feeding may also be used. Keeping the head of the bed elevated at least 30 to 45 degrees while the tube feeding is running is important. The head should remain elevated for 30 to 60 minutes, or according to facility policy, after the feeding is completed. For residents who receive continuous feedings on a pump, the head of the bed must be elevated at all times. This increases the risk of skin breakdown on the hips, buttocks, and coccyx area.

| PROCEDURE 51 | Feeding the Dependent Resident | |

1. Perform your beginning procedure actions.
2. Place the tray on the overbed table and sit at or below the resident's eye level.
3. Inform the resident what is on the tray and ask what he or she would like to eat first.
4. Fill the fork or spoon half-full. If the resident has had a stroke, place food in the unaffected side of the mouth.
5. Alternate liquids and solids.
6. Wipe the resident's mouth as often as necessary.
7. Remove the tray when the resident is finished.
8. Wash the resident's hands and face, if necessary.
9. Assist the resident with oral hygiene and toileting after meals.
10. Record the resident's appetite and fluid intake according to facility policy.
11. Perform your procedure completion actions.

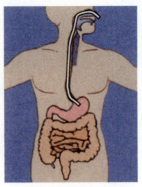
A. Nasogastric route

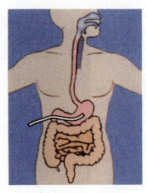
B. Gastrostomy route

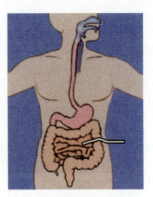
C. Jejunostomy route

FIGURE 13-12 Enteral feeding methods: (A) Nasogastric feeding (B) Gastrostomy feeding (C) Jejunostomy feeding

Anticipate this and plan your care to position the resident correctly and use pressure-relieving devices to avoid breakdown.

The skin around the feeding tube must be kept clean and dry. Sometimes the skin around a gastrostomy tube is covered with gauze. If the resident has a nasogastric tube, it may be clipped to the gown or clothing to prevent pulling.

Residents who are receiving tube feedings are also at nutritional risk. Their medical needs sometimes change, and tube-feeding formula and fluid orders must be adjusted to keep up with their bodies' demands. Inform the nurse promptly if you observe any of these potential problems:

- Nausea
- Vomiting
- Diarrhea
- Swollen stomach
- Constipation
- Excessive flatus, cramping
- Pain, redness, heat, swelling, crusting, or fluid oozing from the site where the feeding tube enters the body
- Coughing, choking
- Wet breathing

- Feeling that something is caught in the throat
- Complaints of dryness or discomfort in the mouth or throat
- Pulling at or removing the feeding tube
- The feeding solution is low or empty
- The pump alarm sounds.

Nursing assistant actions to take when residents are at risk of tube-feeding complications are:

- Keep the head of the bed elevated 30° to 45° **(Figure 13-15)** any time the tube feeding is running, and for one hour after feeding is completed
- Provide frequent oral care
- Follow the nurse's instructions and care plan for care of the skin around the feeding tube
- Move the resident carefully and position to avoid tension or traction on the tube
- Make sure that the tube is not kinked or obstructed
- Give the resident something to hold if he or she is pulling on the feeding tube; notify the nurse promptly
- Turn the resident on the side if coughing or choking
- Report observations and warning signs to the nurse promptly; if the resident is in distress,

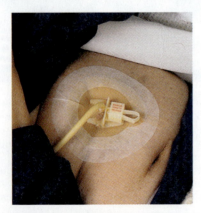

FIGURE 13-13 A gastrostomy tube is surgically inserted into the stomach through the abdominal wall.

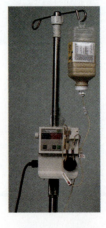

FIGURE 13-14 Most tube feedings are delivered through a pump. The total amount of tube feeding formula is not equivalent to free liquid. Approximately 15 to 20 percent of the formula is considered solid. To prevent dehydration, the dietitian will calculate the free fluid needs based on the resident's weight. Additional water will be given by the nurse.

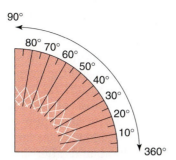

FIGURE 13-15 The head of the bed must be elevated 30 to 45 degrees or as specified on the plan of care whenever the tube feeding is running, and for at least an hour after the feeding is completed. To prevent aspiration, never position the head of the bed lower than 30 degrees.

remain in the room and use the call signal, phone, or other method of getting help

Intravenous Feedings

Intravenous feedings, or **IVs** **(Figure 13-16),** are sterile liquid and nutrient solutions used for many purposes. Sometimes they are used to give the resident extra fluids or medications. The intravenous solution is attached to a needle or plastic cannula in the vein. The intravenous line may be placed in the veins of the arms, legs, neck, or chest. The solution may flow into the vein by gravity or be measured through an electric pump. For some residents, the intravenous feeding is the only source of nutrition. Intravenous solutions are not nutritionally complete, so this will be used for only a short period of time.

Residents who are receiving intravenous feedings may also receive a meal tray. Consult the care plan for instructions regarding a meal tray.

Hyperalimentation

Hyperalimentation, also called *total parenteral nutrition (TPN)*, is another type of intravenous feeding that is sometimes used to provide total nutrition. This type of feeding is discussed in greater detail in Chapter 19.

FLUID INTAKE

An adequate intake of water and other fluids is essential to life. Two-thirds of the body is water. The body uses complex mechanisms to balance the fluid we take in with the fluid eliminated. In sickness and disease, ensuring that the resident drinks enough fluid is important. Fluid eliminated from the body may also be monitored. This will be described in Chapter 14.

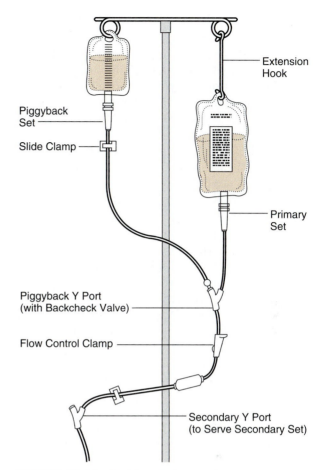

FIGURE 13-16 Residents who receive an intravenous infusion may also be served a meal tray. Oral intake and fluid output will also be monitored.

Dehydration

We normally take in two to three quarts of liquid each day. Most of this is consumed in liquid beverages and water. Some fruits and vegetables also provide water. **Dehydration** is a serious condition resulting from inadequate fluid in the body. It can occur if residents do not drink enough liquid or have excessive output from urine, diarrhea, vomiting, or drainage of other secretions from the body. Signs of dehydration are mental confusion, **lethargy** (abnormal drowsiness), weakness, dry mucous membranes, rapid pulse, scant or concentrated urine, and low blood pressure. Dry skin that "tents" when you pinch it gently is also a sign of dehydration. This is called poor skin **turgor** and indicates lack of fluid in the subcutaneous tissues. Turgor is skin elasticity. Good elasticity indicates good hydration.

Like malnutrition, dehydration can and does occur in long-term care facility residents. This is partially due to decreased thirst in the elderly. Some residents deliberately forgo fluids because they fear incontinence. Some residents do not like to drink water, but willingly accept other liquids when provided. The majority of residents who become dehydrated do so because of medical illness and the physical or mental inability to ask for liquids. For example, they cannot reach for or hold the cup, pour from the pitcher, or drink from a straw without assistance. Extra fluid is needed by all residents in very hot weather.

Dehydration can be a very serious condition in the elderly. Residents who are at high risk for dehydration are those who:

- Have signs and symptoms of dehydration (see preceding paragraph)
- Drink less than six cups of liquid a day
- Do not like to drink water
- Cannot pour water from a pitcher
- Need help drinking from a glass
- Have trouble swallowing liquids
- Have diarrhea, vomiting, infection, or fever
- Have difficulty communicating and cannot make their needs known
- Are weak or tired
- Take medications to remove water from the body
- Do not consume the liquids on meal trays
- Have depression
- Deliberately do not drink liquids for fear of incontinence
- Consume a large amount of caffeine or alcohol
- Have urinary output that exceeds fluid intake
- Have had a recent unplanned weight loss

Nursing Assistant Actions. Nursing assistant actions to prevent dehydration are:

- Offering the resident a drink each time you enter the room; set a goal, such as two to four ounces of liquid each time
- Drinking with the resident, if permitted
- Providing fluids the resident likes, at the preferred temperature, as permitted on the diet
- Making sure fresh water is available, that the resident can reach it, and that the pitcher and cup are light enough to hold
- Providing physical assistance to pour and consume fluids, as needed
- Offering ice chips, if permitted
- Following all swallowing precautions listed on the care plan
- Alternating liquids with solids when feeding meals
- Encouraging the resident to attend activities involving food and fluids
- Accurately monitoring and recording intake and output, when ordered
- Promptly notifying the nurse of your observations

Measuring and Recording Fluid Intake

Because most residents are asleep during the night, most of the liquid taken in should be consumed during the day and the evening. There are two meals on the day shift, so this is usually the time of day when most of the fluids are consumed. Measurements are often taken of how much liquid the resident takes in. Output from urine, vomitus, blood, and other drainage the resident excretes is also measured and recorded. This is called **intake and output (I & O).** Regardless of whether a resident is on intake and output, taking in enough liquid each day is still important. Offer residents liquids each time you are in the room. Pay particular attention to confused and dependent residents who may not be able to drink without your help. Providing extra liquids in hot weather is particularly important, as fluid needs are increased to keep the body cool.

Fluid intake is all liquid that the resident takes into the body. This includes everything the resident drinks and all fluid given in intravenous feedings and tube feedings. The nurse is responsible for keeping track of fluid intake given through tubes and with medications, but the nursing assistant is responsible for monitoring the oral intake. This includes all fluids consumed in the resident's room, with meals in the dining room, and during activity programs.

When monitoring intake and output, certain food items are also considered liquids, and should be recorded. These are things that would become liquid if allowed to stand at room temperature, such as ice cream, sherbet, gelatin, pudding, custard, and popsicles. Pureed foods and items such as applesauce are not counted as fluid intake.

Force Fluids. Residents who require extra fluid often have an order to **force fluids.** This does not mean that you physically force the resident to drink. When this order is written, you will encourage the resident to drink as many fluids as possible. Finding out what beverages the resident likes and providing them may be helpful. Offer the resident a drink every time you are in the room. It may be helpful to offer fluid in small amounts instead of large quantities each time. You will write down the amount the resident drinks. This will be totaled and recorded at the end of your shift. The night shift adds the amounts consumed on all shifts to obtain the 24-hour total **(Figure 13-17).**

Fluid Restrictions. Sometimes residents with heart or kidney disease or other medical

Intake Section of Intake and Output Form

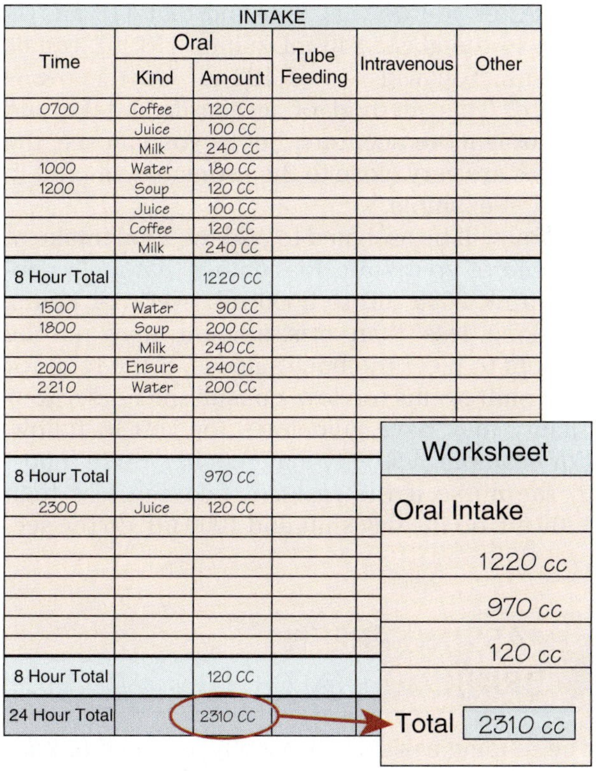

Time	Oral		Tube Feeding	Intravenous	Other
	Kind	Amount			
0700	Coffee	120 CC			
	Juice	100 CC			
	Milk	240 CC			
1000	Water	180 CC			
1200	Soup	120 CC			
	Juice	100 CC			
	Coffee	120 CC			
	Milk	240 CC			
8 Hour Total		1220 CC			
1500	Water	90 CC			
1800	Soup	200 CC			
	Milk	240 CC			
2000	Ensure	240 CC			
2210	Water	200 CC			
8 Hour Total		970 CC			
2300	Juice	120 CC			
8 Hour Total		120 CC			
24 Hour Total		2310 CC			

Worksheet

Oral Intake

1220 cc

970 cc

120 cc

Total   2310 cc

FIGURE 13-17 The oral intake is on the left side of the form. The type of fluid, time, and amount are recorded. The intake is totaled every 8 hours and cumulated every 24 hours.

problems have **fluid restrictions.** Residents with fluid restrictions can take in a very limited amount of fluid each day. The total liquid allowed in a 24-hour period is calculated carefully. Usually, the total is divided by three shifts, and the care plan lists how much fluid each shift may give the resident. The fluid given includes fluid served on meal trays as well as liquids consumed on the nursing unit. The largest quantity is usually given by the day shift. The night shift may be allowed to give only a very small amount of fluid, because the resident is usually asleep during the night. In some facilities, residents who are on fluid restrictions do not get water pitchers.

Measuring Fluid Intake. The metric system is used to measure fluid intake and output. Fluid intake is measured in **milliliters (mL)** or **cubic centimeters (cc).** The two measurements are equivalent. One ounce is the equivalent of 30 mL or 30 cc. Your facility will have a chart that gives the number of milliliters for containers, such as the cups, dishes, and water pitchers (**Table 13-4**). You must understand how to convert the commonly used measurements of ounces, pints, quarts, and gallons into metric measurements. **Table 13-5** lists the common U.S. measurements for liquids and their metric equivalents.

TABLE 13-4	Example container amounts	
Container	**Approximate Number of Ounces**	**Approximate Number of mL (cc)**
Water glass	6 oz	180 mL
Styrofoam cup	6 oz	180 mL
Juice glass	4 oz	120 mL
Large glass	8 oz	240 mL
Water pitcher	32 oz (1 qt)	1000 mL (930 mL)
Coffee or tea pot	10 oz	300 mL
Coffee cup	5 oz	150 mL
Milk carton	8 oz	240 mL
Soup bowl (small)	6 oz	180 mL
Soup bowl (large)	10 oz	300 mL
Gelatin	4 oz	120 mL
Ice cream cup	4 oz	120 mL
Creamer	1 oz	30 mL

Note: This is only an example. Your facility will have a listing of specific amounts.

TABLE 13-5	Metric equivalents for common U.S. measurements
Common U.S. Measurement	**Metric Equivalent**
1 teaspoon	5 mL
1 ounce	30 mL
1/2 pint	250 mL
1 pint	500 mL
1 quart	1000 mL (or 1 liter)
1/2 gallon	2000 mL
1 gallon	4000 mL

ter into a measuring device to see how much is left. After you do this, you find that 118 mL remain in the glass: 240 mL minus 118 mL equals 122 mL. You will record 122 mL on the I & O record. This method of measuring intake and output is more accurate, but as you can see, the figures are very close to the estimated amount in the first example.

You will be assigned to add the total intake at the end of your shift. Remember that most people drink 2000 mL to 3000 mL every 24 hours. Drinking less than this amount may not be enough to meet the body's needs. If the total for your shift seems too low, consult the nurse. Your facility may have guidelines for you to follow. For example, a facility may require you to report to the nurse if the resident takes in less than 1200 mL on the day shift and 1000 mL on the second shift.

When calculating how much liquid a resident drinks, you must first know how much liquid the container holds when full. You will estimate how much the resident drank, then subtract it from the total. For example, a water glass holds 240 mL. The resident drinks half a glass, or 120 mL. 240 mL minus 120 mL equals 120 mL. You will record 120 mL under the intake column of the I & O record.

Usually, an estimation of the amount of fluid the resident drinks is adequate. When we measure intake and output, our figures are very close estimates. Sometimes the doctor will order **strict I & O.** This means that the fluid must be measured exactly. Using the same example, the water glass holds 240 mL. The resident drinks approximately half a glass. You will pour this wa-

PASSING FRESH DRINKING WATER

The nursing assistant is usually assigned to pass fresh drinking water to residents every four to eight hours. Consult the care plan to see if the resident is allowed to have ice. In certain medical conditions, beverages are served without ice. The care plan will also note if the resident needs thickened water. Also check to see if residents are NPO. Most facilities remove the cup and water pitcher from the room while a resident is NPO. The method of passing drinking water and the type of ice dispenser will vary with your facility. However, certain common rules for passing drinking water apply in all facilities.

GUIDELINES FOR
Providing Fresh Drinking Water

- Wash your hands before beginning this procedure. If your hands become contaminated, or if you assist a resident, wash your hands again before continuing. Your hands remain clean if you are touching only clean items.
- Follow facility policy and good infection-control practices.
- Avoid contaminating the ice scoop, ice machine, or supply of clean ice with your hands, a cup, pitcher, or ice scoop. Avoid touching the ice scoop against the pitcher when you are filling the pitcher with ice.

- Do not pour water from a cup back into a water pitcher.
- Avoid filling a pitcher or cup directly over the clean ice supply. Ice from the scoop will hit the outside of the container and fall back into the clean ice supply, causing contamination. Fill the pitcher over a plastic bag, sink, or other container.
- Avoid mixing the pitchers and cups if there is more than one resident in the room. Pitchers that are reused should be labeled with the resident's name. Return the correct pitcher to each resident.

KEY POINTS

- Water, vitamins, minerals, carbohydrates, fats, and proteins are essential for good health.
- The USDA food pyramid recommends a specific number of servings from each of the five food groups each day.
- There are five common categories for diets served in health care facilities.
- Therapeutic diets are planned by the licensed dietitian to meet a resident's specific medical needs.
- The nursing assistant is responsible for preparing residents for meals, serving trays, feeding residents, documenting food intake, and removing trays after residents have eaten.
- Dysphagia is a condition in which the resident has difficulty swallowing and is at risk for aspiration. Special techniques are used to prevent inhalation of food and fluids.
- Tube feeding, intravenous feeding, and hyperalimentation are alternative methods of feeding residents who have special needs.
- Residents in long-term care facilities can and do develop malnutrition and dehydration. The nursing assistant must be aware of at-risk residents and take steps to prevent these conditions.
- Adults need 2000 mL to 3000 mL of liquid each day for their bodies to function properly.
- Measuring fluid intake and output is an important responsibility of the nursing assistant.
- The nurse is responsible for recording intake for tube feedings and medications. The nursing assistant is responsible for recording all other fluid intake, including fluids that residents consume in the dining room and at activities.
- The nursing assistant applies principles of medical asepsis when passing fresh drinking water to residents.

REVIEW

A. Multiple Choice

Select the one best answer.

1. How many nutrients are essential for good health?
   a. two
   b. three
   c. five
   d. six

2. The type of food called "nature's building blocks" is
   a. minerals.
   b. proteins.
   c. carbohydrates.
   d. vitamins.

3. According to the USDA food pyramid, how many servings of fruit should you have each day?
   a. two to four
   b. three to five
   c. one or two
   d. six to eleven

4. According to the USDA food pyramid, how many servings of bread, rice, cereal, or pasta should you have each day?
   a. two to four
   b. three to five
   c. one or two
   d. six to eleven

5. You are assigned to serve a full liquid diet to Mr. Johnson. Which of the following would you expect to find on his tray?
   a. vegetable soup
   b. pureed fish
   c. yogurt
   d. peach cobbler

6. Therapeutic diets
   a. are planned by the dietitian for residents with special medical needs.
   b. are rarely used in the health care facility.
   c. have no effect on residents with heart disease or diabetes.
   d. are always limited in sugar.

7. Foods that are high in sodium include
   a. fresh fruit.
   b. fresh vegetables.
   c. bread and grains.
   d. lunch meat and ham.

8. Guidelines for passing trays to residents include
   a. handwashing and identifying the resident.
   b. preparing the food.
   c. removing the lid after taking the tray off the cart.
   d. serving all trays, then returning to feed residents.

9. If you feel that a food is too hot to feed to a dependent resident, you should
   a. return the food to the tray cart uneaten.
   b. blow on the food to cool it.
   c. leave the food until it cools.
   d. put the food in the refrigerator.

10. When feeding a resident who has a paralyzed side, direct the food
    a. to the unaffected side of the mouth.
    b. to the affected side of the mouth.
    c. in the center of the mouth.
    d. to the back of the throat.

11. Alternative methods of feeding include
    a. therapeutic diets.
    b. tube feeding.
    c. mechanically altered diets.
    d. thickening liquids.

12. When a resident is receiving a tube feeding, the head of the bed should be
    a. flat.
    b. elevated 10 to 20 degrees.
    c. elevated 30 to 45 degrees.
    d. tilted back.

13. When caring for a resident with a gastrostomy feeding, notify the nurse if the
    a. resident is coughing or choking.
    b. head of the bed is elevated more than 45 degrees.
    c. resident needs mouth care.
    d. resident needs to be turned to the side.

14. The normal daily fluid requirement for adults is
    a. 100 to 1000 mL.
    c. 2000 to 3000 mL.
    b. 500 to 2000 mL.
    d. 3500 to 4000 mL.

15. A condition that results from inadequate fluid in the body is
    a. hydration.
    b. dehydration.
    c. mechanical alteration.
    d. dysphagia.

16. Lethargy is
    a. hyperactivity.
    c. abnormal drowsiness.
    b. abnormal thirst.
    d. an indication of overhydration.

17. 1 quart is the same as
    a. 100 mL.
    c. 500 mL.
    b. 250 mL.
    d. 1000 mL.

18. 30 mL is equivalent to
    a. 1 teaspoon.
    c. 1 cup.
    b. 1 ounce.
    d. 1 quart.

19. 8 ounces is equivalent to
    a. 24 mL.
    c. 240 mL.
    b. 80 mL.
    d. 800 mL.

20. 500 mL is equivalent to
    a. 1 pint.
    c. 1 gallon.
    b. 1 quart.
    d. 1 dram.

21. Malnutrition
    a. is a risk in certain residents in long-term care facilities.
    b. is a chronic condition in most elderly individuals.
    c. frequently occurs in residents with diabetes and chronic disease.
    d. never occurs in the long-term care facility.

22. Residents who are at risk of dehydration
    a. drink six cups of fluid each day.
    b. are always confused.
    c. have straw-colored urine.
    d. often have difficulty holding a cup.

23. Food thickeners may be ordered for residents with
    a. malnutrition.
    b. dehydration.
    c. tube feedings.
    d. dysphagia.

24. Residents at risk for dysphagia are those who have had
    a. a stroke.
    b. an amputation.
    c. fluid restriction.
    d. malnutrition.

25. The purpose of a calorie count is to
    a. document the total volume of liquids consumed.
    b. evaluate intake for a 30-day period.
    c. evaluate the intake for one meal.
    d. analyze intake for nutritional adequacy.

26. Sodium-restricted diets
    a. limit concentrated sweets.
    b. contain extra salt.
    c. may be difficult to follow.
    d. are ordered by the nurse.

27. Residents who are on fluid restrictions
    a. must drink 2000 mL to 3000 mL each day.
    b. are on intake and output monitoring.
    c. should not consume more than 500 mL daily.
    d. are usually fed by gastrostomy tube.

28. A nasogastric tube
    a. is threaded through the nose and into the stomach.
    b. is inserted into the mouth and into the lungs.
    c. requires surgical insertion.
    d. enters the stomach through the abdominal wall.

29. When a resident has an order to force fluids, the
    a. nursing assistant should force the resident to drink.
    b. resident must consume at least one pitcher of water each shift.
    c. nurse is responsible for administering fluids.
    d. resident should be encouraged to drink as much as possible.

30. Poor skin turgor may be a sign of
    a. dehydration.
    b. dysphagia.
    c. neurologic disease.
    d. lethargy.

B. Clinical Applications

Answer the following questions.

31. Mr. Long has a complete set of dentures. He is on a regular diet. When you serve his meal trays, he picks at his food. He seldom eats much meat. He always eats his mashed potatoes, pudding, and soft foods. After meals, he commonly removes his dentures and leaves them out. He confides in you that his dentures are loose and make his gums sore when he chews. What should you, the nursing assistant, do?

32. Miss Stewart is an obese diabetic resident who receives insulin injections daily. When you open the drawer of the resident's bedside stand to get her toothbrush, you notice several candy bars. Miss Stewart begs you not to tell anyone about the candy. What should you do?

33. Mrs. Martinez is an elderly resident with a bleeding ulcer. She is on a bland diet. The resident immigrated from Mexico and lived with her daughter in your city for several years before admission. When you pick up her supper tray, you find the food uneaten. Mrs. Martinez tells you that her daughter will be visiting soon and will bring her a special Mexican dinner. She is looking forward to visiting with her daughter and eating her favorite food. What should you do?

34. Will James is a 31-year-old resident. He is on a regular diet, but has been losing weight. He tells you he is tired of institutional food and wants a hamburger, french fries, and a milkshake from the fast-food restaurant. He also says he likes Chinese food. What can a nursing assistant do?

35. Mr. Hall, the nurse, instructs you to encourage fluids for Mrs. Blount. He puts the resident on I & O to evaluate her fluid balance. When you enter the resident's room and offer her water, she tells you that she does not like water. What should you do to make sure Mrs. Blount gets enough liquid on your shift?

36. Mr. Arnold is an underweight resident with pressure ulcers. He is on a regular diet, but his appetite is poor. He receives liquid nutritional supplements several times on your shift. When you serve the supplements, he takes a sip, then puts the container down. He rarely drinks any more after you leave the room. What can you do?

CHAPTER 14

Elimination

OBJECTIVES

After reading this chapter, you will be able to:

- Spell and define key terms.
- Describe the purpose of the urinary system.
- Identify the common problems with urinary elimination associated with aging, trauma, and disease.
- List the responsibilities of the nursing assistant in assisting residents with urinary elimination.
- Describe the purpose of the urinary catheter.
- Describe the ability to accurately measure urinary output.
- Describe the purpose of collecting urine and stool specimens and demonstrate the procedure.
- Identify the common problems with bowel elimination and list the responsibilities of the nursing assistant in assisting residents with bowel elimination.
- Demonstrate procedures related to elimination.

OBSERVATIONS TO MAKE AND REPORT RELATED TO ELIMINATION

Sores or ulcers inside the mouth
Difficulty chewing or swallowing food
Unusual or abnormal appearance of feces
Blood, mucus, parasites, or other unusual substances in stool
Unusual color of feces
Hard stool, difficulty passing stool
Extremely small or extremely large stool
Loose, watery stool
Complaints of pain, constipation, diarrhea, bleeding
Frequent belching
Changes in appetite
Excessive thirst
Fruity smell to breath
Complaints of indigestion
Excessive gas (flatus)
Nausea, vomiting
Choking
Abdominal pain
Abdominal distention (swelling)
Oral or rectal bleeding
Vomitus, stool, or drainage from a nasogastric tube that looks like coffee grounds

Urinary output too low when compared with oral intake
Urinary output greatly exceeds fluid intake
Fluid intake and output not reasonably balanced on your shift
Resident not drinking sufficient fluids
Resident on fluid restriction drinking excessive fluids, exceeding limitations
Abnormal appearance of urine: dark, concentrated, red, cloudy
Unusual substances in urine: blood, pus, particles, sediment
Complaints of difficulty urinating
Foul-smelling urine
Complaints of pain, burning, urgency, frequency, pain in lower back
Urinating frequently in small amounts
Sudden-onset urinary incontinence
Dribbling of urine
Edema; obvious fluid in tissues, particularly face, fingers, legs, ankles, feet
Sudden weight loss or gain
Respiratory distress

OBSERVATIONS TO MAKE AND REPORT RELATED TO ELIMINATION, CONTINUED

Changes in mental status
Resident complains of inability to empty bladder, or cannot empty bladder completely
Signs of dehydration, including low fluid intake; low output of dark urine with strong odor;

weight loss; dry skin; dry mucous membranes of the lips, mouth, tongue, eyes; drowsiness; confusion; poor skin turgor

URINARY SYSTEM

The urinary system removes waste products and regulates water in the body. The parts of the urinary system are shown in **Figure 14-1.** The urinary system consists of the **kidneys, ureters,** **bladder,** and **urethra.** The kidneys are organs that filter and remove waste products from the blood, forming urine. The ureters are two hollow tubes leading from the kidneys to the bladder. Urine passes from the kidneys through the ureters to the bladder. The bladder is a hollow muscle that stores urine until it is eliminated from the body. When urine is eliminated, it leaves the bladder through a hollow tube called the urethra and passes to the outside of the body. Several medical terms are used to describe the elimination of urine from the body. These are **urination, voiding,** and **micturition.** Most people feel the urge to urinate when the bladder contains 100 to 200 mL.

External Organs

The external organs associated with elimination in the female are the **urinary meatus, labia majora,** and **labia minora (Figure 14-2A).** The urinary meatus is the external opening of the urethra to the outside of the body. The labia majora are two large, hair-covered structures on the external female genitalia. The labia minora are smaller, liplike structures on the inside of the labia majora. The external organs in the male are the **penis,** urinary meatus, and **foreskin (Figure 14-2B).** The penis is the external male

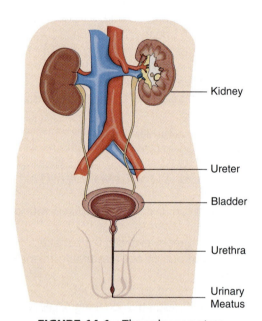

Kidney

Ureter

Bladder

Urethra

Urinary Meatus

FIGURE 14-1   The urinary system

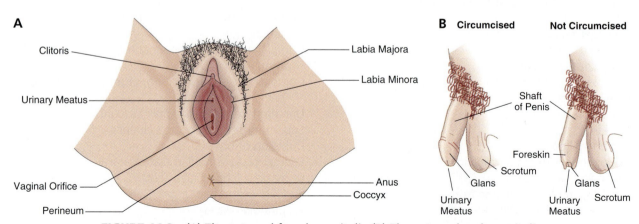

A

Clitoris

Urinary Meatus

Vaginal Orifice

Perineum

Labia Majora

Labia Minora

Anus

Coccyx

B   Circumcised   Not Circumcised

Shaft of Penis

Foreskin

Scrotum

Glans

Urinary Meatus

Glans

Scrotum

Urinary Meatus

FIGURE 14-2   (A) The external female genitalia (B) The external male genitalia

sex organ used for sex and elimination. The foreskin is the loose tissue at the tip of the penis. If the resident has been circumcised, the loose skin has been removed.

Normal Elimination

You have learned that the normal fluid intake for most adults is 2000 to 3000 mL per day. The average adult eliminates about 1500 to 2000 mL of urine a day from the bladder. The remaining liquid is eliminated from the body in sweat (450 to 1050 mL), moisture in respiratory secretions (250 to 500 mL), and liquid in bowel elimination (50 to 200 mL). Many factors influence urine production. Some factors, such as disease, ingestion of salt, and certain medications, reduce urine production and cause the body to retain fluid. Drinking coffee, tea, or alcoholic beverages, and some medications increase urine production.

COMMON PROBLEMS RELATED TO THE URINARY SYSTEM

Problems with elimination have many causes. These are related to aging, medications, and many different diseases. Elimination is very private for most people, and even a change in routine can cause embarrassment. This is particularly true if someone else must assist with this very personal body function. Physical changes in elimination can have a major impact on the resident's self-esteem. Considering the resident's feelings when assisting with urinary elimination procedures is important. The care provider must be sensitive, understanding, and professional.

Incontinence is a medical problem. Health care workers often use underpads, incontinent pads, and briefs to contain urine, prevent skin breakdown, and avoid embarrassment to the resident. Select your words carefully and do not call these medical aids *diapers*, or other words that can be demeaning. Appropriate words to use include *adult brief, garment protector*, and *clothing protector*. Your facility may have specific names for the products you will be using.

Changes in Urinary Function Associated with Aging and Disease

The aging process affects the urinary system. The kidneys do not filter the blood as efficiently as they did previously, so less urine is produced. Muscle tone decreases with aging and some diseases. The bladder is a muscle. Although the bladder is still able to hold urine, the capacity is reduced, and it cannot hold as much as it once did. A common myth is that incontinence is a normal part of aging. This is not true. Incontinence usually indicates a physical problem. It can also occur in mentally confused residents because they cannot express the need to use the bathroom. However, if they are taken to the bathroom and seated on the toilet, they will usually urinate. Most do not forget this basic activity of daily living.

Elderly men often develop **prostate** problems. The prostate is a gland that secretes fluid in semen **(Figure 14-3)**. It surrounds the urethra just below the bladder in the male. As men age, the prostate gland enlarges and applies pressure to the urethra. This causes **urinary retention,** or inability to empty the bladder completely. Other problems related to the prostate are frequent dribbling of urine or inability to urinate at all. Because men are used to urinating while standing, sometimes assisting the male resident to stand will help him empty his bladder more efficiently.

Many diseases also affect the urinary system. In heart disease, the blood is not circulated through the body efficiently, so less urine is produced. Edema often results. High blood pressure causes severe kidney damage over time. Other conditions, such as strokes, trauma, and neurological diseases, affect the resident's sensation. This may cause inability to feel the urge to urinate when the bladder is full. Some residents do not feel the need to urinate until the bladder is very full. When this happens, the need is immediate. If they have to wait, accidents will result.

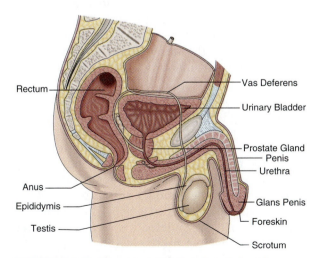

FIGURE 14-3 The prostate gland encircles the urethra. It enlarges in aging, causing partial or complete urinary obstruction.

Urinary Incontinence. You have learned that incontinence is the inability to control the passage of urine from the bladder. Incontinence can be temporary or permanent. In addition to the problems listed earlier, other common causes of incontinence are disease, trauma, surgery, infection, stress, anxiety, tumors, mental confusion, and loss of muscle control. **Constipation,** or passage of hard, dry stool from the lower bowel, may also contribute to incontinence. Some residents are unable to communicate the need to use the bathroom or are physically unable to get to the bathroom. These problems can also cause incontinence. When caring for residents who are incontinent, provide perineal care after each incontinent episode, following the guidelines in Procedures 41 and 42. Some facilities used premixed sprays for this purpose. Some are rinsed off with water. Others are no-rinse solutions or disposable wipes. Follow the directions for the type of product you are using, but apply the principles of peri-care when you perform the procedure. Notify the nurse of any signs of skin redness, irritation, or breakdown.

Types of Incontinence. Some residents have a condition called **stress incontinence.** This is a common problem in women, caused by weak muscles, having multiple children, and aging. In stress incontinence, the bladder leaks urine when the pelvic muscles are strained during activities such as laughing, coughing, sneezing, and lifting.

Urge incontinence is often caused by infection. Other causes of urge incontinence include tumors, neurological problems, reproductive problems, and constipation. Residents with this condition have little warning of the need to use the bathroom. When they feel the urge, the need is immediate. If the urine begins to escape, the resident may be unable to control it, and the bladder empties involuntarily.

Functional incontinence occurs when the resident is physically unable to get to the bathroom on time or is disoriented and unable to find the bathroom. It is easily treated by anticipating residents' needs in advance, answering call signals immediately, and meeting residents' needs responsively. If the resident is in a restraint, he or she will be unable to get to the bathroom without your help. Anticipate the need and offer to toilet the resident routinely.

Mixed incontinence is a combination of urge and stress incontinence. **Overflow incontinence** occurs when the bladder is very full.

When it can hold no more, urine leaks out to ease the pressure. **Reflex incontinence** is loss of urine that occurs without awareness in residents who are paralyzed or have other neurologic problems.

Mental Confusion. Residents who are mentally confused present a special challenge. Most are able to urinate if they are taken to the toilet. Some residents who are mentally confused have behavior problems caused by the discomfort of needing to use the toilet. They are not able to express themselves verbally, so they yell, scream, hit, or cry. After they have eliminated, the behavior problems cease. Some confused residents become restless and will pull at or remove their clothing. Anticipate the need for toileting and take confused residents to the bathroom every two hours. Managing incontinence requires planning and effort on your part. However, preventing accidents makes your work easier. A wet bed is a warm, moist, dark environment, so it presents an ideal breeding ground for bacteria. The risk of skin and bladder infections is increased by incontinence. Preventing incontinence also prevents skin breakdown, discomfort, and other complications for the resident.

Urinary Tract Infections. Urinary tract infections (UTIs) are common in women. The urethra in the female is only 1½ to 2½ inches long **(Figure 14-4)**. Because the urethra is so short, bacteria can easily enter it and travel to the bladder. This is why following the correct procedure for perineal care is so important. The urethra in the male is six to eight inches long. Bacteria can

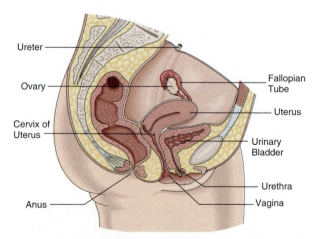

FIGURE 14-4 The female urethra is 1½ to 2½ inches long, providing easy access for invading pathogens to enter a sterile area.

GUIDELINES FOR
Assisting Residents with Urinary Elimination

- Provide adequate fluid intake. Many residents drink less because they believe they will urinate less. The opposite is true. If the resident does not drink enough fluids, the bladder capacity will shrink, and the resident will void more frequently.
- Answer call signals promptly. Take residents to the bathroom, or provide a **bedpan, urinal,** or bedside commode **(Figure 14-5)**, if necessary. The bedpan is a device used for elimination in bed. A urinal is used by some male residents for urination.
- Assist residents to assume an upright position for urination. Emptying the bladder in the supine position is difficult.
- Provide privacy by closing the door, privacy curtain, and window curtain. Cover the resident with a bath blanket when using the bedpan or commode, even if alone in the room. Leave the resident alone if doing so is safe. Return immediately when the resident signals. Remain nearby if the resident is unable to safely be left alone.
- Never restrain a resident on the toilet or commode.
- Allow adequate time for the resident to empty the bladder. Leave toilet paper and the call signal nearby.
- If the resident has difficulty urinating, try running a slow, steady stream of water so the resident can hear it. Placing the hands in warm water, offering the resident a drink of water, or pouring warm water over the genital area may also be helpful.
- After the resident has voided, give perineal care if needed.
- Bedpans and urinals should always be covered when removing them from the bedside. Some agencies use covers designed for this purpose. Others use disposable underpads. Wear gloves when handling the bedpan or urinal. Avoid contaminating side rails, door knobs, and faucets with your gloves. Wearing a glove on one hand **(Figure 14-6)** is a good method of preventing environmental contamination. If removing a glove is not possible, use a paper towel under your gloved hand to avoid touching environmental surfaces.
- Before discarding the specimen, check to see if a urine specimen is needed or if the resident's urinary output must be measured.
- Follow your facility policy for discarding urine and disinfecting the bedpan or urinal after each use.
- Assist the resident to wash hands after emptying the bladder.

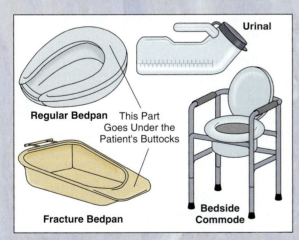

FIGURE 14-5 Devices used to assist residents with elimination

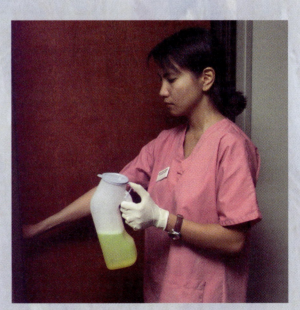

FIGURE 14-6 To avoid environmental contamination, open doors and turn on faucets with your ungloved hand.

travel through the male urethra, but because of the length, the problem is less common than it is in women.

Urine is normally amber or straw colored and clear. There is no mucus or sediment. It has a faint odor. In a urinary tract infection, an unusual color or odor, blood, mucus, or pus may be present in the urine. If you think the urine appears abnormal, save it for the nurse to observe. Pain in the **flank,** or the area of the back immediately above the waist, may indicate an infection. Other signs and symptoms include:

- Voiding frequently in small amounts
- Incontinence or dribbling
- Having an urgent need to void
- Getting up at night to urinate
- New onset of mental confusion
- Burning or pain on urination
- Feeling as if the bladder will not empty
- Being unable to urinate despite having an urge to do so
- Foul odor
- Change from clear to cloudy appearance

If you observe any of these signs in a resident, notify the nurse. If a resident normally has bladder control, and begins to have episodes of incontinence, this is also an important observa-

tion. If the resident has not voided at all on your shift, this could also indicate a problem. Notify the nurse of these findings.

ROLE OF THE NURSING ASSISTANT IN ASSISTING RESIDENTS WITH URINARY ELIMINATION

The nursing assistant has a very important responsibility in assisting residents with elimination. Always apply the principles of standard precautions when assisting residents with elimination. The circumstances of elimination are highly personal. Use good judgment regarding when to apply and remove gloves. Avoid

---

| PROCEDURE 52 | Assisting the Resident with a Bedpan | |

1. Perform your beginning procedure actions.
2. Gather supplies needed: gloves, bedpan, bedpan cover, two bed protectors, toilet tissue, basin of water, soap, washcloth, towel.
3. Cover the top linen with a bath blanket and remove the upper linen without exposing the resident, or fold the upper linen down to expose the buttocks.
4. Optional measures for comfort and convenience:
   a. You may run the bedpan under warm water before placing it, for resident comfort. Dry the outside of the bedpan before placing it under the resident.
   b. Dust the edges of the (dry) bedpan lightly with baby powder, then rub the powder around evenly with your gloved hand. This reduces friction, making the bedpan easier to insert and remove. The powder reduces inadvertent shearing on the resident's skin.
5. Ask the resident to flex the knees, resting weight on the heels, and lift the buttocks off the bed, if able.
6. Help the resident raise the buttocks by:
   a. Putting one hand under the small of the back and gently lifting while the resident pushes with the feet **(Figure 14-7).**
   b. With the other hand, insert the bed protector under the buttocks.
7. If the resident is unable to lift the buttocks:
   a. Assist the resident to turn on the side, with back facing you.
   b. Place the bed protector on the bed.
   c. Place the bedpan flat against the buttocks **(Figure 14-8).**
   d. Assist the resident to roll back while you hold the bedpan in place.

8. Cover the resident with the top sheet or bath blanket.
9. Raise the head of the bed up, for comfort.
10. Remove your gloves.
11. Raise the side rail.
12. Dispose of gloves according to facility policy.
13. Wash your hands.
14. Give the resident the call signal and toilet tissue and leave the room.
15. Return immediately when the resident signals.
16. Put on gloves.
17. Lower the side rail.

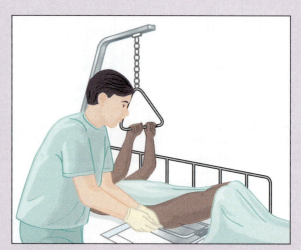

FIGURE 14-7 The resident pulls on the trapeze to lift her hips off the bed. The nursing assistant slides the bedpan under the buttocks.

Continues

PROCEDURE 52 Assisting the Resident with a Bedpan, *Continued*

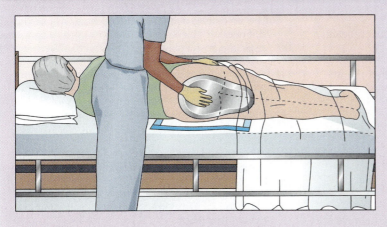

FIGURE 14-8 If the resident cannot lift his or her hips, the resident turns to the side. The nursing assistant places the bedpan against the buttocks, then holds it in place while the resident turns back.

18. Remove the bedpan by asking the resident to raise his or her hips.
19. If the resident is unable to raise the hips, hold the bedpan securely while the resident rolls to the side with his or her back facing you. Remove the bedpan. Cover the pan with a bedpan cover or disposable underpad according to facility policy.
20. Place the bedpan on a bed protector on the chair in the room, or according to facility policy. It is usually not placed on the overbed table or bedside stand.
21. Remove one glove to avoid environmental contamination.
22. Fill the washbasin with water (105°F). Help the resident to clean the perineal area. If you will be

assisting with the procedure, wear two gloves. Follow the guidelines in Procedure 41 or 42 for perineal care.
23. Remove one glove and raise the side rail with the ungloved hand.
24. Take the covered bedpan to the bathroom. Empty and disinfect it according to facility policy. Use the ungloved hand to turn on faucets and flush the toilet. Store the bedpan in its proper location.
25. Assist the resident with handwashing.
26. Perform your procedure completion actions.
27. Report or record output. Note color, amount, or any abnormalities.

contaminating environmental surfaces with your gloves. Wear a gown, eye protection, and face mask if splashing is likely.

Assisting Residents with the Bedpan, Urinal, and Bedside Commode

Residents who are confined to bed must use the bedpan or urinal for elimination. The bedpans used in long-term care facilities are regular bedpans and fracture pans. Adjusting to using a bedpan in bed may be difficult for residents. The urinal is a container the male resident uses for urination. The urinal is a plastic or metal container with a handle and lid. It is usually marked on the side with measurements in milliliters. Male residents use the bedpan for bowel movements.

Assisting Residents with the Bedside Commode. The bedside commode is a raised seat placed over the regular toilet, or is used at the

bedside with a bedpan or other container placed under the seat. It is used for residents who can get out of bed, but are unable to walk to the bathroom. Using the commode positions the resident in a natural position for elimination, and increases resident independence. The bedside commode is more secure for some residents to sit on because it has sturdy arms that help with sitting, rising, and positioning. Some commodes have wheels. If this is the case, they should be locked securely at all times. Most commodes have a cover over the container used for elimination. However, the commode should be emptied each time it is used. The cover is used when transporting the container to the designated area for emptying and disinfecting.

The procedure for transferring a resident to the commode is the same as the procedure used to transfer from bed to chair. Apply the principles of standard precautions when handling the container the resident uses for elimination.

Assisting the Male Resident with a Urinal

1. Perform your beginning procedure actions.
2. Gather supplies: gloves, urinal with cover, basin of water, soap, washcloth, towel.
3. Put on gloves.
4. Lift the top covers and hand the resident the urinal. If the resident is unable to take the urinal, place it between the resident's legs and insert the penis into the opening.
5. Remove your gloves and discard according to facility policy.
6. Raise the side rail.
7. Wash your hands.
8. Give the resident the call signal and leave the room.
9. Return immediately when called.
10. Put on one glove.
11. Ask the resident to hand you the urinal. Remove it if he is unable, using the gloved hand. Close the lid if needed.
12. Assist the resident with perineal care. Wear two gloves, if assisting.
13. Take the covered urinal to the bathroom and empty and disinfect it according to facility policy. Store the urinal in its proper location.
14. Remove the glove(s) and dispose according to facility policy.
15. Wash your hands.
16. Lower the side rail.
17. Help the resident to wash his hands.
18. Raise the side rail.
19. Perform your procedure completion actions.
20. Report or record output. Note color, amount, or any abnormalities.

URINARY CATHETERS

A **catheter** is a hollow tube inserted into the bladder to drain urine. This is a sterile procedure that is done by the nurse. Sometimes a catheter is called a *Foley*, which is a common brand name for **indwelling catheters.** It may also be called a *retention catheter* or *indwelling catheter.* Catheters are inserted through the urethra, and are held in place with a balloon inflated with saline solution or sterile water **(Figure 14-9).** The catheter remains in the body for a period of time. Sometimes the resident will complain of feeling the urge to urinate after the catheter is inserted. This is due to the pressure of the balloon on the internal sphincter of the urethra. The pressure feels the same as the sensation of urine pressing on the sphincter. If the resident with a catheter complains of feeling the urge to void, notify the nurse.

A **suprapubic catheter (Figure 14-10)** is inserted surgically through the abdominal wall directly into the bladder. A **condom catheter**

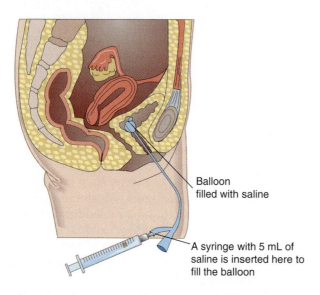

FIGURE 14-9 A small balloon filled with sterile saline solution holds the catheter in the bladder. Pressure from the balloon on the internal sphincter of the urethra may cause the resident to feel the urge to void.

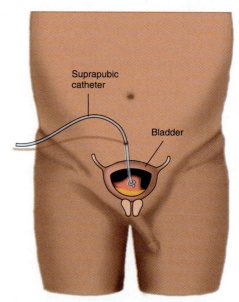

FIGURE 14-10 The suprapubic catheter is surgically inserted through the abdominal wall. The urethra is not functional.

(Figure 14-11) is an **external catheter** used in males. It is applied over the penis and attached to drainage tubing. It is sometimes called a *Texas catheter.* An **intermittent catheter** is inserted into the bladder for emptying the bladder or obtaining a urine specimen. After the bladder is emptied, the catheter is removed.

Purpose of Catheters

Catheters are used for many reasons. Some catheters are intermittent. Some are temporary and others are used permanently. Catheter use is avoided whenever possible because it presents a very high risk of infection. Because the catheter provides a direct opening into the bladder, pathogens can make their way up the tubing and cause serious problems. Residents who are elderly and those with weakened immune systems often become **septic** because of bladder infections. Sepsis is a very serious, sometimes fatal, systemic infection caused by bacteria.

Catheters are never used for staff convenience. Many residents with neurological problems or trauma are catheterized because the condition has affected sensation, and the resident cannot feel the urge to void. Some residents retain urine until the bladder is stretched beyond capacity. This is very painful. Catheters are used to empty the bladder in these cases. Catheters are also used after many surgical procedures. These catheters are used temporarily and are removed when the resident is able to use the toilet again. Residents with severe skin problems may also use catheters temporarily, allowing time for the skin to heal without the irritation of urine on the wound. Some residents routinely catheterize themselves to empty the bladder.

Drainage Systems

Catheters must be ordered by a physician and are inserted by licensed personnel. They must always be secured to the resident's body with a special strap **(Figure 14-12).** Securing the catheter prevents accidental pulling during movement. Pulling can cause damage to the bladder and urethra, and is very uncomfortable for the resident. After the catheter is inserted, it is connected to a **closed drainage system. (Figure 14-13).** The system is connected to the catheter with a long tubing that empties urine into a **drainage bag (Figure 14-14),** where urine is collected. As long as the system is not opened, it remains **sterile,** or free from all microbes. Each time the system is opened, the risk of infection increases. Opening a closed urinary drainage system is usually a licensed nursing responsibility. Do not open a closed system unless you have been taught the proper techniques and are permitted to do so in your facility.

Some facilities use **leg drainage bags (Figure 14-15)** on both indwelling catheters and condom catheters. These are used for ambulatory residents who are up and about during the day. The bag is attached to the leg with elastic straps or Velcro bands. The leg bag holds a smaller amount of urine than a normal drainage bag, and must be emptied more often. Use of the leg bag is avoided whenever possible, because it requires frequent manipulation and opening of the closed system and increases the chance of infection. Some facilities have policies and procedures for disinfecting and reusing them; others use a new bag each day. Know and follow your facility policy. Residents who use the leg

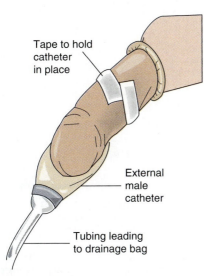

FIGURE 14-11 This male external catheter is secured with spiral-wrapped tape. Another type has a self-adhesive inner surface.

Tape to hold catheter in place

External male catheter

Tubing leading to drainage bag

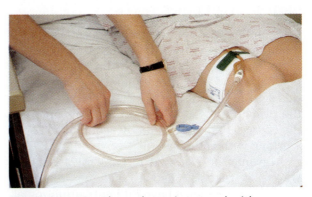

FIGURE 14-12 The catheter is secured with a Velcro strap to prevent pulling and damage to the bladder and urethra. For a male resident, the catheter may be taped to the abdomen.

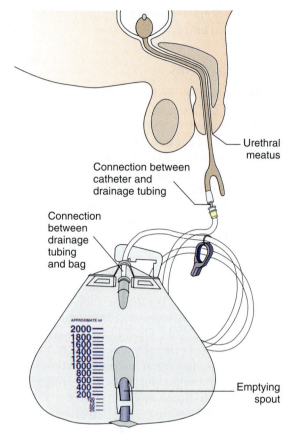

FIGURE 14-13 Handle the closed drainage system carefully to avoid accidental contamination of these areas.

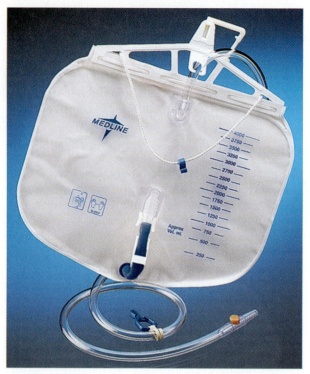

FIGURE 14-14 The catheter bag is attached to the bed frame below the level of the bladder. Handle the bag carefully. It should never be positioned so that urine flows back into the bladder. Note the numbers on the bag. These are approximations only, and are used for monitoring purposes. Do not use these numbers for intake and output measurements. *(Courtesy of Medline Industries, Inc. 1-800-MEDLINE)*

bag are connected to the normal catheter drainage bag when they are in bed. Never put a resident to bed with a leg bag in place. Follow your facility policy for use of the leg bag.

If you are responsible for applying a leg bag or opening a closed system, use aseptic technique. Insert a catheter plug into the end of the catheter **(Figure 14-16A)**. Cover the end of the drainage tube with the sterile cap **(Figure 14-16B)**.

Caring for a Catheter

The nursing assistant is usually responsible for maintaining the closed drainage system. The tubing may be secured to the bed linen with a rubber band and clip. Maintaining the sterility of this system is an important responsibility. Apply the principles of standard precautions, and use the correct personal protective equipment when working with catheters.

You may be assigned to care for a resident who has recently had a catheter removed. Sometimes residents have difficulty urinating after the catheter is removed, or the bladder does not empty completely. After the catheter is

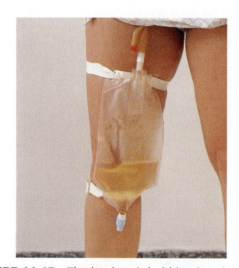

FIGURE 14-15 The leg bag is held in place by adjustable straps. The bag is smaller than a bed collection bag and must be emptied more often. Carefully connect the catheter to the leg bag. Avoid touching anything against the end of the catheter. The drainage tubing on the bed bag is covered with a sterile cap that is left in place until it is reconnected to the catheter.

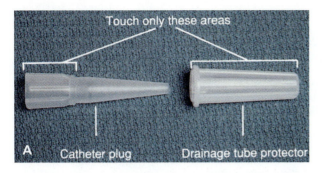

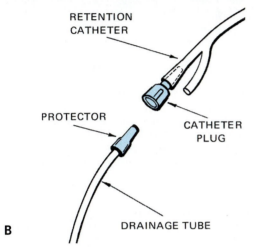

FIGURE 14-16 A, B The sterile plug and drainage tube protector are used to maintain sterility of the closed catheter system. Never touch the inside of the cap or patient end of the plug with your fingers.

removed, monitor the resident and record the time and amount of each voiding for the rest of your shift. If the resident has not voided by the end of your shift, notify the nurse. Monitoring of the resident's urination will continue for at least 24 hours after the catheter has been removed.

Providing Catheter Care

The nursing assistant is responsible for providing catheter care to residents who use catheters. Always apply the principles of standard precautions when caring for the catheter. Use **aseptic technique** when caring for the catheter or the drainage system. Aseptic technique means you will perform the procedure correctly so you do not introduce microbes to the area. The perineum should be as clean as possible, so perform perineal care before caring for the catheter.

Some facilities use specially packaged catheter care kits, but most use soap and water when providing perineal and catheter care. The supplies for performing this procedure will vary depending on which method you use, but the principles of care are the same.

Caring for the External Catheter

The risk of infection is not as great when using an external catheter. However, the catheter must be cared for correctly because infection can occur. Other complications, such as irritation and circulatory problems, can also occur. The external catheter is applied over the penis. It is usually attached with an adhesive strip. The strip should always be wrapped in a spiral. If it completely encircles the penis, severe injury can result. Some external catheters have a self-adhesive film on the inside, making the adhesive strip on the outside unnecessary. About one inch of the catheter should extend beyond the tip of the penis and attach to the drainage tubing. Always apply the principles of standard precautions when caring for an external catheter.

GUIDELINES FOR
Maintaining a Closed Drainage System

- Always wash your hands and apply gloves before handling the catheter and closed drainage system. Avoid contaminating the environment with your gloves.
- Wear a face shield, mask, and gown if you are performing a procedure in which splashing is likely, such as emptying a very full drainage bag.
- The catheter, bag, and tubing are never disconnected unless sterile technique is used.
- When the resident is in bed, the closed drainage bag is attached to the frame of the bed, never the side rail.
- The urinary drainage bag must never touch the floor, as this contaminates the system.

- When the resident is in a chair or wheelchair, the closed drainage bag is attached to the frame of the chair.
- Many facilities use cloth catheter bags for privacy. The cloth bag is connected to the bed or chair frame, and the urinary drainage bag is placed in it. The cloth bag should not touch the floor.
- Avoid elevating the urinary drainage bag and tubing above the level of the bladder. This causes a backflow of urine into the bladder, greatly increasing the risk of infection.

Continues

GUIDELINES FOR

Maintaining a Closed Drainage System, *Continued*

- When the resident is ambulating, the tubing and drainage bag are carried below the level of the bladder.
- Secure the catheter with a strap. Some facilities secure the catheter to the leg in women, and the abdomen, using tape, in men. When securing the catheter to the leg, it is positioned on the top side. Avoid placing the catheter under the leg, as this placement may pinch and obstruct the flow of urine. Know and follow your facility policy.
- Attach the tubing to the bed with a rubber band and plastic clip. The tubing should not hang below the drainage bag.
- Make sure the urine is draining freely through the system and that there are no kinks or obstructions in the tubing.
- Never disconnect the tubing, unless you are trained in this procedure.
- Use care when lifting, moving, and transferring residents with catheters, to avoid accidentally dislodging the catheter by pulling on the tubing.
- When the resident is positioned on his or her back, the catheter should be on top of the leg. The drainage bag is positioned on the bed frame on the same side of the bed as the catheter. (If the catheter is on the left leg, the bag is on the left side of the bed.)

- If the resident is positioned on his or her side, the catheter is positioned between the legs. Make sure the urine flow is not obstructed. The bag is placed on the bed frame on the side the resident is facing (if the resident faces right, the bag hangs on the right side of the bed).
- When transferring the resident to a chair or wheelchair, move the bag first, then the resident. Take care to avoid stepping on the tubing during the transfer.
- Monitor the level of urine in the drainage bag. Most people excrete about 50 to 80 mL of urine each hour. If the level of urine in the bag does not change, if the catheter is leaking, if no urine is present in the bag, or if the urine has an abnormal color, odor, or appearance, inform the nurse.
- Notify the nurse if redness, irritation, drainage, crusting, or open areas are present at the catheter insertion site.
- Notify the nurse if the resident complains of pain, burning, or tenderness, or has other signs or symptoms of urinary tract infection.
- Most facilities routinely measure intake and output on residents who are using a urinary catheter. Follow your facility policy.

Emptying the Urinary Drainage Bag

The nursing assistant is responsible for emptying the urinary drainage bag at the end of the shift, and more often if the bag becomes full. The output is measured and recorded. Apply the principles of standard precautions when performing this procedure. All facilities require you to wear gloves. Some also require the use of a face mask and eye protection, because of the risk of splashing if the drainage bag is full. Know and follow your facility policy.

GUIDELINES FOR

Opening a Closed Drainage System

Note: In some states, nursing assistants are not permitted to perform this procedure. Additionally, the policies of some facilities state that only licensed nurses may open a closed urinary drainage system. Perform this procedure only if you are permitted to do so by state law and facility policies.

- Always wash your hands and apply gloves before handling the catheter and closed drainage system. Avoid contaminating the environment with your gloves. Use sterile technique.
- Position an underpad under the connection between the catheter and drainage tube.
- Open the sterile package containing the catheter plug and cap. Leave it open on the table, but avoid

touching it. Disconnect the catheter and tubing. Hold both ends in your hand. Do not set them down. Insert the catheter plug into the end of the catheter. Avoid touching the tip of the plug. Place the sterile cap over the end of the drainage tube. After covering, both items may be put down.
- If accidental contamination occurs, wipe the ends well with an antiseptic wipe before placing the cap or inserting the plug.
- Empty the drainage bag, if necessary. Secure the tubing to the bed so it does not touch the floor.
- Reverse these steps to reconnect the catheter. If you find an unconnected, disconnected catheter, do not reconnect it. Inform the nurse at once.

GUIDELINES FOR
Applying a Urinary Leg Bag

Note: In some states, nursing assistants are not permitted to perform this procedure. Additionally, the policies of some facilities state that only licensed nurses may open a closed urinary drainage system. Perform this procedure only if you are permitted to do so by state law and facility policies.

- Always wash your hands and apply gloves before handling the catheter and closed drainage system. Avoid contaminating the environment with your gloves. Use sterile technique.
- Position an underpad under the connection between the catheter and drainage tube.
- Open the sterile package containing the leg bag. Leave it open on the table, but avoid touching it.
- Open the sterile package containing the catheter plug and cap. Leave it open on the table, but avoid touching it. Disconnect the catheter and tubing. Hold both ends in your hand. Do not set them down. Insert the catheter plug into the end of the

catheter. Avoid touching the tip of the plug. Place the sterile cap over the end of the drainage tube. After covering, both items may be put down.

- If accidental contamination occurs, wipe the ends well with an antiseptic wipe before placing the cap or inserting the plug.
- Secure the tubing to the bed so it does not fall on the floor.
- Remove the catheter plug. Place it on the open, sterile package.
- Insert the upper connector of the leg bag into the catheter.
- Fasten the leg bag to the resident's leg with the Velcro or vinyl straps. Make sure the catheter is straight and able to drain freely. Check for leaks.
- Empty the drainage bag, if necessary.
- Reverse these steps to reconnect the catheter. If you find an unconnected, disconnected catheter, do not reconnect it. Inform the nurse at once.

GUIDELINES FOR
Drainage Bag Disinfection

Note: Using a new, sterile leg bag each day is the best method of preventing infection. However, some facilities disinfect the bags, using procedures that markedly reduce the risk of infection. If this is the case, follow your facility policies and procedures. These disinfection guidelines apply only to those bags that are opened so that a leg bag can be attached. They do not apply to all drainage bags in the facility.

Caution: Avoid contact of solution with eyes and skin. Irritation can occur. Metal bathroom fixtures can rust or corrosion can occur. Harmful fumes can arise from contact with other cleaning products. Follow facility policies for handling bleach solution. Be familiar with the information on the MSDS for the bleach.

- Continuous drainage bags that are disconnected from the catheter and leg bags that are applied in their place must be decontaminated at least every 24 hours. The bags should be labeled with the resident's name and next date of change.
- Obtain a 500 mL plastic squeeze bottle. Label the bottle with the resident's name and next date of change. (The bottle should be changed each time the catheter bag is changed.) Fill the squeeze bottle with 480 mL of warm tap water. Pour 15 mL of liquid bleach containing 5.25% sodium hypochlorite solution into a medicine cup.

- Wash your hands and apply gloves before handling the drainage system. Avoid contaminating the environment with your gloves. Use sterile technique.
- Empty the bag.
- Using the squeeze bottle, empty half the bottle of tap water into the *top end* of the leg bag or urinary drainage bag. Filling from the top end flushes bacteria out of the bag and away from the connection.
- Close the bag and shake vigorously for 15 seconds. Agitation is necessary to loosen bacteria.
- Empty the bag into the toilet. (For infection control purposes, do not use the sink.)
- Repeat a second time with the remaining water-and-bleach solution in the bottle. Two rinses are necessary to flush bacteria from the bag.
- Fill the squeeze bottle half full with tap water. Pour 15 mL liquid bleach containing 5.25% sodium hypochlorite solution into a medicine cup. Add the bleach to the tap water in the bottle.
- Squirt 30 mL of the solution onto the outer surfaces of the drainage bag or leg bag spigot, bell, sleeve, and cap. These connections hold bacteria, so it is important to direct bleach to these sites.
- Squirt the remaining solution into the bag. Shake gently for at least 30 seconds. Make sure that the solution touches all surfaces inside the bag.
- Empty the solution into the toilet. (For infection control purposes, do not use the sink.). Remove as much

Continues

GUIDELINES FOR
Drainage Bag Disinfection, *Continued*

solution as possible. Bacteria are less likely to grow in a dry environment. Air-dried bags last longer than those stored with bleach solution trapped inside.
- Cover the open upper end with a cap, or use a clean gauze pad secured with a rubber band. Close the drainage port at the bottom of the bag.
- Hang the bag in the designated location in the soiled utility room or resident bathroom.

- Discard the plastic medicine cup. Store the plastic squeeze bottle in a clear plastic bag according to facility policy.

(Adapted from Dille, C., and Kirchoff, K. Decontamination of vinyl urinary drainage bags with bleach. Rehabil Nurs. 1993;18(5):292–5.)

PROCEDURE
54
Providing Indwelling Catheter Care

Note: The guidelines and sequence for this procedure vary slightly from state to state. Your instructor will inform you if the sequence in your state differs from the procedure listed here. Know and follow the required sequence for your state.
1. Perform your beginning procedure actions.
2. Gather supplies needed: catheter care kit or basin, soap, two washcloths, towels, clean gown or clothing, bath blanket, bed protector, hamper or plastic laundry bag, gloves.
3. Place the equipment on the overbed table. Follow your facility policy for covering the overbed table with a barrier.

4. Perform perineal care, following the guidelines in Procedure 41 or 42.
5. Using a clean washcloth, wash the catheter for three to four inches from the insertion site into the body. Begin washing at the urinary meatus and wash downward. Avoid rubbing back and forth on the tubing.
6. Thoroughly rinse and dry the tubing.
7. Secure the tubing to the leg.
8. Perform your procedure completion actions.

GUIDELINES FOR
Caring for an External Catheter

- Wear gloves and apply the principles of standard precautions when caring for an external catheter and drainage system. Avoid contaminating the environment with your gloves.
- Provide perineal care, following the guidelines in Procedure 42, before applying the external catheter.
- Dry the penis well before applying the catheter. Report redness, irritation, discharge, or signs of infection to the nurse.
- Roll the tip of the condom catheter over the tip of the penis and up the shaft. Leave one inch of space at the end.
- Wrap the adhesive strip in a spiral.
- Attach the connecting tube of the catheter to the drainage tubing and urinary drainage bag.

- Change the catheter daily. Discard the external catheter and apply a new one each day, and more often if necessary. Never reuse a catheter after it has been removed.
- To change the catheter, remove the adhesive strip and roll the condom down over the tip of the penis. Discard it in the biohazardous waste, according to facility policy.
- Observe the skin on the penis for redness, irritation, swelling, and open areas. If noted, report your observations to the nurse before applying a new external catheter.
- After the catheter has been removed, perineal care must be done before a new catheter is applied.

PROCEDURE

55

Emptying the Urinary Drainage Bag

Note: The guidelines and sequence for this procedure vary slightly from state to state. Your instructor will inform you if the sequence in your state differs from the procedure listed here. Know and follow the required sequence for your state.

1. Perform your beginning procedure actions.
2. Gather supplies needed: gloves; mask and eye protection, if necessary; graduated pitcher; paper towel; alcohol sponge.
3. Place the paper towel on the floor and place the graduated pitcher on it **(Figure 14-17A)**.
4. Apply gloves.
5. Remove the drainage spout from the bag and center it over the graduate. Avoid touching the tip of the drainage spout with your hands or the side of the graduate.
6. Open the clamp on the drainage spout and drain the urine into the graduate **(Figure 14-17B)**.
7. After the urine has drained into the graduate, wipe the spout with the alcohol sponge, if this is your facility policy. Some facilities do not wipe the tip of the spout unless it has contacted your hands or the graduate.
8. Replace the drainage spout into the holder on the side of the catheter bag. Pick up the graduate and dispose of the paper towel.

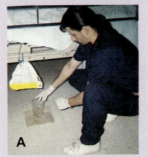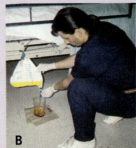

FIGURE 14-17 (A) Place a paper towel on the floor under the graduate. (B) Center the drain spout over the graduate to avoid accidental contamination.

9. Note the amount, color, and character of urine.
10. Discard urine and disinfect the graduate according to facility policy. Store the graduate in its proper location.
11. Report or record output. Note color, amount, or any abnormalities.
12. Perform your procedure completion actions.

MEASURING URINARY OUTPUT

You have learned that most people eliminate about 1500 mL of urine each day and the reasons for recording intake and output. If the resident is incontinent, follow your facility procedure for recording fluid output. Some facilities count the number of episodes of incontinence. Others measure the size of the urine puddle or weigh the underpad. The dry weight of the pad is subtracted from the total weight, and an estimation of the amount of urine eliminated is made. A scale that measures weight in grams is usually used. The most common formula is 1 gram of weight is equivalent to 1 mL of urine.

A **graduate** is a container used for measuring liquids in the health care facility. The graduate is marked on the side in ounces and milliliters (or cubic centimeters). Measuring the urine in a graduate is more accurate than using the markings on a catheter bag or estimating the output.

If you will be measuring urinary output, remind the resident not to drop toilet tissue into the container holding the urine. The toilet tissue is discarded into a plastic bag, or according to facility policy. Apply the principles of standard precautions when measuring urinary output.

COLLECTING A URINE SPECIMEN

The nursing assistant is responsible for collecting routine urine specimens for analysis by the laboratory. The physician will use the information gathered to aid in diagnosis and treatment of the resident. A **laboratory requisition** is completed and attached to each specimen. The requisition contains identifying resident information and specifies the type of test to be performed on the specimen.

Urine is collected in a clean bedpan, urinal, or specimen collection container in the toilet. This container may be called a specimen collection

PROCEDURE 56
Measuring Urinary Output

1. Perform your beginning procedure actions.
2. Gather supplies needed: graduate, intake and output work sheet, gloves.
3. After the resident has voided, apply gloves.
4. Empty the urine into the graduate. Measure the amount of urine in the container at eye level **(Figure 14-18)**.
5. Empty the graduate into the toilet, and rinse and disinfect the container.
6. Rinse, disinfect, dry, and replace the bedpan, urinal, or commode container.
7. Perform your procedure completion actions.
8. Record the output on the intake and output work sheet, or according to facility policy.

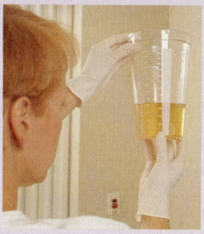

FIGURE 14-18   Hold the graduate at eye level or place it on the counter and view at eye level to measure the output accurately.

"hat," or "nun's hat" **(Figure 14-19)**. The specimen is poured into a closed urine specimen container with a lid. A routine urine specimen is collected using clean technique. The specimen does not have to be sterile, but must be free from outside contamination.

A **midstream (clean-catch) specimen** is collected from the middle of the urinary stream and is as sterile as possible. The specimen cup is sterile. Urine in the bladder is normally sterile. Precautions are taken when obtaining the specimen to avoid contamination. The perineum is washed before collecting the specimen, to eliminate microbes on the skin. The resident starts to void into the toilet or other container, and stops the flow of urine partway through. The sterile

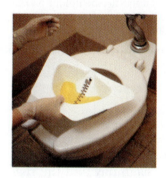

FIGURE 14-19   The specimen collection container may be called a specimen "hat" or "nun's hat."

specimen cup is placed under the urethra, and the resident voids into the container until an adequate amount of urine is obtained. The resident stops voiding again, the cup is removed, and the resident finishes the elimination in the toilet.

GUIDELINES FOR
Collecting a Urine Specimen

- Apply the principles of standard precautions. Avoid contaminating the environment with your gloves.
- *The lid to the specimen container is always placed topside down on the table, so the clean inner side faces up.*
- *Avoid touching the inside of the container or lid with your hands.*

- The specimen container is always labeled with the resident's name and other identifying information. Follow your facility policy for labeling the container.
- Ask the resident not to discard toilet tissue into the specimen. The toilet tissue is discarded into a plastic bag, or according to facility policy.

Continues

GUIDELINES FOR

Collecting a Urine Specimen, *Continued*

- Pour the specimen into the specimen collection container. If you will be placing the container on a counter or other flat surface, place a paper towel under it.
- After you have collected the specimen, put the lid on the container and place it in a sealed **transport bag** labeled with a biohazardous waste label **(Figure 14-20)**. The transport bag is a plastic bag that can be sealed tightly to prevent leaking.
- If the urine specimen cannot be transported to the lab immediately, it can be stored in a designated refrigerator or cooler for lab specimens.

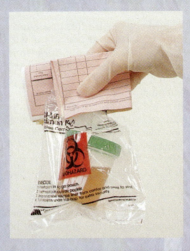

FIGURE 14-20 Specimens are transported to the laboratory in a sealed plastic transport bag with a biohazard label.

| **PROCEDURE** **57** | Collecting a Routine Urine Specimen | |

1. Perform your beginning procedure actions.
2. Gather supplies needed: specimen collection container, label, transport bag, bedpan, urinal, commode or specimen collection device, plastic bag for waste disposal, gloves.
3. Complete the label and put it on the container.
4. Ask the resident to urinate into the collection device. Instruct the resident not to place toilet tissue into the specimen. Provide a plastic bag for this purpose.
5. Provide privacy and make sure the call signal and toilet tissue are within reach.
6. Return immediately when the resident signals.
7. Open the specimen collection container and place the lid on the counter, with the top side down.
8. Apply gloves.
9. Take the container of urine to the toilet and raise the seat.
10. Measure the urine if the resident is on intake and output.
11. Hold the specimen collection container over the toilet. Pour the urine into the collection container. The container should be about three-quarters full. Discard the rest of the urine into the toilet.
12. Put the lid on the specimen container. Place it on a paper towel on the counter **(Figure 14-21)**.
13. Rinse and disinfect the bedpan or other container according to facility policy.
14. Remove one glove and place the specimen into the transport bag with your gloved hand. Avoid touching the outside of the bag with your glove. Handle the transport bag with your ungloved hand.
15. Remove the other glove and discard according to facility policy. (Gloves can be discarded in the plastic bag with toilet tissue.)
16. Wash your hands.
17. Record output, if the resident is on intake and output.
18. Perform your procedure completion actions.
19. Discard the plastic bag containing the waste in the biohazardous waste container.
20. Take the specimen to the designated location.
21. Report that the specimen was collected, and report any abnormalities to the nurse.

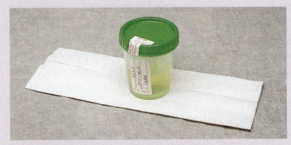

FIGURE 14-21 To prevent environmental contamination, place the specimen collection cup on a paper towel.

PROCEDURE 58

Collecting the Midstream (Clean-Catch) Urine Specimen

Note: The guidelines and sequence for this procedure vary slightly from state to state. Your instructor will inform you if the sequence in your state differs from the procedure listed here. Know and follow the required sequence for your state.

1. Perform your beginning procedure actions.
2. Gather supplies needed: midstream specimen kit, or other equipment used by your facility; bedpan; urinal or commode; transport bag; plastic bag for waste disposal; gloves.
3. Open the specimen collection kit. Remove the specimen collection container. Apply gloves.
4. Remove the towelettes or swabs from the collection kit.
5. Clean the penis or female perineal area with the swabs or towelettes, using the guidelines in Procedure 41 or 42. Use each swab or towelette once, then discard in a plastic bag. Do not place the used swabs near the clean kit. Discard in a plastic bag after use.
6. In a female resident, keep the labia separated until the specimen has been collected. In an uncircumcised male resident, keep the foreskin retracted until the specimen is collected.
7. Explain the procedure to the resident and ask him or her to begin urinating into the toilet or other container. Ask the resident to stop the stream. Hold the collection cup under the urethra without touching the body, and collect the specimen. Ask the resident to stop urinating, and re-

move the container. Instruct the resident to finish urinating in the toilet. Assist the resident to use toilet tissue, if necessary.
8. Put the lid on the specimen container. Place it on a paper towel on the counter.
9. Remove gloves and discard according to facility policy.
10. Wash your hands.
11. Assist the resident to wash his or her hands and return to bed, if necessary.
12. Wash your hands and apply clean gloves.
13. Rinse and disinfect the bedpan or other container, if used, according to facility policy.
14. Remove one glove and place the specimen into the transport bag with your gloved hand. Avoid touching the outside of the bag with your glove. Handle the transport bag with your ungloved hand.
15. Remove the other glove and discard according to facility policy.
16. Wash your hands.
17. Record output, if the resident is on intake and output.
18. Perform your procedure completion actions.
19. Discard the plastic bag containing the waste in the biohazardous waste container.
20. Take the specimen to the designated location.
21. Report that the specimen was collected, and report any abnormalities to the nurse.

GASTROINTESTINAL SYSTEM

Excretion of wastes from the gastrointestinal system **(Figure 14-22)** is called *bowel elimination.* A process called **peristalsis** moves the food from the upper end of the gastrointestinal system to the lower end. Peristalsis is caused by the contraction and relaxation of the muscles in the intestines. As the muscles contract, the food is propelled downward in the system. Food and fluids are taken in orally and partially digested by the stomach. They are mixed with digestive juices, then move from the stomach to the small intestine, where nutrients are absorbed and more digestion takes place. The food mass passes to the large intestine, where extra water is absorbed. After the liquid is absorbed, the solid food mass is called **feces.** The

feces moves from the large intestine to the rectum, where it is stored until it is excreted through the **anus.** Additional water is absorbed from the stool in the rectum. The waste material excreted may be called feces, **fecal material, stool,** or **bowel movement (BM).** The process of eliminating the waste from the anus is called **defecation.**

Bowel Elimination

The frequency of bowel movements varies with the individual. Some people have more than one bowel movement a day. Others have a bowel movement every two or three days. Fecal material is usually brown, but this color can be affected by certain foods, medications, and diseases. The bowel movement is normally soft and

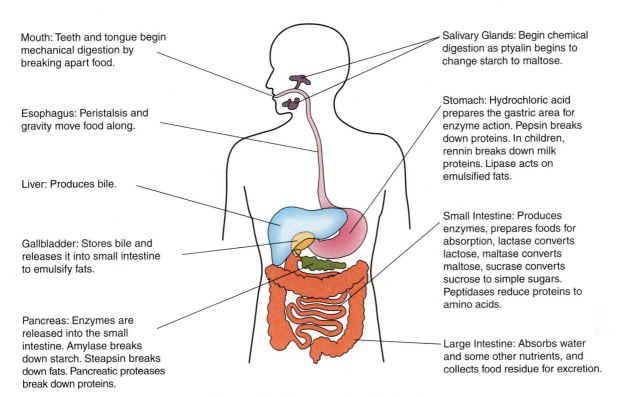

Mouth: Teeth and tongue begin mechanical digestion by breaking apart food.

Esophagus: Peristalsis and gravity move food along.

Liver: Produces bile.

Gallbladder: Stores bile and releases it into small intestine to emulsify fats.

Pancreas: Enzymes are released into the small intestine. Amylase breaks down starch. Steapsin breaks down fats. Pancreatic proteases break down proteins.

Salivary Glands: Begin chemical digestion as ptyalin begins to change starch to maltose.

Stomach: Hydrochloric acid prepares the gastric area for enzyme action. Pepsin breaks down proteins. In children, rennin breaks down milk proteins. Lipase acts on emulsified fats.

Small Intestine: Produces enzymes, prepares foods for absorption, lactase converts lactose, maltase converts maltose, sucrase converts sucrose to simple sugars. Peptidases reduce proteins to amino acids.

Large Intestine: Absorbs water and some other nutrients, and collects food residue for excretion.

FIGURE 14-22 The gastrointestinal system

formed. If it passes through the colon too quickly, the stool is loose and watery. Passage of frequent liquid stools is called **diarrhea.** If it passes through too slowly, the fecal material becomes hard, dry, or sticky and pasty in consistency. This is called constipation. Certain foods, medications, infections, and diseases can cause constipation and diarrhea.

Flatus is intestinal gas. As foods move through the gastrointestinal tract by peristalsis, gas is formed. When the gas is expelled from the body, it is called "passing flatus," or flatulence. If the gas is not passed, it accumulates in the abdomen. The abdomen will enlarge and appear bloated. This is called **abdominal distention,** and is an important observation to report to the nurse. Abdominal distention may also be caused by constipation and urinary retention.

Observations to Make when Assisting Residents with Bowel Elimination. You must observe the color, odor, character, and consistency of the resident's bowel movement before discarding it. Notify the nurse if it has an unusual color, odor, or volume, or if blood, mucus, parasites, or food particles are present (except corn and raisins) in the stool. If you think a stool is abnormal, save the specimen for the nurse to assess.

COMMON PROBLEMS RELATED TO THE GASTROINTESTINAL SYSTEM

The most common problems in the gastrointestinal system are related to constipation, diarrhea, and excessive flatulence. Other problems are caused by cancer, diseases, and trauma.

Constipation and Fecal Impaction

Report problems with constipation to the nurse. If the resident has not had a bowel movement in more than three days, must strain to pass stool, or passes hard, marble-like stools, this is an indication of constipation. **Fecal impaction (Figure 14-23)** is the most serious form of constipation. This is caused by retention of stool in the rectum. Water is absorbed in the rectum, causing the fecal mass to become hard and dry. The resident may be unable to pass it. The resident may complain of abdominal or rectal pain, nausea, or lack of appetite. Sometimes fecal impaction will cause mental confusion and fever. Other signs and symptoms of fecal impaction are passing excessive flatus, bloating, frequent urination, inability to empty the bladder, or leaking around the catheter. Residents may complain of

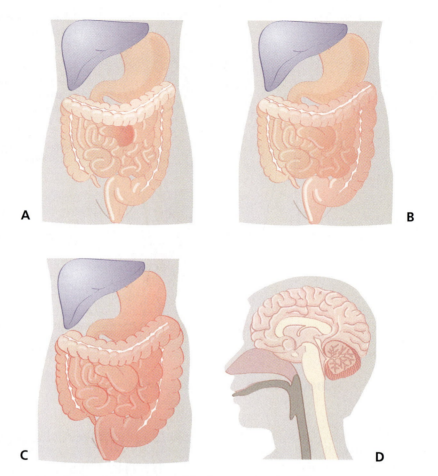

FIGURE 14-23 Progression of a fecal impaction, a life-threatening condition: **A.** A fecal impaction blocks the rectum. The rectum and sigmoid colon become enlarged. **B.** The colon continues to enlarge. **C.** Fecal material fills the colon. Digested and undigested food back up into the small intestines and stomach. The resident has signs and symptoms of acute illness, including lethargy, distention, constipation, and pain that is dull and cramping. **D.** The entire system is full, and the resident vomits fecal material. The feces are commonly aspirated into the lungs. At this point, the condition is life-threatening.

feeling the need to have a bowel movement, but being unable to do so. Eventually, liquid stool begins to seep from the rectum. This is easily mistaken for diarrhea. It occurs because liquid feces pass through the colon to the rectum, but are obstructed by the hard fecal mass. The rectum becomes so full that the fluid escapes around the impaction and is eliminated from the body. Fecal impaction is a very serious condition that is usually treated by manual removal of the mass by the nurse. Laxatives and enemas are also used to treat fecal impaction. The best thing to do is observe the resident's bowel elimination carefully and prevent fecal impaction from occurring.

Diarrhea

Diarrhea occurs when peristalsis in the intestines is very rapid. The need to defecate may be very urgent if the resident has diarrhea. The resident may also complain of abdominal pain and cramping. Some residents may become incontinent because of the force with which the fecal material moves through the intestines.

Diarrhea can cause dehydration and other serious medical problems if undetected or untreated. Most health care facilities do not consider one loose stool to be diarrhea. Diarrhea is usually defined as three or more loose stools in a designated period of time. Remember to be objective in reporting your observations. When reporting loose stools to the nurse, report the color, odor, consistency, character, amount, and frequency of stools. Also report any resident complaints of pain or other discomfort. If the resident is on intake and output, you may be asked to record the output from diarrhea. Use a specimen collection hat or graduate. Select PPE appropriate to the task. Avoid showing disgust for the procedure. Maintain a professional demeanor.

Changes in Function of the Gastrointestinal System Associated with Aging and Disease

Change in bowel function may be caused by aging, disease, surgery, diet, and medications. Lack of privacy may also affect the resident's ability to have a bowel movement. In aging, movement in the colon is decreased. Food absorption is slowed, and fewer digestive juices are produced. Constipation is a common problem. Other factors that affect bowel function are:

- Bed rest
- Inactivity
- Inadequate exercise
- Inability to chew foods properly
- Loose or missing teeth
- Inadequate fluid intake
- Stress
- Change in environment
- Change in diet

A diet that does not contain enough fiber, fruits, or vegetables may cause constipation and other nutritional problems.

Bowel Incontinence

Bowel incontinence is involuntary passage of fecal material from the anus. It has many causes, including trauma, neurological diseases, inability to reach the toilet quickly, and mental confusion. Fecal material is very irritating to the skin, so the resident must be cleansed well after each episode of incontinence. Skin exposed to fecal material will break down quickly. Bowel incontinence may lower the resident's self-esteem. Be professional, compassionate, and understanding when assisting residents with bowel elimination and incontinence.

ROLE OF THE NURSING ASSISTANT IN ASSISTING RESIDENTS WITH BOWEL ELIMINATION

Assisting with bowel elimination is a very important responsibility. Always apply the principles of standard precautions when assisting with

GUIDELINES FOR
Assisting Residents with Bowel Elimination

- Apply the principles of standard precautions when assisting with bowel elimination. Avoid contaminating the environment with your gloves.
- Encourage residents to consume an adequate amount of fluid. Maintaining fluid intake is as important for bowel elimination as it is for urinary elimination.
- Encourage residents to eat a well-balanced diet.
- Allow adequate time for residents to eat meals.
- Encourage residents to chew food well. Cut food into small pieces if necessary. Report chewing problems to the nurse for further assessment.
- If you observe that a resident has not eaten fiber foods, fruits, or vegetables, offer a substitute. The dietitian may have to visit the resident to discuss likes and dislikes and assure that the resident will eat the foods served.
- Encourage exercise and activity as allowed and as tolerated.
- Assist residents with toileting at regular intervals and provide privacy.
- Position residents in a sitting position, if allowed, for bowel elimination.
- Use a bath blanket to cover residents when using the bedpan or commode, for privacy and warmth.
- Leave the call signal and toilet tissue within reach and respond to the call signal immediately.
- Allow adequate time for defecation.

- Provide perineal care as needed, or according to facility policy. Fecal material is very irritating to the skin and promotes skin breakdown and infection.
- Assist residents with cleaning the anal area (this may be called the rectal area by some health care providers).
- Assist residents with handwashing and other personal hygiene after bowel elimination.
- Monitor bowel elimination and report irregularities.
- Record bowel movements on the flow sheet or other designated location. If a resident is independent with bowel elimination, ask if he or she has had a bowel movement each day. In some facilities, the size of the bowel elimination is documented. The most common measurements used are small, medium, large, and extra large. Your facility will have guidelines for these amounts. In general, small is a 3-inch elimination, medium is a 6-inch elimination, large is a 9-inch elimination, and extra large is a 12-inch elimination.
- Report frequent stools, absence of stools, pain, cramping, excessive flatulence, abnormal color or consistency of stool, extremely small amounts of stool, hard, dry stool, or enlargement of the abdomen to the nurse.
- Specific abnormalities in stools to report are presence of blood, pus, mucus, black or other unusual color, undigested food (except corn and raisins), or presence of parasites in the stool.

elimination. Avoid contaminating environmental surfaces with your gloves. Wear a gown, eye protection, and face mask if splashing is likely.

ENEMAS

An **enema** is the introduction of fluid into the lower bowel to cleanse the anus, rectum, and lower colon. Enemas are ordered by the physician and are used to relieve constipation and empty the colon before some tests and surgeries. Occasionally, enemas are given to relieve excessive flatulence. The physician always specifies the type of enema to give and the solution to use. The nursing assistant is responsible for administering enemas in many health care facilities. Always apply the principles of standard precautions when you are performing this procedure. Avoid contaminating environmental surfaces with your gloves.

A **cleansing enema** removes fecal material from the rectum and lower bowel. It also stimulates peristalsis and softens stool. A water-based solution is used in a cleansing enema. The cleansing enema is administered through a special enema bag or other container.

A **retention enema** may be given for constipation or fecal impaction. An oil-based solution, packaged in a small, commercial container, is used for the retention enema. The purpose of this enema is to soften hard stool and gently

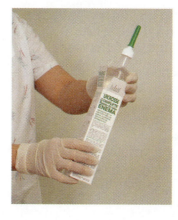

FIGURE 14-24
A commercially prepared enema

stimulate evacuation. The enema lubricates the rectum, making it easier to pass the stool.

Commercially prepared enemas (Figure 14-24) are administered in small, premeasured containers. Commercially prepared enemas are available with either cleansing or retention enema solutions.

The **Sims' position (Figure 14-25)** is a side-lying position used for giving enemas,

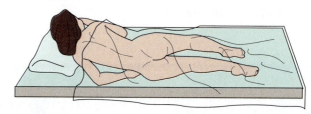

FIGURE 14-25   The Sims' position is used for enema administration and rectal treatments.

GUIDELINES FOR
Enema Administration

- Apply the principles of standard precautions. Avoid contaminating the environment with your gloves.
- Administer an enema only upon the direction of a licensed nurse.
- Avoid giving an enema within an hour after a meal, because the increased peristalsis makes it difficult for the resident to retain the solution. Avoid administering an enema to a resident who is in a sitting position, such as on the toilet. The solution will not flow high into the colon when administered to a resident who is seated. It will cause the rectum to enlarge, causing rapid expulsion of the fluid.
- Consult the care plan or nurse for the amount and type of solution to use and any special instructions.
- Provide privacy. Cover the resident with a bath blanket.
- Check the temperature of a water-based solution with a bath thermometer. The solution temperature should be 105°F.

- Commercially prepared enemas can be administered at room temperature, or warmed by placing the container in a basin of warm water.
- Lubricate the tip of the enema tubing well with a water-based lubricant before inserting it into the rectum. Most disposable units are prelubricated. However, if the tip appears dry, apply additional lubricant before inserting it into the rectum.
- Insert the enema tube gently into the rectum. The tube should be inserted two to four inches. If you meet resistance, do not force the tube. Remove it and consult the nurse.
- An enema in a bag should be raised 12 to 16 inches above the rectum **(Figure 14-26)**. Follow your facility policy.
- Administer the enema solution slowly. Instruct the resident to inhale and breathe in slowly through the nose and exhale through the mouth. If the resident

Continues

GUIDELINES FOR
Enema Administration, *Continued*

complains of pain, stop the solution briefly before proceeding. If the pain is severe or persistent, stop the solution and notify the nurse.

- Hold the enema tubing in place with your gloved hand when administering the solution.
- Instruct the resident to retain the enema solution for the designated time.
- Ensure that the bathroom, bedside commode, or bedpan are readily available.
- Assist the resident to a sitting position on the bedpan, commode, or toilet, if possible, to expel the enema.
- Leave the resident alone to expel the enema solution, if doing so is safe. Place the signal light and toilet tissue within reach.
- Respond promptly when the resident signals.
- Save the enema results for the nurse to observe before discarding.
- Assist the resident to cleanse the perineal area and wash hands after the enema has been expelled.

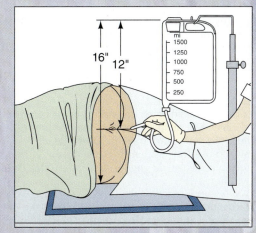

FIGURE 14-26 Hang the enema bag 12 to 16 inches above the rectum.

PROCEDURE **59**	## Administering a Cleansing Enema	

Note: In some states, nursing assistants are not permitted to perform this procedure. Additionally, the policies of some facilities state that only licensed nurses may perform rectal treatments, including enemas. Perform this procedure only if you are permitted to do so by state law and facility policies.

1. Perform your beginning procedure actions.
2. Gather supplies needed: assembled enema kit, prescribed solution, water-soluble lubricant, bath blanket, bath thermometer, bed protector, bedpan, toilet tissue, washcloth, towel, washbasin, paper towel, plastic bag, gloves.
3. Close the clamp on the enema container.
4. Prepare the enema solution in the bathroom or utility room, according to facility policy. Fill the enema container with water in the specified amount. This usually varies from 500 to 1500 mL, but more or less solution can be used. Follow the nurse's instructions. Check the water temperature with a bath thermometer. It should be 105°F.
5. If you are instructed to administer a soapsuds enema, empty the contents of the soap packet into the container *after* the water has been added. Squeeze and agitate the bag slightly to mix the solution.
6. Open the clamp on the tubing and allow the solution to flow through the tubing to the tip, to prevent the injection of air into the body. Close the clamp when the solution begins to flow through the tip.

7. Take the solution to the bedside. Squeeze some water-soluble lubricant onto a paper towel or gauze sponge.
8. Place the bed protector under the buttocks. Cover the upper bedding with a bath blanket, then remove the linen from under the blanket without exposing the resident.
9. Assist the resident into the Sims' position and ensure that he or she is comfortable.
10. Apply gloves.
11. Expose the rectal area.
12. Remove the cap from the end of the tubing, and lubricate the tube if it is not prelubricated. If the tip appears dry, apply extra lubricant.
13. Separate the buttocks to expose the anal area.
14. Tell the resident you are going to insert the tube and ask him or her to take a deep breath and then exhale.
15. Gently insert the enema tubing two to four inches while the resident exhales.
16. Hold the solution 12 to 16 inches above the rectum, or according to facility policy.
17. Unclamp the tubing and allow the solution to flow into the rectum. Instruct the resident to try to relax and retain the solution.
18. Allow the desired amount of solution to flow into the rectum. When the fluid level reaches the bottom of the bag, clamp the tubing to avoid injecting air into the rectum.

Continues

PROCEDURE 59
Administering a Cleansing Enema, *Continued*

19. Remove the tubing and insert the tip into the enema administration container.
20. Instruct the resident to retain the solution for the designated amount of time.
21. Place the enema container in a plastic bag.
22. Remove your gloves and place them in the plastic bag.
23. Assist the resident to the bathroom or commode, or place the bedpan. Instruct the resident not to flush the toilet after expelling the enema.
24. Make sure the resident is safe, warm, and comfortable. Leave the signal light and toilet tissue within reach.
25. Wash your hands.
26. Leave the room if doing so is safe. Take the plastic bag containing the enema container and gloves and discard it in the biohazardous waste.
27. Return immediately when the resident signals.
28. Apply gloves and assist the resident with cleansing and perineal care.
29. Remove one glove or use a paper towel to turn on the faucet, and assist the resident with hand-washing.

30. Remove the bed protector with the gloved hand, and discard according to facility policy.
31. Remove the other glove and discard according to facility policy.
32. Wash your hands.
33. Assist the resident back to bed, or position the resident in bed for comfort and safety.
34. Observe the results of the enema and save them for the nurse, or discard according to facility policy.
35. Perform your procedure completion actions.
36. Observe and report to the nurse:
    - Type of enema and amount of solution
    - Results of the enema, estimated amount of solution returned, amount and consistency of stool
    - Unusual observations (if noted, save the returns for the nurse to assess)
    - Presence of blood, mucus, undigested food (except corn and raisins), or parasites in stool
    - Resident's response to the procedure

PROCEDURE 60
Administering a Commercially Prepared Enema

Note: In some states, nursing assistants are not permitted to perform this procedure. Additionally, the policies of some facilities state that only licensed nurses may perform rectal treatments, including enemas. Perform this procedure only if you are permitted to do so by state law and facility policies.

1. Perform your beginning procedure actions.
2. Gather supplies needed: commercial enema, water-soluble lubricant, bath blanket, bed protector, bedpan, toilet tissue, washcloth, towel, washbasin, plastic bag, paper towel, gloves.
3. Warm the container of enema solution in a basin of warm water, if this is your facility policy. Dry the outside of the container.
4. Take the solution to the bedside.
5. Place the bed protector under the buttocks. Cover the upper bedding with a bath blanket, then remove the linen from under the blanket without exposing the resident.
6. Assist the resident into the Sims' position and ensure that he or she is comfortable.

7. Apply gloves.
8. Expose the rectal area.
9. Remove the cap from the end of the container and lubricate the tip, if it is not prelubricated.
10. Separate the buttocks to expose the anal area.
11. Tell the resident you are going to insert the tube and ask him or her to take a deep breath and then exhale.
12. Gently insert the tip of the container while the resident exhales.
13. Gently squeeze and roll the container until the desired quantity of solution is administered. A small amount of solution will remain in the container. Avoid releasing pressure on the container, or the solution will return.
14. Instruct the resident to hold his or her breath, then gently remove the tip of the container.
15. Place the enema container in a plastic bag to avoid contamination.
16. Remove your gloves and place them in the plastic bag.

Continues

Administering a Commercially Prepared Enema, *Continued*

17. Assist the resident to the bathroom or commode, or place the bedpan. Instruct the resident not to flush the toilet after expelling the enema.
18. Make sure the resident is safe, warm, and comfortable. Leave the signal light and toilet tissue within reach.
19. Wash your hands.
20. Leave the room if doing so is safe. Take the plastic bag containing the enema container and gloves, and discard it in the biohazardous waste.
21. Return immediately when the resident signals.
22. Apply gloves and assist the resident with cleansing and perineal care.
23. Remove one glove or use a paper towel to turn on the faucet, and assist the resident with handwashing.
24. Remove the bed protector with the gloved hand and discard it according to facility policy.

25. Remove the other glove and discard it according to facility policy.
26. Wash your hands.
27. Assist the resident back to bed, or position the resident in bed for comfort and safety.
28. Observe the results of the enema and save for the nurse, or discard according to facility policy.
29. Perform your procedure completion actions.
30. Observe and report to the nurse:
    - Type of enema and amount of solution
    - Results of the enema, estimated amount of solution returned, and amount and consistency of stool
    - Unusual observations (if noted, save the returns for the nurse to assess)
    - Presence of blood, mucus, undigested food (except corn and raisins), or parasites in stool
    - Resident's response to the procedure

rectal examinations, and other rectal treatments. This position promotes evacuation of the bowel. To assist a resident into the Sims' position, turn him or her onto the left side. Position the shoulder, arm, and hip for comfort. Bend the right leg at the knee and flex the leg forward slightly.

COLLECTING A STOOL SPECIMEN

Stool specimens are collected and analyzed by the laboratory for presence of blood, parasites, fat, bacteria, and other abnormalities. Analysis of the stool assists the physician with diagnosis and treatment. The resident is instructed to defecate in a specimen collection device, commode, or bedpan. The stool is then transferred into the specimen collection container and packaged according to facility policy prior to transport to the laboratory. The resident should be instructed not to urinate into the stool specimen. Follow the general guidelines for collecting a urine specimen when collecting a stool specimen. Apply the principles of standard precautions. Some stool specimens must be analyzed while warm, so they must be transported to the laboratory immediately. Check with the care plan or nurse for special directions for the type of specimen you are collecting.

CARING FOR RESIDENTS WITH OSTOMIES

An **ostomy** is a surgically created opening into the body. There are many types of ostomies **(Figure 14-27)**. Some are performed for bowel elimination. These are usually done because of cancer, bowel disease, and trauma. The opening to the outside of the body is called a **stoma.** An ostomy may be temporary or permanent. The location of the ostomy is determined by the part of the colon that is injured or diseased.

In most facilities, a licensed nurse will care for a newly created ostomy. However, in residents with well-established ostomies, the nursing assistant is usually responsible for caring for the area. Know and follow your facility policy.

Colostomies

The **colostomy** is the most common type of ostomy. This ostomy is located between the colon and the abdomen. The intestines are brought to the outside of the body to create the stoma. A bag is attached to the stoma to collect fecal material. When the ostomy is first performed, the stool is loose and watery, but becomes soft and formed over time. The amount of liquid in the stool is also determined by how much of the colon remains after surgery. If a large amount of colon is left, the

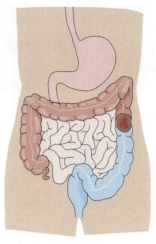
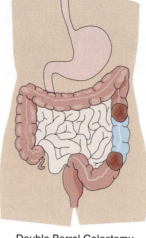
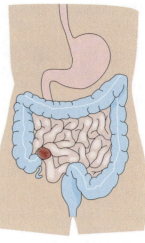

Colostomy   Double Barrel Colostomy   Ileostomy

FIGURE 14-27 The location of the ostomy determines the amount of water in the stool. The double-barrel colostomy is usually temporary. After the digestive system rests, the intestines are surgically reconnected.

colon will absorb water and the stools will be formed. If most of the colon has been removed, the body will be unable to absorb the water in the stool, so the stools in the ostomy are more liquid. Flatus is also passed through the stoma.

Many people live successfully for years with an ostomy, but this type of surgery is very difficult for the resident to adjust to psychologically. Residents are often upset by this change in normal function. They worry about the appliance

---

PROCEDURE 61

Collecting a Stool Specimen

1. Perform your beginning procedure actions.
2. Gather needed supplies: bedpan and cover, commode, or specimen collection pan; specimen container with lid; transport bag; tongue blade; toilet tissue; plastic bag; gloves.
3. Complete the label and put it on the container.
4. Ask the resident to defecate into the designated collection device. Instruct him or her not to discard toilet tissue into the collection device. Provide a plastic bag for this purpose.
5. Provide privacy and make sure the call signal and toilet tissue are within reach.
6. Return immediately when the resident signals.
7. Apply gloves and remove the stool specimen collection container.
8. Provide a clean container or bedpan for urination, if necessary. Allow the resident to urinate. Provide privacy.
9. Cover the specimen collection container and assist the resident with cleansing, returning to bed, or positioning. Wear gloves and apply the principles of standard precautions if appropriate to the activity.
10. Take the collection device to the bathroom or other designated location according to facility policy.
11. Open the specimen collection cup and place the lid on the counter, with the top side down.
12. Apply gloves.
13. Uncover the container. Use the tongue blade to remove the feces from the collection device and place it in the specimen container. About two tablespoons of stool are necessary. Taking a small sample from each part of the stool is best. Discard the tongue blade in the plastic bag.
14. Put the lid on the specimen container. Place the container on a paper towel on the counter.
15. Rinse and disinfect the bedpan or collection container according to facility policy.
16. Remove one glove and place the specimen into the transport bag with your gloved hand. Avoid touching the outside of the bag with your glove. Handle the transport bag with your ungloved hand.
17. Remove the other glove and discard according to facility policy.
18. Wash your hands.
19. Perform your procedure completion actions.
20. Discard the plastic bag containing the waste in the biohazardous waste container.
21. Take the specimen to the designated location.
22. Report that the specimen was collected, and report any abnormalities to the nurse.

showing under their clothing. They also worry about odors and sounds that are offensive. The resident may have to adjust the diet to avoid gas-forming foods. Adjusting a dietary pattern that a person has established over a lifetime may be difficult. The resident with an ostomy requires you to be very professional, tactful, patient, and understanding.

The Ostomy Appliance. The ostomy **appliance (Figure 14-28)** is the plastic container into which the contents of the bowel are emptied. It is fastened to the body with a belt or a self-adhesive seal around the bag. Remember that fecal material is very irritating to the skin. A new ostomy is sore and tender. The fecal material, particularly liquid stool, causes additional irritation. Even established ostomies become irritated from the combination of fecal material and adhesive on the skin. The care plan will guide you in caring for the ostomy. Report redness or skin irritation to the nurse. Always apply the principles of standard precautions when caring for the ostomy appliance.

Odors from ostomies are a particular problem. Good personal hygiene is essential. The skin around the stoma is washed and dried well each time the bag is removed. A special skin bar-

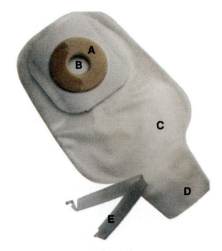

A. Adhesive ring seals around stoma to prevent leakage
B. Opening placed over stoma
C. Collection bag
D. Drainage end of bag
E. Secures drainage end of bag to prevent leakage

FIGURE 14-28 A disposable ostomy appliance

rier product may also be used. The used bag is discarded in the biohazardous waste. Various deodorizing products are available to place inside the bag to reduce or eliminate odors.

GUIDELINES FOR
Caring for an Ostomy

- Apply the principles of standard precautions. Avoid contaminating the environment with your gloves.
- Remove and apply the ostomy appliance gently to prevent irritation to the skin. It may help to apply gentle traction to the skin next to the appliance when you are removing the adhesive.
- Empty the reusable bag and wash it thoroughly with soap and water after each bowel movement. Secure the clamp at the bottom of the bag to prevent leaking. Discard a disposable bag in the biohazardous waste and replace it with a new bag.
- Observe the skin around the stoma for redness, irritation, and skin breakdown, and report to the nurse.
- After the appliance has been removed, gently wipe the area surrounding the stoma with toilet tissue. Discard the tissue in the toilet or a plastic bag. If a

plastic bag is used, discard it in the biohazardous waste.
- Wash the skin around the stoma with mild soap when the appliance is removed. Rinse well and gently pat dry.
- Apply skin barriers, lubricants, or medicated creams to the area surrounding the stoma as stated on the care plan. Apply only a thin layer. Avoid caking the products on the skin.
- You may be required to cut an opening into the appliance before applying it to the skin. Cut the area about ⅛-inch larger than the size of the stoma.
- When reapplying a new appliance, seal the entire area surrounding the stoma to prevent leaking.
- Observe the color, character, amount, and frequency of stools, and report abnormalities to the nurse.

KEY POINTS

- The urinary system regulates water in the body and filters waste products from the blood and eliminates them from the body.
- The average adult eliminates 1500 mL of urine from the body each day. Additional fluid is lost in respiration, perspiration, and bowel elimination.
- The nursing assistant must be professional, sensitive, and understanding when assisting residents with elimination needs.
- Incontinence is a medical problem.
- Urinary tract infections are more common in women than in men because the female urethra is shorter.
- Residents with catheters are at high risk of infection because the catheter provides an opening directly into the bladder.
- Maintaining sterility of the catheter by using aseptic technique is a very important responsibility.
- A graduate is used to accurately measure urinary output.
- Feces is a solid waste product eliminated through the digestive system.
- Constipation, fecal impaction, and diarrhea are common problems that the nursing assistant will assist with.
- The resident's self-esteem is affected by problems with elimination, and the nursing assistant must be professional, sensitive, and compassionate in meeting the resident's needs.
- An enema is an injection of fluid into the rectum to cleanse the lower bowel.
- An ostomy is a surgically created opening into the body. Several different types of ostomies are used to treat disorders of bowel elimination.

REVIEW

A. Multiple Choice

Select the one best answer.

1. The urinary system
   a. removes solid waste from the digestive tract.
   b. removes waste from the blood and regulates water in the body.
   c. recirculates waste products through the system.
   d. removes waste from the pancreas and intestines.

2. The average adult eliminates
   a. 500 mL of urine per day.
   b. 1000 mL of urine per day.
   c. 1500 mL of urine per day.
   d. 4500 mL of urine per day.

3. Which of the following affect urinary elimination?
   a. starches
   b. salt
   c. sugars
   d. high-fiber foods

4. Incontinence
   a. occurs naturally in aging.
   b. is always a psychological problem.
   c. is a medical problem.
   d. always occurs when residents are confused.

5. Aging and disease may affect
   a. length of the urethra.
   b. the kidney's ability to filter efficiently.
   c. color of urine.
   d. clarity of urine.

6. A common cause of urge incontinence is
   a. infection.
   b. multiple childbirths.
   c. physical inability to get to the bathroom.
   d. lifting heavy objects.

7. Which of the following are signs or symptoms of urinary tract infection?
   a. diarrhea
   b. voiding frequently in small amounts
   c. vomiting
   d. profuse sweating

8. A container that the male resident uses for urination in bed is the
   a. urinal.
   b. regular bedpan.
   c. fracture bedpan.
   d. indwelling catheter.

9. A catheter is used
   a. for staff convenience.
   b. to drain urine from the bladder.
   c. to obstruct the bladder so urine cannot escape.
   d. only for diagnostic tests.

10. The inside of the unopened closed drainage system is
    a. clean.
    b. contaminated.
    c. septic.
    d. sterile.

11. When a resident is in bed, the catheter drainage bag should be positioned
    a. above the level of the bladder.
    b. on the bed frame above the floor.
    c. on the side rail above the floor.
    d. on the floor.

12. When caring for a catheter, you should practice
    a. contact precautions.
    b. airborne precautions.
    c. medical asepsis.
    d. isolation technique.

13. The catheter should always be
    a. secured to the resident's body.
    b. opened and cleaned twice a day.
    c. washed from bottom to top with alcohol.
    d. drained every two hours.

14. The adhesive strip that secures the external catheter to the penis should be wrapped
    a. in a circle.
    b. diagonally.
    c. in a spiral.
    d. very tightly.

15. Condom catheters should be disposed of in the
    a. trash can in the resident's room.
    b. biohazardous waste.
    c. puncture-resistant container.
    d. sanitary sewer.

16. You are assigned to measure urinary output on Mr. Davis, a resident with an indwelling catheter. To obtain an accurate measurement, you should
    a. record the level of urine according to the markings on the catheter bag.
    b. empty the catheter bag into a bedpan.
    c. withdraw the urine with a syringe.
    d. empty the catheter bag into a graduate.

17. When preparing to collect a midstream urine specimen from a female resident, you should wipe the labia
    a. from front to back.
    b. from back to front.
    c. back and forth.
    d. from side to side.

18. Water is absorbed from fecal material in the
    a. stomach.
    b. small intestine.
    c. large intestine.
    d. liver.

19. The medical term for passing gas is
    a. impaction.
    b. distention.
    c. flatulence.
    d. obstruction.

20. The most serious form of constipation is
    a. flatulence.
    b. impaction.
    c. distention.
    d. diarrhea.

21. Which of the following affect normal bowel elimination?
    a. sugar in food
    b. inadequate fluid intake
    c. confusion
    d. skin breakdown

22. The enema tubing is inserted into the rectum
    a. 1 to 2 inches.
    b. 2 to 4 inches.
    c. 4 to 6 inches.
    d. 6 to 8 inches.

23. The opening of a colostomy to the outside of the body is called the
    a. rectum.
    b. insertion site.
    c. stoma.
    d. appliance.

24. Fecal material is
    a. very irritating to the skin.
    b. normally liquid.
    c. excreted through the urethra.
    d. hard and pasty.

25. The ostomy appliance is
    a. an irrigating device.
    b. similar to a catheter.
    c. difficult to apply.
    d. a plastic bag.

B. Clinical Applications

Answer the following questions.

26. Mr. Hoover is a 76-year-old confused resident. He ambulates in his room and is normally pleasant and talkative, even though he does not always make sense. He recognizes you as his primary caregiver. Mr. Hoover uses the urinal for elimination. When you enter his room to give AM care, you find him sleeping in the chair, which is unusual. His skin is hot to the touch and he is lethargic. He does not speak or answer your questions. You notice his urinal on the floor next to his chair. The urine in the urinal is reddish in color with mucus threads in it. What should you do?

27. Mrs. Sanders tells you that she has burning on urination. You notice that she is voiding every 30 to 45 minutes in small amounts. What do you think is wrong? What should you do?

28. Miss Gonzalez has just started eating her breakfast. The nurse instructs you to give the resident an enema this morning. What should you do?

29. Mr. Deck has a colostomy. You change the bag and care for the stoma each day. When you remove the self-adhesive bag, Mr. Deck flinches as if in pain. The area around the stoma is very red. What should you do?

30. You are assigned to collect a stat midstream urine specimen from Mrs. King. The resident accidentally contaminates the specimen with BM. What should you do?

CHAPTER 15

Restraints and Restraint Alternatives

OBJECTIVES

After reading this chapter, you will be able to:

- Spell and define key terms.
- Define restraints and list six reasons for using restraints.
- Describe when and how restraints are used as enablers.
- List the guidelines for using restraints.
- List the complications of restraint use.
- Define restraint alternative and describe when to use an alternative device.
- Demonstrate procedures related to restraints and restraint alternatives.

OBSERVATIONS TO MAKE AND REPORT RELATED TO RESTRAINTS AND RESTRAINT ALTERNATIVES

Need for Restraints or Restraint Alternatives

Decreased ability to see or hear
Lack of connection to or awareness of environment
Use of corrective devices and aids
Lack of communication ability
Agitation

Situation-specific problem behaviors
Discomfort
Loneliness, isolation, boredom
Need for assistance in standing or ambulation
Falls

During Restraint Use

Decreased independence, increased dependence on staff
Impaired circulation, skin breakdown
Pressure ulcers
Weakness
Decreased range of motion
Muscle atrophy (wasting)
Contractures
Decreased ability to ambulate
Edema
Decreased appetite
Weight loss
Distended abdomen

Incontinence
Constipation or fecal impaction
Increased or new-onset mental confusion
Lethargy
Restlessness
Crying, screaming, yelling
Depression
Irritability
Agitation, combativeness
Withdrawal
Forgetfulness
Ritualistic behavior

RESTRAINTS

Restraints are safety devices attached to or adjacent to the resident's body. Reasons for using restraints include:

- To prevent injury and falls.
- To prevent the resident from injuring himself or herself, or others.
- To prevent pulling on tubes, drains, wound coverings, or other forms of treatment.
- To maintain position when the resident is in bed or in a chair. Some residents are repositioned by staff, but quickly reposition themselves, causing complications or skin problems. Use of a restraint helps maintain position in some situations.
- To support the resident in good anatomical alignment to prevent discomfort and deformity.

Restraints are most commonly used to prevent falls and wandering, and to protect residents from injury. Some residents are unaware of hazards in the environment and unknowingly jeopardize their own safety as well as the safety of others.

Definition of Restraints

Restraints are physical, manual, or mechanical devices attached or adjacent to the resident's body. They cannot be removed easily by the resident and prevent access to the body. Restraints restrict freedom of movement. They are used to prevent injury to the resident and others, and allow medical treatment when the resident is confused and uncooperative. Restraints *may not* be used to force alert residents to accept specific treatments. Refusing a treatment is the resident's right, and a restraint is not used to administer treatment that an alert resident does not want. A physician's order is always needed for the use of restraints.

   Physical restraints (**Figure 15-1**) are devices applied to the resident's body or chairs that prevent the resident from standing. Side rails are physical restraints. Many devices can be considered restraints, even those that are marketed as

restraint alternatives. A device is considered a restraint if:

- It restricts access to the resident's body
- It restricts movement

or

- The resident does not have the physical or mental ability to remove it easily

Examples of restraints, using this definition, are:

- Raising side rails to prevent a resident from voluntarily getting out of bed
- Tucking in or using Velcro to hold a sheet, fabric, lap blanket, or clothing tightly so that a resident's movement is restricted
- Using devices in conjunction with a chair, such as overbed tables, trays, tables, pads, bars, or belts, that the resident cannot remove easily and that prevent the resident from rising
- Placing a resident in a chair that prevents the resident from rising, such as a beanbag chair, reclining chair, or geriatric chair
- Placing a chair or bed so close to a wall that the wall prevents the resident from rising out of the chair or voluntarily getting out of bed

Chemical restraints are drugs used for discipline and staff convenience and not required to treat a resident's medical symptoms. Tranquilizers and mood-altering drugs are chemical restraints. In some residents these drugs have the opposite effect from that intended. Instead of calming the resident, they may cause agitation. They also may make the resident very lethargic. Side effects from long-term use of these drugs can be very serious. Licensed nurses and advanced care providers are responsible for medication administration. This chapter will focus on the use of physical restraints.

   Enablers are devices that empower residents and assist them to function at their highest possible level. For example, a resident in a wheelchair is unable to sit up straight to feed himself or herself, so he or she is fed by staff. If a supportive device is applied to correct his or her posture and allow the resident to feed himself or herself, the device is an enabler. Devices used as enablers that maintain body position and alignment are commonly called **postural supports.** Used correctly, they give residents a higher degree of independence and enable them to perform tasks they were previously unable to do. In this case, using the restraint improves the resident's self-esteem.

   The wheelchair lap tray (**Figure 15-2**) is a simple-to-use restraint alternative that is also used as an enabler. The tray is attached to the

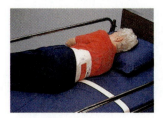

FIGURE 15-1 Physical restraints limit the resident's movement and access to her body. *(Courtesy of Skil-Care Corporation, Yonkers, NY, (800) 431-2972)*

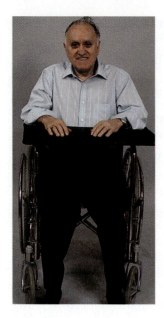

FIGURE 15-2 The Velcro lap tray is used as an enabler, restraint alternative, or restraint, depending on the resident's physical and mental ability. Some residents will push on the tray, releasing the Velcro straps. Because of this, using a lightweight tray is best. Heavy trays may cause injury to the legs and feet. *(Courtesy of Skil-Care Corporation, Yonkers, NY, (800) 431-2972)*

back of the wheelchair with Velcro straps. It can be used for residents to lean on, and it provides a surface to hold personal items and reading and writing supplies. A tray may enable the resident to feed himself or herself by moving the food closer so the resident can reach it. The tray serves as a reminder to the resident not to stand up. If the tray allows the resident to perform a task, it is an enabler. If it is used strictly to keep the resident in the chair, and the resident does not have the physical or mental ability to remove the tray, it is considered a restraint. If the tray can be removed by the resident, it is a restraint alternative.

Using Restraints

Unfortunately, most restraints are not used as enablers. They are commonly used to manage behavior problems, prevent wandering, and prevent falls. Several studies have shown that injuries related to falls are more severe in residents who are under restraint, compared with residents who are not restrained. Because residents tend to fight restraints, their behavior may be more aggressive than it was before the restraint was applied.

Before restraints are used, the staff must evaluate the resident's capabilities and the reasons for the restraint. If the reason for the resident's problem can be determined and corrected, the need for a restraint can be eliminated. For example, if use of restraints is being considered to prevent the resident from falling, all risk factors associated with falls are assessed. If some risk factors can be eliminated,

this reduces the risk of falls, and restraint use may not be necessary. For example, the evaluation reveals that the resident rushes to the bathroom and loses his balance, falling along the way. A urinalysis reveals a urinary tract infection, which is treated. A care plan is developed based on the resident's needs and risk factors. The care plan states:

- The urinal must always be within reach
- Staff must check the resident hourly and offer to take him to the bathroom
- A second urinal must be placed in a cabinet next to the chair where the resident sits to watch television
- A hand bell must be placed by the resident's chair so he can call for help easily

Eliminating these risk factors reduces the risk of falls. Once the care plan is initiated, the resident stops trying to go to the bathroom by himself and the falls stop. The need for restraints has been eliminated by meeting the resident's individual needs. No single approach will be effective in eliminating the use of restraints for all residents. The answer lies in identifying and meeting each resident's needs.

If a resident is a danger to himself or herself, or to others, or requires emergency medical treatment, restraints may be appropriate. However, less restrictive alternatives to restraints must be considered first. Sometimes the environment can be modified to avoid restraint use. Many alternative devices are available for use instead of restraints. If a restraint is determined to be the best approach, it is applied. However, the factors necessitating use of the restraint are continuously reevaluated, and the interdisciplinary team works to reduce or eliminate the need for the restraint.

If the interdisciplinary team determines that restraints are needed, the least restrictive restraint required to keep the resident safe should be selected. The restraint should be used as infrequently as possible. Using restraints requires careful assessment, care planning, and monitoring by members of the interdisciplinary team. Studies have proven that it takes more time to care for residents in restraints compared with residents who are not restrained. The physician must agree to the use of restraints and write an order before they can be used. The care plan will specify the type of restraint to use, the time the restraint is to be applied, and other special information and instructions.

Although a physician's order is needed for the use of restraints, there must be a medical reason for their use. The decision to use restraints is a joint one made by facility staff, the resident (if alert), responsible family members, and the physician. Family members cannot demand that a facility use restraints unless the resident has a valid, documented medical problem that necessitates the restraint. Restraint assessment must be done except in an emergency. Dealing with family members' emotions and threats may take the skills of the entire interdisciplinary team. Restraint requests can present a very delicate situation for the facility. The outcome can be negative if this request is not handled correctly. If a family member asks you to apply a restraint to a resident, inform the nurse promptly.

Factors to Evaluate and Risk Factors to Eliminate

The nursing assistant makes a valuable contribution to the interdisciplinary team's restraint assessment. Because you have the most direct contact with the residents, you may be in the best position to know what does and doesn't work in managing the problem that creates the need for the restraint.

Many commercial devices are available to use in place of restraints. Sometimes clothing or other items can be used as restraint alternatives. For example, a male resident who pulls at his urinary catheter can be fitted with boxer shorts. A resident with a feeding tube can be covered with a t-shirt or abdominal binder. A resident with an intravenous infusion in the arm can wear a long-sleeved shirt or skin sleeve. Covering the medical device may be all that is necessary to keep the resident from pulling on it. Previously, wrist restraints would have been used routinely to keep the resident from dislodging tubes. Giving the resident something to hold, such as a Nerf ball, will occupy the hands and serve as a distraction. The nursing assistant plays an important role in knowing the residents' needs and making recommendations for restraint alternatives. Making sure the resident is in touch with his or her environment reduces agitation and confusion. Simply ensuring that the resident can see or hear well may improve mental orientation. Other observations that will help eliminate the need for restraints are:

- Does the resident see and hear well? Does the resident normally wear glasses? Is he or she wearing them now? Are they clean? Does the hearing aid work? Are the resident's ears plugged with wax? Sometimes behavior problems, balance problems, and other safety issues are caused because the resident is out of touch with the environment. Applying these simple corrective devices may eliminate the need for a restraint.
- Is the resident able to make his or her needs known? Unsafe behavior is often caused by fears or unmet needs. Discovering the unmet need and meeting it may help you avoid using a restraint.
- Does noise or confusion in the environment cause the resident to become agitated? Noise can be caused by other residents or staff, the public address system, radios, or television. Eliminating the noise may stop the behavior.
- Does the behavior occur during a certain time of day, during a certain activity, or when a specific person is providing care?
- Does the resident seem uncomfortable? Physical pain, hunger, thirst, or the need to use the bathroom can cause unsafe behavior.
- Does the resident seem lonely or isolated? Bored? Boredom, loneliness, or looking for a misplaced item can cause unsafe behavior.
- Does the resident try to get out of bed or the chair without help? Is the resident steady on his or her feet? Does the resident normally use a cane or walker? Is he or she using it now? Is the call signal available, and does the resident know how to use it? Would the resident benefit from the use of an alarm that sounds when he or she stands up? Would use of an alarm remind the resident to sit down, alert the staff, and eliminate the need for a restraint?

Complications of Restraints

Caution is used in making the decision to use restraints, because many complications and side effects are associated with their use. Residents have been severely injured and have died struggling to free themselves from restraints, so restraint use must be taken very seriously. Many burn injuries and burn-related deaths have occurred as a result of residents trying to burn off restraint straps to free themselves. In doing so, the residents themselves have caught on fire, sustaining serious burns. Several residents have died as a result of such injuries. Residents have also been injured by scissors, nail files, and other sharp objects that they used to try to cut restraint straps. If a resident is seriously injured or dies as the result of being restrained, the Safe Medical Device Reporting Act requires that the incident be reported to the government for investigation. Accrediting and licensing organizations require health care facilities to reduce

TABLE 15-1   Complications of restraints

Potential Physical Problems	Potential Psychosocial Problems	Potential Physical Problems	Potential Psychosocial Problems
Decreased independence	Worsening of behavior problems	Urge to void frequently, dribbling	Sense of abandonment
Increased dependence on staff		Incontinence	Loss of self-esteem
Pressure ulcers	Withdrawal, loss of social contact	Urinary tract infection	Crying
Weakness	Depression	Constipation	Screaming, yelling, calling out
Decreased range of motion	Forgetfulness	Fecal impaction	
Muscle wasting	Fear	Lethargy	Loss of dignity
Contractures (frozen, deformed joints)	Anger	Shortness of breath	Boredom
	Shame	Pneumonia	Feelings of hopelessness
Loss of ability to ambulate	Agitation	Bruising, redness, cuts	
Edema of ankles, lower legs, feet, fingers	Mental confusion	Falls	Feelings of helplessness
Decreased appetite, weight loss	Combativeness	Impaired circulation	Irritability
Dehydration	Restlessness	Blood clots	Ritualistic behavior
Acute mental confusion		Choking	
Distended abdomen		Death	

physical restraint use and track all restraint-related incidents. Complications related to the use of restraints are listed in **Table 15-1.**

APPLYING RESTRAINTS

Despite the efforts of staff, restraints are sometimes necessary. The law is very clear regarding the use of restraints. It specifies that restraints must be applied according to manufacturers' directions. Each manufacturer determines the best way to apply its restraints. The directions for restraint application are sent to the government, which approves the instructions. There are many restraint manufacturers, so you must become familiar with the directions for applying the types of restraints used in your facility.

Consideration must also be given to the size of the restraints. Restraints come in different sizes. Each manufacturer lists weight and size guidelines for its restraints. Some restraints are color-coded so you can determine the size at a glance. Using a restraint that does not fit the res-

ident correctly is dangerous. Applying the correct size is very important.

Restraint straps are tied where the resident is unable to reach them. This is usually under the frame of the chair or to the springs of a hospital bed. Many types of hospital beds are used in long-term care facilities. When applying a restraint to a resident who is in bed, fasten the straps to the moveable part of the bed frame, so that if the bed is repositioned the restraint moves with the resident. Tying the restraint to the stationary part of the bed frame can cause serious injury. Avoid tying restraints to the side rails. When applying restraints to a resident in a chair, the straps are usually inserted between the seat and the armrest. A common mistake is threading the straps *through the armrest.* Residents in wheelchairs frequently try to stand or slide their hips toward the front of the seat while restrained, causing injury. Threading the straps through the armrest places the restraint straps around the abdomen and fails to keep the hips down. If the resident attempts to stand or slides forward, the chair may tip or another injury may occur. Attention to manufacturer's directions

GUIDELINES FOR
Using Restraints

- Each facility has policies and procedures for the use and application of restraints. Know and follow your facility policies.
- Restraints are never used for staff convenience. They are used for the safety of the resident and others.
- Restraints are applied only with a physician's order and for a specific medical reason.
- The resident and family should clearly understand the purpose of the restraint. Emphasize safety; restraints are not used for punishment.
- The need for restraints is assessed by members of the interdisciplinary team, and alternatives are considered.
- The least restrictive type of restraint is used to keep the resident safe.
- The restraint is applied for the least time possible.
- Restraints are applied only according to manufacturers' directions.
- The proper size restraint must be used for the resident's weight and body size.
- Check the care plan for instructions on using restraints. The care plan will specify the type of restraint to use, the length of time it is to be applied, the reason for the restraint, when to release the restraint, and any special information.
- Check the restraint before using it. If it is worn, torn, cut, or frayed, discard it and obtain another restraint that is in good repair.
- Restraints used on the torso area of the body are always applied over clothing. They should not be applied directly against the skin. Extremity restraints are applied either over or under clothing on the arms and legs, but are padded to prevent restriction of circulation.
- The restraint straps should be smooth. Avoid twisting.
- When applying a restraint to a female resident, make sure the breasts are not under the strap to the restraint.
- After a restraint is applied, check the fit by slipping two or three fingers under the strap to be sure it is not too loose or too tight.
- The skin under the restraint is closely monitored to observe for signs of redness, irritation, or breakdown from the restraint.
- Check the skin above and below the restraint for signs of impaired circulation, such as blue or abnormal color and swelling.
- If the resident is restrained in the chair, the feet must be supported to prevent pain and circulatory problems.
- Restraints are tied in slipknots or bows so the health care provider can release them quickly in an emergency.
- The resident should be positioned using good body mechanics and good posture while in a restraint. Props and supports may also be necessary to keep the resident in good alignment.
- When the resident is restrained in a chair, the hips should be kept back. The purpose of the restraint is to keep the hips down. Restraint straps applied to the waist area instead of the hips may be incorrectly applied. Check the manufacturer's recommendations. The restraint should be at a 45° angle to keep the hips back.
- Most restraints are tied under the chair to the frame. Avoid tying them around the back of the chair, unless the manufacturer's directions clearly give this direction.
- When the resident is restrained in a wheelchair, the brakes should be locked when the chair is parked. The large part of the small front wheels of the chair should face forward. This changes the center of gravity of the chair, making the chair more stable and preventing tipping. The resident's feet should be supported.
- Facility policies vary on visual checks of residents in restraints, but a general rule is that the resident should be visually checked every 15 to 30 minutes while restrained.
- The resident should have the call signal, water, and other needed items within reach while restrained. Provide an alternative type of call signal, such as a manual bell, if the resident cannot use the regular call signal.
- The restraint is released every 2 hours for 10 full minutes. During this time the resident is repositioned, exercised, ambulated, and taken to the bathroom.
- Report any changes in behavior or side effects from the restraint.
- Restraint use must be recorded on the medical record. A flow sheet is commonly used for this purpose.

for strap placement in the wheelchair is very important for preventing injuries.

Most restraints are tied in a slipknot. This allows for quick release in case of choking, fire, or other emergency.

After restraints have been applied, you must visually check the resident every 15 to 30 minutes, or according to your facility policy. The restraint must be completely released every 2 hours for 10 minutes. During this time, the resident should be repositioned, ambulated, offered fluids, taken to the bathroom, and exercised. The restraint may be reapplied after the 10-minute release.

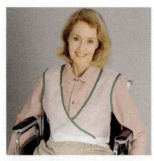

FIGURE 15-3   Vest restraints must be applied as pictured here, with the straps crossed over in front of the resident. Selecting the correct size is also very important. When the resident is in the chair, the straps should be positioned to keep the hips down. They should not encircle the waist. *(Courtesy of Skil-Care Corporation, Yonkers, NY, (800) 431-2972)*

Common Restraints

Although many types of restraints are available from different manufacturers, similar restraints are used in most health care facilities. They are all applied in a similar manner. The **vest restraint (Figure 15-3)** is applied to the upper body to prevent movement and sliding. The **belt restraint (Figure 15-4)** encircles the waist or hips and prevents rising. **Extremity restraints** encircle the arm or leg and prevent movement.

Vest Restraints.   The vest restraint is a very secure restraint used for residents who are at high risk of injury. The restraint looks like a vest and crosses over in the front. Other similar restraints are pulled over the head **(Figure 15-5)**. These are called by different names, such as jacket or poncho, but the principles of application are the same for all three devices. Years ago, health care providers were taught to cross the vest restraint over the resident's back. This is no longer acceptable and should never be done. Crossing the vest in the back can cause choking

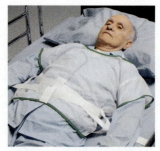

FIGURE 15-5   The jacket restraint is not interchangeable with the vest. This restraint is more secure than a vest, and requires a specific physician's order. *(Courtesy of Skil-Care Corporation, Yonkers, NY, (800) 431-2972)*

and other serious injury. A properly fitting vest restraint, crossed in front according to the manufacturer's directions and tied correctly out of reach, will safely and securely hold the resident.

The vest restraint is applied by placing the resident's arms through the sleeves, then crossing the vest over itself in the front. The straps thread through the vest on the side. The vest is pulled down as low as possible on the resident's torso. The straps are drawn behind the resident and fastened to the bed or chair frame.

Belt Restraints.   A belt restraint may also be called a waist restraint or a soft tie. It is a wide, padded strap that encircles the resident's waist and attaches to the chair at a 45° angle to keep the hips down. Belts are usually used to remind the resident not to stand up.

Extremity Restraints.   Extremity restraints **(Figure 15-6)** are used to hold the resident's arms and legs. They are usually used to prevent the resident from pulling at tubes or dressings, and to keep the resident still during a medical procedure. Many different extremity restraints are available. Most of these are padded with

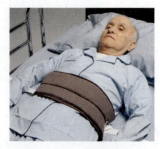

FIGURE 15-4   When the resident is in bed, the belt restraint permits him to turn from side to side. When the belt is used in the chair, it should be positioned to keep the hips down, preventing the resident from standing. *(Courtesy of Skil-Care Corporation, Yonkers, NY, (800) 431-2972)*

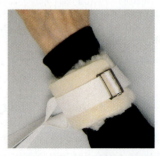

FIGURE 15-6   Extremity restraints are commonly used to keep the resident from pulling on tubes. Make sure the restraint is well padded. *(Courtesy of Skil-Care Corporation, Yonkers, NY, (800) 431-2972)*

PROCEDURE 62

Applying a Vest Restraint

1. Perform your beginning procedure actions.
2. Get help from another nursing assistant if necessary.
3. Slip the resident's arms through the armholes of the vest.
4. Straighten the clothing to be sure it is not wrinkled under the vest.
5. Pull the vest down and smooth it over the clothing.
6. Cross the vest in the front and thread the straps through the slots on the sides.

7. Thread the straps *between* the seat and the armrest or *between* the back of the seat and back of the chair, according to the manufacturer's directions. If the resident is in bed, attach the straps to the moveable part of the bed frame.
8. Pull the straps securely and tie them in a slipknot under the chair or to the moveable part of the bed frame, according to the manufacturer's directions.
9. Insert three fingers under the restraint and check to be sure that it is not too tight.
10. Perform your procedure completion actions.

PROCEDURE 63

Applying a Belt Restraint

1. Perform your beginning procedure actions.
2. Get help from another nursing assistant, if necessary.
3. If the resident is in a wheelchair, lock the brakes, move the hips as far back as possible, and position the footrests to support the feet.
4. Place the belt around the waist. Cross the straps through the loops behind the resident.
5. After the straps are threaded through the loops, tighten the belt securely around the waist.

6. Insert three fingers under the restraint and check to be sure that it is not too tight.
7. Insert the straps between the seat and armrest, or between the seat and backrest, according to the manufacturer's recommendations for the type of restraint you are using.
8. Bring the straps down and tie them to the kick-spurs of the wheelchair, using a quick-release knot, according to the manufacturer's directions.
9. Perform your procedure completion actions.

PROCEDURE 64

Applying an Extremity Restraint

1. Perform your beginning procedure actions.
2. Get help from another nursing assistant if necessary.
3. Position the resident's extremity in good alignment. The joints should be bent slightly inward, in a state of **flexion.**
4. Pad the skin with a washcloth or other padding, if necessary.
5. Insert hand rolls into the hands.
6. Encircle the extremity with the restraint, and loop it over itself according to the manufacturer's directions.

7. Place two fingers under the restraint to check for tightness. Observe the toes or fingers farthest away from the center of the body, or **distal** to the restraint, to be sure circulation is adequate.
8. Tie the ends of the restraint to the bed frame or springs, according to facility policy.
9. Check the resident's circulation and pulse in the restrained extremity every 15 minutes.
10. Perform your procedure completion actions.

sheepskin or foam, so no additional padding is necessary. If your facility uses unpadded restraints, wrap a washcloth or other padding around the extremity before applying the restraint, to prevent circulatory problems. Some facilities require that hand rolls be placed in the resident's hands when wrist restraints are used. Commercial devices should be used. Do not use rolled washcloths as hand rolls, because they promote squeezing and can cause deformities. The resident's skin must be kept clean and dry under the hand roll. Use of hand rolls is discussed in Chapter 18.

For residents who hit, scratch, or pull at tubes even if restrained, several types of mitten restraints are available. The fingers are inserted into the mitten **(Figure 15-7)**. The bottom is padded to maintain alignment, prevent pulling at tubes, and prevent injury. Mittens with mesh on top are common and convenient because you can see through them to check the resident's circulation.

When caring for residents who are in wrist restraints, remember that the restraint renders the resident helpless. You must feed the resident and offer fluids frequently. The call signal should be positioned close to the dominant hand. If the resident cannot push the call signal because of a mitten, an alternative type of signal, such as a manually operated bell, should be provided.

Side Rails as Restraints. According to the definition of restraints at the beginning of the chapter, side rails are a restraint. They can also be an enabler. Many residents pull on them to position and turn themselves in bed. Some residents may feel more secure if the rails are up. Side rails must always be up when the resident who is in bed is restrained in a vest, belt, or extremity restraint.

Studies have shown that serious injuries can occur if residents attempt to climb over side rails and fall. This is a common cause of hip fractures in confused elderly residents. Leaving the rails down may be safer. Each resident's care plan will provide instructions regarding the use of side rails or alternative devices. Know and follow your facility policy.

When side rails are used, it is important to check the space between the rail and the mattress. Hospital beds are permanent pieces of equipment that are used for years. Mattresses wear out and are replaced. There have been cases of injury and death when residents became trapped between the mattress and side rails because the replacement mattress was not the same size as the original. Residents at high risk for entrapment include those with conditions such as confusion, restlessness, lack of muscle control, or a combination of these factors. *Make sure that the gap between the mattress and the side rail is not large enough to cause injury.* This is an important safety issue. **Figure 15-8** shows potential areas of entrapment. Padded foam barriers may be used to close the space between the mattress, side rails, and bed frame **(Figure 15-9)**. Limiting the space reduces the risk of choking, entrapment, and other injuries.

Facilities and commercial manufacturers have developed many excellent alternatives to the use of side rails. Each resident's care plan will provide instructions regarding the use of restraints, side rails, or alternative devices. Before applying restraints or raising the rails, ask yourself if the risks associated with their use presents less danger than other available options, including making the environment as safe and

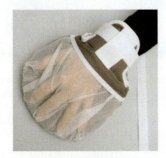

FIGURE 15-7 Mitten restraints are used to prevent self-injury from scratching, picking at the skin and hair, hitting, and pulling on tubes. They may be secured to the bed, like a wrist restraint, or the mitten may be worn alone, depending on the resident's needs. *(Courtesy of Skil-Care Corporation, Yonkers, NY, (800) 431-2972)*

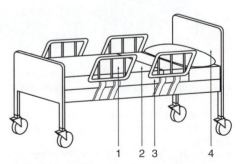

FIGURE 15-8 Entrapment occurs in one of the following ways: (numbered 1-4 in the diagram): (1) through the bars of an individual side rail; (2) through the space between split side rails; (3) between the side rail and mattress; or (4) between the headboard or footboard, side rail, and mattress.

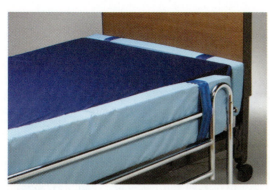

FIGURE 15-9 Various foam wedges and pads may be used to close the space between the side rails, bed frame, and mattress, reducing the risk of injury. *(Courtesy of Skil-Care Corporation, Yonkers, NY, (800) 431-2972)*

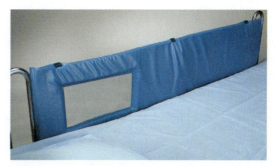

FIGURE 15-12 Side rail pads prevent injury and skin tears from contact with the side rails. They cover the side rail, eliminating the feeling that the resident is looking at the world through bars. *(Courtesy of Skil-Care Corporation, Yonkers, NY, (800) 431-2972)*

user-friendly as possible. Other possible alternatives to the use of side rails are:

- Keeping the bed in the lowest possible position with the wheels locked.
- Using a bed that can be raised and lowered close to the floor.
- Placing mats on the floor next to the bed **(Figure 15-10)** so that if a fall occurs, the resident will fall on a padded surface instead of the hard floor.
- Anticipating reasons the resident will use to get up, including need to use the bathroom, hunger, thirst, restlessness, and pain. Meet these needs promptly and provide calm interventions when you are in the room.
- Using side-rail bolster cushions **(Figure 15-11)** and side-rail pads **(Figure 15-12)**.

- Using pressure-sensitive alarms that sound when a resident attempts to get up **(Figures 15-13A–C)**.

Each health care facility has policies addressing when side rails may be used. Know and follow your facility policies.

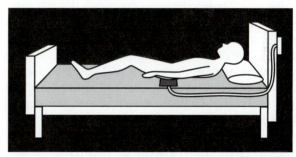

FIGURE 15-13A The pressure-sensitive pad is placed under the sheet. When the resident attempts to stand, an alarm sounds. The pad may also be used in a chair. *(Courtesy of RN+ Systems/Tactilitics, Inc.)*

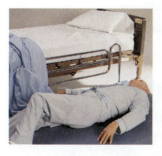

FIGURE 15-10 Placing foam mats on the floor reduces the risk of injury if the resident falls from the bed. *(Courtesy of Skil-Care Corporation, Yonkers, NY, (800) 431-2972)*

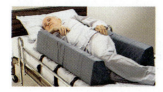

FIGURE 15-11 Bed control bolsters are a good option to use in place of side rails. *(Courtesy of Skil-Care Corporation, Yonkers, NY, (800) 431-2972)*

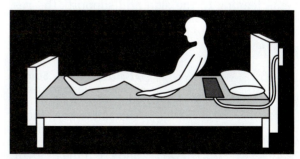

FIGURE 15-13B This pressure-sensitive pad is placed under the sheet beneath the resident's shoulders. When he lifts his upper body off the pad, the alarm will sound. *(Courtesy of RN+ Systems/ Tactilitics, Inc.)*

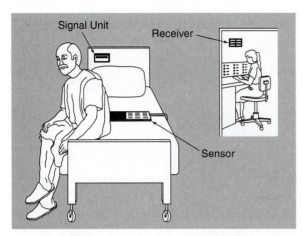

FIGURE 15-13C The pressure-sensitive pad is placed under the sheet. The sensor box is placed in the room. When the resident relieves pressure from the pad, a distinctive alarm sounds. The alarm may be set to sound only at the desk, at both the desk and the resident's room, or in the room only. *(Courtesy of RN+ Systems/Tactilitics, Inc.)*

ALTERNATIVES TO RESTRAINTS

Ideally, alternative devices will be used before the resident is placed in restraints. However, this does not always happen, because health care workers are not always aware of the wide variety of alternatives available. Some can be made from common items. Others are available from commercial manufacturers and are reasonably priced. If you know of a restraint alternative that you feel would be useful to a resident, inform the nurse.

Types of Restraint Alternatives

Lateral body supports **(Figure 15-14)** improve sitting posture for residents who lean to the side. They are commonly used for residents who have paralysis on one side of the body. The foam prevents leaning to the side and supports the resi-

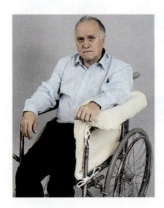

FIGURE 15-14 Some residents lean to the side, necessitating restraint to keep them upright in the chair. The lateral armrest supports and keeps the resident upright, making restraint unnecessary. *(Courtesy of Skil-Care Corporation, Yonkers, NY, (800) 431-2972)*

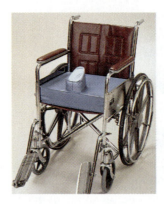

FIGURE 15-15 The pommel cushion keeps the resident from sliding and thrusting the hips forward. *(Courtesy of Skil-Care Corporation, Yonkers, NY, (800) 431-2972)*

dent's arm to prevent discomfort and swelling. Lateral stabilizer armrest bolsters are also used to correct leaning. These are commonly used for residents who have problems with motor control or balance.

The slide guard wedge **(Figure 15-15)** may also be called a pommel or saddle cushion. The wedge shifts the resident's weight to the back of the seat. The shape of the cushion and the pommel in the center prevent the resident from sliding. It is used for residents who slide forward on the seat of their chairs. Monitor the skin between the legs for redness and irritation.

The vinyl wedge cushion **(Figure 15-16)** is used for residents who slide forward in their chairs. The cushion also makes it more difficult for residents to stand, because the hips are lower than the knees. Wedges come in different sizes. The front of the wedge should be high enough to prevent the resident from rising, but

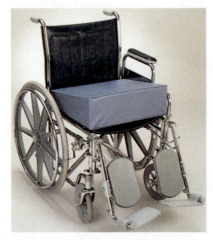

FIGURE 15-16 Some residents slide forward to the edge of the chair, and must be restrained to keep their hips back. The wedge cushion prevents sliding. A piece of gripper can be placed on top of and underneath the wedge for additional security. *(Courtesy of Skil-Care Corporation, Yonkers, NY, (800) 431-2972)*

should not raise the feet off the floor or footrests. When using a wedge cushion, make sure that the resident's legs are not dangling.

Nonslip matting **(Figure 15-17)** is sometimes called "gripper" or Dycem. This is a useful restraint alternative. It can be used as a place mat to enable residents to feed themselves. Some residents scoop their food away from the body, causing the plate to slide. The matting prevents dishes from sliding away. It can be used alone on the seat of a wheelchair to prevent rising, or placed under a wedge cushion for extra security. Gripper comes on a roll, and you cut off a section of the correct size. It may be rinsed with water if it becomes soiled. Hang the matting to dry. The surface is slippery when wet, so do not use it until it is completely dry.

Supporting the feet when the resident is seated in the chair is very important. Dangling the legs is painful and may allow complications such as blood clots to develop. The resident's legs may be too short to reach the floor or footrests of the chair. In this case, a footrest extender pad **(Figure 15-18)** is useful. The pad provides a firm base of support and makes it difficult to tip the chair.

Bed control bolsters (see Figure 5-11) are a good alternative to side rails. The bolsters can be used alone or in pairs. They protect the resident from rolling over the edge and serve as a reminder not to get up. The bolsters are half the length of the bed. They can also be used as a support to

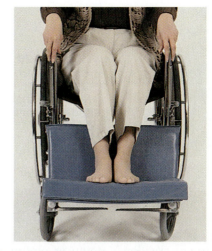

FIGURE 15-18 The resident's feet must be supported when she is sitting in a chair. The footrest elevator keeps the resident's legs from dangling and prevents sliding forward in the chair. *(Courtesy of Skil-Care Corporation, Yonkers, NY, (800) 431-2972)*

maintain good body alignment. They can be used for residents who are restless to prevent injury caused by striking or bumping the side rails.

Other Restraint Alternatives

- Magnetic sensor bracelets **(Figure 15-19)** set off alarms if the resident enters a dangerous area or tries to leave the premises. These work on the same principle as the magnetic detectors used in stores to prevent shoplifting. They are applied to the dominant hand to make them difficult to remove.

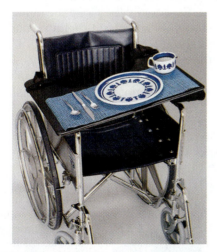

FIGURE 15-17 Gripper is a versatile product with many uses as an enabler and restraint alternative. It makes an excellent place mat, making cutting easier and preventing the dishes from sliding. Gripper may become slippery when wet. It may be rinsed if it becomes soiled, but should not be used until it is dry. *(Courtesy of Skil-Care Corporation, Yonkers, NY, (800) 431-2972)*

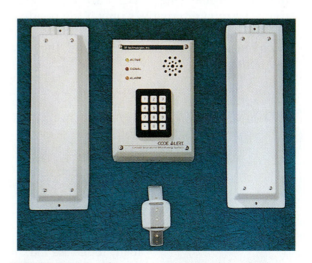

FIGURE 15-19 The magnetic sensor bracelet is used to allow cognitively impaired residents to wander within the unit. The door alarm will sound if the resident tries to exit. *(©1996, RF Technologies. Used by permission)*

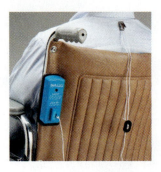

FIGURE 15-20 The personal alarm is a versatile restraint alternative that may be used in the bed or chair. *(Courtesy of Skil-Care Corporation, Yonkers, NY, (800) 431-2972)*

- Alarm cushions are available; these sound an alarm when the resident stands up or tries to get out of bed. Some facilities attach the signal cord to the resident's gown or clothing, so if the resident rises, it pulls the call signal. Various other personal alarms are also used, in which one end of the signal cord is attached to the resident's clothing. The alarm box is fastened to the bed or chair **(Figure 15-20).** When the resident stands, the signal cord pulls the alarm, sounding a very loud signal. These devices are used after careful resident evaluation. Some residents respond to the alarm by sitting down immediately. However, the noise from the alarm may startle some residents, increasing the risk of falls. In any event, you must respond to personal alarms immediately. Other personal alarms are used on doors for stairwells and other dangerous areas. There are many potential uses for this device.
- Self-releasing seat belts **(Figure 15-21)** are similar to the lap belts used in a car. Some belts have buckles and some have Velcro fasteners. Self-releasing devices are considered to be restraint alternatives only if the resident has the ability to remove them. If the resident does not know how to release them, they are restraints.

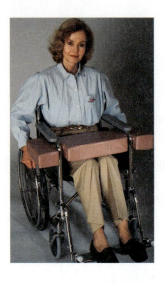

FIGURE 15-22 The lap buddy is foam covered with vinyl. It is lightweight and comfortable and may be used in place of a heavier tray. It is a restraint if the resident cannot remove it. *(Courtesy of Skil-Care Corporation, Yonkers, NY, (800) 431-2972)*

- "Lap buddies" **(Figure 15-22),** or foam cushions placed on the lap, keep the resident from rising.
- Special chairs are designed to make it more difficult for the resident to get up. Many chairs are available for residents with special positioning needs **(Figure 15-23).** Use caution, however. A common restraint alternative is a commercial reclining chair designed for health care facilities. Although some residents benefit from this device, it causes complications in others. Residents who stay in this type of chair for prolonged periods develop weakness in the neck muscles and lose the ability to hold their heads up. They are unable to feed themselves in the reclining position, so they are fed by staff. Eventually they lose the ability to feed themselves. Residents in reclining chairs look at the ceiling all day and may be out of touch with the environment because they cannot see it. Headrests are available to position the head forward and promote eye contact. Using these

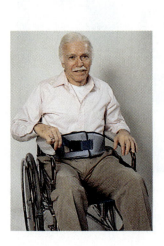

FIGURE 15-21 The self-release belt serves as a reminder to call for help before rising. It is not a restraint if the resident has the physical and mental ability to release the Velcro fastener. *(Courtesy of Skil-Care Corporation, Yonkers, NY, (800) 431-2972)*

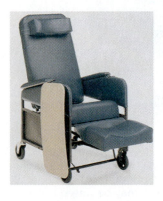

FIGURE 15-23 The geriatric chair can be used as a recliner for resident comfort. If the resident cannot stand, the chair is a restraint when in the reclining position. The tray is locked across the lap to prevent rising. It cannot be removed independently, and is considered a restraint. *(Photo courtesy of Hill-Rom Long Term Care Division)*

chairs as a restraint alternative must be considered cautiously, because although they solve one problem, they have the potential to create others.

• The **Vail bed** (**Figure 15-24**) is a useful alternative for confused adult residents who try to climb over the side rails. It is not used for mentally alert residents. This bed looks somewhat like a canopy bed or adult crib. The top and sides are surrounded by netting. From the inside, the netting seems to fade out and is not perceived as a barrier. The resident views the room as though looking through a screen door. The resident can move about in the bed without becoming entangled or falling out of bed. The netting protects the caregiver if the resident becomes aggressive. The bed is accessible from all sides through special zippers in the netting that open only from the outside. Residents should not be left unattended with the covers unzipped. Pediatric versions of this bed are also available for infant and child residents.

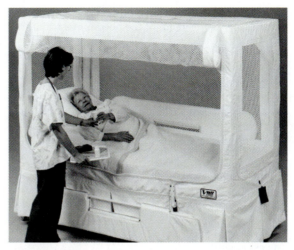

FIGURE 15-24 The Vail bed is a good alternative to physical restraints and side rails. *(Courtesy of Vail Products, Inc.)*

KEY POINTS

- Restraints are safety devices.
- Restraints can be dangerous if used incorrectly or inappropriately.
- The least amount of restraint required to keep the resident safe should be used.
- Restraints may be used as enablers to empower the resident and improve independence.
- Risk factors in the environment should be eliminated to reduce the need for restraints.
- The use of alternatives to restraints should be considered and continually reevaluated.

REVIEW

A. Multiple Choice

Select the one best answer.

1. Restraints are
   a. always used to prevent residents from wandering.
   b. enablers.
   c. devices that restrict freedom of movement.
   d. used when requested by the resident's family.

2. An enabler is
   a. a type of drug therapy.
   b. something that improves independent functioning.
   c. a mechanical device to manage behavior problems.
   d. a form of punishment.

3. Restraints may be used
   a. if the care provider feels they are needed.
   b. to punish the resident.
   c. with a physician's order.
   d. for convenience when the facility is short of staff.

4. Modifying the environment involves
   a. eliminating risk factors that contribute to the need for a restraint.
   b. assessing the resident for the proper size restraint.
   c. always restraining unsafe residents when out of bed.
   d. applying restraints correctly.

5. Which of the following will guide you in the type of restraint to use and the length of time the restraint should be applied?
   a. the resident
   b. the care plan
   c. the family
   d. the progress notes

6. Which of the following are complications of restraints?
   a. dehydration
   b. aphasia
   c. dysphagia
   d. independence

7. Which of the following should be considered when evaluating the resident for the need for restraints?
   a. age
   b. gender
   c. ability to see and hear
   d. staffing needs

8. Which of the following should be considered when obtaining a restraint from the linen closet to put on a resident?
   a. restraint size and condition
   b. the resident's age
   c. the resident's ability to ambulate
   d. the resident's mental status

9. Restraints should be released
   a. every 15 to 30 minutes.
   b. every 2 hours.
   c. every 4 hours.
   d. every shift.

10. When the resident is restrained in a chair, the hips should be
    a. as far forward as possible.
    b. flexed as much as possible.
    c. as far back as possible.
    d. extended as much as possible.

11. When applying a vest restraint to a resident,
    a. apply the restraint directly against the resident's skin.
    b. cross the vest in the front.
    c. thread the straps through the armrests of the chair.
    d. cross the vest in the back.

12. Restraint alternatives are
    a. devices that hold residents very securely.
    b. devices to use instead of restraints.
    c. always postural supports.
    d. used only if the resident cannot remove the device.

B. Clinical Applications

Answer the following questions.

13. Mr. Black has an order for a vest restraint when he is up in the chair. He wears an extra-large vest. You are preparing to transfer him from the bed to the chair. When you go to the linen room, you find only one extra-large vest on the shelf. The vest is frayed around the edges. It appears that the straps have been cut. Both straps are very short. There are several size medium and large restraints on the shelf, all in good condition. What should you do?

14. Mr. Black has been restrained in the chair. You notice that when he is wearing a vest restraint, he yells, pulls at the restraint, and asks others for scissors to cut the straps. Sometimes he throws his food and water. When Mr. Black is unrestrained in bed, he does not behave this way. What do you think is the cause of the agitation? What can the nursing assistant do to help?

15. Mr. Long is a confused resident. He ambulates in the facility. Occasionally he goes into other residents' rooms and takes things. Mr. Long fell recently, but was not injured. Since the fall, he has been unsteady on his feet. Staff is concerned for his safety, and you know that restraints are being considered. The nurse has called a team conference and asked your opinion about how to keep the resident safe. David, your coworker, states that he thinks Mr. Long should be restrained. What suggestions do you have for nursing assistant measures to avoid the use of restraints?

16. Mrs. Stone uses a belt restraint when in bed to keep her from climbing over the side rails. You applied the restraint and correctly tied it to the moveable part of the bed frame. Mrs. Stone's daughters visited today. After they left, you noticed that the restraint straps were tied to the side rails. What action should you take?

17. Mrs. Decker is an alert resident with multiple sclerosis. She has poor motor control of her body. Mrs. Decker leans forward or to the side when she is seated in a chair. She is afraid of falling. What can the nursing assistant do to help her feel secure and prevent injury?

CHAPTER 16

Measuring Vital Signs, Height, and Weight

OBJECTIVES

After reading this chapter, you will be able to:

- Spell and define key terms.
- Define vital signs and explain why accurate measurements are important.
- Identify abnormal vital signs.
- Demonstrate procedures related to measuring vital signs, height, and weight.

OBSERVATIONS TO MAKE AND REPORT RELATED TO MEASURING VITAL SIGNS, HEIGHT, AND WEIGHT

Elevated or subnormal temperature

Pulse rate below 60 or above 100

Pulse irregular, weak, or bounding

Blood pressure below 100/60 or above 140/90

Unable to hear blood pressure or palpate pulse

Pain over center, left, or right chest

Chest pain that radiates to shoulder, neck, jaw, or arm

Shortness of breath, dyspnea, or any abnormal respirations

Headache, dizziness, weakness, paralysis, vomiting

Cold, blue, or gray appearance

Cold, blue, numb, painful feet or hands

Feeling faint or lightheaded, losing consciousness

Respiratory rate below 12 or above 20

Irregular respirations

Noisy, labored, respirations

Dyspnea

Shortness of breath

Gasping for breath

Cheyne-Stokes respirations

Wheezing

Coughing (dry or moist/productive)

Retractions

Blue color of lips or nail beds, mucous membranes

Change in weight of 5 or more pounds (increase or decrease) compared with previous month

VITAL SIGNS

Vital signs are an indication of body function. Vital signs are measurements of **temperature, pulse, respiration,** and **blood pressure.** They are called vital signs because they are measurements of the most vital functions of the body. Temperature is a measurement of heat within the body. The pulse measures how fast the heart is beating. The pulse is checked by feeling the expansion and contraction of an artery with your fingertips. The blood pressure is a measurement of how hard the heart is working. This pressure is measured using the walls of the artery in the upper arm. Measuring respirations is an indication of how fast the person is breathing. Vital signs fall within certain normal ranges. Readings above or below these values may be symptoms of illness and disease. Measurement of vital signs provides an indication of whether a resident's condition is improving, worsening, or staying the same. The physician depends on these readings to order diagnostic tests and make changes in the treatment regimen.

Accurate measurement of vital signs is an important responsibility.

Vital Signs in Pediatric Residents

Many long-term care facilities have infant and child residents. Policies and procedures for taking vital signs in these residents may be different than they are for the adult population. Temperature values are less stable in children. Normal values for vital signs are different as well. The values vary with the age of the child.

TEMPERATURE

Temperature indicates how much heat is in the body and is measured with an instrument called a **thermometer.** In some conditions, such as infection, the temperature will be elevated. In other conditions, the temperature will be low. These are important findings. The body attempts to regulate temperature on its own. If you feel hot, your body will sweat and you will feel thirsty. If you feel cold, you will shiver to stimulate circulation and increase your temperature. Diseases and medications affect temperature within the body. Many other factors can also affect the body temperature. Some changes in temperature require immediate attention from the nurse or physician.

Long-term care facilities use many different types of thermometers. Temperature is measured by different methods, depending on the needs of the resident. Your facility will teach you how to use its equipment, which recording scale to use, and how to document your findings.

The nursing assistant must use good judgment in deciding which method to use for taking the temperature. You must evaluate the resident's condition and other safety factors, and select the method that is safe for the resident and will give you the most accurate reading. Four methods are used to measure body temperature:

1. **Oral temperature** is taken by inserting a thermometer in the mouth under the tongue. This is the most common method.
2. **Rectal temperature** is taken by inserting the thermometer into the anus. This method is used for adults only when the temperature cannot be taken orally. In some facilities, this procedure is done only by licensed nurses. Know and follow your facility policies.
3. The **axillary temperature** is taken by placing the thermometer under the arm. An alternate site to use is the groin. This is the least accurate method and is used only when taking the temperature by other methods is not possible.
4. The **aural** or **tympanic temperature** is taken in the ear. This method is controversial. It is an accurate, safe method of taking temperature and is faster than other methods. However, variations in equipment and technique can affect the reading. Some facilities previously used this method, but have now eliminated it because the technique used may affect the accuracy of the reading.

Temperature Values

Health care facilities use different methods of recording temperatures. The **Fahrenheit scale** is the method used most commonly. In the Fahrenheit scale, the boiling point of water is 212 degrees. Writing an F after the temperature value indicates a Fahrenheit reading. Writing a C after the value indicates the **Celsius,** or **centigrade, scale.** In the Celsius scale, the boiling point is 100 degrees. In the United States, we commonly use figures in the Fahrenheit scale. The formulas used to convert temperature readings between the two scales are found in **Table 16-1.** Both scales are recorded in degrees. The symbol for degree is "°," so a properly recorded temperature would be written *98.6°F* or *37°C.*

The normal temperature range for adults is listed in **Table 16-2.** Memorize these values. If a resident's temperature falls outside the values, report to the nurse immediately.

Reporting. It is important to report abnormally high or low temperatures to the nurse promptly. Elevated temperature usually occurs as a result of infection. Elderly individuals do not mount a strong immune response because of normal aging changes. Because of this, even a small elevation in temperature can indicate serious illness. Other common causes of temperature elevation are dehydration and hot environmental temperature.

Abnormally low body temperature (below 95°F) can also be very significant in the elderly. This condition is called **hypothermia.** Some elderly persons do not adjust well to environmental temperature changes and do not tolerate cold environments well. Many feel cold in room temperatures that are comfortable for younger persons. Hypothermia develops as a result of exposure to cold, ingestion of alcohol and some medications, sepsis, and shock. This can be extremely serious. In fact, abnormally low body temperature can cause death in

TABLE 16-1 Formulas for converting Fahrenheit and Celsius temperature readings	Celsius (C)	Fahrenheit (F)
Conversion Formulas	F to C $\quad C = \dfrac{5}{9}(F - 32)$	C to F $\quad F = \dfrac{9}{5}C + 32$

For example: To convert a Celsius temperature of 100 to Fahrenheit, follow the procedure:

$$\frac{9}{5} \times 100 + 32 = \frac{900}{5} + 32 = 180 + 32 = 212°F$$

For example: To convert a Fahrenheit temperature of 212 to Celsius, follow the procedure:

$$\frac{5}{9} \times (212 - 32) = \frac{5}{9} \times 180 = 100°C$$

elderly individuals. Signs and symptoms of hypothermia are not specific to this condition, so having an accurate temperature reading is very important. Symptoms worsen as temperature decreases. Once hypothermia is identified, special treatment is necessary to prevent further complications. Keeping residents warm and reporting abnormally low temperature values promptly is the best means of prevention.

Documentation. Facilities have different methods of recording temperatures. Some facilities list the method by which the temperature was taken in parentheses next to the reading. Writing the letter O indicates an oral reading. If recording in this manner is your facility policy, you would record the oral temperature value listed above as *98.6°F (O)*. The common abbreviations for vital signs, height, and weight are listed in **Table 16-3**.

Gloves. Facility policies vary greatly regarding whether gloves should be worn for measuring

temperature. The principles of standard precautions should be followed at all times. Gloves are always worn when taking a rectal temperature with either glass or electronic thermometers. Many agencies require gloves for the oral temperature procedure with a glass thermometer because of the possibility of contacting saliva, which is a body fluid, and the mucous membranes in the mouth. Use of gloves with an oral electronic thermometer is usually not necessary. Standard precautions do not call for the use of gloves for contact with perspiration (sweat), so your agency may not require glove use for taking an axillary temperature. However, if you are using this method to take the temperature in the groin, gloves are worn. Wearing gloves when using a tympanic thermometer is not necessary. Know and follow your facility policy, but remember that there may be exceptions to the rule. Your facility may not require gloves for oral temperatures. However, if the resident has open lesions in or

TABLE 16-2 Normal vital sign ranges for adults				
Temperature	Normal	Range	Report Changes Above	Report Changes Below
Axillary temperature	97.6°F	96.6-98.6°F	99°F	96°F
Oral temperature	98.6°F	97.6-99.6°F	100°F	97°F
Rectal temperature	99.6°F	98.6-100.6°F	101°F	98°F
Pulse	76	60-100	100	60
Respiration	16	14-20	20	12
Blood pressure	120/80	100/60-140/90	140/90	100/60

Note: These values are guidelines only. Your instructor will inform you if facility reporting values are different in your area. Know and follow your facility reporting guidelines.

TABLE 16-3 Abbreviations used in documentation of vital signs

Abbreviation	Vital Sign
VS	Vital signs, vitals
TPR	Temperature, pulse, and respiration
BP or B/P	Blood pressure
(O) or (PO)	Oral temperature
(R)	Rectal temperature
(Ax) or (A)	Axillary temperature
No abbreviation, (AU), (A), or (T), depending on agency policy	Aural (tympanic) temperature
F	Fahrenheit
C	Celsius or Centigrade
°	Degrees
T	Temperature
P	Pulse
R	Respiration
Ht	Height
Wt	Weight
mm Hg	Millimeters of mercury

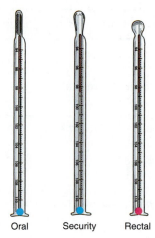

FIGURE 16-1 Clinical thermometers from left to right: oral, security, rectal.

Glass Thermometers. Glass thermometers are thin, hollow tubes with a column of liquid inside that provides the temperature reading. Three types of glass thermometers are used: oral, security, and rectal. **Figure 16-1** compares glass thermometers. As you can see, the sizes and shapes of the bulbs are different. Oral thermometers are marked with a blue or clear dot on the end. Rectal thermometers are marked with a red dot. Security thermometers are commonly used in health care facilities.

Facilities that use glass thermometers usually cover them with plastic, disposable **sheaths** (**Figure 16-2**). Although glass thermometers are normally disinfected between each use, the sheath provides further protection against pathogens. It also protects the resident by containing the glass if the thermometer is accidentally cracked or broken.

Reading the Glass Thermometer. The glass thermometer is read by measuring the level of liquid on the inner column. The liquid rises and falls to indicate the temperature value. Most thermometers begin with 94°F. Each long line on the thermometer is one degree. Every other long line (or degree) is marked with a number. There are four short lines between each long line. Each short line indicates ²⁄₁₀ of a degree, or 0.2 degrees.

To read the thermometer, hold it at eye level. Rotate it gently between your thumb and index

around the mouth or is drooling excessively, use good judgment and apply gloves. You are taught the principles of standard precautions so that you can apply them as needed in procedures to protect yourself. In health care, there are so many variables that the rules must be flexible. Using the one-glove technique is convenient for taking temperatures. If your ungloved hands accidentally contact a body fluid or mucous membrane during this, or any, procedure, wash them immediately.

Types of Thermometers

Three basic types of thermometers are used in long-term care facilities. The nursing assistant must be able to operate and read all three types. Although variations exist among thermometers and manufacturers, they all operate in basically the same way.

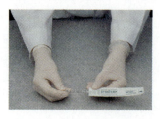

FIGURE 16-2 The disposable sheath is used for safety and infection control.

finger until you can clearly see the liquid column. Find the sharp edge where the liquid ends. Take the temperature reading at this point **(Figure 16-3)**. When taking temperatures with a glass thermometer, the value is recorded as an even number. If the reading falls between the lines, use the higher number.

Mercury. Mercury thermometers have been used for many years. However, the recent trend in health care has been to avoid the use of products containing mercury, because they can be very toxic to humans and wildlife if broken. This is true even if mercury exposure occurs in very small amounts.

A mercury thermometer is a small glass tube containing liquid mercury, a silvery-white substance that registers body heat. Alternative products are being used in many glass thermometers because of mercury's potential for toxicity. Some thermometers contain a red or blue liquid. These are alcohol thermometers and contain no mercury. Another, less common thermometer contains galinstan, a substance that is similar to mercury in appearance. These thermometers are mercury-free, however, and are generally marked as such.

Mercury can be toxic in small amounts, particularly if it vaporizes and is inhaled. Even small mercury spills must be cleaned up properly to prevent contamination and illness. If you accidentally break a mercury thermometer or other device containing mercury, inform the nurse promptly. Follow facility policies and procedures for picking up mercury. If no procedures are available, apply gloves, face mask, and eye protection. Pick up broken glass and other debris and place in a puncture-resistant container. Use an index card to consolidate the mercury droplets, then seal them in a plastic bag or covered container. Small droplets can be picked up with adhesive tape or wet paper towels. Seal the container and affix a label identifying the material as "mercury spill debris." Consult the nurse for information regarding where to discard this material.

Electronic Thermometers. Many facilities use electronic thermometers **(Figure 16-4)**. These thermometers are battery operated and stored in a charger when not in use. They are quick, easy to use, and accurate. Electronic thermometers usually have a plastic neck strap on the end. This is worn around your neck when taking temperatures or walking in the hallway. The unit is very sensitive and can be damaged if it is dropped or bumped. Wearing it around your neck frees your hands and helps avoid accidents. The electronic thermometer displays the temperature digitally on a screen. The unit will beep or blink when the temperature reading is completed.

The electronic thermometer consists of a main thermometer unit. You will attach an oral or rectal **probe** to record the temperature. The oral probe is colored blue and the rectal probe is red. The probe is covered by a heavy plastic disposable **probe cover** that is used for one resident and then discarded **(Figure 16-5)**. The unit can be used for many different residents by changing the probe cover.

Tympanic Membrane Thermometers. The **tympanic thermometer (Figure 16-6)** is a battery-operated unit. It is held in your hand and inserted into the resident's ear. The ear piece of the thermometer is covered with a protective sheath to prevent infection. The sheath is discarded after each use. The temperature reading is displayed digitally on the handset. Tympanic thermometers can be set to provide the equivalent of either an oral or a rectal reading. They can also be set for a Fahrenheit or Celsius value.

Other Types of Thermometers. Other types of thermometers are available, but they are not as

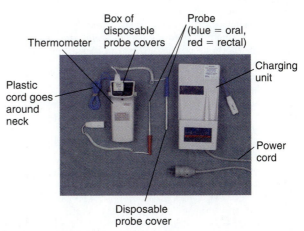

FIGURE 16-4 The electronic thermometer is fast and accurate.

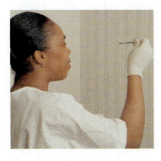

FIGURE 16-3 Hold the thermometer at eye level, then rotate it until you can read the column of liquid.

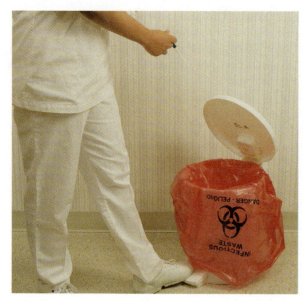

FIGURE 16-5 Dispose of the probe cover properly.

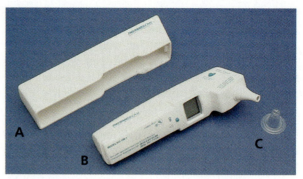

FIGURE 16-6 When positioned correctly, the tympanic thermometer is the fastest and most accurate method of taking the temperature. (A) Holder (B) Tympanic thermometer (C) Disposable speculum or cover

widely used or as accurate as the instruments and methods listed earlier. Another type of thermometer is a paper or plastic, chemically treated, disposable unit **(Figure 16-7)**. Dots on the thermometer are read to obtain the temperature value. This thermometer is used following the guidelines for taking an oral temperature with a glass thermometer. A disposable sheath is not necessary, because the

thermometer is discarded after use. This thermometer is commonly used for residents who are in isolation. The disposable thermometer is made of rigid plastic. Remove the thermometer from the resident's mouth *slowly*. Pulling the thermometer out rapidly from between closed lips can cause painful tears of the lips and mucous membranes in the mouth. Small, handheld, battery-operated thermometers are also available **(Figure 16-8)**. These are covered with plastic sheaths. The guidelines for taking the temperature with this thermometer are the same as those for using an electronic

GUIDELINES FOR
Measuring Temperature

- Apply the principles of standard precautions.
- Check glass thermometers for chips and cracks.
- Make sure electronic thermometers are fully charged and that you have the correct probe for the type of temperature you are taking.
- If a glass thermometer is accidentally broken, follow your facility policy for cleaning and disposing of it. Mercury is poisonous and glass must be discarded in a puncture-resistant container. Wear gloves.
- When using a glass thermometer, shake the liquid down below 96°F before inserting the thermometer. Stand away from the resident or surfaces you might hit when shaking the thermometer.
- Use a probe cover or disposable sheath, depending on the type of thermometer you are using.
- Use a clean probe cover for each resident.
- Lubricate the rectal thermometer before inserting it.
- Hold the oral electronic thermometer probe in place, as the probe is heavy and the resident may not be able to hold it between the lips.

- When using the tympanic thermometer, make sure it is securely inside the ear canal. If it is not placed correctly, the reading will not be accurate.
- Hold a rectal thermometer in place with your gloved hand. Hold an axillary thermometer in place (use your judgment and apply the principles of standard precautions as to use of gloves).
- Leave the glass thermometer in place for the length of time specified by your facility for the type of temperature you are taking.
- Follow your facility policy for cleaning, disinfecting, and storing glass thermometers.
- A glass thermometer is used for one resident only, then is disinfected. This is true even if a plastic thermometer sheath was used. Electronic thermometers with probe covers may be used for more than one resident if the cover is changed.
- Use cold water to clean glass thermometers. Hot water may cause breakage.
- The containers used for clean and soiled glass thermometers must be disinfected regularly. Your facility will have policies and procedures for cleaning them.

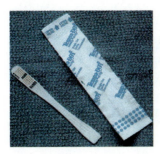

FIGURE 16-7 The chemical-dot thermometer is used only for oral temperatures. It is used once, then discarded.

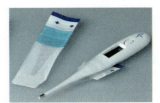

FIGURE 16-8 The battery-operated digital thermometer is commonly used in long-term care facilities. Always cover the thermometer with a disposable probe cover before use. *(Courtesy of Medline Industries, Inc. 1-800-MEDLINE)*

thermometer. Follow facility policies for disinfecting the thermometer between residents.

Oral Temperature

Oral temperature is taken by placing the thermometer in the resident's mouth. If the resident has recently had something to eat or drink, this may affect the temperature reading. Temperature is also affected by smoking. If the resident has had something to eat, drink, or smoke, instruct the resident not to have anything further, and return in 15 minutes to check the temperature.

Oral temperatures are usually taken in alert, cooperative adults. Oral temperatures should not be taken in residents who are:

- Mentally confused
- Uncooperative
- Combative
- Chilled or shivering
- Coughing or sneezing
- Unconscious
- Restless
- Receiving heat or cold treatments about the neck or face
- Mouth-breathing or cannot keep the mouth closed around the thermometer
- Short of breath or having difficulty breathing
- Unable to breathe through the nose
- Receiving oxygen by mask
- On seizure precautions
- Recovering from surgery on or an injury to the nose or mouth
- Using a nasogastric tube
- Under the age of six

If you are in doubt, check with the nurse. The oral thermometer is left in place for a minimum of three minutes.

PROCEDURE

65

Measuring an Oral Temperature with a Glass Thermometer

Note: The guidelines and sequence for this procedure vary slightly from state to state, and from one facility to another. Your instructor will inform you if the sequence in your state or facility differs from the procedure listed here. Know and follow the required sequence for your state and facility.

1. Perform your beginning procedure actions.
2. Gather supplies needed: glass thermometer, disposable plastic sheath, notepad and pen, gloves, container for used thermometers.
3. Rinse the disinfectant off the thermometer and dry it.
4. Shake the thermometer down to 96°F.
5. Cover the thermometer with a plastic sheath.
6. Apply gloves.
7. Place the bulb under the resident's tongue and instruct the resident to close his or her lips.

8. Leave the thermometer in place for three minutes, or according to facility policy.
9. Remove the thermometer.
10. Discard the sheath according to facility policy.
11. Hold the thermometer at eye level and read the liquid column. Note the reading.
12. Shake the thermometer down to 96°F.
13. Place the thermometer in the container for used thermometers or disinfect it according to facility policy.
14. Remove gloves and discard them according to facility policy. Wash your hands.
15. Record the reading.
16. Perform your procedure completion actions.

PROCEDURE 66

Measuring an Oral Temperature with an Electronic Thermometer

1. Perform your beginning procedure actions.
2. Gather supplies needed: electronic thermometer, oral probe, plastic probe cover, notepad and pen.
3. Insert the probe into the probe cover.
4. Place the tip of the probe under the resident's tongue and instruct the resident to close his or her lips.
5. Hold the end of the probe in place.
6. When the alarm sounds, note the reading and remove the probe.
7. Dispose of the probe cover according to facility policy.
8. Insert the probe into the side of the thermometer.
9. Record the reading.
10. Perform your procedure completion actions.

Oxygen. Each facility has policies and procedures for taking an oral temperature when the resident is using oxygen. In general, if the resident is using oxygen by mask, you should avoid taking an oral temperature. If the resident uses oxygen through a nasal cannula, the temperature reading may be slightly (approximately 0.3 degrees) lower because of the oxygen. Consult the nurse if you are unsure of how to take the temperature of a resident who is using oxygen.

Rectal Temperature

Rectal temperature is commonly taken when oral methods cannot be used. It is also routinely used for taking the temperature of chil-

PROCEDURE 67

Measuring a Rectal Temperature with a Glass Thermometer

Note: The guidelines and sequence for this procedure vary slightly from state to state, and from one facility to another. Your instructor will inform you if the sequence in your state or facility differs from the procedure listed here. Know and follow the required sequence for your state or facility.

Note: In some states, nursing assistants are not permitted to perform this procedure. Additionally, the policies of some facilities state that only licensed nurses may perform rectal treatments, including taking temperatures. Perform this procedure only if you are permitted to do so by state law and facility policies.

1. Perform your beginning procedure actions.
2. Gather supplies needed: glass (rectal) thermometer, disposable plastic sheath, lubricant, notepad and pen, gloves, container for used thermometers.
3. Rinse the disinfectant off the thermometer, and dry it.
4. Shake the thermometer down to 96°F.
5. Cover the thermometer with a plastic sheath.
6. Position the resident in the Sims' position.
7. Apply gloves.
8. Place a small amount of lubricant on a tissue or paper towel. Use the tissue to lubricate the bulb of the thermometer **(Figure 16-9).** Some plastic sheaths are prelubricated.
9. Separate the buttocks with one hand.
10. Insert the bulb into the rectum one inch **(Figure 16-10).**
11. Hold the thermometer in place for three minutes, or according to facility policy.
12. Remove the thermometer.
13. Discard the sheath according to facility policy.
14. Hold the thermometer at eye level and read the liquid column. Note the reading.
15. Place the thermometer in a container for used thermometers or disinfect it according to facility policy.
16. Remove gloves and discard them according to facility policy. Wash your hands.
17. Record the temperature reading.
18. Perform your procedure completion actions.

Continues

OBRA

PROCEDURE 67

Measuring a Rectal Temperature with a Glass Thermometer, *Continued*

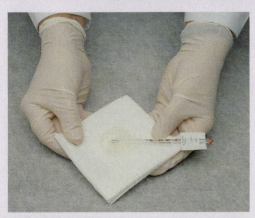

FIGURE 16-9 Lubricate the rectal thermometer well.

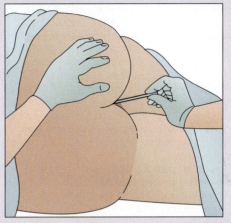

FIGURE 16-10 Spread the buttocks, then gently insert the lubricated thermometer one inch into the rectum.

PROCEDURE 68

Measuring a Rectal Temperature with an Electronic Thermometer

OBRA

Note: The guidelines and sequence for this procedure vary slightly from state to state, and from one facility to another. Your instructor will inform you if the sequence in your state or facility differs from the procedure listed here. Know and follow the required sequence for your state or facility.

Note: In some states, nursing assistants are not permitted to perform this procedure. Additionally, the policies of some facilities state that only licensed nurses may perform rectal treatments, including taking temperatures. Perform this procedure only if you are permitted to do so by state law and facility policies.

1. Perform your beginning procedure actions.
2. Gather supplies needed: electronic thermometer, rectal probe, plastic probe cover, lubricant, notepad and pen, gloves.
3. Position the resident in the Sims' position.
4. Apply gloves.

5. Place a small amount of lubricant on a tissue or paper towel. Use the tissue to lubricate the bulb of the thermometer.
6. Separate the buttocks with one hand.
7. Insert the probe into the probe cover. Lubricate the end.
8. Insert the tip of the probe cover into the rectum one inch, or according to manufacturers' directions. (Some manufacturers recommend inserting it ¼ to ½ inch.)
9. Hold the probe in place until the alarm sounds.
10. Note the reading and remove the probe.
11. Discard the probe cover according to facility policy.
12. Insert the probe into the side of the thermometer.
13. Wipe excess lubricant from the anal area.
14. Remove gloves and discard according to facility policy. Wash your hands.
15. Record the reading.
16. Perform your procedure completion actions.

PROCEDURE 69
Measuring an Axillary Temperature with a Glass Thermometer

 OBRA

Note: The guidelines and sequence for this procedure vary slightly from state to state, and from one facility to another. Your instructor will inform you if the sequence in your state or facility differs from the procedure listed here. Know and follow the required sequence for your state and facility.

1. Perform your beginning procedure actions.
2. Gather supplies needed: glass thermometer, disposable plastic sheath, towel, notepad and pen, gloves, container for used thermometers.
3. Rinse the disinfectant off the thermometer, and dry it.
4. Shake the thermometer down to 96°F.
5. Cover the thermometer with a plastic sheath.
6. Apply gloves, if this is your facility policy.
7. Dry the axilla with the towel.
8. Insert the thermometer into the center of the axilla, then lower the resident's arm and bend it across the abdomen. Hold the thermometer in place, if this is your facility policy.
9. Leave the thermometer in place for 10 full minutes.
10. Remove the thermometer.
11. Discard the sheath according to facility policy.
12. Hold the thermometer at eye level and read the liquid column. Note the reading.
13. Remove gloves, if worn, and discard them according to facility policy. Wash your hands.
14. Record the reading.
15. Place the thermometer in a container for used thermometers or disinfect it according to facility policy.
16. Perform your procedure completion actions.

dren below the age of six. The rectal temperature registers one degree higher than the oral value. If the oral temperature is 98.6°F, the rectal temperature in the same resident would be 99.6°F.

Times when a rectal temperature *should not* be taken are:

- If the resident is having diarrhea
- If the resident has constipation or fecal impaction
- If the resident has had a colostomy
- If the resident is combative
- If the resident has rectal bleeding, hemorrhoids, or some other rectal condition, or has had rectal surgery
- If the resident has recently had prostate surgery
- If the resident has severe heart disease or has recently had a heart attack

Gloves are always worn when taking a rectal temperature. The thermometer is lubricated before insertion. The glass thermometer must be held in place for three full minutes, or according to facility policy.

Axillary Temperature

Axillary temperatures are not taken as commonly as oral and rectal temperatures because they are not as accurate. They are used only when the temperature cannot be obtained by other methods. The axilla must be dry. An oral thermometer is used. The thermometer is placed in the center of the armpit and must remain in place for 10 full minutes. The axillary value is normally one degree less than the oral reading. If the oral temperature in a resident is 98.6°F, the axillary temperature in the same resident would be 97.6°F.

Tympanic Membrane Temperature

The temperature inside the ear is the most accurate temperature in the body. It is often preferred by health care workers because it is quick and convenient. The temperature reading is taken by holding the thermometer next to the tympanic membrane, which is close to the core of the body. It takes one to three seconds to obtain a tympanic temperature. The end of the thermometer is covered with a plastic sheath or cover before it is inserted into the ear.

The tympanic, or aural, thermometer is inserted into the ear by gently lifting the top of the outer ear up and back. This straightens the ear canal. Insert the end of the thermometer as far as it will go. For the temperature to be accurate, the detector at the end of the thermometer must be flat against the tympanic membrane. The reading will not be accurate if it is tipped to the side. The thermometer is held in place until the display flashes. The thermometer is removed and the protective cover discarded.

PROCEDURE 70

Measuring an Axillary Temperature with an Electronic Thermometer

Note: The guidelines and sequence for this procedure vary slightly from state to state, and from one facility to another. Your instructor will inform you if the sequence in your state or facility differs from the procedure listed here. Know and follow the required sequence for your state and facility.

1. Perform your beginning procedure actions.
2. Gather supplies needed: electronic thermometer, oral probe, plastic probe cover, notepad and pen, gloves.
3. Insert the oral probe into the probe cover.
4. Apply gloves, if this is your facility policy.
5. Dry the axilla with the towel.
6. Insert the probe into the center of the axilla, then lower the resident's arm and bend it across the abdomen. Hold the probe in place, if this is your facility policy.
7. When the alarm sounds, remove the probe. Note the reading.
8. Dispose of the probe cover according to facility policy.
9. Insert the probe into the side of the thermometer.
10. Remove gloves, if worn, and discard them according to facility policy. Wash your hands.
11. Record the reading.
12. Perform your procedure completion actions.

The tympanic temperature is the fastest and most convenient method, but it can also provide inaccurate readings if the user's technique is not precise. To ensure an accurate reading, insert the probe tip into the ear as far as it will go.

Next, rotate the probe handle until it is aligned with the jaw, as though it were a telephone handset. Quickly press the "scan" button. Using this method will help ensure accurate temperature readings.

GUIDELINES FOR

Using a Tympanic (Ear) Thermometer

- Make sure the thermometer lens is clean and there is no dirt or debris on the lens at the end of the probe tip.
- Use each probe cover only once. Make sure the cover is on snugly, without ripples.
- Store the thermometer out of the path of cold air flow. If the thermometer is in a cold area, allow it to warm up before use, or it may read low.
- Make sure the resident is not directly in the path of cold air or being fanned. This action cools the ears, which can cause a low temperature reading.
- The tympanic thermometer can be set to oral, core, or rectal mode. In most cases, oral is appropriate. The mode will be shown in the readout screen. If the screen says "CAL," the thermometer is in the unadjusted mode, which is used only for calibration and other bench work.
- If the resident is lying on one side, use the opposite ear to take the temperature. If this is not possible, turn the resident's head so the ear is uncovered. Wait several minutes before taking the temperature.
- Remove hearing aids from the resident's ears. Wait several minutes before taking the temperature.

(Lying on the ear or having a hearing aid retains heat in the ear canal. Repositioning the resident or removing the hearing aid is similar to taking the lid off a pan on the stove to allow heat to escape.)

- Insert the probe tip into the ear as far as possible, then rotate the handle to the correct position, in alignment with the jaw. This step is very important for ensuring an accurate temperature reading.

Ear thermometers are similar to cameras. They provide the temperature of what you point them at. If the thermometer is not used correctly, you will get an inaccurate reading. Common causes of inaccurate tympanic temperatures are:

- Pressing the scan button before the probe is fully inserted
- Using a probe cover more than once
- Using a thermometer without a probe cover
- Improper cleaning of the thermometer lens
- Not following manufacturer's instructions for placing the probe tip into the ear; following instructions for the thermometer you are using is important
- Using a thermometer with a broken or missing lens (the shiny disk at the end of the probe tip through which the infrared energy must pass to be processed)

<table>
<tr><td>PROCEDURE
71</td><td>Measuring a Tympanic
Temperature</td><td>OBRA</td><td></td></tr>
</table>

1. Perform your beginning procedure actions.
2. Gather supplies needed: tympanic thermometer, probe cover, gloves if needed.
3. Check the lens of the thermometer to make sure it is clean.
4. Cover the thermometer lens with a clean probe cover.
5. Select the appropriate mode on the thermometer.
6. Gently pull the outer ear up and back to straighten the ear canal **(Figure 16-11).**
7. Insert the thermometer, aiming it toward the tym-

panic membrane (ear drum). Insert until the tip seals in the ear canal. Rotate the probe handle slightly until it is aligned with the jaw, as though speaking on the telephone **(Figure 16-12).**
8. Press the activation (scan) button. Hold the thermometer in place until the display flashes or the thermometer indicates that you have a reading.
9. Remove the thermometer and discard the probe cover according to facility policy.
10. Document the reading.
11. Perform your procedure completion actions.

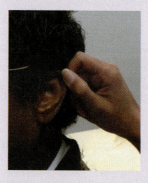

FIGURE 16-11 Gently pull the pinna up to straighten the ear canal.

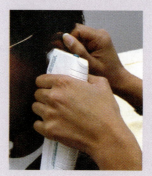

FIGURE 16-12 Insert the thermometer until it seals in the ear canal, then rotate it until it is positioned like a telephone receiver.

PULSE

The pulse is a measurement of how fast the heart is beating. Each time the heart beats, the arteries in the body expand and contract, forcing blood through the system. The pulse is taken in locations where arteries can be easily compressed against the bones underneath, called **pulse points. Figure 16-13** shows common pulse points. The **radial pulse** at the wrist is used by most health care workers for counting the pulse. The pulse can also be heard by placing a **stethoscope** directly over the heart. The stethoscope is an instrument used to listen to sounds in the body. The **apical pulse** in the heart is usually taken by the licensed nurse or advanced care provider.

Observations of the Pulse

Counting the pulse reveals things about the condition of the heart and circulatory system. When we "take the pulse," we are doing more than counting the number of beats per minute. We are also gathering other information that is impor-

tant in treating the resident's condition. Some electronic blood pressure devices count the pulse and display the rate. Feeling the pulse is still necessary, however, to make other important observations.

Pulse Rate. We count the number of beats in the pulse to determine how fast the heart is beating. The number of beats per minute is called the **pulse rate.** The normal pulse rate in an adult is between approximately 60 and 100 beats per minute. Pulse rates outside this range may indicate a problem and should be reported to the nurse immediately. Pulse rates lower than 60 beats per minute are called **bradycardia.** Pulse rates above 100 beats per minute are called **tachycardia.**

Pulse Rhythm and Force. The **rhythm** of the pulse is an indication of how regularly the heart is beating. The rhythm should always be regular. Pulse beats should repeat at approximately the same time interval. Beats should not be missed, skipped, or come early in the cycle. If you observe that the pulse is irregular, count it for one full minute and report your findings to the nurse immediately for assessment.

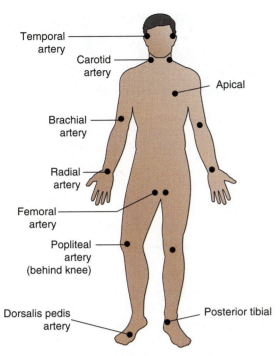

Temporal artery
Carotid artery
Apical
Brachial artery
Radial artery
Femoral artery
Popliteal artery (behind knee)
Dorsalis pedis artery
Posterior tibial

FIGURE 16-13 Pulse locations

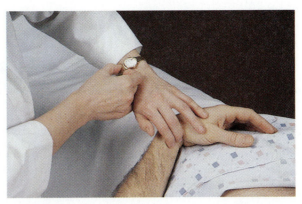

FIGURE 16-14 The radial pulse is on the thumb side of the wrist.

The **force** of the pulse is the strength of the beat. The pulse beat is normally strong and full. If the pulse is weak and hard to feel, this may indicate a problem that should be reported to the nurse. Pulses that feel thready or bounding (full) should also be reported promptly.

Counting the Pulse

The radial pulse is located on the thumb side of the wrist **(Figure 16-14)**. It is easily accessible and commonly used to take vital signs. To count the radial pulse, gently put the first three fingers of your hand on top of the pulse. Avoid pressing too hard or you will obliterate the pulse. Never count the pulse beat with your thumb, which has a pulse of its own. With the second hand of your watch, count the beat for 30 seconds. If the pulse is strong and regular, stop after 30 seconds. Multiply the number of beats counted in 30 seconds by two to obtain the pulse rate for one minute. The pulse rate documented on the medical record is always recorded in number of beats per minute. If the pulse is weak, irregular, very slow, or very rapid, or if counting for a full minute is your facility policy, count for one full minute and do not multiply the number. Report the abnormality to the nurse.

PROCEDURE 72	Taking the Radial Pulse	

Note: The guidelines and reportable values for this procedure vary slightly from state to state, and from one facility to another. Your instructor will inform you if the guidelines or reportable values in your state or facility differ from those listed here. Know and follow the required guidelines for your state and facility.

1. Perform your beginning procedure actions.
2. Gather needed supplies: watch with second hand, notepad and pen.
3. Support the resident's arm on a secure surface.
4. Locate the radial pulse and place the first three fingers of your hand on it. Position your thumb on the other side of the wrist to keep it from moving.
5. Look at your watch and begin counting.
6. Count the number of pulse beats for 30 seconds.
7. Multiply the number of beats in 30 seconds by two. Record this figure.
8. If you are taking respirations, you will leave your fingers on the pulse. If you are also counting the respirations, do not stop to record the pulse rate. Remember the number and document it when you are finished.
9. If you are not counting the respirations, perform your procedure completion actions.

PROCEDURE 73 — Counting Respirations

Note: The guidelines and reportable values for this procedure vary slightly from state to state, and from one facility to another. Your instructor will inform you if the guidelines or reportable values in your state or facility differ from those listed here. Know and follow the required guidelines for your state and facility.

1. Perform your beginning procedure actions.
2. Count the resident's pulse and remember the number.
3. After you have counted the pulse, glance at the chest, while continuing to look at your watch.
4. Count one inhalation and one exhalation as one respiration.
5. Count the number of respirations in 30 seconds and multiply this number by two.
6. Record the resident's pulse and respirations on your note pad.
7. Perform your procedure completion actions.

RESPIRATIONS

Respiration is the act of breathing. **Inhalation,** or **inspiration,** is the act of taking air in. **Exhalation,** or **expiration,** is the act of breathing air out. One respiration is counted as one inhalation and one exhalation. Normal adult respirations are smooth, regular, and unlabored. The normal respiratory rate in adults is about 14 to 20 per minute. If you observe a resident with a respiratory rate under 12 or over 20, report this information to the nurse.

Respiratory Distress

Difficulty breathing, or **dyspnea,** means labored respirations. **Cheyne-Stokes respirations** are seen in critically ill and dying residents. They are irregular and are followed by periods of **apnea,** or no respirations, before the resident starts breathing again. If you observe abnormal or difficult respirations, notify the nurse immediately.

Because respiration involves bringing fresh oxygen into the body, the skin of a Caucasian resident who is breathing normally is pink. A dark bluish or purplish discoloration of the skin and mucous membranes is called **cyanosis.** This condition is caused by inadequate oxygen in the blood. If the skin or nail beds appear cyanotic (blue, gray, or dusky in appearance), the resident is having a serious problem with the intake and use of oxygen. In dark-skinned residents, problems with oxygenation are noted by looking at the nail beds, lips, and mucous membranes inside the mouth. If the color is abnormal, notify the nurse immediately.

Counting Respirations

Respiration is under voluntary control. The resident should not be aware that you are counting

GUIDELINES FOR
Using a Stethoscope

- Clean the ear pieces and diaphragm of the stethoscope before using it.
- Clean the stethoscope tubing if it contacts the resident or bed linen.
- Check the ear pieces of the stethoscope for wax, and remove it if present.
- Check the stethoscope tubing. Do not use if it has cracks or holes in it.
- The ear pieces of the stethoscope should face forward.
- The diaphragm of the stethoscope should not come in contact with the resident's clothing, blood pressure cuff, or other device.
- Place the diaphragm of the stethoscope flat against the resident's skin and hold it in place. If the diaphragm is at an angle, you will not be able to hear the sounds.
- Apply firm but gentle pressure when holding the diaphragm in place. If you press too hard, you may be unable to hear the sound.

the respirations. Placing the resident's arm across the chest or abdomen when counting the pulse is helpful. After you have counted the pulse for 30 seconds, glance at the resident's chest to count respirations. Continue looking at your watch while you count. Remember, one respiration consists of one inhalation and one exhalation. If you are unable to see the resident breathing, count how many times the abdomen rises and falls.

When counting respirations, you may count for 30 seconds and multiply this number by two. Like the pulse, the respiratory rate recorded is for one full minute. If the respirations are slow, labored, irregular, or unusual, count them for one full minute and report this information.

USING A STETHOSCOPE

A stethoscope is a medical instrument used to listen to sounds inside the body. It intensifies sounds so they can be heard clearly. The parts of the stethoscope are seen in **Figure 16-15.** Many health care workers use stethoscopes on many residents. This creates the potential for infection to be passed to both workers and residents. Before and after using the stethoscope, wipe the ear pieces and diaphragm with an alcohol sponge or other disinfectant. If the tubing of the stethoscope contacts the resident or bed linen, wipe the tubing as well.

You will use the stethoscope to take blood pressures. Your health care facility may teach you other procedures with the stethoscope, including taking an apical pulse.

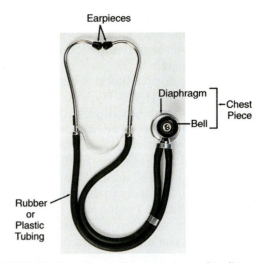

FIGURE 16-15 The stethoscope is used to listen to sounds inside the body.

BLOOD PRESSURE

The blood pressure is a measurement of how the heart is working. It measures the force of the blood on the inside of the arteries. The **systolic blood pressure** is a sound you hear during the working phase of the heart cycle. The systolic sound is the first sound heard when the heart contracts and forces blood through the body. The **diastolic blood pressure** is the sound you hear when the heart is resting. This sound is heard when the heart relaxes and refills with blood. Blood pressure is often called the fourth vital sign. If the nurse instructs you to obtain the vital signs, you will take the resident's TPR and blood pressure. Sometimes the doctor will order

---

PROCEDURE 74 | **Using the Stethoscope**

1. Perform your beginning procedure actions.
2. Gather needed equipment: stethoscope, alcohol sponges, notepad and pen, watch with second hand.
3. Wipe the ear pieces and diaphragm of the stethoscope with the alcohol sponge.
4. If the diaphragm is cold to touch, rub it against your clothing to warm it.
5. Feel the pulse you will be listening to with your fingers.
6. Place the ear pieces of the stethoscope in your ears.
7. Place the diaphragm of the stethoscope over the pulse.
8. Listen to the sound and count if necessary.
9. Remove the stethoscope from your ears and record your findings.
10. Wipe the ear pieces and diaphragm of the stethoscope with the alcohol sponge.
11. Perform your procedure completion actions.

blood pressure readings when the resident is both sitting and standing. Most of the time, the resident should be seated and relaxed when the blood pressure is taken.

In adults, the normal blood pressure range is between 100/60 and 119/79. **Hypertension** is the medical term for high blood pressure, or values over 140/90. Blood pressure values above this value should be reported to the nurse. **Prehypertension** is a blood pressure reading between 120/80 mmHg and 139/89 mmHg. Having this condition means you are likely to develop high blood pressure in the future. People with prehypertension should take steps to decrease their risk. **Hypotension** is the medical term for low blood pressure, or values below 100/60.

Blood pressure classifications are listed in **Table 16-4.** When systolic and diastolic blood pressures fall into different categories, the higher category is used to classify blood pressure level. For example, 172/78 mmHg would be stage 2 hypertension (high blood pressure).

Measuring Blood Pressure

Blood pressure is measured with an instrument called a **sphygmomanometer.** Several different types of sphygmomanometers are used in long-term care facilities **(Figure 16-16).** The technique for measuring blood pressure is the same with most of the units. Many blood pressure units use an **aneroid gauge.** This is a spring-loaded dial

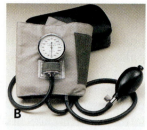
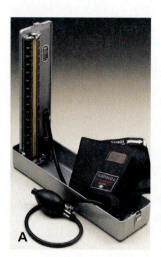
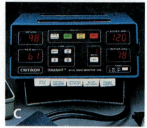

FIGURE 16-16 Different types of sphygmomanometers. (A) Mercury sphygmomanometer (B) Dial (aneroid) sphygmomanometer (C) Electronic sphygmomanometer

marked with numbers to display the reading. The mercury blood pressure cuff also has numbers marked on it. With this unit, the blood pressure is measured by reading the level of a column of mercury. A mercury unit must be placed on a flat surface and read at eye level for readings to be accurate. Some facilities use electronic units. However, no truly satisfactory alternative has been found for mercury in blood pressure devices, so these are still in use in health care facilities. Use mercury devices carefully to avoid breakage.

The fabric blood pressure cuff is wrapped around the resident's upper arm about one inch above the brachial artery. After the cuff is wrapped around the arm, a stethoscope is placed over the **brachial artery** in front of the elbow to obtain the reading.

Reading the Blood Pressure Gauge. The gauge on the sphygmomanometer is marked with a series of lines. A number is marked on the gauge in increments of 10 or 20, depending on the unit you are using. If the gauge is marked in increments of 20, a long line appears in the center of each 20 units. The long line represents a value of 10. Each short line on the gauge represents a value of 2. **Figure 16-17** demonstrates how to read the gauge on both an aneroid and a mercury blood pressure unit. The number on the gauge is 80 for both units. If the dial or mercury was one small line above 80, the reading would be 82. If the dial or mercury was one small line below 80, the value would be 78. Blood pressure is always recorded in even numbers.

TABLE 16-4	National Heart, Lung, and Blood Institute blood pressure definitions 2003		
	Blood Pressure Level (mmHg)		
Category	**Systolic**	*****	**Diastolic**
Normal	< 120	and	< 80
Prehypertension	120-139	or	< 80
High Blood Pressure			
Stage I Hypertension	140-159	or	90-99
Stage II Hypertension	≥ 160	or	≥ 100

Legend:
< means less than
≥ means greater than or equal to
Source: National Heart, Lung, and Blood Institute, National Institutes of Health 2003.
For additional information, see
http://www.nhlbi.nih.gov/hbp/index.html

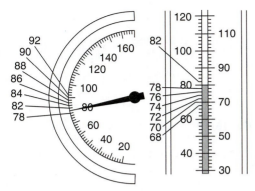

FIGURE 16-17   Read the pressure at the closest line. The pressure on both these gauges is 80.

When measuring blood pressure, you use your vision and hearing. You inflate the cuff, then release it slowly, so the gauge falls in increments of 2 mmHg. The stethoscope is placed over the brachial artery and you listen for a sound while simultaneously looking at the gauge. The first sound you hear is the systolic value. The last sound you hear is the diastolic value. The difference between the two numbers is called the **pulse pressure.** In healthy adults, the differ-

ence is about 40 mmHg. The normal range is between 30 and 50 mmHg. For example, if the systolic pressure is 118 and the systolic pressure is 78, 118 minus 78 equals 40. The pulse pressure in this case is 40.

Accuracy of Blood Pressure.   The blood pressure value is a very important measurement that the physician uses to measure the resident's progress and determine treatment. It is important that blood pressure values be accurate. Blood pressure should not be measured in an arm with a **shunt.** A shunt is a surgically implanted passage between two blood vessels. It is used for **dialysis,** which is a process of removing waste products from the blood for residents with kidney disease.

Do not take a blood pressure on an arm with:

- Paralysis
- An intravenous infusion
- Impaired circulation
- Fracture
- Burns
- Edema
- A recent mastectomy (breast removal) or other surgical procedure on that side

GUIDELINES FOR
Taking Blood Pressure

Blood Pressure Cuff
- Be sure the cuff is the correct size to fit the resident.
- Check the screw valve to be sure it opens and closes easily.
- Close the valve and pump the cuff. Make sure the gauge rises.
- Place the center of the bladder in the cuff over the brachial artery, or use the arrows on the cuff to guide you.

Aneroid Sphygmomanometer
- Check the placement of the needle on the gauge. It should be exactly at zero. The needle is very delicate and will change position if the gauge is bumped or dropped. If the needle is not on zero, the reading will not be accurate.
- Place the gauge flat against the cuff where you can see it.

Mercury Sphygmomanometer
- Check to be sure you can see the mercury in the glass tube.
- Make sure the glass tube is not cloudy.
- Check the mercury level. It should be at zero.
- Place the unit on a flat surface where you can read it at eye level.
- When you inflate the cuff, the mercury should rise readily. If it is slow to respond, this indicates a

problem with the unit, and the reading may not be accurate.

Resident
- Have the resident sit and relax.
- Some facilities prefer to measure the blood pressure in the left arm, if possible, because it is closest to the heart.
- Remove the resident's blouse or shirt, or pull up the sleeve. Do not roll up the sleeve so tightly that it constricts the arm, which will alter the reading. *The cuff must be wrapped around the bare skin.*
- Ask the resident not to talk and to turn the radio or television off while you are taking the blood pressure.
- Notify the nurse if the resident was in pain or uncomfortable when the reading was taken. Pain, anxiety, and discomfort may affect the reading.
- Flex the resident's arm slightly and support it at the level of the heart while you are taking the blood pressure. If the arm is not supported, or is above or below heart level, the accuracy of the reading will be affected.

The Environment
- The temperature should be comfortable.
- Environmental noise should be eliminated whenever possible.

- A dialysis access device on that side (Chapter 19)
- A pulse oximeter on that side (Chapter 19)

Causes of inaccurate blood pressure readings include:

- Use of the wrong size cuff
- An improperly wrapped cuff
- Incorrect arm position
- Not using the same arm for all readings
- Not viewing the gauge at eye level
- Deflating the cuff too rapidly or too slowly
- Being distracted by noise in the room, such as the resident talking, a radio, or a television
- Rapidly inflating and deflating the cuff several times in a row

Ask the resident not to talk, which makes it difficult for you to hear, and may change the reading. The temperature in the room should be comfortable. Changes in temperature may alter the reading.

The technique you use for measuring the blood pressure affects the accuracy of the reading. The cuff must fit the resident correctly. Cuffs come in many different sizes **(Figure 16-18)**. Although there is a standard size adult cuff, some residents require an extra-large cuff. Very small residents require a pediatric cuff. If the cuff is too large or small, the reading will be incorrect. To check the size of the cuff, compare the length of the rubber bladder **(Figure 16-19)** with the resident's arm circumference. The bladder should be at least 80% of the circumference of the arm. If it is larger or smaller, obtain a different size cuff.

Wrap the cuff snugly around the resident's arm. If it is too loose or too tight, the reading will be affected. Most cuffs have arrows marked on the fab-

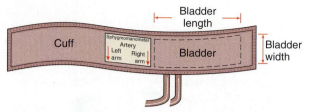

FIGURE 16-19   For an accurate reading, the bladder inside the cuff should be 80% the circumference of the resident's arm.

ric near the tubing. The arrows and markings show you where to place the cuff in relation to the brachial artery. When reading the value on the blood pressure gauge, be sure the gauge is flat and not tipped. Always read the gauge at eye level.

Documenting Blood Pressure.   Blood pressure is recorded in millimeters of mercury. The abbreviation for this is *mmHg*. Blood pressure is recorded in fraction form. Because the systolic sound is the first sound you hear, it is the first number recorded. The diastolic reading is the second number recorded. An example of how to record the blood pressure is 118/78. The systolic value is 118. The diastolic value is 78.

Facility policies vary as to the order in which to record vital signs. For example, some facilities require you to record the blood pressure first. In these facilities, the vital signs would be recorded in this order:

- blood pressure
- temperature
- pulse
- respirations

In this facility, the vital signs would be recorded as *120/80-98.6°F(O)-88-16*. Some facilities document the blood pressure last. Know and follow your facility policy.

MEASURING AND RECORDING HEIGHT AND WEIGHT

Measuring the resident's height and weight is often the responsibility of the nursing assistant. Many members of the interdisciplinary team need to know the resident's height and weight to perform their assessments and plan care. The dietitian uses the information to plan the diet. The physician uses the information to calculate doses of medications. Most facilities measure the height and weight of residents upon admission, then weigh residents monthly thereafter.

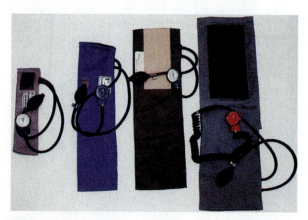

FIGURE 16-18   Select a cuff that fits the resident's arm.

Measuring the Blood Pressure

Note: This is the "two-step" procedure recommended by the American Heart Association (AHA) as of 1993. The AHA considers the two-step procedure the most reliable for normal blood pressure measurement. (The most accurate values are obtained by internal monitoring, in which a catheter is placed in an artery. The internal method is not practical for most clinical situations.) In some states, nursing assistants use a one-step procedure for measuring blood pressure. For your convenience, the one-step procedure is listed in Appendix A of this book. In some facilities, electronic blood pressure monitoring equipment is used. Procedure 82 (Unit 19) describes the procedure for taking a blood pressure using an electronic monitoring device.

Note: The guidelines and reportable values for this procedure vary slightly from state to state, and from one facility to another. Your instructor will inform you if the guidelines or reportable values in your state or facility differ from those listed here. Know and follow the required guidelines for your state and facility.

1. Perform your beginning procedure actions.
2. Gather supplies needed: sphygmomanometer, stethoscope, alcohol sponges, notepad and pen.
3. Wipe the ear pieces and diaphragm of the stethoscope with the alcohol sponge.
4. Locate the brachial artery on the thumb side of the inner upper arm.
5. Wrap the cuff around the arm, centering the arrow over the brachial artery. The cuff should be one inch above the artery in the **antecubital space,** in front of the elbow.
6. Locate the radial pulse on the thumb side of the wrist. Keep your fingers on it.
7. Close the screw on the hand set and inflate the bulb until you can no longer feel the radial pulse. Mentally add 30 to the number on the gauge.
8. Open the screw and deflate the cuff.
9. Wait 30 seconds.
10. Place the stethoscope in your ears. Place the diaphragm of the stethoscope over the brachial artery. (You will not hear a sound until you inflate the cuff and open the valve.)
11. Close the screw and rapidly and steadily inflate the cuff to 30 points higher than where the radial pulse was last palpated.
12. Slowly release the screw so the pressure in the cuff falls at 2 mmHg increments.
13. Listen for a sound. When you hear it, note the closest number on the gauge. This is the systolic pressure.
14. Continue to listen until the sound stops. Note the closest number on the gauge. This is the diastolic pressure. Continue to listen for 10 mmHg below this sound.
15. Open the screw completely and deflate the cuff.
16. Remove the stethoscope from your ears.
17. Remove the cuff from the resident's arm.
18. Record your findings.
19. If you are unsure of the blood pressure, wait one to two minutes, then check it again.
20. Wipe the ear pieces and diaphragm of the stethoscope with the alcohol sponge.
21. Perform your procedure completion actions.

This gives the team members baseline information to compare with. Residents who have heart and kidney disease may be weighed daily to monitor for rapid weight gain, which indicates a fluid balance problem. Residents who are underweight are usually weighed weekly.

Weight loss can be a serious problem in the elderly. Weight loss is a risk factor for skin breakdown and other conditions. Progressive, unplanned weight loss may be a symptom of a more serious problem. Aggressive measures are taken when unplanned weight loss is detected. Accurate measurement and recording of weight is an important responsibility that you must take very seriously. The physician is notified of unplanned weight loss, and steps are taken to prevent additional loss. Know and follow your facility policies for reporting weight loss or gains.

Methods of Weighing Residents

Many different scales are available. Some are mechanical balance scales. Others are electronically operated. Most of the balance scales must be leveled or balanced before they are used, to assure an accurate reading. Check your facility policy and learn how to balance the type of scale you are using.

Standing Balance Scale. The standing balance scale **(Figure 16-20)** is commonly used if residents are able to stand and balance unassisted. Shoes are usually removed and the resident stands on a paper towel.

To weigh a resident on the balance scale, you must understand how to calculate the weight by adding the reading on the two bars. The lower bar is marked with lines every 50 pounds. The

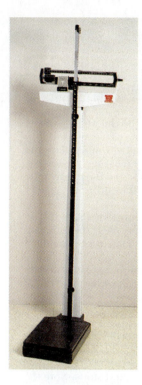

FIGURE 16-20 The balance scale is used for ambulatory residents who can stand unassisted.

Wheelchair Scale. When using the wheelchair scale **(Figure 16-22)**, three steps are required to obtain an accurate weight. First, the wheelchair is weighed empty. The weight of the chair is recorded. The resident is transferred to the chair and weighed. The weight is recorded. The empty weight of the chair is subtracted from the total weight. This figure gives you the resident's weight. Most wheelchair scales are balance scales. Some facilities have removable ramps that are placed over the standing balance scale so it can be used for wheelchairs. Some wheelchair scales are electronically operated.

If the resident uses a lap tray on the wheelchair, remove the tray before weighing the resident. If the tray cannot be removed, weigh the tray and the wheelchair together during the first step of the procedure, then subtract the combined weight from the total. Lap trays can add as much as five pounds to the total weight.

Bed Scale. There are several types of bed scales. The electronic bed scale has a sling attached. The resident is placed in the sling, which is suspended from the bed. Both the resident and the sling must be lifted completely off the surface of the bed for the weight to be accurate. After the resident is suspended above the bed, the scale electronically records the weight.

Another type of bed scale is attached to the mechanical lifting device. The resident is transferred to the mechanical lift, using the guidelines in Procedure 23. The lift is elevated until the resident is above the surface of the bed. This type of scale usually has a detachable dial, balance mechanism, or electronic gauge to record the weight. A similar electronic bed scale **(Figure 16-23)** uses a canvas sling for residents who must remain supine.

upper bar has single pound readings. Even numbers are marked on the bar every 2 pounds. Each long line indicates an odd-numbered pound. Each short line on the upper bar is ¼ of a pound. You will adjust the weights on each balance bar until the rod hangs free on the end. To obtain the total weight, add the number of pounds on each bar **(Figure 16-21).**

Chair Scale. The chair scale has a chair permanently attached to it. The resident is transferred to the chair to be weighed. Some chair scales use a balancing mechanism, similar to the standing balance scale. Others read the weight electronically and display a digital readout on a screen.

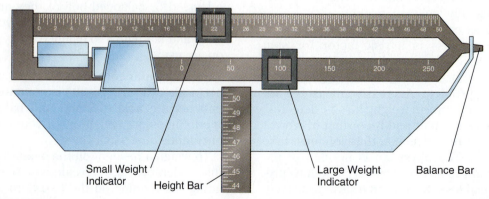

Small Weight Indicator   Height Bar   Large Weight Indicator   Balance Bar

FIGURE 16-21 Add the number of pounds on the upper bar to the weight on the lower bar to obtain the resident's total weight.

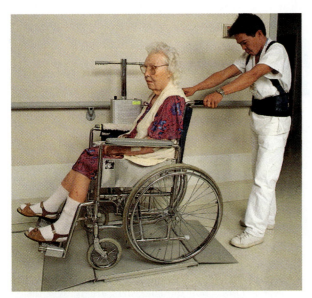

FIGURE 16-22 This wheelchair scale uses a ramp over the balance scale. The wheelchair weight is subtracted from the total weight.

Methods of Measuring Height

Knowing the resident's height is important for determining if the resident is within the ideal weight range. The height is usually taken on admission. It is not checked again because it does

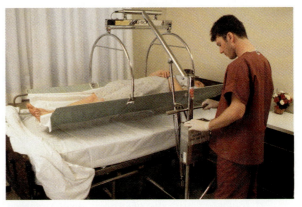

FIGURE 16-23 The bed scale is used for nonambulatory residents who cannot sit in a chair. Make sure the sling is not touching the bed when you take the weight reading.

not change. You must learn several methods of measuring the resident's height.

Height may be measured in either centimeters or inches, depending on your facility policy. One centimeter equals 2.5 inches. If your facility uses a centimeter measurement, multiply the number of inches by 2.5.

Standing Height. The standing balance scale has a height bar that can be used for residents

---

PROCEDURE 76	Measuring Weight and Height	OBRA 🔀

Note: These procedures are generic and apply principles used for common types of scales. Follow the instructions for the specific scale you are using. The operating instructions are slightly different for each. Your instructor will inform you if the directions for the equipment you are using differ from those listed here.

1. Perform your beginning procedure actions.
2. Gather supplies needed: scale, paper towels, notepad and pen.
3. Standing scale
   a. Balance the scale.
   b. Place a paper towel on the scale platform.
   c. Assist the resident to remove shoes and stand on the platform.
   d. Adjust the weights on the scale until the bar hangs freely on the end.
   e. Add the weight on the two bars to determine the weight. Write this down on your notepad or remember it.
   f. Assist the resident to turn around, facing away from the scale.
   g. Raise the height bar until it is level with the top of the head.

h. Record the measurement in the center of the height bar **(Figure 16-24)**.
i. Help the resident down from the scale and assist him or her to put on shoes, if necessary.
j. Remove and discard the paper towel.

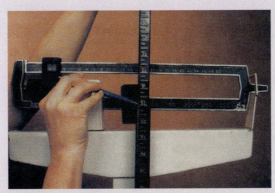

FIGURE 16-24 Read the height at the movable part of the ruler bar.

Continues

PROCEDURE 76	Measuring Weight and Height, *Continued*	OBRA

4. Chair scale
   a. Balance the scale.
   b. Assist the resident to transfer from the wheelchair to the chair scale.
   c. Place the resident's feet on the footrest of the chair.
   d. Move the weights until the balance bar hangs freely, or read the electronic display screen. Remember this number or write it down on your notepad.
   e. Transfer the resident back to the wheelchair.
5. Wheelchair scale
   a. Balance the scale.
   b. Obtain a wheelchair and take it to the scale and weigh it. Write down the weight.
   c. Take the wheelchair to the resident's room and assist the resident to transfer into it.
   d. Take the resident to the scale. Roll the wheelchair up the ramp and lock the brakes.
   e. Adjust the weights until the balance bar hangs freely on the end. Write down this number on your notepad.
   f. Unlock the brakes and slowly guide the wheelchair down the ramp.

   g. Return to the resident's room and assist the resident to transfer out of the wheelchair.
   h. Subtract the weight of the empty wheelchair from the total weight of the resident and chair and record this number.
6. Bed scale (follow the guidelines in Procedure 23 for assisting the resident into the lift seat or sling).
   a. Balance the scale. The scale should be balanced with the canvas seat, chains, or straps attached.
   b. Remove the sling from the scale and position the resident on the sling.
   c. Connect the straps and elevate the lift above the level of the bed. Raise the sling so the resident's body and the sling hang freely over the bed.
   d. Adjust the weights until the balance bar hangs freely on the end, or read the electronic display screen. Remember this number or write it on your notepad.
   e. Lower the resident back into the bed and remove the sling.
7. Perform your procedure completion actions.

who can stand. An adjustable height bar is lifted up from the scale and the height is measured.

Measuring Height in Nonambulatory Residents. There are several methods of measuring a resident who cannot stand. The simplest is to use a tape measure while the resident is lying supine in bed. Before beginning, smooth and straighten the bottom sheet so it is tucked in tightly and is wrinkle-free. Straighten the resident's back, arms, and legs so he or she is lying as straight as possible. Make a small mark on the sheet with your pen at the top of the resident's head. Make another mark at the level of the resident's heels. Measuring the distance between the two marks with the tape measure will give you the height.

GUIDELINES FOR
Weight and Height Measurements

- Weigh residents at the same time of day.
- Use the same scale each time.
- Balance the scale before weighing the resident.
- Have the resident wear similar clothing each time he or she is weighed.
- Have the resident empty the bladder before being weighed.
- If the resident is wearing an incontinent brief, make sure it is dry before weighing.
- If the resident has an indwelling catheter, make sure the bag is empty before weighing.
- If the resident has a cast, has recently had a cast re-

moved, or has new-onset edema, consult the nurse about possible weight discrepancies.
- If you are taking a standing weight and height on a balance scale, have the resident remove his or her shoes and stand on a paper towel.
- If you are responsible for documenting the weight on the resident's chart, compare it to the previous weight. If there is a difference of five pounds or more (or according to facility policy), recheck the resident's weight. If, after rechecking the weight, there continues to be a difference, inform the nurse.

KEY POINTS

- Vital signs tell you how well the body's vital organs are working.
- Body temperature can be measured orally, rectally, axillary, or at the tympanic membrane.
- The site used most often for taking the pulse is the radial artery.
- Because respirations are under voluntary control, the resident should not know when you are counting them.
- The systolic blood pressure is the first sound heard when the heart is contracting.
- The diastolic blood pressure is the last sound heard when the heart is resting.
- Abnormal vital signs must be reported to the nurse immediately.
- Accuracy is very important when taking and recording vital signs.
- The nursing assistant is responsible for obtaining and accurately recording the resident's height and weight.

REVIEW

A. Multiple Choice

Select the one best answer.

1. The nurse assigns you to take vital signs on Mr. Vasquez. You know this means you will take the
   a. TPR.
   b. B/P.
   c. TPR and B/P.
   d. B/P and mmHg.

2. The aural (tympanic) temperature is taken
   a. in the ear.
   b. rectally.
   c. under the arm.
   d. in the mouth.

3. The normal rectal temperature is
   a. 97.6°F.
   b. 98.6°F.
   c. 99.6°F.
   d. 100.6°F.

4. The normal oral temperature is
   a. 97.6°F.
   b. 98.6°F.
   c. 99.6°F.
   d. 100.6°F.

5. The normal axillary temperature is
   a. 97.6°F.
   b. 98.6°F.
   c. 99.6°F.
   d. 100.6°F.

6. You are assigned to take Mr. Washington's temperature rectally with a glass thermometer. After lubricating the thermometer, you will insert it into the anus
   a. ¼ inch.
   b. ½ inch.
   c. 1 inch.
   d. 2 inches.

7. The oral thermometer is marked with a
   a. blue dot.
   b. red dot.
   c. green dot.
   d. yellow dot.

8. The rectal thermometer is marked with a
   a. blue dot.
   b. red dot.
   c. green dot.
   d. yellow dot.

9. When taking an axillary temperature, you should use a/an
   a. green probe.
   b. red probe.
   c. rectal thermometer.
   d. oral thermometer.

10. Before taking a temperature with a glass thermometer, shake the thermometer down to
    a. 96°F.
    b. 97°F.
    c. 98°F.
    d. 99°F.

11. The most commonly used site for taking the pulse in adults is the
    a. temporal artery.
    b. apex of the heart.
    c. brachial artery.
    d. radial artery.

12. When palpating the pulse, always use your
    a. thumb.
    b. stethoscope.
    c. first three fingers.
    d. third and fourth fingers.

13. Which of the following pulse rates should you report to the nurse?
    a. 60
    b. 72
    c. 96
    d. 112

14. A pulse rate that is abnormally slow is called
    a. tachycardia.
    b. hypotension.
    c. bradycardia.
    d. pulse pressure.

15. The normal respiratory rate in adults is
    a. 14 to 20.
    b. 16 to 24.
    c. 10 to 20.
    d. 20 to 30.

16. You are assigned to take vital signs on Team A. Which of the following would you report to the nurse?
    a. 98.4°F (O)-80-18
    b. 97.6°F (Ax)-64-16
    c. 100.2°F (R)-110-24
    d. 99.2°F (O)-96-20

17. Which artery is used for taking blood pressure?
    a. carotid
    b. brachial
    c. radial
    d. femoral

18. Hypertension is blood pressure
    a. under 140/90.
    b. over 140/90.
    c. under 100/60.
    d. over 120/80.

19. Hypotension is blood pressure
    a. under 140/90.
    b. over 140/90.
    c. under 100/60.
    d. over 120/80.

20. The instrument used to take a blood pressure is the
    a. sphygmomanometer.
    b. thermometer.
    c. aneroid dial.
    d. mercury probe.

21. When weighing a resident on the balance scale, you know that each marking on the large bar represents
    a. 1 pound.
    b. 5 pounds.
    c. 25 pounds.
    d. 50 pounds.

22. Oral temperatures should not be taken on residents
    a. over the age of 80.
    b. with colostomies.
    c. with seizure disorders.
    d. who are alert.

23. Rectal temperatures should not be taken on residents
    a. with respiratory disease.
    b. with fecal impaction.
    c. using oxygen.
    d. who are confused.

24. The normal pulse rate in adults is
    a. 40-60.   c. 60-100.
    b. 20-80.   d. 70-90.

25. Which of the following is the *least accurate* method of taking the temperature?
    a. rectal   c. oral
    b. tympanic   d. axillary

B. Clinical Applications

Answer the following questions.

You are assigned to take vital signs on the north hallway. Your facility uses glass thermometers that are covered with disposable sheaths.

26. You obtained Mrs. White's TPR, but cannot hear her blood pressure. What should you do?

27. Mr. Camp is a new admission. He is using oxygen by mask at six liters per minute. Mr. Camp has an old, well-established colostomy. What method should you use to take his temperature? What type of personal protective equipment should you wear when taking a temperature using this method?

28. You have taken Mr. Camp's temperature. It is 103.2°F. You still have to take vital signs on four more residents. What action should you take?

29. You are assigned to do monthly weights on east wing. After obtaining the weights, you go to the nurses' station to document them. Mr. Lyer weighed 154 pounds last month. Today's weight is 138 pounds. What action should you take?

30. Mrs. Roosevelt is a new admission who has a doctor's order for bed rest. As part of the admission process, you must obtain her height and weight. Mrs. Roosevelt is an obese resident. Her left leg has been amputated above the knee. How will you obtain her height and weight?

CHAPTER 17

Admission, Transfer, and Discharge

OBJECTIVES

After reading this chapter, you will be able to:

- Spell and define key terms.
- Explain why first impressions are important and describe how they set the tone for the resident's stay.
- Describe family dynamics and emotions that occur when a loved one is admitted to a long-term care facility.
- List ways in which the nursing assistant can develop positive relationships with family members.
- Describe the nursing assistant's responsibilities in the admission, transfer, and discharge processes.
- Demonstrate procedures related to admission, transfer, and discharge.

OBSERVATIONS TO MAKE AND REPORT RELATED TO ADMISSION, TRANSFER, AND DISCHARGE

Pay particular attention to the patient's skin condition:
Rashes
Bruises
Pressure ulcers
Any other abnormalities
The nurse will assess the resident on admission and begin a care plan. Likewise, the nurse will assess the resident's discharge needs. Your

observations and measurements of vital signs, height, and weight contribute to this assessment. Note and report:
Vision problems
Hearing problems
Communication problems, including ability to make needs known and call for help
Ability to ambulate and transfer safely
Ability to use the bathroom safely

ADMITTING, TRANSFERRING, AND DISCHARGING A RESIDENT

One responsibility of the nursing assistant is to assist residents with **admission, transfer,** and **discharge** in the health care facility. You are expected to gather information, meet the resident's basic needs, and make the process as smooth and comfortable as possible. Your pleasant and courteous manner sets the tone for the admission process. During transfer, being calm and understanding will ease any fears the resident may have. Upon discharge, the professionalism you

have shown throughout the resident's stay will be remembered and appreciated.

ADMISSION

The nursing assistant is frequently the person who admits residents to the long-term care facility. This may be a difficult, frightening time for the resident. There is a common expression that "first impressions are usually lasting ones." The resident's perception of what is happening may be affected by illness, pain, and fear. Making a good first impression on the resident and family

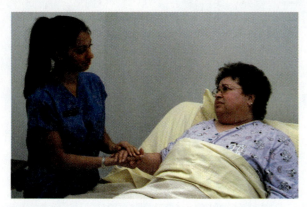

FIGURE 17-1 A positive first impression is long lasting, and will help relieve the resident's fear and anxiety.

members is important. If the first impression of the nursing assistant is negative, it will affect the resident's impression of all health care providers, and even the long-term care facility. Think about this, remember the resident's fears during the admission process, and do your best to provide a positive, professional impression **(Figure 17-1).**

Each facility has policies and procedures for resident admissions. Usually, you will be aware of the admission in advance and should prepare the room. If the resident will be admitted by ambulance and put to bed, elevate the bed to the highest horizontal height and open the bed. Move furnishings if necessary, so that the stretcher can be positioned next to the bed. If the resident will require special equipment, such as an **IV standard (Figure 17-2A)** or bed

trapeze **(Figure 17-2B),** the equipment should be taken to the room prior to admission. If the resident is ambulatory or will be up in a chair, prepare the room so that it looks clean, comfortable, and inviting. Leave the bed closed. If the family has dropped off personal items, arrange them in the room in an attractive manner **(Figure 17-2C).** Having personal items from home will help the resident make the transition to facility living. Make sure that all lights, electrical items, and outlets are in working order. Check the call signals at the bed and in the bathroom to make sure they are in working order.

When you meet the resident, introduce yourself by name and title. Ask the resident what he or she prefers to be called. Avoid addressing adults by the first name without permission. Your responsibility is to make the resident feel secure and welcome. You will begin gathering information that will be used by other members of the interdisciplinary team. You may be responsible for gathering information for the admission checklist, checking and listing the resident's belongings **(Figure 17-3),** and obtaining vital signs, height, and weight. Provide information about the health

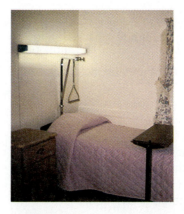

FIGURE 17-2B The trapeze is a heavy piece of equipment that should be installed on the bed before the resident arrives.

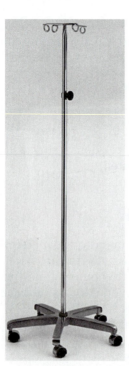

FIGURE 17-2A The intravenous standard is used for hanging IV solutions, IV pumps, tube-feeding solutions, and tube-feeding pumps. Occasionally, it is used to help elevate a resident's arm after an injury. *(Courtesy of Medline Industries, Inc. 1-800-MEDLINE)*

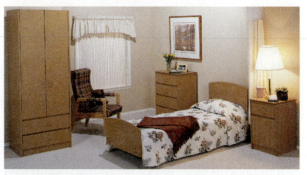

FIGURE 17-2C Arrange the room so it is comfortable and inviting. Placing the resident's personal belongings in prominent positions will make the resident feel more at home. *(Courtesy of Medline Industries, Inc. 1-800-MEDLINE)*

INVENTORY OF PERSONAL EFFECTS
(Reference tag: F252)

INSTRUCTIONS: Upon admission, identify the resident's personal belongings by indicating quantity of those items listed. Use the space allowed to write in additional items as necessary. The original copy shall be kept in the resident's chart. The copy is given to the resident or resident representative. Update as necessary throughout the resident's stay by using the space provided. Upon discharge, use the "√" columns to indicate that all personal belongings are accounted for.

QTY.	ARTICLES	√
	Belts	
	Blouses	
	Coats	
	Dresses	
	Gloves	
	Handkerchiefs	
	Hats	
	Housecoats/robes	
	Jackets	
	Nightgowns/pajamas	
	Purses	
	Shaving kit	
	Shoes	
	Shorts	
	Slacks	
	Slippers	
	Slips	
	Shirts	
	Socks/hose	
	Suitcases	
	Suits	
	Suspenders	
	Sweaters	
	Ties	
	Undershirts	
	Underwear	
	Hearing aid	
	Dentures: ☐ Up ☐ Low ☐ Part	
	Eyewear	
	Cane	
	Walker	
	Wheelchair	
	Brace	
	Prosthesis	

ITEMS OF SPECIFIC VALUE (JEWELRY, APPLIANCES, FURNITURE)

QTY	DESCRIPTION	VALUE	√
		$	

ITEMS ACQUIRED AFTER ORIGINAL ENTRY

DATE	ITEM	HOW RECEIVED	INITIAL	√

USE THIS SPACE TO RECORD MISCELLANEOUS INFORMATION
(i.e. LOST, STOLEN, RETURNED/GIVEN TO FAMILY, ETC.)

DATE	DESCRIPTION / EXPLANATION	INITIAL	√

CERTIFICATION OF RECEIPT

ON ADMISSION	ON DISCHARGE
Signed **X** _____ Date _____ *Resident or resident representative*	Signed **X** _____ Date _____ *Resident or resident representative*
Signed _____ Title _____ Date _____ *Facility representative*	Signed _____ Title _____ Date _____ *Facility representative*
If resident unable to sign, state reason:	If resident unable to sign, state reason:
Signed _____ Date _____ *Witness*	Signed _____ Date _____ *Witness*

NAME—Last	First	Middle	Attending Physician	Chart No.

INVENTORY OF PERSONAL EFFECTS

FIGURE 17-3 The nursing assistant is responsible for completing the personal effects inventory form. *(Courtesy of Briggs Corporation, Des Moines, IA (800) 247-2343)*

care facility to the resident and visitors. Before you leave the room, provide fresh drinking water, if allowed, and make sure the resident knows how to use the call signal, telephone, television, and electric bed controls. Label disposable equipment such as the water pitcher, drinking glass, bedpan, urinal, emesis basin, and other personal care items with the resident's name according to facility policy. Mark resident clothing and personal items with a permanent marker, according to facility policy. When marking clothing, take care to mark the name on the inside of the garment, where it is not visible from the outside. Mark items in a location where the marker will not bleed through to the outside of the garment. If this is not possible, consult the nurse for an alternate method of labeling the garment. Ask the resident if he or she needs anything else, and do what he or she asks, if possible.

After you have completed your part of the admission, the nurse will **assess,** or evaluate, the resident. This helps identify the resident's problems and needs. Assessment is the first step of the **nursing process.** The nursing process is a four-step process that provides the structure for nursing action. The nursing assistant is an active participant in the nursing process. **Planning** is the second step. Assessment and planning involve gathering information to determine the resident's problems and needs, and then planning care to meet them. The nurse will begin to develop the care plan based on his or her assessment and the information you provide. **Implementation** is the next step. The interdisciplinary team will implement the care plan. **Evaluation** is the final step of the nursing process. The resident's response to the care plan is evaluated and the plan is revised continuously throughout the resident's stay to ensure that his or her needs are met.

FAMILY DYNAMICS

The family is an extension of the resident. Like the resident, they must make many adjustments during the transition to the long-term care facility. Admitting a loved one to a long-term care facility is usually a very emotional time. Emotions range from relief in getting help with the resident's care to guilt for being unable to care for the loved one. Other common emotions family members experience are:

- Fear. Some family members feel fearful about leaving their relative in the facility. They may have preconceived or incorrect notions about long-term care based on news reports, rumors, or other sources.

- Anger. Some families become angry about the admission. They feel as if they are losing control and are being replaced. They may take their anger out on the staff.
- Uncertainty. The family may feel uncertain about placing a loved one in a facility. They worry that they have made the wrong decision. They may seem afraid, worried, nervous, and tense.
- Sadness. The family may have difficulty coping with being separated from the resident.
- Guilt. The family may feel guilty for turning the care of the resident over to complete strangers.
- Helplessness. Family members may feel helpless because the resident's physical and/or mental condition has worsened, and despite their best efforts, they cannot change the situation.
- Worry. Family members may worry about their loved one's well-being. They may worry about how to pay the bills, or what to do with the house or pets. They often feel overwhelmed with decisions and responsibilities.

Understanding the emotions that families experience should give you an appreciation of why making a good first impression is so important. In addition, you must use good communication skills and show that you care. Greet each family member with warmth, courtesy, kindness, and respect. Introduce yourself and explain your responsibilities as a nursing assistant in the care of their loved one **(Figure 17-4).** Introduce the resident and family to roommates and other staff members. Make them feel welcome, and show that you are sincerely interested in the resident. If appropriate, make comments such as, "I know this must be very difficult for you."

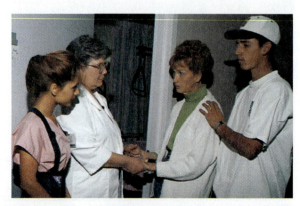

FIGURE 17-4 Families experience a wide range of emotions when a loved one is admitted to a long-term care facility. Introduce yourself and explain the nursing assistant's responsibilities in the care of the residents. Be sincere, and show that you are honestly interested in the resident's well-being.

GUIDELINES FOR
Family Dynamics

- Get to know family members. Greet them warmly when they come to the facility.
- Wear a name badge. Introduce yourself by name and position.
- Work to build a positive and trusting relationship with the family.
- Be available to talk to the family. Listen carefully to what they have to say and respond appropriately.
- Let the family know that you respect and support their role as their loved one's caregivers.
- Provide information about the resident's activities and daily routines, if requested.
- Familiarize the family with facility routines and services.
- Refer questions of a medical or personal nature to the nurse.

- Listen to family members' suggestions, complaints, and comments. Inform the nurse of family complaints or concerns, or refer the family to the nurse, as appropriate.
- Listen closely to family members' advice about resident care. If the family has been caring for the resident at home, they often know what works best. Pass the information on to the nurse.
- Inform the nurse if a visit is stressful or tiring to a resident.
- Avoid judging the family and decisions they make. Stay out of family disagreements.
- Avoid gossiping with the family, and do not discuss facility business with family members.
- Allow the family to participate in the resident's care, if the resident does not object. Avoid making the family feel as if they must provide care for the resident.

PROCEDURE 77 — Admitting the Resident

1. Perform your beginning procedure actions.
2. Gather supplies needed: admission checklist, pen and paper, gloves, hospital gown (if needed), clothing inventory list, scale, tape measure for height, sphygmomanometer, stethoscope, thermometer, standard agency admission kit **(Figure 17-5),** if used.
3. Remove the contents of the admission kit, mark them with the resident's name, and put them away.
4. Bring permanent equipment to the room, if needed for resident care.
5. Upon resident arrival, introduce yourself by name and title.
6. Introduce the resident to roommates.
7. Provide privacy, and inform family members where they can wait.
8. Obtain the resident's height and weight, following the guidelines in Procedure 73.
9. Obtain the vital signs. Follow the guidelines in Procedures 62 through 72.
10. Complete the information on the admission checklist and personal inventory.

11. Assist the resident to put personal articles and toilet items away, if necessary. Mark items with the resident's name, if needed.
12. Familiarize the resident with his or her surroundings. Show the resident how to use the call signal, and explain the intercom system. Explain the use of the telephone, bed controls, and any other equipment in the room.
13. Provide water, if allowed **(Figure 17-6).**
14. Make the resident comfortable.
15. Perform your procedure completion actions. Do not leave the room until the resident is settled and has no more questions or requests.

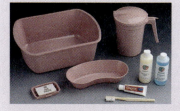

FIGURE 17-5 A standard admission kit. *(Courtesy of Medline Industries, Inc. 1-800-MEDLINE)*

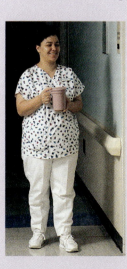

FIGURE 17-6 After admitting the resident, provide fresh water, if allowed.

PROCEDURE 78

Transferring the Resident

1. Perform your beginning procedure actions.
2. Gather supplies needed: wheelchair or stretcher, cart for resident's belongings, chart, other medical supplies as instructed by the nurse.
3. Gather the resident's belongings and other items to be transferred and place them on the cart **(Figure 17-7).** Make sure you have the resident's dentures, glasses, and hearing aid, if used.
4. Assist the resident to transfer to the wheelchair or stretcher for transportation to the new unit. Reassure the resident that family and visitors will be given information about the new location.
5. Transport the resident and belongings to the new unit **(Figure 17-8).**
6. Introduce the resident to the roommate and nursing staff.
7. Put away the resident's belongings, if this is your facility policy.
8. Make the resident comfortable.
9. Before leaving the unit, make sure that the call signal is within reach and that the resident knows how to use it.
10. Return to your unit.
11. Inform the nurse that the transfer has been completed, and report the resident's reaction and any other observations.
12. Strip the resident's unit and remove any permanent equipment from the room, according to facility policy. Notify the **environmental services department** that the unit is ready to be cleaned. Environmental services is the department responsible for cleanliness and sanitation in the long-term care facility.
13. Perform your procedure completion actions.

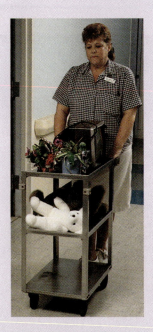

FIGURE 17-7 Use good body mechanics by moving the resident's belongings to the receiving unit on a cart.

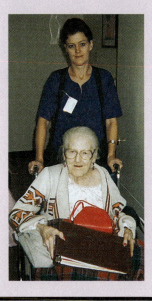

FIGURE 17-8 Transport the resident to her new room in a wheelchair and make her feel comfortable.

Offer to assist in unpacking and storing the resident's belongings. Mark personal items with the resident's name in an inconspicuous location, such as the labels of clothing. Make sure the marker does not bleed through to the outside of the garment. Encourage the family to bring in items from home to personalize the room and make it comfortable for the resident.

Knowing when to ask a visitor to leave the room takes tact and diplomacy. Try to schedule your care when the resident is alone, if this is possible. If not, ask visitors to leave any time the resident's body will be exposed or a procedure will be performed. If the resident requests that the visitor be allowed to stay, honor the request. However, do not ask the resident in the presence of others if he or she would like the visitor to stay. Consult the nurse if you are unsure of how to handle a visitor situation.

Admission to the long-term care facility need not be a negative experience. A competent, caring, professional staff will calm residents' and family members' fears and turn a potentially negative experience into a positive one.

PROCEDURE 79 — Discharging the Resident

1. Perform your beginning procedure actions.
2. Gather supplies needed: wheelchair, cart for resident's belongings, discharge slip (if used by your agency), clothing list or personal inventory, instructions and supplies provided by the nurse.
3. Collect the resident's belongings.
4. Check the belongings against the personal inventory or clothing list to ensure that the resident has all belongings.
5. Complete and have the resident sign the clothing inventory.
6. Assist with packing, if necessary.
7. Assist the resident to dress, if necessary.
8. Assist the resident to transfer to the wheelchair.
9. Check with the nurse to see if prescriptions, medications, or other supplies will be given to the resident before he or she leaves.
10. Transport the resident to the car. Assist the resident into the car.
11. Say goodbye to the resident.
12. Return to your unit.
13. Inform the nurse that the discharge has been completed, and report the resident's reaction and any other observations.
14. Strip the resident's unit and remove any permanent equipment from the room according to facility policy. Notify the environmental services department that the unit is ready to be cleaned.
15. Perform your procedure completion actions.

TRANSFER

There are two types of health care facility transfers. The nursing assistant usually assists with both types. Performing this procedure correctly will ease the resident's fears about going to a new, unfamiliar unit or location. You are responsible for moving the resident and belongings, making the resident comfortable in the new unit, and introducing the staff who will be caring for him or her.

After the initial admission to the health care facility, the resident's needs may change. This may require a transfer to another unit within the facility. For example, the resident is admitted to a skilled nursing unit for intensive rehabilitation therapy. The resident makes good progress and is discharged from therapy. The resident is not receiving any other skilled services and does not need the high level of care provided in the skilled unit. The resident is transferred to another unit in the nursing facility.

Residents may become acutely ill and require transfer to the hospital for acute care. For example, a resident who has suffered a stroke is admitted to the acute care hospital. After the medical symptoms of the stroke have stabilized, the resident is transferred to a subacute care unit, rehabilitation center, or skilled nursing facility to complete the recovery. In this case the resident is discharged from one facility and admitted to another facility. This process is also called a "transfer," although you will be performing the procedure in the same manner as a discharge.

DISCHARGE

Discharge planning begins at the time of admission. Many members of the interdisciplinary team are involved with this process. In long-term care, the social worker also functions as a **discharge planner.** The social worker plans for discharge and is responsible for making arrangements with other community agencies, assisting with social and financial concerns, and providing continuity of care between the long-term care facility and the community. The social worker fills an important role throughout the resident's stay and during the discharge process.

When a resident is ready to leave the facility, you will perform the discharge procedure. This involves assisting the resident to gather personal belongings and escorting him or her to a waiting car or ambulance outside the facility. The nurse is responsible for resident teaching and providing discharge instructions before the resident leaves. You may be asked to assist with this process during routine care to ensure that the resident understands the instructions. For example, the resident who has a paralyzed arm will need to learn how to perform basic activities of daily living using the nonparalyzed arm. You will assist the resident to perform these procedures when you are assisting with bathing and other personal care. A correctly performed discharge will increase the resident's confidence in his or her ability to manage and adjust in the new location.

The physician must write an order for discharge. If the resident advises you that he or she is leaving without a physician order, inform the nurse immediately.

KEY POINTS

- The first impression that the resident has of the health care agency and its workers is a lasting one.
- The resident's perception of the admission process may be clouded by pain, illness, and fear.
- The nursing assistant is responsible for admitting the resident, gathering information, and making the resident comfortable.
- The nursing process involves assessment, planning, implementation, and evaluation.
- The nursing assistant makes valuable contributions to the nursing process.
- The family is an extension of the resident and will experience many emotions upon the resident's admission to a long-term care facility. A professional demeanor and good communication skills will help make the admission a positive experience.
- The nursing assistant is responsible for transferring the resident to a new unit within the health care facility and ensuring the resident's comfort before leaving the unit.
- A physician's order is required for discharge from the health care facility.
- The nursing assistant is responsible for gathering the resident's belongings and safely escorting the resident to the car.

REVIEW

A. Multiple Choice

Select the one best answer.

1. Which of the following statements is true?
   a. Sick residents do not care about first impressions.
   b. First impressions are important for family members only.
   c. First impressions are often lasting ones.
   d. Illness does not affect the resident's fear of admission.

2. An IV standard is the
   a. pump used to administer an intravenous feeding.
   b. metal pole that supports the IV pump, bottle, or bag.
   c. standard of care for administering IVs.
   d. bag that contains the intravenous fluid.

3. During the admission process, the nursing assistant is responsible for gathering the following assessment information
   a. vital signs, height, weight.
   b. food likes and dislikes.
   c. disease diagnoses.
   d. the resident's bedtime.

4. After you have admitted a resident, what should you do before leaving the room?
   a. Show the resident how to use the call signal.
   b. Call the nurse to the room.
   c. Always provide fresh water.
   d. Always put the resident to bed.

5. Which step of the nursing process involves gathering information?
   a. planning
   b. implementation
   c. assessment
   d. evaluation

6. Which step of the nursing process involves providing care to meet the resident's needs?
   a. planning
   b. implementation
   c. assessment
   d. evaluation

7. Which step of the nursing process involves analyzing information and developing a care plan?
   a. planning
   b. implementation
   c. assessment
   d. evaluation

8. Which step of the nursing process involves determining whether the care plan is working?
   a. planning
   b. implementation
   c. assessment
   d. evaluation

9. Discharge planning begins
   a. at admission.
   b. at discharge.
   c. several days before discharge.
   d. a month before discharge.

10. When discharging the resident, the nursing assistant is responsible for
    a. taking vital signs, height, and weight.
    b. safely escorting the resident to the car.
    c. providing instructions on medications to use at home.
    d. designing a discharge teaching plan.

11. Admitting a loved one to a long-term care facility
    a. is usually an emotional time for family members.
    b. is usually not an emotional experience.
    c. often signifies unstable family relationships.
    d. is not a significant event for stable families.

12. Which of the following is *not* an important characteristic when working with resident's families?
    a. warmth and courtesy
    b. having all the answers
    c. kindness and respect
    d. showing that you care

B. Clinical Applications

Answer the following questions.

13. Mrs. Davis has been a resident on the skilled nursing unit for three months. She has reached her maximum potential in therapy, and Medicare will no longer pay for her care. Mrs. Davis's daughter is transferring her to an assisted living facility for financial reasons. Mrs. Davis confides in you that she is nervous and scared about the transfer, because she does not know anyone at the assisted living facility. How can you assist the resident?

14. Mr. Truehart fell and fractured his hip. He has been transferred to the hospital in an ambulance. The nurse informs you that he will remain in the hospital for surgical hip repair. Mr. Truehart has a lock box containing some papers, a bank passbook, a few inexpensive rings, a watch, and $7.32. The box is unlocked on the nightstand in his room. What should you do?

15. The nurse informs you that a new resident will be admitted to room 732. The female resident will be on bed rest. She has a gastrostomy tube feeding. The nurse informs you that the resident is underweight and is at risk for pressure ulcers. How will you prepare the room for admission?

16. The new resident, Mrs. Brady, arrives in an ambulance at 1:15 p.m. Mrs. Brady is mentally confused, weak, and quiet. She is accompanied by her daughter. The EMTs transfer the resident to bed and leave the room. Mrs. Brady's daughter immediately starts complaining that she doesn't like the view out the window. She says she wanted her mother admitted to another nursing facility. However, her brother is the mother's legal guardian, and this is the facility he selected. What should the nursing assistant do?

17. Mr. Harris is being discharged from the nursing facility this afternoon. After you help him pack his clothing, he gives you a $20 bill for "being so nice" during his stay at the facility. What should you do?

CHAPTER 18

Restorative Care

OBJECTIVES

After reading this chapter, you will be able to:

- Spell and define key terms.
- Describe restorative care and the restorative environment.
- Describe restorative care for at least 10 common conditions seen in long-term care facilities.
- Explain why promoting independence is important in restorative care.
- List and describe common restorative programs.
- List three types of range-of-motion exercises and describe how each is different.
- Describe how a bowel and bladder management program is established and list the nursing assistant's responsibilities.
- Describe the nursing assistant's role in using restorative equipment.
- Demonstrate the procedures related to restorative care.

OBSERVATIONS TO MAKE AND REPORT RELATED TO RESTORATIVE CARE

Change in level of consciousness, orientation, awareness, or alertness

Feeling faint or lightheaded, losing consciousness

New-onset inability to recognize familiar persons or objects

New-onset disorientation; does not know person, place, time

Increasing memory loss or mental confusion, worsening confusion

Progressive lethargy

Loss of sensation

Numbness, tingling

Change in pupil size; unequal pupils

Abnormal or involuntary motor function

Spasticity (sudden, frequent, involuntary muscle contractions that impair function)

Loss of ability to move a body part

Incoordination (uncoordinated, irregular voluntary muscle movement)

Changes in speech

Changes in ability to swallow

Drooping of one side of the face

New-onset weakness or paralysis on one side of the body

Pain

Deformity

Edema

Immobility

Inability to move arms and legs

Inability to move one or more joints

Limited/abnormal range of motion

Shortening and external rotation of one leg in resident with history of fall

Sudden onset of falls, difficulty balancing

Jerking, tremors, shaky movements, muscle spasms

Weakness

Sensory changes

Changes in ability to sit, stand, move, or walk

Pain upon movement

INTRODUCTION TO RESTORATION

Restorative care is given to assist the resident to attain and maintain the highest level of function possible in the resident's individual situation. A **restorative environment** is one in which the resident can function as independently as possible. The environment may require modification to meet the resident's need for independence. Being **dependent** on others has a negative effect on self-esteem. Dependence means you are unable to care for or do things for yourself, and that others must care for you. You learned in Chapter 6 that disabled persons do not want to be treated differently than anyone else. They worked hard to become **independent,** or self-reliant and able to care for themselves. Most can do the same things you do, but they may do them differently. Their bodies work differently. Being independent is important for most people. This is especially true with personal care. Imagine how you would feel if someone had to bathe you and feed you. This would be very frustrating. Your self-esteem might suffer. Feeling helpless causes feelings of hopelessness.

The Restorative Team

Many departments assist in providing restorative care to residents **(Figure 18-1).** All members of the interdisciplinary team provide restorative care. The therapy departments usually take the lead role in resident restoration. **Rehabilitation** is a program designed by a therapist to help residents regain lost skills, or to teach new skills. Therapists teach residents, families, and staff members techniques for reinforcing and maintaining what the residents have learned. When you follow the restorative program established by the therapist to accompany the rehabilitation program, this reinforces what the therapists are teaching, and the resident masters the skill more quickly. This process is called **restoration.** Restorative nursing involves using basic measures to assist the resident to attain the highest degree of independence and self-care possible. Some facilities use the terms *rehabilitation* and *restoration* interchangeably, but rehabilitation really refers to a higher level of care provided by licensed therapy personnel. Restoration is delivered by both unlicensed and licensed caregivers in many departments. A restorative nurse may also develop restorative programs. The interdisciplinary approach provides continuity of care, because all staff members are working on the same goals 24 hours a day to benefit the resident.

Complications of Bed Rest

Years ago, people who were sick stayed in bed for long periods. After childbirth, women were kept on bed rest for at least seven days. We now know that early activity is best for the resident. Rest is essential to the treatment of many illnesses. Nevertheless, the physician and other members of the interdisciplinary team will assess the resident and determine how much activity the resident can tolerate. This assessment forms the basis for the restorative program. Like the nursing process, the resident's response to the program is continuously evaluated, and the program modified to meet the resident's individual needs. Remember, **bed rest, inactivity,** and **immobility** affect every system in the body. Bed rest is a medically prescribed treatment in which the resident cannot get out of bed. A resident who is inactive is quiet and still. Immobility means the resident is motionless and unable to move. A summary of the major complications of immobility on each body system is found in **Table 18-1.**

COMMON CONDITIONS

Some chronic conditions are commonly seen in the long-term care facility. Residents with these conditions usually receive restorative care to maintain independence, prevent declines, and prevent injuries.

Arthritis

Arthritis is a common condition in long-term care facility residents. There are many different

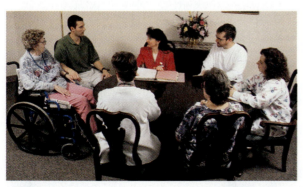

FIGURE 18-1 The interdisciplinary team meets to find out which skills are most important to the resident and develop a plan to assist her.

TABLE 18-1	Major complications of immobility
System	**Complication**
Respiratory	The resident has more difficulty expanding the lungs. Fluid and secretions collect in the lungs. This increases the risk of pneumonia and other lung infections.
Circulatory	Blood clots are caused by pooling of blood and pressure on the legs. Edema may be caused by lack of movement. The heart must work harder to pump blood through the body. Changes in the blood vessels may cause dizziness and fainting when the resident is placed in an upright position.
Integumentary (skin)	Pressure sores may develop in a short time from lack of oxygen to the tissues. Pressure ulcers may worsen quickly and be difficult or impossible to reverse.
Muscular	Weakness and atrophy develop from lack of use. Contractures (deformities) develop because of the resident's position. Contractures may be painful and are difficult or impossible to reverse. Contractures also promote pressure ulcer development, and make treating pressure ulcers more difficult. The contractures cause reduced capillary blood flow to bony prominences, and estimates are that up to 60% of all pressure ulcers involve some sort of unattended contracture. Voluntary movement of the contracted joint becomes difficult or impossible as the contracture worsens.
Skeletal	Calcium drains from the bones when they are inactive. This contributes to fractures, non-healing, osteoporosis, and other complications.
Genitourinary	The extra calcium in the system from the bones promotes the development of kidney stones. Retention of urine is common, and is often caused by the resident's position in bed. Overflow of a full bladder leads to incontinence. The resident is at high risk of urinary tract infection.
Gastrointestinal	Indigestion and heartburn may result if the resident is not positioned properly for meals. The resident is at risk for choking unless positioned upright during and after meals. Loss of appetite may occur from lack of activity, illness, and boredom. Constipation and fecal impaction result from immobility.
Nervous	Weakness and limited mobility develop. Insomnia may result from sleeping too much during the day, then being unable to sleep at night.
Mental changes	Irritability, boredom, lethargy, and depression result from the resident's frustration and feelings of helplessness.

types of arthritis. The most common are osteoarthritis, rheumatoid arthritis, and gout, or gouty arthritis. The most common symptom of arthritis is pain. Arthritis can cause mild discomfort to severe deformities and disability **(Figure 18-2).** The pain is usually described as a deep, aching pain that occurs after exercise, weight bearing, or exertion. It is often relieved by rest. Changes in the weather may also cause pain. Other symptoms include limited ability to move and stiffness, particularly upon arising in the morning. This also may occur after strenuous exercise or physical over activity. In some individuals, an audible grating sound can be heard in the joints during movement. Arthritis may cause redness and swelling in the joints. Conditions such as obesity and stress aggravate the symptoms.

Residents with arthritis are at high risk of contractures. The care plan may instruct you to place residents with this condition in the prone position periodically. This reduces the risk of contractures of the hips and knees. Avoid placing pillows under the knees or elevating the knee area of the bed. Using a small, flat pillow under the head and neck is best. A large pillow pushes the neck into a position of flexion. You will perform range of motion procedures on residents

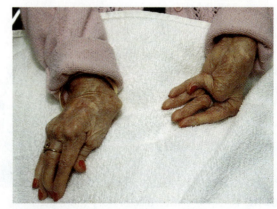

FIGURE 18-2 Signs and symptoms of arthritis can range from mild discomfort to severe deformity, making joint movement difficult or impossible.

with arthritis. Be very gentle. Avoid moving joints past the point of resistance.

Osteoporosis

Osteoporosis is a metabolic disorder of the bones. It is most common in elderly females. Bone mass is lost, causing the bones to become porous and spongy **(Figure 18-3)**. Bones affected are at very high risk of fracture. Fractures can occur spontaneously, such as when the resident is walking. They can also occur when the resident is turned in bed or during transfers.

The cause of osteoporosis is unknown. It is thought to result from years of inadequate calcium intake. Other potential causes are declining adrenal function, faulty protein metabolism, estrogen deficiency, and lack of exercise or activity. The first sign of osteoporosis is usually a fracture. Commonly, the resident moves or lifts something. He or she hears a "pop" or snapping sound in a bone. This frequently occurs in the lower back or hip. Sometimes the resident is walking and falls because of a fracture. (In most falls, the opposite is true.) After the initial incident, the area is very painful, particularly upon movement. Sometimes the onset of osteoporosis begins with a curvature of the spine and loss of height. The back progressively weakens, straining the neck, hips, and low back. Spontaneous fractures may occur on movement or as a result of a minor injury. The care plan may instruct you to use a turning sheet and two assistants for moving the resident in bed. Handle the resident gently.

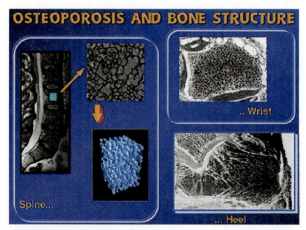

FIGURE 18-3 Bone loss from osteoporosis causes painful, disabling fractures in both genders. About 40% percent of women and 13% of men will suffer a bone fracture in their lifetime due to osteoporosis. *(Courtesy of Sharmila Majumdar, Ph.D., Professor, University of California, San Francisco)*

Hip Surgery

Hip fractures are the most common type of fracture in the elderly. The most common cause of hip fractures is falls, but they may also occur because of osteoporosis. The term "hip fracture" really is not accurate. This term refers to a fracture anywhere in the upper third or head of the femur.

Caring for the Resident Who Has Had Hip Surgery. Hip fracture is almost always treated with surgery. Depending on the condition of the bone, the fracture may be repaired, or the hip completely replaced. Hip replacement surgery may also be done when the joint is painful and damaged, but not fractured. When the resident is admitted or readmitted to the long-term care facility following hip surgery, the following general hip precautions will be ordered:

- A trapeze is attached to the bed to assist with movement. The resident is instructed not to press down on the foot of the affected leg when using the trapeze.
- Antiembolism stockings are applied.
- A fracture bedpan or urinal is used initially for elimination. When the resident is able to use the toilet, an elevated toilet seat is used.
- The head of the bed is not elevated more than 45 degrees.
- Acute flexion of the hip and legs is avoided. The therapist will give directions for positioning and the degree of flexion permitted. Generally, the resident should never flex the hip more than 90 degrees.
- A special pillow, called an **abduction pillow,** will be used to keep the legs apart **(Figure 18-4)** after the resident has had hip replacement surgery. This is particularly important when the resident is turned on the side.
- The resident will be instructed to avoid crossing the legs, which can cause a dislocation.

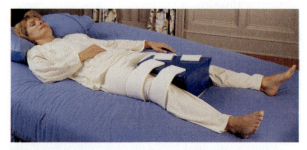

FIGURE 18-4 An abduction pillow is commonly used after hip surgery to keep the legs from adducting or crossing at the ankles. *(Photo courtesy of Sammons Preston)*

- The affected leg should not be internally or externally rotated. Maintain good alignment without internal or external rotation.

The physician will specify how long the resident must avoid weight bearing after surgery. The physical therapist will work with the resident to restore mobility. Some residents are able to ambulate soon after surgery. A walker is commonly used for a period of time after surgery. Some physicians do not permit full weight bearing for as long as four to six weeks. Initially, you will assist with procedures to prevent the complications of immobility. Restorative care of a resident who has had hip surgery will include:

- Range-of-motion exercises on the unaffected extremities
- Turning and repositioning
- Coughing and deep breathing exercises if the resident is bedfast
- Pressure ulcer prevention

Residents with hip surgery are at very high risk of developing heel pressure ulcers. Follow the care plan and get specific instructions from the nurse for positions and techniques to use for turning and repositioning the resident. Relieve pressure from the heels and check the resident's skin carefully each day for signs of red or open areas.

Cerebrovascular Accident

Cerebrovascular accident (CVA) is a common condition in the long-term care facility. A CVA may also be called a *stroke.* A newer term is *brain attack.* A CVA is caused by a sudden interruption of blood to the brain. This can be caused by a blood clot, which blocks a small vessel. Sometimes a vessel bursts, causing blood to spill out into the brain cavity. Both conditions decrease blood supply and often cause permanent damage **(Figure 18-5)**.

CVA is the third leading cause of death in the United States, affecting about 500,000 people annually. About half of these die. About half of the survivors develop a permanent disability. Survivors often experience a recurrence some time later in life. This could be days or weeks later. It could also be many years after the initial CVA. The resident is usually hospitalized for aggressive treatment as soon as the signs and symptoms of CVA are recognized. Some treatments will reverse the damage from the CVA. However, the treatment must be given within the first four hours.

When a resident has a stroke, one side of the body becomes weak or paralyzed. These conditions may be temporary or permanent. **Hemiparesis** is weakness on one side of the body.

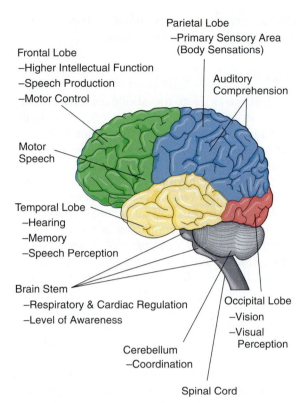

FIGURE 18-5 A stroke or head injury in the areas of the brain shown will result in loss of ability.

Hemiplegia is paralysis on one side of the body. The ability to speak or understand the spoken word may be affected, depending on the location of the attack in the brain. The resident may develop loss of half of a visual field. Recognizing the effects of a CVA on vision is important.

Some residents lose the ability to differentiate right from left, or up from down. Some residents have a condition that causes them to ignore the affected side of the body. Stroke may also affect emotions. The resident may cry, laugh, or become angry for no apparent reason. This is very embarrassing for the resident. He or she is aware of the behavior but cannot control it.

Restorative Care. Rehabilitation and restorative nursing are started soon after admission or readmission to the facility. The resident will usually require physical, occupational, and speech therapy. The goals of care are to:

- Maintain or improve the resident's condition
- Prevent contractures and deformities
- Restore as much self-care ability as possible
- Prevent injury
- Prevent complications of immobility

Rehabilitation and restoration programs focus on activities such as ADLs and bowel and bladder control. Restoration of residents with CVA takes a long time. It is a great deal of work for the resident. Several restorative programs may be ordered for residents with CVA. Allow the resident to rest between treatments. Fatigue is a common problem.

The care plan usually list these approaches:

- Monitor the position of affected extremities during positioning, transfers, and ambulation, to prevent injury.
- Use a transfer belt for transfers and ambulation.
- Position the resident in good alignment to prevent contractures and deformities, using pillows and props if necessary.
- Use pressure ulcer prevention measures, including special mattresses, turning, repositioning, props, and skin care.

Care of a resident who has had a stroke is highly individual, depending on the area of the brain affected. Residents who have had a CVA on either side of the brain may have memory and behavior problems. These may interfere with the restorative program. Remember that the problems are beyond the resident's control. If the resident ignores one side of the body, the care plan will direct you to approach the resident from the affected side. You will encourage the resident to look at the affected side so he or she knows where it is. Touch the extremity gently, but firmly, periodically. Residents with CVA often have an impaired sense of balance. Assist the resident to develop an awareness of good posture and balance.

Residents with hemiplegia may complain of pain in the affected arm and shoulder. This occurs because the force of gravity pulls it downward. Avoid pulling on the arm or shoulder during transfers. A sling may be ordered to help support the arm. Other devices, such as a lap board or table, may also be used to provide support and relieve pressure on the shoulder joint.

Transient Ischemic Attack

A **transient ischemic attack (TIA)** is a temporary period of diminished blood flow to the brain. The attack occurs suddenly and may last from 2 to 15 minutes. Rarely, an attack will last as long as 24 hours. Signs and symptoms are similar to those of a stroke, but are reversible and temporary. Persons who experience TIAs are at high risk for eventually suffering a stroke.

Parkinson's Disease

Parkinson's disease (PD) is a neurological disease. Symptoms usually begin between the ages of 40 and 60. Occasionally they begin as early as the late teens or early twenties. About 1% of individuals over age 50 have the disease. Self-care in the home becomes difficult or impossible because the disease increases the risk of injury. Residents with Parkinson's disease have many restorative care needs.

In the early stages of the disease, the individual is slow when completing ADLs. He or she will also experience:

- Muscle stiffness
- Mild pain
- Tremors of the upper extremities
- Difficulty walking

The tremors are very embarrassing for some residents. The disease is progressive and symptoms gradually worsen with age. As symptoms progress, voluntary movement becomes difficult **(Figure 18-6).** As the condition worsens, the resident develops:

- Pill-rolling motions in the fingers (in this condition, the fingers move involuntarily in a circular motion as though the resident were rolling a pill between the thumb and fingers)
- Stooped posture
- Shuffling gait; falls are common
- Mask-like expression
- Low-pitched, monotonous speech
- Difficulty controlling oral secretions
- Dementia (only in some individuals)

The effects of the disease can be controlled to a degree with drug therapy. There is no known treatment for Parkinson's dementia.

Restorative Care. Licensed nurses will administer medication to control the tremors. Restorative nursing care includes:

- Range-of-motion exercises and other activities to prevent contractures
- Safety measures to prevent falls and injuries
- Using a gait belt and/or walker for ambulation
- Encouraging the resident to maintain good posture when walking
- Avoiding flexion of the neck and shoulders
- Using assistive devices for ADLs
- Being very patient; the tremors cause the resident to be very slow with ADLs and movement
- Allowing adequate time for residents to complete tasks independently

Some residents with Parkinson's disease have difficulty feeding themselves. The tremors may be so severe that the food spills before it gets to the mouth. In this situation, the therapist may evaluate the resident and establish a restorative program. Weights are often used to control the tremors **(Figure 18-7).** Some therapists prescribe weights to the backs of the hands. Others use weighted silverware. You will assist the

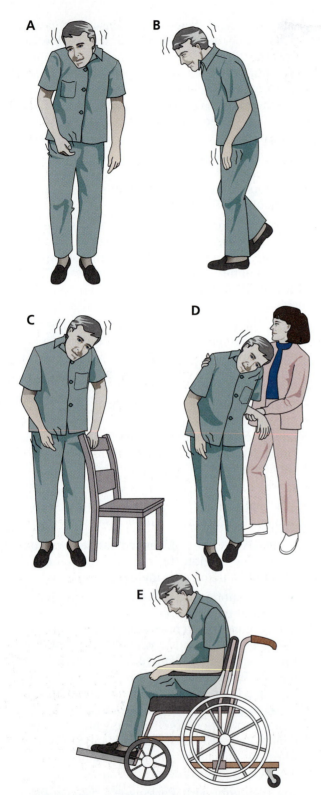

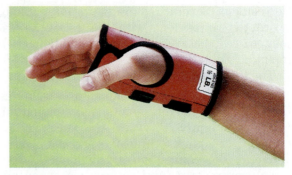

FIGURE 18-7 Various weights are available to reduce tremors of the hands and arms, enabling the resident to maintain greater independence. *(Photo courtesy of Sammons Preston)*

resident to become proficient in eating while using the weights or weighted utensils. Special cups with lids are also used to prevent spilling. Feeding the resident is not desirable, if it can be avoided. However, the resident's weight must be monitored closely. The tremors of Parkinson's consume extra calories. The resident is at very high risk for weight loss. This is because of the extra caloric need, combined with problems such as spilling. Residents are often given nutritional supplements or nourishing snacks to help maintain their weight.

Huntington's Disease

Huntington's disease (HD) is also called *Huntington's chorea.* This is a hereditary disease. In recent years, a genetic test has become available to show if individuals with a family history of the disorder have the Huntington's gene. If the gene is present, development of the disease is inevitable.

Clinical signs of the disease usually begin when individuals are in their 40s or 50s. In some individuals, symptoms of the disease first appear in childhood or young adulthood. The disease is progressive and there is no cure. Disability and death occur within 15 to 20 years. Abnormal movements, called **chorea,** are the primary sign of Huntington's disease. The movements are subtle early in the course of the illness. The individual will appear anxious or restless. He or she appears to move frequently. Most people are aware of this movement. The resident may try to disguise the activity with voluntary movements, such as scratching the head or crossing the legs. As the disease progresses, rapid, jerking choreiform movements develop. These movements involve the entire body. The individual eventually loses voluntary control of all movement. He

FIGURE 18-6 Progression of Parkinson's disease. (A) The resident leans slightly forward and develops flexion of the affected arm. (B) The resident stoops forward slightly and walks with a shuffling gait. (C) As the disease progresses, the resident needs support to prevent falling. The resident tends to shuffle faster and faster, leaning farther forward until he falls on his face. (D) The disease progresses to the point of needing assistance for ambulation. (E) The resident has profound weakness and severe tremors. Ambulation becomes impossible.

or she also loses control of the bowel and bladder. The **spasticity** (involuntary movement) increases with stress and attempts to control the choreiform motions. The resident becomes totally dependent on others. The risk of skin breakdown is high in the later stages. Individuals with Huntington's disease develop mental changes that progress to dementia.

Restorative Care. Residents with Huntington's disease are commonly admitted to the long-term care facility because they cannot function safely at home. There is no known treatment or cure. Care is designed to:

- Keep the resident as independent as possible for as long as possible
- Prevent injury
- Maintain nutrition and prevent weight loss

The rapid movements consume many extra calories. The resident is at very high risk for weight loss. Extra nutrition and hydration will be ordered. Restorative nursing programs for residents with chorea usually involve ambulation with a gait belt. Some residents can walk independently by pushing an empty wheelchair.

Residents with HD will develop difficulty swallowing and are at very high risk for choking. When residents with Huntington's disease are eating, they must sit completely upright to prevent choking. The care plan will specify other special feeding techniques.

Poor muscular control makes communication difficult. The speech-language pathologist will assess the resident and establish a communication program. The resident will be taught to use either hand signals, cards **(Figure 18-8),** or a communication board. Give the resident feedback when he or she speaks. Repeating what the resident says is a good way to show that the communication was successful.

Multiple Sclerosis

Multiple sclerosis (MS) is another neurological disorder commonly seen in long-term care. Sadly, many young adults are affected **(Figure 18-9).** This progressive disease causes a degeneration of the nervous system that interferes with conduction of nerve impulses. The exact cause is not known. It is thought to be an **autoimmune disorder.** In this type of condition, the individual makes antibodies that work against his or her own body. Recent research suggests that a virus may cause MS. The signs and symptoms of MS vary widely. They include:

- Weakness
- Numbness and tingling in one or more extremities, with eventual progression to complete loss of sensation
- Visual disturbances
- **Incoordination** (uncoordinated, irregular voluntary muscle movement)
- Poor muscular control, muscle spasms, and tremors
- Paralysis
- Uncontrolled emotions
- Slow, scanning speech
- Short attention span
- Incontinence
- Urinary retention
- Fatigue that worsens as the day progresses
- Seizures
- Depression

Residents with MS often develop a **neurogenic bladder.** In this condition, the resident cannot feel the sensation of urine in the bladder. The bladder will become very full, retaining urine.

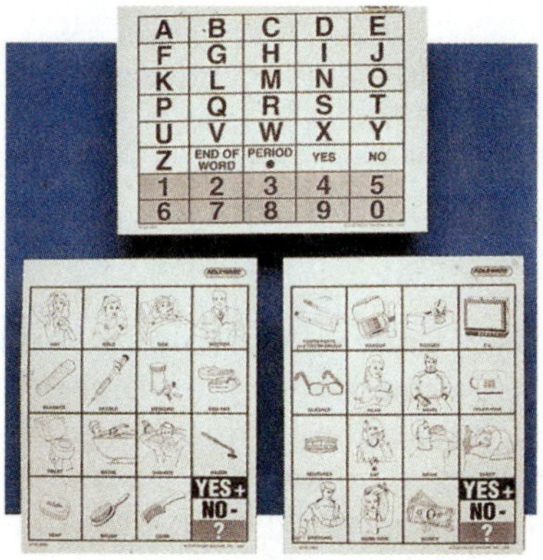

FIGURE 18-8 Alternate methods of communication may be used by residents who have difficulty speaking. *(Permission given for reprint/reproduction courtesy of Maddak, Inc.)*

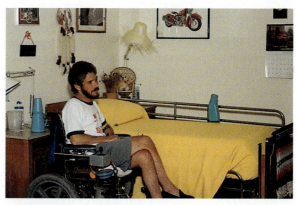

FIGURE 18-9 Multiple sclerosis often affects young adults. This resident is independent with ambulation because he uses a motorized wheelchair.

The resident may have to be catheterized to relieve the problem.

Multiple sclerosis is a condition in which there are **exacerbations** and **remissions.** During an exacerbation, signs and symptoms worsen. Stress, infection, and injury are risk factors for exacerbations. Some residents are relatively stable for long periods of time. Others deteriorate rapidly. They quickly become dependent on staff for care. Residents in remission appear stable and relatively symptom-free.

Restorative Care. Preventive skin care is important for the resident with MS. Residents with this condition are at high risk for breakdown. MS causes impairment in the resident's sensation. He or she may not notice the discomfort of an early pressure ulcer. Pressure-relieving mattresses and other preventive devices are used routinely. The care plan will also list measures to prevent contractures and maintain independence.

Post Polio Syndrome (PPS)

Polio is a very serious neurological disease caused by a virus. It has been with us since at least 1350 BC. The virus attacks the motor neurons in the brain and spinal cord. Muscles affected by these neurons no longer function properly. Some individuals had respiratory paralysis and required a special ventilator to breathe. Others had speech and swallowing problems. Most had paralysis and weakness in the arms and legs. Many people died as a result of polio. Most of those who survived learned to overcome their disabilities and lead productive lives.

Post polio syndrome (PPS) is a neurologic condition marked by increased weakness and abnormal muscle fatigue in persons who had polio many years earlier **(Figure 18-10).**

Post Polio Syndrome Diagnostic Criteria

- Prior episode of polio with residual motor neuron loss.
- A period of neurologic recovery followed by neurologic and functional stability (usually lasts 15 years or more).
- Gradual or abrupt onset of new weakness and/or abnormal muscle fatigue.
- May also have generalized fatigue, muscle atrophy, pain.
- Exclusion of other conditions that may cause symptoms similar to post polio syndrome.

FIGURE 18-10 Post polio syndrome is diagnosed in persons who had polio many years previously, based on identification of new signs and symptoms. Many other conditions are ruled out before this diagnosis is made.

Estimates are that 30% to 70% of all polio survivors will develop this condition. There are several theories about the cause of PPS. The most common involves the motor neurons. Most polio survivors have about half as many motor neurons as others who were not affected by polio. It is believed that motor neurons that were not destroyed by the initial polio infection compensated by sprouting new connections. Some of the new neurons adapted to innervate areas that are five to seven times larger than normal. These neurons may be slowly dying, perhaps because of years of overuse. As the neurons die, they lose their muscle connections, and muscles stop responding when a nerve signals them.

Signs and symptoms of PPS range from annoying to debilitating. Onset may be sudden, following trauma, infection, surgery, a fall, or a stressful event. The new injury stresses the remaining motor neurons, causing new reduction in function and increased pain and fatigue. Signs and symptoms of PPS include:

- Fatigue that may be debilitating and worsens as the day progresses
- New joint and muscle pain
- New weakness in muscles affected by polio; unaffected muscles are also affected. (The new weakness may be more prominent on one side of the body.)
- New dyspnea and other respiratory problems
- Severe cold intolerance, even with mild cold exposure. This causes the muscle weakness to worsen, the arms or legs to become pale or cyanotic, and the extremities to feel cold to touch. The resident may say," It's so cold it hurts."
- Muscle spasms and cramps that are sometimes severe and painful
- Difficulty swallowing and increased risk of choking
- Difficulty falling asleep and waking frequently during the night
- Anxiety, anger, frustration, and emotional outbursts due to loss of ability
- Disturbed sleep, sleep apnea

Restorative Care. Most polio survivors are fiercely independent, making them difficult to care for. PPS residents fear becoming dependent on others. Coping with the new problems from PPS is often very difficult for the resident. Residents may not complain because most were taught that they had to appear normal as part of their recovery. They have spent their lives trying to appear normal. Asking for and accepting help is very difficult. Because of this, pay attention if the resident says he or she cannot do something. Anticipate the resident's needs, and ask if assistance is needed. Even if the resident refuses your help, stand by to see if he or she can perform the task safely. Adapt the environment, whenever possible, for independent function. You may do this by moving furniture, or bringing a bedside commode, for example. Goals of restorative care are designed to:

- Maintain maximum independence
- Prevent falls and injury
- Prevent pain, pressure ulcers, and deformities
- Conserve energy

Residents with PPS have serious problems with cold because the nerves that control blood vessel size were destroyed by the virus. The legs and feet are commonly affected. One theory is that people with PPS function as if it were 20 degrees colder than the actual temperature. Their legs and feet turn bright red following a hot bath. When the resident stands to get up, she may become dizzy or faint as blood pools in the legs, causing her blood pressure to drop. If the resident complains of cold, assist her with socks or extra blankets. You may be instructed to soak the feet in warm water, or assist with a warm bath. Caution the resident to call for help before getting out of the tub.

Brain Damage

Some individuals are admitted to the long-term care facility because of head injuries. These usually result from trauma, falls, or automobile accidents. The injury often results in severe, permanent brain damage. Many young adults are admitted to long-term care facilities with this condition.

Signs and symptoms of brain damage vary widely. Most residents admitted to the nursing facility show signs and symptoms of severe damage. They are often dependent on staff for care. Common signs and symptoms of severe brain damage are:

- Ability to open eyes, but unaware or minimally aware of the surroundings
- Inability to follow commands, make decisions, or participate in care
- Loss of bowel and bladder control
- Inability to speak or communicate
- Paralysis of the extremities
- Lack of safety awareness
- Impaired sensation

Restorative Care. The goal of restorative care is to prevent complications. The care plan will list measures to:

- Prevent skin breakdown
- Prevent contractures, which are common
- Prevent deformities
- Prevent injuries

Spinal Cord Injuries

Some residents are admitted to the facility because of injuries or other conditions of the spinal cord resulting in paralysis. Paralysis affects sensation and voluntary movement below the level of injury **(Figure 18-11)**. The most common cause is trauma, but medical problems and birth defects can also cause paralysis.

Restorative Care. Restorative nursing depends on the level of injury. Overall, treatment is directed at:

- Preventing pressure ulcers and other complications of immobility
- Preventing contractures and deformities
- Restoring the resident to the highest degree of independence possible

PROMOTING INDEPENDENCE

Promoting independence is part of restorative care. Independence is relative to the resident. No one is 100% independent. We all depend on others for some things. Independence for the resident, then, means being as self-sufficient as possible. Preventing total dependence on others is important both physically and psychologically. It is better for the resident to complete part of a task than it is for you to perform the task. Allowing the resident to do what he or she is able makes the resident feel useful and worthwhile. It may take longer for the resident to complete a task than it takes you **(Figure 18-12)**. However, maintaining the resident's ability to perform the skill and the effect of personal independence on the resident's self-esteem are worth the investment of your time.

Some residents have medical problems that cause physical dependence. For example, a resident who suffered a neck injury in an accident may be paralyzed from the neck down. This resident is physically dependent. However, if the resident is allowed to set the care routine, and tell you what he or she wants, the resident is psychologically independent. Psychological independence is also very important.

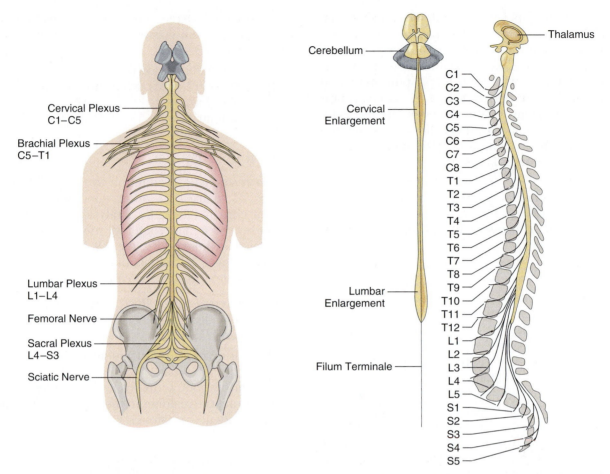

FIGURE 18-11   The type of paralysis is determined by the level of injury to the spinal cord.

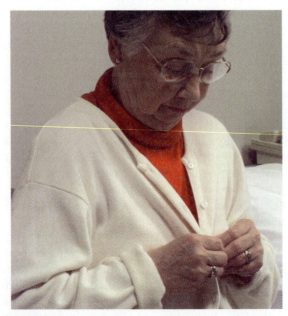

FIGURE 18-12   Although it may take a long time for the resident to button her buttons, you are helping her by encouraging independence.

Principles of Restoration

The principles of restoration and rehabilitation are the same, and apply to all residents:

- *Begin treatment early.* If restorative care is started early in the resident's disease, the outcome will be better.
- *Activity strengthens and inactivity weakens.* The goal should be to keep the resident as active as possible, considering the medical condition. The resident should do an activity whenever possible. For example, passive range-of-motion exercises given by the nursing assistant will prevent deformity and complications. However, active range-of-motion exercises done by the resident will prevent deformity and strengthen muscles.
- *Prevent further disability.* Follow the care plan to prevent injury and deformity. Practice safety.
- *Stress what the resident can do.* Minimize what the resident cannot do. Emphasizing

what the resident can do is better than telling the resident he or she can't do something.

- *Treat the whole person.* Restorative care works on the principle that residents are complex individuals. Each individual has many strengths and needs. You cannot isolate the medical problem from the rest of the person. Consider all of the resident's strengths and needs when delivering restorative care. Use and build on the resident's strengths to overcome the needs. The program must be individualized for the resident. The care plan will guide you in the approaches to use. If you discover something that works for the resident, share this information with the nurse and other team members so it can be included on the care plan.

Providing Restorative Care

When providing restorative care, always follow the care plan. The amount and type of activity al-lowed are ordered by the physician. The care is supervised by the licensed nurse. The care plan will guide you in the type of restorative care to deliver.

Providing restorative care takes a great deal of patience. We did not learn to care for ourselves overnight. Think about how long it takes a small child to learn to take a bath and get dressed. When adults lose the ability for self-care, it takes time to restore. The process can be frustrating for both the resident and the nursing assistant. Being patient, positive, and supportive is the best approach.

Monitoring the Resident's Response to Restorative Care

It is important to observe how the restorative program affects the resident. This is particularly true in the early stages of illness. The resident may become easily frustrated. Allow the resident to struggle, but intervene before he or she

GUIDELINES FOR
Restorative Care

- Practice good body mechanics for yourself and the resident.
- Provide restorative care at the usual time of day for the activity.
- Remember that all ADLs have many steps. If the resident cannot complete one step, he or she will not be able to do the activity.
- Do not rush the resident.
- Give verbal **cues,** if necessary. Cues are brief verbal hints that indicate what you want the resident to do. Make your directions as clear and simple as possible. If the resident does not understand, demonstrate.
- If the resident does not respond to verbal cues, use hand-over-hand technique **(Figure 18-13)** by placing your hand on top of the resident's hand and performing the activity.
- Practice safety and teach the resident safety measures.
- Allow the resident to do as much self-care as possible. Show the resident that you are confident in his or her ability.
- Use adaptive devices, if necessary.
- Apply **orthotic** and **prosthetic** devices as ordered by the therapist and described on the care plan. Orthotic devices improve function and prevent deformities. Prosthetic devices are replacements for body parts, such as the eye, breast, hand, leg, or foot.

- Modify the environment to promote independence, if necessary.
- If the resident cannot complete an ADL, praise his or her accomplishment and complete the task for the resident.

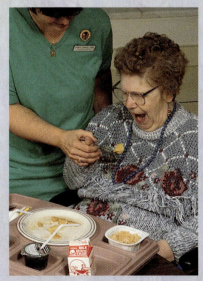

FIGURE 18-13 Use hand-over-hand technique if the resident does not respond to verbal cues.

reaches the point of frustration. Encourage the resident and remind him or her that learning takes time. Practice empathy. Tell the resident you understand how frustrated he or she feels. Be aware of the resident's fears. Sometimes fear of falling or spilling will prevent the resident from participating in the restorative program.

Early in the restorative program, the resident may also have a physical response. Bed rest, even for a short period, can have a negative effect on the body. Any movement or exertion may cause a change in the resident's physical condition. Monitor for signs of fatigue. Be alert for changes, and report them to the nurse. A good practice is to take the resident's pulse before you begin restorative care. Then perform the activity. Monitor the pulse every five minutes during the activity. Normally, the pulse will increase. If the rate is more than 100, or if the resident shows signs of other problems, such as pain, shortness of breath, nausea, or perspiration, stop the activity and notify the nurse. After you complete the activity, check the pulse again. It should return to within 10 beats of the resting pulse rate within 5 minutes.

Maintaining a Restorative Attitude

Your attitude affects the resident and has a major effect on the care you deliver. You must believe that restorative care works and that it is good for the resident. Do not judge the value of restorative care by the results you see tomorrow. It takes a long time for the effects to become evident. Restorative care should be viewed as a positive process that is best for the resident, but results are usually slow in coming. Understanding this in advance will help you to avoid discouragement. Be patient, sincere, tactful, sensitive, and empathetic. Explain the importance of the program to the resident and provide encouragement. Good communication is part of restorative care.

APPLYING THE PRINCIPLES OF RESTORATIVE CARE TO ACTIVITIES OF DAILY LIVING

Most of the restorative care you provide will be done when you assist residents with activities of daily living. Observe the resident carefully. Learn which activity of daily living the resident is most interested in accomplishing. Share this information with the nurse. The information you contribute to the interdisciplinary team based on your observations of the resident is very important.

Role of the Nursing Assistant in Assisting with Restorative Programs

Many residents have nursing diagnoses listed on the care plans that include the words **self-care deficit.** A self-care deficit is an inability to perform an activity of daily living. The care plan will guide you in implementing restorative programs. Each program is designed specifically by the therapist or restorative nurse to meet the resident's needs. You must develop a sensitivity to the resident's abilities. Provide what the resident needs, but do not do more than necessary. Be available to assist, but do not help until you are certain the resident cannot accomplish the task. This may be difficult, but the only way the resident will relearn the skill is by doing it.

Bathing and Personal Hygiene Programs. Residents with many different illnesses lose the ability to bathe themselves and perform routine hygienic measures. This is very difficult and frustrating for the resident. The occupational therapist often develops restorative programs to assist in this area. The care plan will provide directions for each program. The therapist does a **task analysis, Table 18-2,** of the steps in each procedure. The task analysis analyzes a procedure to determine which steps the resident can do independently. For example, part of the task analysis for brushing your teeth includes turning on the faucet, wetting the toothbrush, removing the cap from the toothpaste, and squeezing the toothpaste onto the brush. If the resident cannot do any of these steps, he or she will be unable to brush his or her teeth. The therapist will assess the resident to determine which steps he or she can do, then instruct you to work on the next step. After the resident accomplishes this step, the therapist will instruct you to add another step until the resident can accomplish the entire task. As you can see from the number of steps involved, this takes time, but is a very worthwhile process.

Common hygiene and grooming ADL programs include bathing and dressing skills, applying makeup, styling hair, and shaving. You will assist the resident to perform small parts of a skill, then build on his or her accomplishments. For example, a resident may be unable to wash his or her face. You will assist the resident to wash one cheek. When he or she accomplishes this, assist the resident to wash the other cheek. Build on this ability until the resident is able to wash his or her entire face. All ADL skills start with small tasks. Like building blocks, each new step is built on mastery of the previous step.

TABLE 18-2	Toothbrushing task analysis

Key: 1 = Resident can complete task
0 = Resident cannot complete task
N/A = Not applicable

Date	Key	Initial	Step
			1. Identifies equipment for toothbrushing.
			2. Gathers equipment.
			3. Removes cap from toothpaste.
			4. Turns on cold water.
			5. Wets toothbrush.
			6. Squeezes tube slowly and applies toothpaste to toothbrush.
			7. Places cap on toothpaste.
			8. Fills a cup with water for rinsing mouth.
			9. Turns off water.
			10. Grasps toothbrush handle.
			11. Turns bristles upward and brushes chewing surface of upper teeth.
			12. Brushes upper teeth beginning at one side, moving across front teeth, and ending on opposite side.
			13. Turns toothbrush and brushes inside of upper teeth.
			14. Brushes lower teeth beginning at one side, moving across front teeth, and ending on opposite side.
			15. Turns toothbrush and brushes inside of lower teeth.
			16. Brushes tongue.
			17. Turns bristles upward and gently brushes roof of mouth.
			18. Takes a sip of water from the cup.
			19. Rinses mouth.
			20. Spits water from mouth.
			21. Turns on cold water.
			22. Rinses toothbrush.
			23. Turns water off.
			24. Dries face with towel.
			25. Returns toothbrushing supplies to storage area.

Feeding Programs. Eating is a social activity. Residents who eat alone may not eat as well as those who eat with others. Being spoon-fed also takes some of the pleasure out of eating. The resident may be able to eat finger foods, but will need to be spoon-fed the remainder of the meal.

Restorative feeding programs frequently involve teaching the resident to use adaptive feeding equipment. The goal of restorative feeding is to assist the resident to be as independent as possible with meals. Your responsibility is to set up the tray by uncovering containers, opening milk cartons, buttering bread, cutting meat, or seasoning foods. Do only what the resident needs. If the resident is able to do some of these things for himself or herself, allow the resident to do so. You will also help the resident use adaptive dishes, silverware, and cups.

Restorative Mobility Programs. Mobility means the ability to move about. The restorative program may start out by teaching the resident how to move about independently in bed. The program then progresses to transfers from bed to wheelchair. Eventually, the program will progress to ambulation, if the resident is able.

Restorative mobility programs are prescribed for many residents. You may be asked to assist residents to move themselves in bed by using the side rails, trapeze, or other equipment. Teaching a resident to use a wheelchair is also a mobility program. Residents in wheelchairs may be taught to lean over, shift their weight, or do pushups in the chair to relieve pressure and prevent skin breakdown.

Restorative Ambulation Programs. These programs are designed for residents who have completed an intensive therapy rehabilitation program. Restorative ambulation further strengthens the resident and ensures that he or she will maintain the ability to ambulate. In most cases, you will support the resident by using a gait belt. You may also assist with the use of a cane, crutches, or walker.

RANGE OF MOTION

Maintaining a resident's **range of motion** is a very important part of restorative care. Range of motion is the normal movement of the joints. Joint motion is affected by age, body size, genetics, and the presence or absence of disease. We do range of motion many times each day during our normal activities of daily living, and at work.

Reasons for Range-of-Motion Exercises

People who are ill or who have been confined to bed do not move as actively, so the joints are not exercised normally. Weakness occurs quickly. Weakness and muscle wasting from lack of use is called **atrophy.** Over time, the muscles become rigid, and the joints do not move as freely as they once did. Joint movement may become painful because the muscles have become short from lack of use. When the joint is moved, the muscle is stretched, and this is uncomfortable or painful.

Contractures and **deformities** develop (**Figure 18-14**). Contractures are usually permanent distortions of the body, caused by muscle shortening from lack of use. Contractures cause deformities, or disfigurement. These are serious complications of inactivity, and are painful for the resident. They make bathing, dressing, and caring for the resident more difficult. Every muscle has an antagonist that works in the opposite direction. If a muscle group is not moved for a period of time, or if the resident is not positioned in good body alignment, the stronger muscles will control the weaker ones, causing contractures. Residents with existing contractures are at high risk of developing additional contractures. Contractures can begin to develop in as little as four days of immobility and inactivity. After 15 days, the resident will lose range of motion.

Doing range-of-motion exercises stimulates circulation and improves the resident's sense of well-being. Residents' joints must be moved regularly to prevent complications. If residents cannot move independently, the nursing assistant is responsible for exercising the joints several times each day.

If you are assigned to assist residents with range-of-motion exercises, take this responsibility very seriously. Sometimes the physical or occupational therapist will prescribe a special routine. The care plan will describe your responsibilities. All residents, including those with no potential for rehabilitation, should be exercised regularly to prevent deformities. Like pressure ulcers, contractures and deformities are much easier to prevent than to reverse. Sometimes, contractures become permanent and cannot be

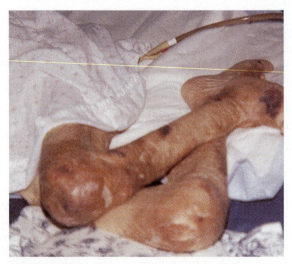

FIGURE 18-14 Contractures are deformities that result from immobility and lack of exercise.

reversed. Your facility will have a policy for how often to perform range-of-motion exercises on residents. Most facilities exercise residents two to three times a day. Each joint is taken through its normal range of motion three to five times. Know and follow your facility policy.

Precautions and Special Situations

Residents with certain conditions require special care and handling. Avoid exercising extremities with fractures or dislocations. Residents with osteoporosis or bone cancer have bones that break very easily. Osteoporosis is a condition in which bone mass decreases, leading to fractures with little or no trauma. Check with the nurse and care plan before proceeding. If the resident has a wound or open area on the joint you are exercising, check with the nurse to see if exercise will be harmful to the healing tissue. If a resident is combative or resists exercise, try to explain why it is important and coax him or her into participating. However, do not force the resident. Notify the nurse if the resident continues to refuse.

Active Range of Motion

Active range-of-motion exercises are done by the resident each day during movement and

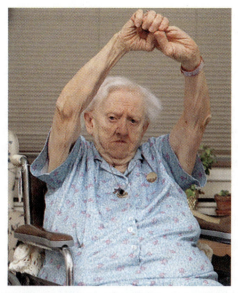

FIGURE 18-15 The resident's left arm is paralyzed from a stroke. She uses her right arm to exercise it several times each day, preventing contractures and deformities.

ADLs. Some residents cannot move all of their joints independently. However, they may be able to use a strong extremity to exercise a weaker extremity. For example, a resident who has had a stroke has a strong right arm and a weak left arm. The resident can be taught to move the weak arm with the stronger right arm **(Figure 18-15).**

GUIDELINES FOR
Assisting Residents with Range-of-Motion Exercises

- Check the care plan for limitations and guidelines for each resident.
- In many facilities, the neck is not exercised without a physician's order. Know and follow your facility policy.
- Perform each joint motion three to five times, or according to facility policy.
- Make sure you have enough space for full movement of the extremities.
- Use good body mechanics and position the resident on the back, in good body alignment, before beginning.
- Expose only the part of the body you are exercising.
- Work systematically from the top of the body to the bottom.
- Never push the resident past the point of joint resistance. Move each joint as far as it will comfortably go.

- Stop the exercise and report to the nurse if the resident complains of pain. Watch the resident's face for an indication of pain or discomfort.
- Support each joint while you exercise it by placing one hand above and one hand below the joint.
- Move each joint slowly and consistently. Stop briefly at the end of each motion before repeating it again.
- Be alert for any changes in the resident's condition during the activity. If you feel that the activity is harming the resident, stop the exercise and notify the nurse. Changes that indicate a potential problem are pain, shortness of breath, sweating, and change in color.
- Help the resident relax during exercise.
- Use the time spent during range-of-motion exercises as quality time to communicate with the resident.
- For residents who are stiff or combative, performing range-of-motion exercises in the bathtub or whirlpool may be helpful. Check with the nurse.

Active range of motion maintains movement, prevents deformity, and strengthens muscles.

Active Assistive Range of Motion

Active assistive range-of-motion exercises are either started or completed by the resident. The nursing assistant assists with the exercise. Sometimes a piece of equipment, such as a pulley, is used to exercise the joint. This is another form of active assistive range of motion.

Passive Range of Motion

Passive range-of-motion exercises are performed by the nursing assistant. The joint is taken through the normal range of movement. Passive range-of-motion exercises maintain movement and prevent deformities, but do not strengthen the muscles.

Range-of-Motion Terminology

Range of motion involves taking the joint through its normal movements. Some important terms describing common joint movements are listed in **Table 18-3.**

BOWEL AND BLADDER MANAGEMENT

The OBRA legislation specifically requires the prevention of declines. Incontinence is a decline. Acute illness and deterioration in mental status may cause a loss of bowel or bladder control. Remember, incontinence is not a normal consequence of aging. Incontinence should be prevented and treated aggressively. Managing incontinence is difficult and unpleasant for the nursing assistant and affects the resident's self-esteem. Incontinence greatly increases the risk for skin breakdown. Apply the principles of standard precautions when assisting residents with incontinence and bowel and bladder management programs.

Incontinence Management Programs

Incontinence management programs are not active restorative programs. These programs are designed for residents who are mentally confused and unable to communicate the need to use the toilet. However, if the resident is placed on the toilet, he or she will use it correctly. The resident is taken to the bathroom at regular intervals,

---

TABLE 18-3 Range-of-motion terminology

- **Abduction (Figure 18-16)** is moving an extremity *away from* the body.

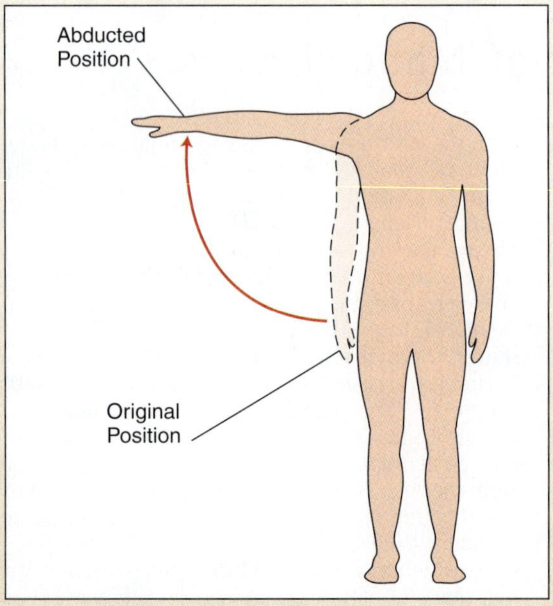

- **Adduction (Figure 18-17)** is moving an extremity *toward* the body.

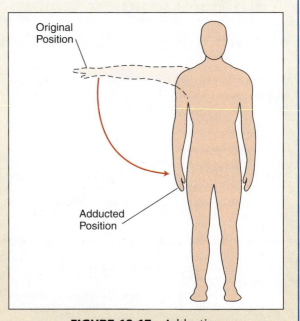

FIGURE 18-16 Abduction

FIGURE 18-17 Adduction

Continues

TABLE 18-3 Range-of-motion terminology, Continued

- **Circumduction** is a circular movement of a joint, such as the thumb or wrist.
- **Dorsal flexion,** or **dorsiflexion,** is pulling the foot upward toward the head.
- **Eversion** is turning a joint outward.
- **Extension** **(Figure 18-18)** is straightening a joint.

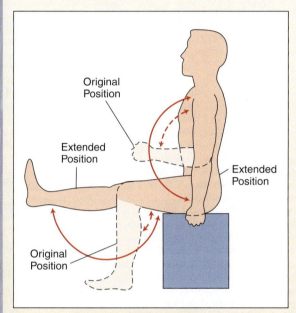

FIGURE 18-18 Extension

- **External rotation** is turning a joint outward away from the median line.
- **Flexion** **(Figure 18-19)** is bending a joint.

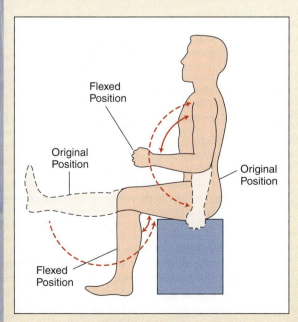

FIGURE 18-19 Flexion

- **Hyperextension** is gentle, excessive extension of a joint, slightly past the point of resistance.
- **Internal rotation** is turning a joint inward toward the median line.
- **Inversion** is turning a joint inward.
- **Medial** pertains to or is situated toward the midline of the body.
- **Median** means situated in the median plane or in the midline of the body.
- **Opposition** is touching each of the fingers against the thumb.
- **Palmar flexion** is the act of bending the hand down toward the palm.
- **Plantar flexion** is bending the foot downward, away from the body.
- **Pronation** is moving a joint to face downward.
- **Radial deviation** is turning the wrist inward, toward the radius.
- **Retraction** is drawing back, away from the body.
- **Rotation** **(Figure 18-20)** means moving a joint in, out, and around.

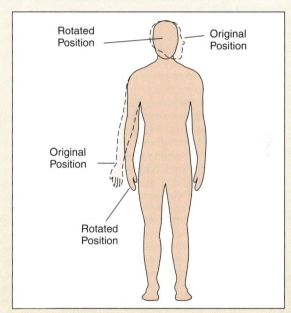

FIGURE 18-20 Rotation

- **Supination** is moving a joint so it faces upward.
- **Ulnar deviation** is turning the wrist outward, toward the ulna.

PROCEDURE 80

Passive Range-of-Motion Exercises

1. Position the resident in good alignment in the supine position.
2. Exercise each extremity as indicated on the care plan, supporting the extremity above and below the joint. Repeat each motion 5 times.
   A. Head and neck (if this is your facility policy or if you have a physician's order)
      1. Tip the head forward, bringing the chin to the chest.
      2. Tip the head backward, with the chin up.
      3. Move the head from side to side.
      4. Move the head back and forth in a circular motion.
   B. Shoulders, arms, and elbows
      1. Raise the arm over the head, then return the arm to the side.
      2. Move the arm from side to side, as far away from the body as possible, then return to the side.
      3. Move the arm across the chest until the fingers touch the opposite shoulder. Return the arm to the side.
      4. With the arm straight out at the side, bend at the elbow and rotate the shoulder. Return the arm to the side.
      5. Bend at the elbow and bring the hand to the chin or shoulder. Return the arm to the side.
   C. Wrists, fingers, and forearms
      1. Support the elbow.
      2. Grasp the hand as in a handshake. Turn the palm up, then down.
      3. Bend the hand backward at the wrist, then return to the neutral position.
   4. Bend the hand forward at the wrist, then return to the neutral position.
   5. Move the hand from side to side, first toward the thumb, then outward.
   6. Move the hand in a circle.
   7. Clench the fingers and thumb as if making a fist.
   8. Extend the fingers and thumb.
   9. Move fingers and thumb together and then apart.
   10. Flex and extend joints in the thumb and fingers.
   11. Move the thumb in a circular motion.
   D. Legs, hips, and knees
      1. Keeping the knee straight, raise the leg up and down.
      2. Bend and straighten the knee.
      3. With the leg resting on the bed, roll it inward and outward.
      4. Stretch the leg out from the body. Return the leg to touch the other leg.
   E. Ankles, foot, and toes
      1. With the leg straight on the bed, push the foot and toes toward the knee, then back down.
      2. Push the foot and toes out straight, pointing toward the foot of the bed.
      3. With the leg straight, turn the foot and ankle from side to side.
      4. Bend the toes downward and upward.
      5. Spread each toe apart, then back together again.

typically every two hours. This prevents incontinence most of the time. A trial of incontinence management should be used on all mentally confused residents who are physically able to use a toilet or commode. Although the resident is not actually "trained" to use the toilet, a successful incontinence management program benefits the resident and facility staff in many ways.

Bowel and Bladder Retraining Programs

Bowel and bladder retraining programs are individually designed for residents who have become incontinent due to acute illness, trauma, infection, medications, and other factors. Residents do not have to be mentally alert to participate. However, they must have some ability to follow directions and cooperate with the program. For the best results, bowel and bladder programs should be developed as early in the illness as possible. Members of the interdisciplinary team assess the resident's physical condition, mental status, and ability to participate. An environmental assessment is also completed to determine access and distance to the toilet, whether the resident can get out of the bed or chair independently, and so forth. The nursing assistant contributes important information to this assessment. After all data are collected, an individual program is developed to meet the resident's specific needs.

Part of the bowel and bladder assessment involves identifying factors that contribute to or cause incontinence. After these factors are identified, the nurse will develop a plan to eliminate them. The nurse will take a history of the resident's previous bowel and bladder habits. A detailed analysis of the resident's incontinent episodes over a period of 7 to 14 days will be completed. The nursing assistant is usually responsible for checking the resident hourly and recording information about incontinence or resident requests to use the toilet **(Figure 18-21)**. Accurate completion of this analysis is very important, because the resident's individual toileting schedule will be developed based largely on this information. Because you are more aware of the resident's habits and patterns than many other care providers, notify the nurse if you believe the resident shows a pattern of urge incontinence, stress incontinence, or overflow incontinence.

Following the initial assessment period, the nurse will analyze all the information collected and develop a plan for the resident. The plan is based on the resident's previous routines and habits and information about times when the resident was incontinent during the assessment. The nurse will write a specific schedule with times to toilet the resident. There may or may not be a pattern to this schedule. It is based on the resident's individual needs. Some people can wait for six hours before urinating. Others urinate every hour or two. The resident's medical condition, specific habits, and needs are considered when the schedule is written. Some environmental modification may be necessary. The schedule will be implemented and reassessed by the nurse every few days. During this time, you will continue to record each time the resident eliminates. The nurse will review the information and readjust the schedule as necessary until success is achieved. Treat the resident with dignity at all times. Flexibility in your schedule, consistency, and punctuality in being available at the scheduled toileting times will help guarantee success. In addition, believe that the program will succeed and maintain your motivation to help the resident.

Scheduled Toileting. **Scheduled toileting** is used for residents who require physical assistance to get to the bathroom. You will be assigned to assist the resident to the bathroom according to a fixed schedule, usually every two to four hours.

Prompted Voiding. Some residents know that their bladders are full, but do not communicate the need to use the toilet. The nurse may instruct you to use **prompted voiding** for these residents. In a prompted voiding program, you will check the resident frequently to determine if he or she is wet or dry. Each time you are in the room, you will ask the resident if he or she needs to use the toilet. Assist the resident to the bathroom or to use the commode, bedpan, or urinal. Praise the resident for remaining dry and for trying to use the toilet. Inform the resident when you will return to take him or her to the bathroom again.

Habit Training. **Habit training** is done for residents who are mentally confused and urinate at fairly predictable times. The resident is taken to the toilet at those times. Praise the resident for being dry and for using the toilet.

Special Situations. Some residents are placed on bladder retraining programs because they have an indwelling catheter. Facilities manage these programs differently. Some facilities completely remove the catheter and begin the retraining assessment. Other facilities clamp and

GUIDELINES FOR
Assisting Residents with Bowel and Bladder Retraining Programs

- Follow the care plan exactly.
- Answer the call signal promptly.
- Do not rush the resident when toileting.
- Provide privacy by closing the door and privacy curtain. Close the bathroom door even if you must remain in the bathroom with the resident for safety.
- Avoid scolding the resident for accidents. Tell the resident that he or she can try again next time. Praise the resident for using the toilet and for staying dry.

- If the resident cannot physically use the toilet, assist with the bedpan, urinal, or commode.
- Keep the path to the bathroom well lit and free from obstacles.
- If used, keep the wheelchair, walker, or cane close to the bed.
- Keep the resident's skin clean and dry.

ASSESSMENT FOR BOWEL & BLADDER TRAINING

PATIENT: _Frank Martin_   ROOM NO: _629C_

	DAY 1	DAY 2	DAY 3	DAY 4	DAY 5	DAY 6	DAY 7
DATE	10/2/XX	10/3/XX	10/4/XX	10/5/XX	10/6/XX	10/7/XX	10/8/XX
7 AM	D	IU	IU	D			
8 AM	IU	D	D	D			
9 AM	D	IU	D	IU			
10 AM	D	D	D	D			
11 AM	D	D	IU	IU			
12 AM	IU	D	D	D			
1 PM	IU	IU	IU	IU			
2 PM	D	D	D	D			
3 PM	D	D	D	D			
4 PM	IBM	D	D	IU			
5 PM	IU	IBM	D	IBM			
6 PM	D	IU	IU	D			
7 PM	D	D	D	IU			
8 PM	IU	IU	IU	D			
9 PM	D	D	D	D			
10 PM	D	D	D	IU			
11 PM	D	IU	IU	D			
12 AM	D	D	D	D			
1 AM	IU	D	D	D			
2 AM	D	IU	IU	IU			
3 AM	IU	D	D	IU			
4 AM	D	D	D	D			
5 AM	D	D	IU	D			
6 AM	IU	IU	D	D			
CODE:	D = DRY IBM = INCONTINENT BM IU = INCONTINENT URINE		TBM = TOILET BM TU = TOILET URINE				

FIGURE 18-21 The resident is checked hourly, but no retraining is done. If the resident asks to use the bathroom, honor the request. At the end of the assessment period, the nurse will develop an individualized toileting schedule based on this information.

unclamp the catheter at intervals so the resident gets used to the sensation of urine in the bladder. You may be asked to clamp and unclamp the catheter during the retraining process. This does not involve opening the closed system. While the catheter is clamped, urine remains in the bladder. Report resident complaints of pain or discomfort to the nurse. Be punctual in the scheduled times to unclamp the catheter to prevent discomfort from the bladder overfilling.

Kegel Exercises. Some residents must do exercises to make the bladder muscles stronger. These exercises are called **Kegel exercises.** Restorative nurses work with these residents initially. Later in the program, you may be instructed to assist and remind the resident to perform the Kegel exercises. Kegel exercises are helpful in preventing incontinence. Over time, they strengthen the muscles of the pelvic floor and the muscles surrounding the urethra and vagina. These muscles contribute to the closing of the urethra and support the pelvic structures. The resident is taught to draw in, or lift up, the muscles surrounding the vagina and anus. This is the same as the action used for controlling urination and defecation. Residents are instructed to contract the muscles, then hold the contraction for at least 10 seconds, then release for 10 seconds. The exercises are done regularly, many times a day, for at least eight weeks. They may have to be continued indefinitely. More time may be required in the elderly before results are seen. Over time, the exercises condition the muscles to contract when abdominal pressure increases. Residents are reminded to contract the pelvic muscles in situations when leakage may occur.

Intake and Output. You may also be asked to record the resident's intake and output during the retraining period. The overall fluid intake for the resident may be increased during retraining. In some facilities, fluids are limited during the evening and night hours. The retraining program may take several months. You must be empathetic, patient, and supportive, and encourage the resident's success.

RESTORATIVE EQUIPMENT

Special restorative equipment is used for many residents to prevent contractures and deformities. These can develop very quickly as a result of immobility. Follow the care plan and use common sense in using restorative equipment. The nursing assistant is usually responsible for plac-

ing and applying the equipment. Some items, such as splints, are worn according to a schedule. Other equipment, such as handrolls, are used at all times. If the equipment is fastened to the resident's body, you are responsible for keeping the skin clean and dry under the device. Usually, the equipment is removed when range-of-motion exercises are being performed, then replaced. Follow the care plan and your facility policy.

Handrolls

Handrolls are used to prevent the fingers from contracting into a tight fist. Although some devices can be fashioned from common items in the health care facility, using commercially manufactured handrolls is best. Years ago, rolled washcloths were used for handrolls. We now know that the softness and texture of a rolled washcloth promotes squeezing and actually worsens contractures! Handrolls should be used by all dependent residents. Soft handrolls **(Figure 18-22A)** are the most comfortable and commonly used. Most commercial varieties have a Velcro® strip attached that is fastened to the hand. Semi-rigid, cone-shaped handrolls **(Figure 18-22B)** are also available. These are used by residents who may have early contractures and those whose fingers are rigid. The cones are fastened to the hand with the large end by the little finger.

Splints

Splints **(Figure 18-23)** are rigid devices used on the hands, arms, legs, and feet. They are used to maintain good alignment, prevent and reverse early contractures, and maintain the extremity in a fixed position. Sometimes splints are used to maintain good alignment of a fracture until the

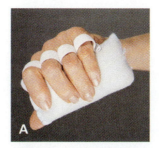 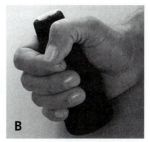

FIGURE 18-22 (A) The soft handroll is comfortable and prevents deformity. (B) The small end of the cone is placed on the thumb side of the hand. The nursing assistant is responsible for keeping the hands clean and the nails trimmed. *(Courtesy of Skil-Care Corporation, Yonkers, NY (800) 431-2972)*

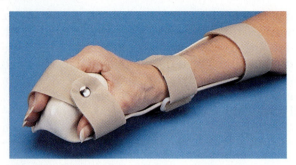

FIGURE 18-23 Apply the splint according to the individual use schedule on the care plan. The nursing assistant is responsible for keeping the resident's hand clean under the splint. Inform the nurse if the splint does not fit correctly. *(Neutral Position wrist/hand orthosis is provided by Sammons Preston, Inc., a Bissell® HealthCare Company. Reprinted with permission.)*

area is casted or an operation is performed. The physical or occupational therapist usually fabricates splints or orders splints for a specific medical purpose. The care plan will describe the reason for the splint and provide instructions for applying and removing the splint. Splints used to support broken bones are not removed by the nursing assistant. Splints used to prevent or reverse contractures are worn according to a schedule. For example, the splint may be worn during the day and removed at night. Keeping the extremity under the splint clean and dry is very important. The splint must be removed at least once each 24 hours for bathing. Check the area under the splint for signs of redness, irritation, and breakdown. Report your observations to the nurse.

Trochanter Rolls

The **trochanter roll (Figure 18-24)** is used to prevent external rotation of the hip. Trochanter

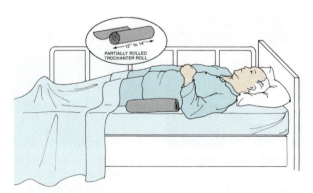

FIGURE 18-24 The trochanter roll is used to prevent the hips from contracting in a position of external rotation.

rolls should be used routinely for bedfast residents to prevent deformities. Unless the resident has a specific medical condition, such as a hip fracture, no special order is necessary. To hold the trochanter roll in place, roll it away from the resident's body. Rolling the trochanter roll toward the body will cause it to slip, making it ineffective.

Foot Boards

Foot boards **(Figure 18-25A)** are used to prevent foot drop **(Figure 18-25B)**. Foot drop is a severe contracture that is difficult or impossible to reverse. It occurs quickly in residents who are confined to bed. The toes of a resident with foot drop point downward, similar to the position of a woman's foot in high heels. The muscles in the foot become stiff and rigid, and the resident is unable to pull the ball of the foot and toes toward the body. This prevents the resident from standing normally on the foot with the heel flat on the floor. Residents with contractures of the feet and ankles are unable to walk.

Some foot boards are positioned at the end of the mattress. The heels hang over the end of the mattress so there is no pressure on them. The ball and sole of the foot are positioned flat against the foot board to prevent the toes from pointing downward. An alternative is to position the foot board on the bed and then to place a pillow in front of the foot board for the feet to rest against. A small pillow under the ankles keeps the heels off the mattress.

No matter which position is used, monitor the resident's heels frequently, relieve pressure as much as possible, and alert the nurse to signs

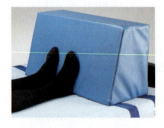

FIGURE 18-25A Foot boards are used to prevent foot drop, a severe contracture of the feet. *(Courtesy of Skil-Care Corporation, Yonkers, NY (800) 431-2972)*

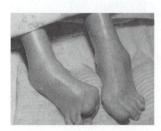

FIGURE 18-25B Foot drop is a serious contracture deformity that prevents the resident from standing or ambulating. Foot drop may be released surgically in some residents, but may become severe and irreversible.

PROCEDURE

81

Making a Trochanter Roll

1. Perform your beginning procedure actions.
2. Gather your equipment: bath blanket, gloves if contact with blood or body fluids is likely.
3. Place the bath blanket on a flat surface. Fold it in thirds lengthwise.
4. Place the blanket on the bed, extending from the waist to the mid-thigh area.
5. Position the resident in the center of the blanket.
6. Roll the center of the blanket outward (away from the resident) until it is firmly against the femur area.
7. Tuck the roll inward to maintain position.
8. Perform your procedure completion actions.

and symptoms of skin irritation or breakdown. Heel breakdown often begins with an area that appears black, brown, purple, or bruised under the skin. It may look like a large blood blister. The heels are a high-pressure area, and the skin may be thinner than on other areas of the body. The risk of heel breakdown is very high, and because of the anatomy, heel ulcers will develop quickly and worsen rapidly, invading underlying structures. Many elderly individuals have diabetes and other conditions that cause reduced circulation to the feet. Because of decreased blood flow, the risk of complications and amputation from heel ulcers is very high.

Other commercial devices that fasten to the foot may be used as substitutes for the foot board **(Figure 18-26)**. Preventing contractures of the feet is an important responsibility.

Other Positioning Devices

Sometimes it is hard to differentiate positioning devices from restraint alternatives. Many devices are used for both purposes. Restraints are commonly used because the resident has a particular positioning problem. When trying to decide how to meet the resident's positioning needs, consider restraint alternatives mentioned in Chapter 15. The devices listed can be used for support and to keep residents positioned comfortably in good body alignment.

Adaptive Devices

Adaptive devices are pieces of equipment used to perform everyday tasks **(Figure 18-27)**. A person with a disability may be unable to perform

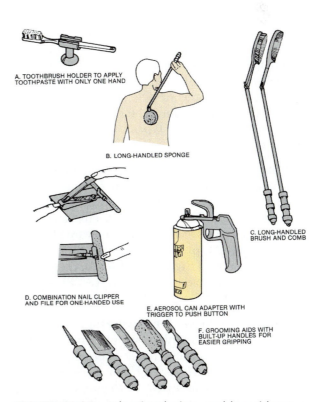

FIGURE 18-26 This heel float boot reduces pressure to the heel, and also keeps the sole of the foot in good alignment to prevent foot drop. *(Courtesy of Skil-Care Corporation, Yonkers, NY (800) 431-2972)*

A. TOOTHBRUSH HOLDER TO APPLY TOOTHPASTE WITH ONLY ONE HAND

B. LONG-HANDLED SPONGE

C. LONG-HANDLED BRUSH AND COMB

D. COMBINATION NAIL CLIPPER AND FILE FOR ONE-HANDED USE

E. AEROSOL CAN ADAPTER WITH TRIGGER TO PUSH BUTTON

F. GROOMING AIDS WITH BUILT-UP HANDLES FOR EASIER GRIPPING

FIGURE 18-27 Adaptive devices enable residents to be independent.

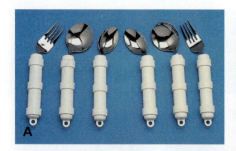

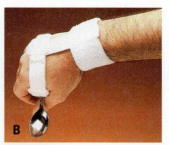

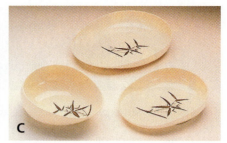

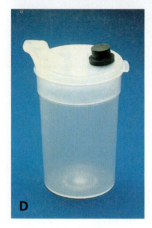

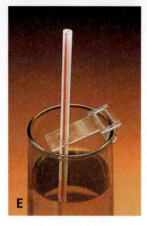

FIGURE 18-28 (A) Many types of adaptive utensils are available to meet individual needs and enable residents to feed themselves. (B) The wrist cuff enables the resident to hold silverware and eat independently. (C) Adaptive plates and bowls have raised edges so residents can scoop food easily. (D) An adaptive cup. (E) The straw holder centers the straw and holds it in place. *(Courtesy of Maddak, Inc.)*

activities of daily living. Sometimes adding a device that changes the way the task is done will enable the resident to perform it independently. Adaptive devices are usually prescribed by the occupational therapist or restorative nurse based on an evaluation of the resident's individual needs. The resident is taught how to use the device for everyday tasks. Your role as a nursing assistant is to make sure the device is clean, available, and used by the resident. The care plan will provide instructions in the types of devices used by residents.

Adaptive Devices for Eating. The most common adaptive devices are used to enable residents to feed themselves. Many individual devices are available to meet residents' needs. The most common devices are adaptive silverware **(Figure 18-28A and B)**, plates **(Figure 18-28C)**, plate guards, and cups **(Figure 18-28D)**. Other items, such as straw holders **(Figure 18-28E)**, may also be necessary.

Adaptive Devices for Dressing. Dressing aids are also commonly used **(Figure 18-29A and B)**. These devices make it easier for residents to dress themselves. Using these adaptive devices may appear awkward to you, but for the resident, being able to dress himself or herself is important for self-esteem.

Adaptive Devices for Grooming and Hygiene. Bathing and grooming are important skills. Each person has a personal hygienic routine. Grooming and hygiene are very private activities. Using adaptive devices permits the resident to perform these skills and increases self-esteem and comfort.

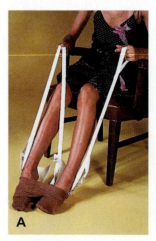

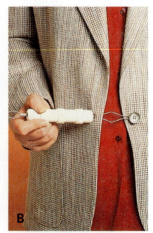

FIGURE 18-29 (A) Various adaptive devices are used by residents to put on socks and hosiery. (B) The hook is threaded through the button hole. The resident grabs the button and pulls it through the hole. *(Courtesy of Maddak, Inc.)*

KEY POINTS

- Restorative care is given to assist residents to attain and maintain their highest level of function.
- Promoting independence is part of restorative care.
- Restorative care is most effective if it is started early in the resident's illness.
- Activity strengthens residents and inactivity weakens.
- When providing restorative care, stress what the resident can do.
- When providing restorative care, the nursing assistant should look at the entire person and not just the illness.
- Many restorative programs involve assisting residents to relearn ADL skills.
- Range of motion is normal movement of joints.
- If a resident's joints do not move through the normal range of motion each day, contractures and deformities may develop.
- Contractures promote pressure ulcer development, and make treating pressure ulcers more difficult.
- Residents with existing contractures are at high risk of developing additional contractures. Contractures can begin to develop in as little as four days of immobility and inactivity. After 15 days, the resident will lose range of motion.
- Arthritis can cause mild discomfort to severe deformities and disability; the most common symptom is pain.
- Osteoporosis is a metabolic disorder in which bone mass is lost, causing bones to become porous and spongy. Residents with this condition are at very high risk for fracture.
- Hip fracture is the most common fracture in the elderly. The term "hip fracture" refers to a fracture anywhere in the upper third or head of the femur.
- A cerebrovascular accident is caused by a sudden interruption of blood to the brain. Residents with this condition will experience weakness or paralysis on one side of the body; other complications such as speech and vision problems may also occur.
- A transient ischemic attack is a temporary period of diminished blood flow to the brain that occurs suddenly and usually lasts from 2 to 15 minutes. Residents with this condition are at risk of stroke.
- Parkinson's disease is an incurable neurological disease that causes tremors and shuffling gait, and increases the risk of injury.
- Huntington's disease is an incurable neurologic disease that is hereditary. The resident develops choreiform movements, loss of voluntary movement, and dementia.
- Multiple sclerosis is a progressive neurological disorder that causes a degeneration of the nervous system and interferes with conduction of nerve impulses.
- Post polio syndrome is a neurologic condition marked by increased weakness and abnormal muscle fatigue in persons who had polio many years earlier. Estimates are that 30% to 70% of all polio survivors will develop this condition.
- Head injuries usually result from trauma, falls, or automobile accidents. The injury often causes severe, permanent brain damage. Residents with brain injury are often totally dependent on staff for care.
- Spinal cord injuries commonly cause paralysis that affects sensation and voluntary movement below the level of injury.
- A self-care deficit is an inability to perform an activity of daily living.
- Bowel and bladder retraining programs are individualized to the resident's needs based on an assessment.
- Kegel exercises strengthen pelvic floor muscles, and the muscles surrounding the urethra and vagina; they are helpful in preventing incontinence.
- The nursing assistant is responsible for applying and removing many types of restorative equipment.
- Trochanter rolls should be used routinely for bedfast residents to prevent deformities caused by external rotation of the hip.

REVIEW

A. Multiple Choice

Select the one best answer.

1. Being dependent on others may cause feelings of
   a. security.
   b. helplessness.
   c. self-esteem.
   d. hopefulness.

2. Restorative care is
   a. highly skilled.
   b. designed to maintain and improve residents.
   c. always given by licensed personnel.
   d. very technical and complex.

3. Continuity of care involves
   a. being assigned to different residents each day.
   b. providing total care to all residents.
   c. all caregivers using the same approaches.
   d. working independently.

4. Which of the following is true?
   a. Bed rest, immobility, and inactivity affect every system of the body.
   b. All sick residents should remain on bed rest.
   c. The cardiopulmonary system is not affected by bed rest.
   d. Most elderly residents need bed rest.

5. You are assigned to care for an alert resident who is paralyzed and cannot perform self-care. You should
   a. perform total care as quietly as possible.
   b. allow the resident to determine the care routine.
   c. provide the care you think is best.
   d. ask the resident's family what to do.

6. Principles of restoration include
   a. beginning treatment early.
   b. inactivity strengthens the resident.
   c. stress what the resident cannot do.
   d. do as much as possible to help the resident.

7. You are assisting a resident with a restorative ADL program. The resident is struggling to squeeze the water out of the washcloth. You should
   a. allow the resident to struggle for a few seconds.
   b. intervene immediately.
   c. complete the procedure for the resident.
   d. get the nurse right away.

8. The therapist who develops bathing, hygiene, and grooming programs is the
   a. physical therapist.
   b. occupational therapist.
   c. speech-language pathologist.
   d. respiratory care practitioner.

9. The weakness and muscle wasting caused by immobility are called
   a. range of motion.
   b. edema.
   c. atrophy.
   d. adduction.

10. Contractures are
    a. extensions of the joints.
    b. pressure ulcers.
    c. blood clots.
    d. painful deformities.

11. You are assigned to do passive range-of-motion exercises on Mr. King. He had knee surgery yesterday and his left knee is bandaged. You should
    a. consult the nurse before performing range of motion on the left knee.
    b. not do the range-of-motion exercises because of the surgery.
    c. exercise all of Mr. King's joints.
    d. perform only flexion and extension exercises on the left knee.

12. When performing range-of-motion exercises, you should
    a. stretch all joints as far as you can.
    b. move each joint as far as it comfortably will go.
    c. ask the resident to tolerate discomfort.
    d. exercise extremities with fractures only.

13. An incontinence management program
    a. is an individual bladder retraining program.
    b. is an assessment of the resident's ability to void.
    c. involves toileting residents on a fixed schedule.
    d. involves using diapers to prevent skin problems.

14. You will assist with the assessment for a bowel and bladder retraining program by
    a. taking the resident to the bathroom every two hours.
    b. writing down the times the resident is incontinent.
    c. administering suppositories and enemas daily.
    d. telling the nurse when the resident requests toileting.

15. Handrolls are used to
    a. prevent contractures of the hands.
    b. promote squeezing.
    c. increase strength.
    d. improve range of motion.

B. Matching.

Choose the correct word from Column II to match the phrases in Column I. Write the letter of the matching term in the appropriate blank.

Column I

16. _____ 60% of all pressure ulcers involve some type of this problem

17. _____ the most common symptom of arthritis

18. _____ metabolic condition in which bones become porous and spongy

19. _____ avoid elevating head of bed more than 45 degrees

20. _____ interruption of blood to the brain

21. _____ choreiform movements

22. _____ fracture anywhere in the upper third or head of the femur

23. _____ cannot feel sensation of urine

24. _____ worsening of symptoms

25. _____ symptoms are stable

26. _____ tremors, shuffling gait

27. _____ degeneration that interferes with conduction of nerve impulses

28. _____ unaware or minimally aware of the surroundings

29. _____ increased weakness, abnormal muscle fatigue, cold intolerance

30. _____ affects sensation and voluntary movement below level of injury

31. _____ inability to perform an activity of daily living

32. _____ exercises to help prevent incontinence

33. _____ prevents external rotation of hips

Column II

a. post polio syndrome
b. hip fracture
c. Parkinson's disease
d. Kegel
e. neurogenic bladder
f. remission
g. brain damage
h. Huntington's disease
i. self-care deficit
j. paralysis
k. hip precautions
l. trochanter roll
m. contracture
n. cerebrovascular accident
o. osteoporosis
p. exacerbation
q. pain
r. multiple sclerosis

C. Short Answer

Answer the following.

34–37. List the principles of rehabilitation.

34. _____   35. _____
36. _____   37. _____

D. Clinical Application

Answer the following questions.

38. Mrs. Lincoln is on a restorative ambulation program. Her goal is to walk from her room to the dining room. Before beginning the walk, you check the resident's pulse. The rate is 64. You ambulate Mrs. Lincoln to the dining room and assist her to sit in a chair. You return to check her pulse 5 minutes later and discover that her pulse is 74. What does this indicate? What action should you take?

39. Mr. Lee is a newly admitted resident. He seems to understand what you say to him, but has aphasia and cannot speak. As part of your routine care, the care plan instructs you to perform passive range-of-motion exercises, five repetitions for each joint. Mr. Lee's joints seem stiff. He makes a face and grimaces when you abduct his right shoulder. You ask him if he is in pain and he looks at you with a blank expression on his face. What should you do?

The restorative nurse is conducting an assessment for bowel and bladder retraining on Miss Rogers. You know that the resident has a bowel movement daily about 30 minutes after eating lunch. You also know that the resident has increased motor activity shortly before she is incontinent of urine. The resident does not appear restless at any other time. She does not urinate often. When she does void, it is usually a large quantity.

40. Is any of this information important to the bladder retraining assessment? Which information is important?

41. List each observation you will share with the nurse and explain why it is important.

42. What are the nursing assistant's responsibilities during the assessment phase of the retraining program? Why is it important to conscientiously fulfill these responsibilities?

CHAPTER 19

The Nursing Assistant in Subacute Care

OBJECTIVES

After reading this chapter, you will be able to:

- Spell and define key terms.
- List the four types of subacute units and describe the services provided in each.
- Describe nursing assistant responsibilities in the care of residents who are receiving subacute care.
- Describe nursing assistant care of residents who are receiving chemotherapy and radiation therapy.
- Demonstrate procedures related to the nursing assistant in subacute care.

OBSERVATIONS TO MAKE AND REPORT RELATED TO THE NURSING ASSISTANT IN SUBACUTE CARE

Chest pain
Shortness of breath
Difficulty breathing
Weakness or dizziness
Headache
Pain or body language suggesting pain
Nausea or vomiting
Diarrhea (multiple loose stools; one loose stool is not diarrhea)
Cough
Cyanosis or change in color
Change in mental status
Excessive thirst
Lethargy
Unusual drainage from the skin, a wound, or a body cavity

Abnormal appearance of urine or feces
Unable to hear blood pressure or palpate pulse
Blood pressure is different in right arm than in left arm
Changes in vital signs
Abnormal behavior, including crying
Requests for medication for an acute problem
Pain
Elevated temperature
Sweating
Chills
Skin hot or cold to touch
Skin color abnormal: flushed, red, gray, or blue
Inflammation of skin (redness, swelling, heat, pain)
Drainage from any skin opening or body cavity
Any unusual body discharge, such as mucus or pus

INTRODUCTION TO SUBACUTE CARE

Many long-term care facilities provide a subacute level of care to residents. A subacute unit is usually separate from other areas of the facility. Equipment and staffing are different on this unit because the needs of the residents and services provided are very different from those of the general nursing facility population.

A subacute unit is a temporary place to stay. If the resident recovers sufficiently, he or she will be discharged home. If the resident's condition becomes chronic and more stable, he or she will go to a long-term care facility to complete the recovery. If the resident becomes unstable or acutely ill, he or she is transferred to the hospital.

Role of the Nursing Assistant in Subacute Care

You will work as a team member on a highly skilled interdisciplinary team. The ability to co-operate with others and follow directions is especially important in the subacute unit. The nursing assistant is a very important team member because the residents require a great deal of personal care, monitoring, and good observational skills. Residents in subacute care often require many diagnostic tests. The nursing assistant is usually responsible for collecting laboratory specimens.

Residents in subacute care have had an acute illness or an acute episode related to a chronic problem. Their condition can change very quickly, and you must be alert to small changes. Be prepared to take rapid action. Residents have complex care needs related to medical problems and surgical procedures. They may be connected to several electronic monitoring or caregiving devices and may have tubes in different areas of the body. Residents in a subacute unit are commonly dependent on the nursing assistant to help them with many of their activities of daily living.

Staff working in the subacute unit must attend extra staff development sessions and classes to learn about individual resident needs, medical conditions, and special equipment. The technology and skills required of workers in this unit change rapidly, and it is your responsibility to keep up. The nursing assistant in subacute care is an important team member who must have excellent communication, technical and observational skills.

Caring for Residents who are Connected to Special Equipment

Residents in the subacute unit frequently are connected to electronic monitoring and caregiving devices. Many of these devices are used by residents 24 hours a day and cannot be disconnected while personal care is provided. The nursing assistant must be careful not to accidentally move, bump, or disconnect the equipment. Make sure the equipment does not restrain the resident. For example, an electronic blood pressure monitor on the left arm, a pulse oximeter on the right hand, and an abductor pillow between the legs immobilizes the resident completely. Inform the nurse if a resident is immobilized as a result of caregiving or monitoring devices. In most cases, you will not be permitted to adjust or regulate the equipment. If an equipment alarm sounds, respond immediately. Notify the nurse without delay.

GUIDELINES FOR
Electronic Blood Pressure Monitoring

Resident Selection

- This procedure can be done on residents of all ages and sizes, but appropriately sized cuffs must be used.
- At least one blood pressure reading should be taken using the auscultation method before using the electronic blood pressure device. The auscultation reading is used as a baseline with which to compare electronic values.

The procedure is contraindicated in residents with:

- Extreme hypertension or hypotension
- Very rapid heart rates
- Irregular heart rhythms or atrial **dysrhythmia** (an abnormal heart rhythm)
- Excessive body movement, tremors

Residents for whom electronic blood pressure monitoring is not acceptable should be known to all caregivers and identified on the care plan or Kardex. If in doubt, check with the nurse for instructions as to residents with very high blood pressure or rapid or irregular heart (pulse) rates.

Do not place the cuff on an arm with:

- Paralysis
- An intravenous infusion
- A pulse oximeter
- Impaired circulation
- A dialysis access device
- Fracture
- Burns
- Edema
- A recent mastectomy or other surgical procedure

Application of the Cuff

- Select the proper cuff size. The width should be equal to 40% of the arm circumference.
- The upper arm is the preferred location, but the forearm or ankle may also be used. However, using these areas may result in inaccurate readings, so they should be used only when measuring pressure in the upper arms is not possible.

Documentation of Care in the Subacute Unit

Reimbursement for care in subacute units is often provided by insurance companies and managed care organizations. These agencies will only pay for care that matches the treatment plan prescribed for the resident. Documentation must reflect the resident's progress toward stated care plan goals and response to treatment provided. You will be responsible for documenting the services you provided. You may also be required to document the resident's response to these services. If you are working with residents on a restorative program, you may be required to document additional information. Your facility will provide training on special documentation requirements related to reimbursement.

Taking Vital Signs in the Subacute Unit

Vital signs of residents in the subacute unit must be closely monitored. Carefully review the information in Chapter 16. Vital signs must be taken in a timely manner, and must be accurate. They must be documented promptly, because many individuals will refer to these values. Report abnormal vital signs to the nurse promptly. If a resident is connected to electronic vital sign monitoring equipment, respond to alarms immediately. Never turn an alarm off. An electronic blood pressure monitoring unit **(Figure 19-1)** is commonly used in the subacute care unit because of the frequency of checks and the need for accuracy.

SERVICES PROVIDED IN SUBACUTE UNITS

Subacute units provide many different types of services. Rules and regulations vary according to the type of services the subacute unit offers and the setting in which it is located. Five basic types of subacute units and a summary of the services provided in each are listed in **Table 19-1** on p. 386.

PROCEDURE 82

Taking Blood Pressure with an Electronic Blood Pressure Apparatus

 OBRA

Note: The guidelines and reportable values for this procedure vary slightly from state to state, and from one facility to another. Your instructor will inform you if the guidelines or reportable values in your state or facility differ from those listed here. Know and follow the required guidelines for your state and facility.

Note: This procedure is generic and applies principles used for common types of electronic blood pressure monitoring devices. Follow the instructions for the specific device you are using. The operating instructions are slightly different for each. Your instructor will inform you if the directions for the equipment you are using differ from those listed here.

1. Perform your beginning procedure actions.
2. Assemble needed equipment: electronic blood pressure device, assortment of cuffs and tubes.
3. Bring the electronic blood pressure unit to the bedside. Place it near the resident and plug it into a source of electricity.
4. Locate the on/off switch and turn the machine on.
5. Select the appropriate cuff for the machine and size for the resident's extremity.

6. Remove restrictive clothing.
7. Squeeze excess air out of the cuff.
8. Connect the cuff to the connector hose.
9. Wrap the cuff snugly around the resident's extremity, verifying that only one finger can fit between the cuff and the resident's skin. Make sure the "artery" arrow marked on the outside of the cuff is correctly placed over the brachial artery.
10. Verify that the hose connecting the cuff and the machine is not kinked.
11. Set the frequency control for automatic or manual.
12. Press the start button.
13. If the cuff will take periodic, automatic measurements, set the designated frequency of measurement.
14. Set upper and lower alarm limits for systolic, diastolic, and mean blood pressure readings.
15. Remove the cuff at least every two hours and alternate sites, if possible. Evaluate the skin for redness and irritation. Report abnormalities to the nurse.
16. Perform your procedure completion actions.

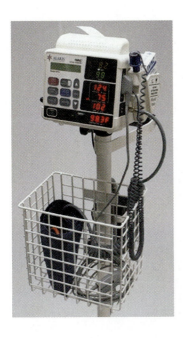

FIGURE 19-1 All vital signs may be checked with a single instrument. *(Vital•Check patient monitor; photo courtesy of ALARIS Medical Systems, Inc., San Diego, CA)*

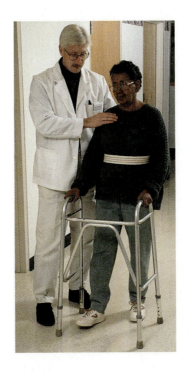

FIGURE 19-2 Residents with subacute rehabilitation needs receive intensive therapy services to help them regain their mobility skills.

Rehabilitation Services

Some subacute care units provide intensive rehabilitation services. Residents often receive more than one type of therapy. Physical, occupational, speech, and respiratory therapy may be provided **(Figure 19-2)**. Therapy is provided 6 or 7 days a week. The resident usually participates for 3 to 5 hours each day.

Chemotherapy

Residents with cancer may receive **chemotherapy,** or use of chemicals and drugs to destroy cancer cells. These drugs are administered by a nurse or physician. The resident receiving chemotherapy may have many fears about the outcome of the disease. The nursing assistant must practice empathy and be emotionally supportive of the resident. Be a good listener. Assist with modesty, head coverings, caps, or scarves as the resident desires.

Chemotherapy is given by many different routes. Some residents are able to take oral medications. Others must receive the drugs in the muscles, veins, or other organs and body cavities. If the drugs are given intravenously, a central intravenous catheter **(Figure 19-3,** p. 389) is often inserted to avoid repeated needlesticks and reduce the risk of vein irritation and collapse. The drugs are very potent and can irritate the skin, eyes, and mucous membranes of caregivers. Because of this, special measures are used to handle the drugs. Never eat, drink, or chew gum in an area where chemotherapy drugs are being prepared. If you accidentally contact a chemother-

apy drug with your hands or mucous membranes, flush well with water and seek medical attention. These drugs and the containers they are dispensed in require special handling and disposal.

Side Effects of Chemotherapy. Chemotherapy targets rapidly regenerating cells, such as cancer cells. The drugs cannot differentiate cancer cells from normal cells, so other cells are also affected. Side effects of cancer drugs can range from mild to life-threatening. Residents who are receiving these drugs need special monitoring. Sometimes the dose and scheduling must be changed to reduce side effects. Inform the nurse promptly if:

- There are signs of intravenous (IV) infiltration, such as redness, swelling, or pain at the needle insertion site
- The resident's mental status changes
- Vital signs change

Common side effects of chemotherapy are:

- Alopecia, or hair loss.
- Nausea and vomiting.
- Anorexia, or loss of appetite.
- Depression, or feeling sad, scared, nervous over the illness, and fearful of what the future holds.
- Fatigue.
- Increased risk of infection.
- Increased risk of bleeding.
- Destruction of the mucous membranes of the mouth.

TABLE 19-1 Types of subacute care units

Type of Subacute Facility	Description	Typical Medical Problems of Residents Admitted	Goals of Care	Average Length of Resident's Stay
Transitional subacute unit	• A less expensive setting than the acute care hospital • Provides 24-hour-a-day RN coverage • RNs in this unit have special acute care education, experience, and certifications • Rehabilitation therapies are seven days a week • Respiratory therapy is available 24 hours a day • A dietitian is regularly available	• Severe wounds or Stage III or IV pressure ulcers • Strokes • Residents who have had open heart surgery, heart attack, acute congestive heart failure, or other heart conditions • Residents with tracheostomies that require respiratory management • Cancer, including chemotherapy and radiation therapy • Need for intensive rehabilitation programs • Medically complex diabetes, digestive problems, or renal disorders	• Manage care and therapy in a less expensive setting than the acute care hospital • Discharge resident to home, an assisted living facility, or a skilled nursing facility	5–40 days
General medical-surgical subacute unit	• Care for residents with complex medical and monitoring needs, rehabilitation therapy, nursing assessment, and intervention • RN coverage is provided 24 hours a day • RNs working in this unit have special acute care education, experience, and certifications • Rehabilitation therapies are available seven days a week • Respiratory therapy is available 24 hours a day • A registered dietitian is regularly available	• Long-term IV therapy for infection, nutrition, or other medical problems without other significant complications • Stable medical problems, including cardiac, digestive, renal problems, or diabetes • Stroke for which the resident requires one to three hours of therapy (PT, OT, and/or speech) daily • Neurologic or orthopedic condition for which the resident requires one to three hours of therapy each day • HIV disease/AIDS	• Manage care and therapy in a less expensive setting than an acute care hospital, in a cost-effective manner • Discharge resident to home, an assisted living facility, or a skilled nursing facility	7–21 days

Continues

TABLE 19-1 Types of subacute care units, *Continued*

Type of Subacute Facility	Description	Typical Medical Problems of Residents Admitted	Goals of Care	Average Length of Resident's Stay
Chronic subacute unit	• Care for residents with little hope of recovery or return to functional independence • RN on duty at least eight hours a day • If an RN is not on duty, an LPN or LVN is in charge • Restorative nursing care is provided for comfort, to prevent deformities, and to maintain self-esteem • Physical, occupational, speech, and respiratory therapies are available	• Dependence on ventilator for breathing • Long-term coma • Progressive neurologic conditions • Need for restorative care from nursing staff with guidance, teaching, or assistance from therapy personnel	• Provide care in the most cost-effective manner, considering medical problems and needs	60–90 days
Long-term transitional subacute unit	• Care for residents with medically complex problems or dependence on an acute ventilator • Many different types of physician specialists must be available to care for residents in this type of unit • Unit director is a highly skilled, educated, and qualified RN with acute care experience • Residents require a high degree of RN intervention because of their acute medical problems • Respiratory therapists usually provide daily services • Dietitian available, if needed	• Acute ventilator dependence for which the resident requires complex daily care and management of respiratory problems • At least two medical or surgical diagnoses requiring special medical services and daily RN assessment and intervention	• Manage care and therapy in a less expensive setting than an acute care hospital	More than 25 days

Continues

TABLE 19-1   Types of subacute care units, *Continued*

Type of Subacute Facility	Description	Typical Medical Problems of Residents Admitted	Goals of Care	Average Length of Resident's Stay
Specialized subacute unit	• Care of specialized groups of residents, such as pediatric residents • Many different types of physicians and other specialists must be available to care for residents in this unit • Unit director is a highly skilled, educated, and qualified RN with experience in the unit specialty • Residents often require a high degree of RN intervention because of their acute medical problems • RN staffing determined by the specialty nature of the unit; most provide RN services 24 hours a day • Residents require daily RN assessment and intervention • Respiratory therapists usually provide daily services • Rehabilitation therapies are available seven days a week • Dietitian available, if needed	• Medically complex problems grouped together according to need or medical diagnosis	• Manage care and therapy in a less expensive setting than an acute care hospital • Discharge resident to home, an assisted living facility, or a skilled nursing facility	Varies with the type of unit; commonly 60–90 days.

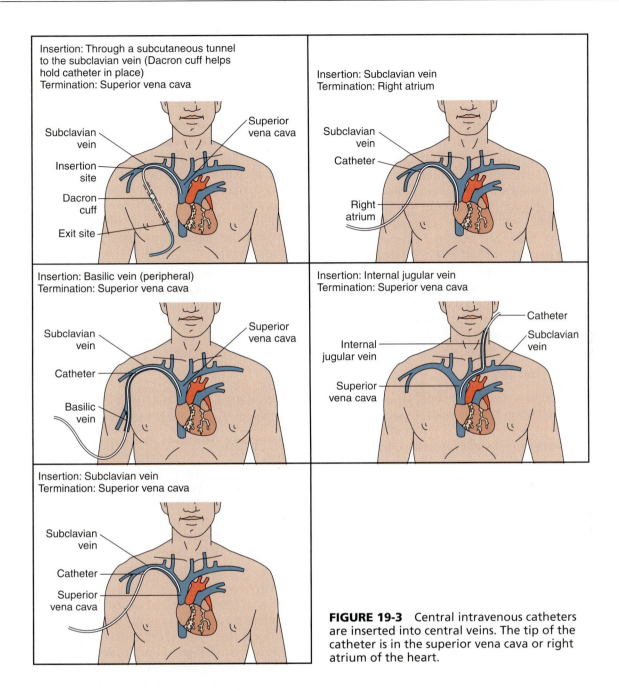

Insertion: Through a subcutaneous tunnel to the subclavian vein (Dacron cuff helps hold catheter in place)
Termination: Superior vena cava

Subclavian vein
Superior vena cava
Insertion site
Dacron cuff
Exit site

Insertion: Subclavian vein
Termination: Right atrium

Subclavian vein
Catheter
Right atrium

Insertion: Basilic vein (peripheral)
Termination: Superior vena cava

Subclavian vein
Superior vena cava
Catheter
Basilic vein

Insertion: Internal jugular vein
Termination: Superior vena cava

Catheter
Subclavian vein
Internal jugular vein
Superior vena cava

Insertion: Subclavian vein
Termination: Superior vena cava

Subclavian vein
Catheter
Superior vena cava

FIGURE 19-3 Central intravenous catheters are inserted into central veins. The tip of the catheter is in the superior vena cava or right atrium of the heart.

Many other side effects are also caused by chemotherapy drugs. The nurse will advise you what to watch for in each resident.

Special Care of the Resident Who is Receiving Chemotherapy. Observe chemotherapy residents for side effects of the drugs and report them to the nurse promptly. Provide nursing comfort measures, such as good mouth care and daily bathing. Routinely take precautions to prevent injuries and infection. For example, you may be instructed to remind the resident to cough and deep-breathe to keep the lungs clear. You may be asked to take vital signs frequently. Rectal temper-

atures should not be taken in some residents. Check with the nurse before taking a rectal temperature. Report a fever over 101°F, chilling, or other signs of infection to the nurse immediately.

Because of the risk of bleeding, residents may have to take special precautions, such as blowing the nose gently, or using an electric razor. A very soft toothbrush will probably be necessary. Special mouthwash products may be ordered. The care plan and the nurse will provide special directions.

Promoting good nutrition and hydration is very important. You may be asked to serve the resident six small meals a day. High-protein drinks may also be ordered. Encourage fluids, and record intake and output, including emesis. Alternate periods of rest with periods of activity to reduce fatigue. Plan your care to allow for frequent rest periods.

Disposal of Body Fluids and Wastes. Residents who are receiving chemotherapy may excrete the drugs in their waste and body fluids. Discard gloves and other protective apparel, if worn, in a leakproof container. Follow facility policies for discarding materials in the biohazardous waste or other contaminated area. Because the drugs are excreted in body waste, linens that have contacted blood, body fluids, or excretions also require special handling. Wear gloves when handling linen, and always apply the principles of standard precautions. Soiled items should be bagged in specially marked bags before you send them to the laundry.

Radiation Therapy

Some types of cancer respond to **radiation therapy.** Radiation treatments are performed in the outpatient department of the hospital. After the treatment, the resident returns to the nursing facility.

Radiation therapy involves the use of high-energy, ionizing beams to the site of the cancer **(Figure 19-4).** The objective is to destroy the cancerous tissue without damaging healthy tissue. Several different types of radiation therapy may be used. Common side effects of radiation that should be reported to the nurse are:

- Fatigue
- Nausea, vomiting
- Diarrhea
- Skin redness, irritation, peeling
- Change in ability to taste
- Irritation of mucous membranes
- Cough
- Shortness of breath

Special Care of the Resident Who is Receiving Radiation Therapy. The resident may have markings on the skin at the site where radiation is delivered. Do not wash these off. The radiation may be very irritating to the resident's skin. Check the skin daily for problems and report them to the nurse, if found. Special skin care may be listed on the care plan. You may be instructed to:

- Wash the resident with lukewarm water and mild soap; in some situations soap is not used
- Avoid rubbing or creating friction on the skin
- Avoid shaving areas near the treatment field
- Avoid putting tape on the resident's skin near the treatment field
- Avoid lotions and cosmetics near the treatment field
- Avoid tight-fitting garments; dress the resident in loose, comfortable clothing

Protecting Yourself from Radiation Exposure. Sources of radiation are sometimes implanted inside the resident's body. If this is the case, you will be instructed in special precautions to follow to reduce your risk of radiation exposure. A list of precautions will be placed on the chart or elsewhere. Follow these instructions carefully. In general, you should:

- Not remain in the resident's room any longer than necessary.
- Stay at least three feet away from the resident unless direct care is being delivered.
- Inform the nurse if an implant comes out of a body cavity (if so, do not touch it).
- Find out if special precautions are necessary for handling soiled linens, tissues, or dressings.
- Inform the nurse if you are pregnant, or suspect you may be pregnant.

Pulse Oximetry

Many residents in the subacute unit are monitored with a device called a **pulse oximeter** **(Figure 19-5)** that measures the amount of oxygen in the arterial blood. Having these data readily available enables the nurse to treat the resident quickly. Pulse oximetry will detect critical changes in the resident's oxygen levels before the skin color changes. This makes it a valuable tool that provides details about changes in the resident's condition as soon as they occur. The

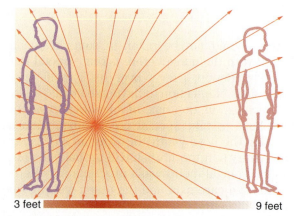

3 feet   9 feet

FIGURE 19-4 Radiation therapy destroys cancer cells by directing high-energy ionizing beams to the site of the tumor.

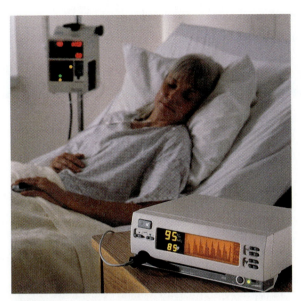

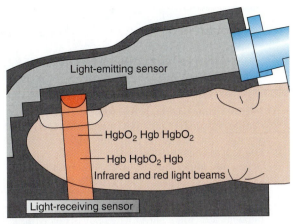

FIGURE 19-7 As light passes through the tissue, a photodetector measures the amount of oxygen in the arterial blood.

FIGURE 19-5 The pulse oximeter measures oxygen in the resident's arterial blood. *(Courtesy of Ohmeda, Louisville, CO)*

resident's outcome is usually better when early treatment is provided. Before applying the pulse oximeter, check the resident's oxygen, if being used. Document the liter flow.

The pulse oximeter is attached to the resident's skin with a sensor. Several different sensors are available. These can be placed on the finger **(Figure 19-6)**, toe, earlobe, foot, forehead, or the bridge of the nose. The tip of the finger and the earlobe are most commonly used. In these areas, a clothespin-like sensor is attached to both sides. The finger and toe sensors work best with dark-skinned residents. Poor circulation interferes with use of the pulse oximeter.

The unit has two light emitting diodes (LEDs). The sensor contains a photodetector that measures the light as it passes through the tissue. This measures the amount of oxygen in the resident's arterial blood **(Figure 19-7)**. The pulse oximeter converts this into a percentage, which can be viewed on the digital display. The physician will

order what he or she wants the minimum oxygen saturation to be. The nurse will give you this information. A measurement of 95% to 100% is considered normal. Readings below 90% suggest complications. When the reading reaches 85%, there may not be enough oxygen for the tissues. Readings below 70% are life-threatening. The pulse oximeter is not used for residents with known or suspected carbon monoxide poisoning.

The pulse oximeter has an alarm, which is usually preset by the manufacturer to normal limits. Make sure that the alarm is in the "on" position, and is set as ordered. Never turn the alarm off.

Monitoring the Resident. You must monitor the resident regularly when the pulse oximeter is used. Reporting to the nurse is part of your procedure completion actions. In this situation, make sure to report the resident's initial pulse oximeter reading and vital signs. This is important information on which the nurse will act. He or she will further assess the resident and provide care for abnormal values. The nurse must know the initial values as a basis for comparison.

If the resident's vital signs or appearance change significantly from your baseline values, notify the nurse promptly. Also inform the nurse immediately if the resident's pulse oximetry value is less than the level ordered by the physician. Monitor the resident's oxygen, if used, each time you are in the room. Make sure it is set at the liter flow ordered by the physician.

Rotate the position of the finger sensor at least every four hours. A spring-clip sensor should be moved every two hours. Rotating the location of the sensor reduces the risk of skin breakdown and complications related to pressure.

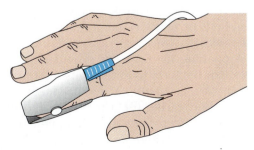

FIGURE 19-6 The fingertip sensor is most commonly used.

PROCEDURE 83 — Using a Pulse Oximeter

1. Perform your beginning procedure actions.
2. Gather needed equipment: pulse oximeter unit; sensor appropriate to the site; adhesive tape, if needed, to secure the sensor.
3. Select and apply the sensor. If the sensor has position markings, align them opposite each other to ensure an accurate reading.
4. Fasten the sensor securely, or the reading will not be accurate. Make sure the sensor is not wrapped so tightly with tape that it restricts blood flow.
5. Attach the sensor to the resident cable on the pulse oximeter.
6. Turn the unit on. You will hear a beep with each pulse beat. Adjust the volume as desired. Some units also have light bars, indicating the strength of the pulse. Note the percentage of oxygen saturation. Inform the nurse, and document according to facility policy.
7. Monitor the resident's pulse rate, if the unit provides this reading. Compare with the resident's actual pulse to make sure the unit is picking up each beat. Inform the nurse, and document according to facility policy.
8. Monitor the resident's respirations and general appearance. Inform the nurse, and document according to facility policy. If the resident's general condition changes at any time, notify the nurse.
9. Perform your procedure completion actions.

Ventilator Support

Some residents require **ventilator** support. A ventilator is a device to control or assist breathing. It is connected to a tube inserted into the lungs. Residents who are ventilator-dependent are unable to breathe normally through the nose and mouth. A surgical procedure called a **tracheostomy,** in which an incision is made in the trachea, is performed. A plastic or metal **cannula** is inserted into the trachea through which the resident breathes **(Figure 19-8).** This will interfere with the resident's ability to speak, and he or she will communicate by an alternate method of communication. Avoid getting soap, water, lint, powder, or other substances near the tracheostomy, as it is a direct passageway to the lungs. Residents with a tracheostomy can be bathed, but the stoma must be covered, and you must take care to avoid getting the area wet.

Notify the nurse if a resident with a tracheostomy:

- Is short of breath
- Is cyanotic
- Has changes in level of consciousness or mental status
- Produces rattling or bubbling noises from the chest

Also notify the nurse if:

- The alarm sounds on the ventilator
- The ties are loose or any part of the device comes apart or is removed
- The ties are too tight. You should be able to slide your finger underneath the tie on either side of the neck. If you cannot, it is too tight, and you need to notify the nurse immediately.
- The tube becomes blocked, dislodged, disconnected, or disrupted

Be especially careful when turning and bathing the resident. Monitor the resident's skin color closely. Watch for cyanosis, changes in color of the nail beds or mucous membranes, or respiratory distress.

The opening in the neck provides an open pathway for bacteria to enter, causing infection. Use standard precautions and frequent handwashing when caring for a resident who has a tracheostomy. Secretions may be expelled from the tracheostomy when the resident coughs. The resident has no control over this. If he or she is expelling secretions, you will also need to wear a

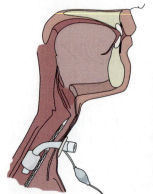
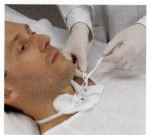

FIGURE 19-8 A cannula is inserted into the tracheostomy to keep the stoma open. Keep water, powder, dust, lint, and other substances away from the opening.

gown, mask, and eye protection when caring for the resident.

Wound Management

Some residents require wound management for severe pressure ulcers **(Figure 19-9),** burns, or surgical wounds. The resident may have special positioning needs related to the injured area of the skin, or may be on a low air loss therapy bed or other type of specialty bed. Notify the nurse if any of the following occur:

- The wound appears red or swollen, or has increased drainage
- A dressing becomes saturated with drainage from the wound
- Wound drainage has a foul odor
- The resident complains of increased pain in the wound
- The wound dressing becomes wet or falls off
- The wound dressing accidentally becomes contaminated with urine or stool

The nurse or physical therapist will perform frequent dressing changes on these areas using sterile technique. You may be required to assist with dressing changes, so a basic knowledge of sterile technique is necessary.

Sterile Technique

Sterile technique is a pathogen-free technique used whenever you are performing procedures within body cavities and during certain dressing changes. Only sterile supplies come into contact with the body during sterile procedures. Sterile gloves are worn. Supplies that are used are either wrapped and autoclaved, or are purchased in disposable sterile packages. As long as the outer wrapper to the package is intact, the items inside are considered sterile. Prior to sterilizing

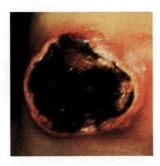

FIGURE 19-9 This necrotic pressure ulcer requires debridement and intensive wound management. *(Courtesy of Emory University Hospital, Atlanta, GA)*

supplies in an autoclave, the outer wrapper is sealed with tape. The tape changes color during the process, indicating that the contents of the package are sterile **(Figure 19-10).**

Total Parenteral Nutrition

Total parenteral nutrition (TPN) is also called **hyperalimentation.** The solution is administered through an intravenous catheter

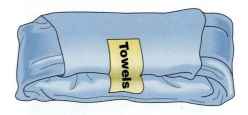

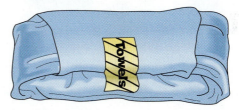

FIGURE 19-10 The tape on the top package is plain, indicating that the contents are not sterile. The tape on the bottom package is striped, indicating that the contents of the package are sterile.

GUIDELINES FOR
Assisting with Sterile Procedures

- If the sterility of any item is in doubt, consider it unsterile and avoid using it.
- If a sterile item contacts an unsterile item, both articles are considered contaminated.
- If a sterile package is cracked, cut, or torn, it is contaminated and should not be used.
- The outside of a sterile wrapper is not sterile. It may be handled with your hands. Avoid touching

the inside of the wrapper or items inside the package with your hands.
- If a sterile item becomes wet, it is contaminated.
- Avoid crossing over or touching the sterile field. If you must add an item to the sterile field, drop it onto the field from the sterile package.
- If you are wearing sterile gloves, avoid touching unsterile articles. Keep your hands above your waist.

PROCEDURE 84

Opening a Sterile Package

1. Perform your beginning procedure actions.
2. Check the seal on the package to ensure that it is sterile.
3. Remove the tape or package seal.
4. Touch only the outside of the package.
5. Open the package away from your body.
6. Open the distal flap of the package by touching only the corner **(Figure 19-11A)**.
7. Open the right-hand flap by touching only the corner.
8. Open the left-hand flap by touching only the corner.
9. Open the proximal flap by touching only the corner, then lifting the flap up and pulling it toward you, allowing it to drop over the edge of the counter or table. Avoid touching the inside of the wrapper or the contents of the package.
10. To add the item to the sterile field, open the sterile package using steps 1-9 above, or peel back the edges of the sterile package.
11. With your dominant hand, grasp the package from the bottom. With your free hand, pull the sides of the package away from the sterile field.
12. Drop the sterile item onto the sterile field **(Figure 19-11B)**. Avoid touching the sterile field with the package wrapper.
13. Discard the wrapper.
14. Perform your procedure completion actions.

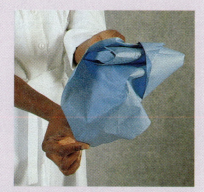

FIGURE 19-11A Holding the package away from your body, unfold the distal flap by lifting the corner of the package.

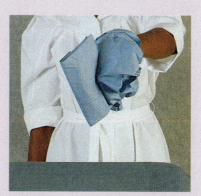

FIGURE 19-11B Wrap the outer package over your hand to avoid contaminating the sterile field, then drop the inner package onto the sterile drape.

PROCEDURE 85

Applying Sterile Gloves

1. Perform your beginning procedure actions.
2. Check the glove package for sterility.
3. Open the outer package by peeling the upper edges back.
4. Remove the inner package containing the gloves and place it on the inside of the outer package.
5. Open the inner package, handling it only by the corners on the outside **(Figure 19-12A)**.
6. Pick up the cuff of the right-hand glove, using your left hand. Avoid touching the area below the cuff **(Figure 19-12B)**.
7. Insert your right hand into the glove. Spread your fingers slightly to insert them into the fingers of the glove. If the glove is not on correctly, do not attempt to straighten it at this time.
8. Insert the gloved fingers of your right hand under the cuff of the left glove **(Figure 19-12C)**.
9. Adjust the fingers of the gloves for comfort. Because both gloves are sterile, they may touch each other. Avoid touching the cuffs of the gloves.
10. Insert your right hand under the cuff of the left glove and push the cuff up over your wrist **(Figure 19-12D)**. Avoid touching your wrist or the outside of the cuff with your glove.
11. Insert your left hand under the cuff of the right glove and push the cuff up over your wrist. Avoid touching your wrist or the outside of the cuff with your glove.
12. You may now touch sterile items with your sterile gloves. Avoid touching unsterile items.

Continues

Applying Sterile Gloves, *Continued*

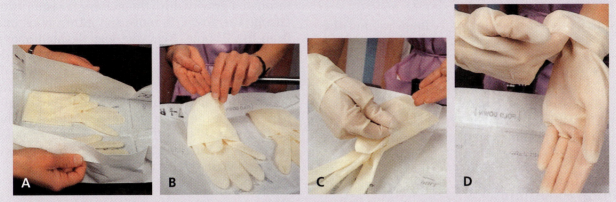

FIGURE 19-12   (A) Fold the edges of the package back without touching the inside of the wrapper or the gloves. (B) Lifting the edges of the cuff, slide your hand into the glove. (C) Insert the fingers of your right hand under the cuff of the left glove. (D) Adjust the cuffs for comfort without touching your wrists.

inserted into the subclavian vein in the chest. A special intravenous catheter in the arm, called a **peripherally inserted central catheter (PICC)** **(Figure 19-13)**, may also be used. The tip of both catheters is threaded through the veins to the superior vena cava of the heart. TPN feedings bypass the organs of the digestive system entirely, allowing them to rest and heal. The nurse will care for the insertion site. Be sure the tubing is not obstructed or kinked. Be very careful to avoid dislodging the tubing when moving or caring for the resident. Many health care facilities keep a special clamp, called a **Kelly** **(Figure 19-14),** at the bedside of residents who have intravenous lines in the subclavian vein. Serious complications occur if the tubing breaks or becomes dislodged. The Kelly is used to clamp the tubing close to the resident's body if the line breaks or is accidentally pulled loose. If air is allowed to enter the line, it could be fatal. The Kelly should be readily available at all times. Avoid storing it in a drawer or removing it from the room.

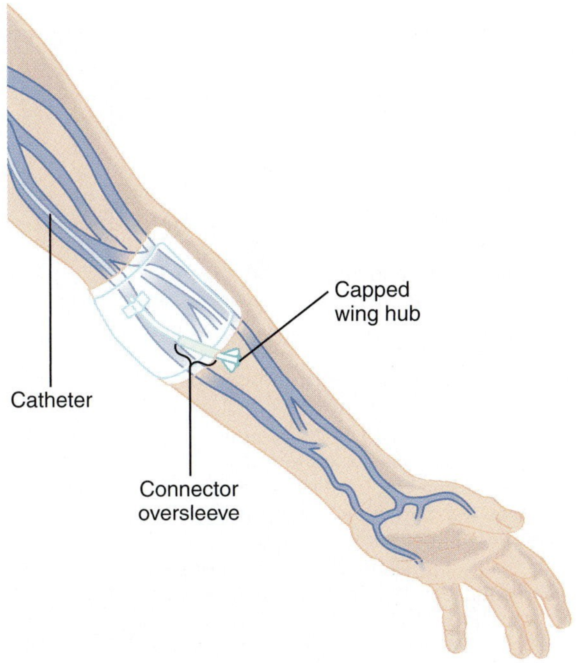

Capped wing hub

Catheter

Connector oversleeve

FIGURE 19-13   The peripherally inserted central catheter (PICC) is inserted into the arm and threaded through the veins to the superior vena cava of the heart.

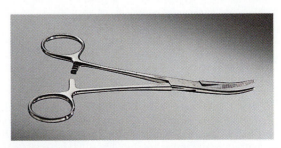

FIGURE 19-14   The Kelly clamp is used to clamp the central catheter close to the body in case of breakage. *(Courtesy of Medline Industries, Inc. 1-800-MEDLINE)*

You may be required to assist the nurse with sterile dressing changes over the intravenous infusion site. When caring for residents with a subclavian line, notify the nurse immediately if:

- You see blood in the intravenous tubing
- The resident has an elevated temperature or experiences chills
- You observe swelling or redness around the collarbone or near the infusion site
- The resident complains of pain in the neck or chest
- The resident becomes short of breath, or experiences elevated blood pressure, or edema
- The catheter is broken or cracked
- The alarm sounds on the intravenous infusion pump

Intravenous Infusions

Many residents in the subacute unit have intravenous infusions running. These are used for providing medications and fluids. The nurse is responsible for the infusion. However, you will be required to monitor the intravenous infusion when you are providing care. Use caution when moving the resident, to avoid dislodging the line.

Changing the Gown on a Resident with an Intravenous Infusion. The nursing assistant must change the gown on residents with intravenous infusions when personal care is provided. If the resident is receiving intravenous fluids through a pump, a gown that snaps at the shoulders should be used. If this type of gown is not available, the nurse must change the gown. If the resident is receiving an intravenous infusion through a gravity drip, the nursing assistant will change the gown. Remove the intravenous bag from the IV pole. Keep the bag elevated above the infusion site. Remove both of the resident's arms from the gown, keeping the chest covered. Pull the sleeve of the gown over the IV tubing and bag to remove it. Insert the IV tubing and bag through the back side of the sleeve of the clean gown. Return the IV bag to the IV pole. Continue to change the remainder of the resident's gown in the normal manner.

Dialysis

Many residents in long-term care receive **dialysis** treatments. Dialysis is performed to cleanse the blood of impurities when the resident's kidneys have failed. It is usually a temporary measure while the resident awaits a kidney transplant. Residents who are receiving dialysis are served a special diet and have fluid restrictions. They are usually on strict intake and output. Most residents on dialysis are weighed daily to monitor for fluid gains.

GUIDELINES FOR
Caring for Residents with Intravenous Infusions

- Make sure that the solution is flowing. Check the drip rate, if this is your facility policy and if you have been trained in this procedure. The nursing assistant is responsible for monitoring the flow only. Never try to adjust the rate of flow of the solution.
- Handle the **infusion site** carefully. The infusion site is the location where the intravenous needle or cannula enters the body.
- Do not adjust the clamps on the tubing.
- Avoid pulling on the tubing when moving the resident.
- Always keep the intravenous solution above the needle insertion site.
- Avoid taking a blood pressure in the arm with an intravenous infusion.
- Never disconnect the tubing. If the tubing or needle accidentally separate, put firm pressure on the needle insertion site with a gloved hand and call for the nurse immediately.
- Avoid kinks and obstructions in the tubing.

Report these observations to the nurse immediately:
- The alarm sounds on an intravenous pump
- Blood backs up into the intravenous tubing
- Redness, swelling, or complaints of pain at the needle insertion site
- Wetness or moisture at the insertion site or where the tubing connects to the intravenous catheter
- If the solution in the intravenous bag or bottle is empty or low; the container should never run dry
- The IV is not dripping or seems to be dripping too fast, or the drip chamber is completely full
- The needle becomes dislodged
- The tubing pulls apart from the needle
- The solution appears to be leaking

Hemodialysis. Residents who are receiving **hemodialysis** go out to a dialysis center several times a week for their dialysis treatment. Residents are gone most of the day. Many facilities prepare a sack lunch to send with residents to the dialysis center.

Residents receiving hemodialysis have a **shunt, graft** (Figure 19-15A), or **fistula** (Figure 19-15B) through which they receive treatment. The dialysis solution is infused at this site. Avoid taking the blood pressure in the arm used for dialysis.

When residents return from hemodialysis treatment, they may be weak. Monitor them closely when they ambulate. Watch for dizziness and syncope. Monitor the vital signs frequently after dialysis, as directed by the nurse.

Peritoneal Dialysis. A type of dialysis procedure performed in the long-term care facility is called **peritoneal dialysis.** It involves inserting dialysis solution through a cannula into the resident's abdominal cavity. The dialysate is usually warmed in a basin of warm water for 20 to 30 minutes prior to its use. The solution hangs on an IV pole and flows into the abdomen to filter impurities, then drains from the body through another tube. Peritoneal dialysis is a sterile pro-

cedure that is performed by the nurse. The type of dialysis used in the subacute unit is usually **continuous ambulatory peritoneal dialysis (CAPD)** (Figure 19-16).

The nursing assistant may be asked to assist the nurse with sterile dressing changes. You will also take vital signs as directed during the dialysis procedure. Notify the nurse if:

- The dialysate that returns appears bloody or has blood clots in the solution
- The resident complains of abdominal pain
- Fluid leaks around the insertion site
- The tubing or catheter is disconnected
- The solution does not appear to be running, or is running very slowly
- The drainage container is almost full
- The resident has low blood pressure or complains of dizziness
- The dressing becomes wet or soiled
- The resident is weak or unsteady
- The resident is short of breath or complains of difficulty breathing

Pain Management

Residents are often admitted to the subacute care unit for pain management. Intermittent and continuous medication infusion may be used to manage pain after major surgery, when the resident has cancer, or another chronic, painful condition. Pain management may be provided by a combination of methods:

- Oral medications
- Injectable medications
- Intravenous medications

A   Graft

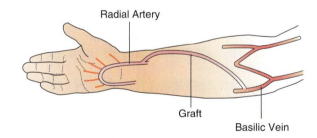

B   A.V. Fistula

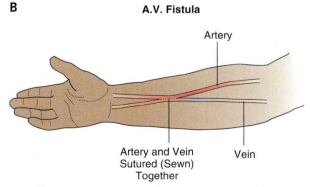

FIGURE 19-15 (A) A dialysis graft (B) A dialysis fistula

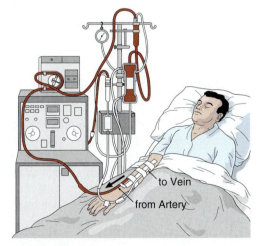

FIGURE 19-16 Dialysis removes wastes and impurities from the resident's blood. Blood leaves the body through an artery, is filtered by the machine, then returns through a vein.

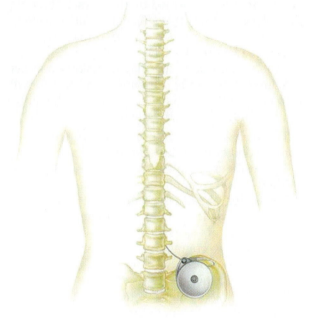

FIGURE 19-17 Implantable medication pumps are sometimes used for long-term medication delivery. The pumps are surgically placed under the abdominal skin. A tiny catheter is threaded under the skin from the pump to the spine. Medications are infused directly into the cerebrospinal fluid. This type of therapy has become common for patients with chronic, severe pain, severe spasticity (sudden, frequent, involuntary muscle contractions that impair function), and some types of cancer. Avoid using a transfer belt for moving the resident until the operative site is well healed. *(Courtesy of Medtronic, Minneapolis, MN; (800) 505-5000)*

- Implanted medication pumps **(Figure 19-17)**
- Other implanted devices
- Transcutaneous electrical nerve stimulation (TENS)

Other approaches, such as massage, physical therapy, and alternative treatments, may also be provided in combination with nursing comfort

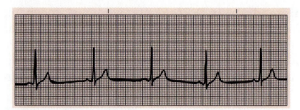

FIGURE 19-18 Some residents require cardiac monitoring.

measures. Residents receive regular pain medications, and the medication regimen is adjusted until the resident receives the maximum benefit. Residents are more willing to participate in their care plans when they are not having pain, and are usually more satisfied with their care.

Other Conditions

As you can see, subacute units care for residents with a wide variety of conditions. In addition to those listed, some subacute units care for:
- Residents who have had surgery and need care and close monitoring until they recover from the effects of the anesthesia; this is called **postoperative care**
- Residents who have had major surgical procedures and require care and rehabilitation
- Residents who require cardiac monitoring **(Figure 19-18)**
- Residents who have injuries from auto accidents and other trauma
- Residents who have had strokes or have other neurological disorders
- Residents who have had orthopedic surgery
- Persons with AIDS who are in the terminal stages of the disease
- Residents who are dying and require the services of a hospice

KEY POINTS

- Residents in the subacute unit have complex needs, and their conditions can change very quickly.
- The nursing assistant in subacute care must have excellent technical, observational, and communication skills.
- The five types of subacute units are transitional, general medical-surgical, chronic subacute, long-term transitional subacute, and specialty subacute.
- Many residents in the subacute unit are monitored with a pulse oximeter to measure the amount of oxygen in their arterial blood.
- A basic knowledge of sterile technique is necessary for the nursing assistant working in the subacute care unit.

REVIEW

A. Multiple Choice

Select the one best answer.

1. The subacute unit is
   a. similar to intensive care.
   b. a temporary place to stay.
   c. a unit that cares for very unstable residents.
   d. an intermediate care area.

2. The nursing assistant in the subacute care unit provides
   a. personal care, monitoring, and observation.
   b. highly technical procedures and psychological care.
   c. laboratory testing and other diagnostic tests.
   d. skilled treatments and oral medications.

3. Chemotherapy is
   a. poisoning with hazardous chemicals.
   b. a treatment for residents with kidney failure.
   c. the use of chemicals to destroy cancer cells.
   d. a form of radiation treatment to the skin.

4. A pulse oximeter measures the
   a. amount of oxygen in arterial blood.
   b. amount of oxygen in venous blood.
   c. blood pressure.
   d. pressure in the superior vena cava.

5. The tube inserted into the trachea through which a resident breathes is called the
   a. incision.
   b. stoma.
   c. cannula.
   d. ventilator.

6. Notify the nurse if a resident with a tracheostomy
   a. smiles.
   b. is short of breath.
   c. coughs.
   d. needs a shower.

7. You are assisting the nurse with a sterile dressing change on Mrs. Lee's pressure sore. You accidentally spill normal saline on the sterile field. The field is now
   a. sterile.
   b. soiled.
   c. aseptic.
   d. contaminated.

8. Hyperalimentation is also called
   a. PICC.
   b. HPA.
   c. TPN.
   d. TENS.

9. You are caring for a resident with a subclavian line. When you enter the room, you should check for the location of the
   a. Kelly.
   b. scissors.
   c. tweezers.
   d. forceps.

10. Mrs. King goes out to the dialysis center three times a week for hemodialysis. When she returns from her treatment, you will
    a. put her to bed.
    b. check her blood pressure.
    c. provide plenty of fluids.
    d. take her to the bathroom.

11. The nursing assistant should avoid taking blood pressure
    a. on the unaffected arm of a resident who has had a stroke.
    b. with an electronic blood pressure unit.
    c. on an arm with an intravenous infusion.
    d. on the arm with the identification band.

12. Always keep the bag or bottle of intravenous solution
    a. below the needle insertion site.
    b. exactly six feet off the floor.
    c. parallel to the needle insertion site.
    d. above the needle insertion site.

13. The normal oxygen saturation is
    a. 95% to 100%.
    b. 85% to 95%.
    c. 80% to 90%.
    d. 70% to 80%.

14. When changing the bed of a resident who is receiving chemotherapy, the nursing assistant should
    a. wear gloves only for contact with blood or body fluids.
    b. apply gown, gloves, a mask, and eye protection.
    c. wear a gown and discard linen in the hamper in the hallway.
    d. wear gloves and discard linen in specially marked bags.

15. When caring for a resident who is receiving radiation therapy, the nursing assistant should
    a. avoid using lotions and cosmetics near the treatment field.
    b. wash the markings on the skin off with soap and hot water.
    c. cover the treatment area with a dressing and tape to avoid getting it wet.
    d. shave the area surrounding the treatment field each day.

16. When entering the room of a resident who has an implanted radiation device, the nursing assistant should
    a. wear a gown, gloves, and face mask.
    b. remain as long as possible to provide emotional support.
    c. stay at least three feet from the resident unless direct care is being given.
    d. encourage the resident to eat high-fiber foods and high-carbohydrate snacks.

B.   True/False

Answer each question true (T) or false (F).

17. _____ It is all right to use a torn sterile package.

18. _____ You may touch unsterile supplies as long as you are wearing sterile gloves.

19. _____ If the sterility of an item is in doubt, do not use it.

20. _____ You may reach over a sterile field if necessary.

21. _____ When applying sterile gloves, hold them by the cuffs.

22. _____ A wet sterile field is contaminated.

23. _____ A sterile article can safely contact an unsterile item.

24. _____ The outer wrapper of the sterile glove package is not sterile.

25. _____ Avoid touching sterile items with ungloved hands.

26. _____ Avoid touching a sterile field with the wrapper to a sterile package.

C.   Clinical Applications

Answer the following questions.

27. Mrs. Allison has cancer and is receiving chemotherapy treatments. Mrs. Allison has taken a shower and washed her hair. She wraps her hair in a towel, dries, and dresses. When she removes the towel from her head, it contains a great deal of hair. Mrs. Allison begins to cry loudly. What can the nursing assistant do?

28. Mr. Gray has been admitted to your subacute unit for care of pressure ulcers. The resident has Stage IV ulcers on the right hip and left buttock. He is on a low air loss therapy bed. Mr. Gray moans in pain when he is moved. How can the nursing assistant position the resident to keep pressure off the existing areas and prevent further breakdown?

29. Mrs. Jewel is alert and ambulatory with assistance. She has an intravenous infusion. The resident requests that you help her to the bathroom. After she is seated on the toilet, you advise her that you will return immediately when she signals. Shortly after leaving the room, you hear a loud crash in Mrs. Jewel's room. When you enter, you find the resident seated on the toilet. The IV pole is lying on its side on the floor. The tubing has become disconnected from the catheter at the infusion site and the resident is bleeding heavily. Mrs. Jewel tells you that she accidentally knocked the pole over. What action will you take?

30. Mrs. Rains is a 56-year-old resident with renal failure. She is receiving dialysis treatments while waiting for a kidney transplant. Mrs. Rains has an ulcer on her left lower leg. She is normally alert, pleasant, and cooperative. She confides in you that she is frustrated and thinks she will die before receiving a donor kidney. When the nurse enters Mrs. Rains's room to change the dressing on her leg, Mrs. Rains yells at her and throws the water pitcher. What do you think the problem is? What can the nursing assistant do to assist the resident?

31. Ray Walters is a 27-year-old resident who has been admitted to your subacute unit with end-stage AIDS. He is 6 feet tall and weighs 105 pounds. Mr. Walters has frequent diarrhea. He seldom has visitors. Staff say that they have a hard time caring for him because it is difficult to watch a young person waste away and die. Mr. Walters tells you that he is very lonely. What can the nursing assistant do to assist him?

CHAPTER 20

Special Behavioral Problems

OBJECTIVES

After reading this chapter, you will be able to:

- Spell and define key terms.
- Identify common causes of behavior problems in alert and confused residents.
- Explain why physical and chemical restraints are not desirable in the management of behavior problems.
- Describe the effect of losses and unmet needs on residents' behavior.
- List the three steps in the ABC method of behavior management and explain how this method is used to eliminate undesirable behavior.
- Describe how to assist residents with specific behavior problems.
- Differentiate cognitive impairment from dementia and delirium.
- Describe methods of caring for and communicating with residents with cognitive impairment and dementia.
- List the three stages of Alzheimer's disease and describe signs and symptoms of each stage.

OBSERVATIONS TO MAKE AND REPORT RELATED TO SPECIAL BEHAVIORAL PROBLEMS

Change in consciousness, awareness, or alertness

Changes in mood, behavior, or emotional status

Changes in orientation to person, place, time, season

Change in communication

Changes in memory

Excessive drowsiness

Changes in ability to respond verbally or nonverbally

Sleepiness for no apparent reason

Sudden onset of mental confusion

Threats of suicide or harm to self or others

Signs or symptoms of illness or infection

BEHAVIOR PROBLEMS

Behavior problems frequently have medical, social, or emotional causes that create great stress. Typical behavior problems include physical or verbal aggression, wandering, yelling or calling out, and other socially inappropriate behaviors. Some behavior problems are related to a decline in intellectual functioning called **cognitive impairment.** Problem behaviors may present a danger to the resident, staff, and other residents on the unit. Other behaviors may be annoying or distressing to the staff, but are harmless. Facility staff often have difficulty caring for residents who have behavior problems. Sometimes this results in overuse of physical restraints or sedation with chemical restraints. Both interventions may have serious consequences and do not always solve the underlying problem. They often worsen physical dependence, and may increase confusion and behavior problems. Although physical and chemical restraints are useful sometimes, other methods of dealing with the behavior should be tried first. If they are ineffective, treatments involving restraints are used as the last resort. Behavior management is a technique commonly used to modify the resident's behavior. Dealing with residents with behavior problems requires using patience, common sense, good communication skills, and a great deal of empathy. Health care professionals have taken positive steps, and the current trend is moving away from using physical and chemical restraints. Other methods of managing behavior have been found to be more effective and beneficial to residents.

The Effect of Losses on Behavior

When people are sick or injured, they suffer losses. The most obvious loss is their health. Loss of health causes loss of independence. Loss of health and independence causes loss of income and security. The loss of health, independence, income, and security may affect the resident's relationships with others. Family and friends may be lost. The resident may feel like a bother, unloved, or both. The resident may feel as if he or she has lost control. Changes in relationships and losses affect the resident's self-esteem. Although the losses may be only temporary, the resident may be afraid the loss will become permanent.

The resident in the long-term care facility has lost his or her home and the comfort of belongings. The loss may be temporary, but this is a difficult adjustment to make. When loss of home is combined with other losses, the resident may feel overwhelmed. Many people go through the grieving process (see Chapter 21) when they suffer the types of losses described here. You will be caring for residents in various stages of the grieving process. Sadness and grief are normal when people suffer a loss. The resident may also be fearful and anxious. This is caused in part by fear of the unknown. The resident does not know what the outcome of the illness will be. He or she may fear a negative outcome. The resident may be afraid of treatments and procedures used to manage his or her illness. Over time, the resident begins to feel helpless and hopeless. He or she may feel frustrated and angry. The anger may be internal, or directed toward oneself. It is difficult to maintain your self-esteem when you are angry with yourself. The anger may also be external. The resident may direct anger toward family, friends, and caregivers. If anger is directed at you, try to understand that the real cause of the resident's anger is fear and anger at the situation. The resident is not mad at you personally.

Unmet Needs

Behavior problems usually develop in response to stress, loss, or unmet needs that exceed the resident's coping ability. Think about the needs in Maslow's hierarchy. Residents with behavior problems who are mentally alert are often responding to an unmet psychosocial need. They also may be responding to a feeling of lack of control over their bodies, their situations, or the environment. Get to know the resident and respect his or her uniqueness as a person. Offer the resident control and choices, showing that you respect him or her as a person. Promote and reward independence, decision making, and assertive behavior. If you are able to identify the resident's unmet needs, share the information with the nurse and other members of the interdisciplinary team. This will help in developing a care plan to meet the needs and minimize or eliminate the behavior problems.

Residents who are mentally confused often demonstrate problem behavior in response to fear, loneliness, boredom, too much stimulation in the environment, or an unmet physical need. The behavior may be the only way the resident has to express himself or herself. For example, a mentally confused resident screams frequently throughout the day. The resident is alone in bed in her room. This presents a challenge because there are so many potential reasons for the screaming. She may be hungry or thirsty, in pain, scared, lonely, bored, too hot, or too cold. She may need to use the bathroom, but is unable to tell you. There may be too much noise or stimulation in the environment, causing her to be agitated. The only way to find out why the resident is screaming is by using common sense and experimenting with different approaches. Offer her a drink or something to eat. Take her to the bathroom. Sit quietly with her and hold her hand. Rubbing lotion on the resident's hands and arms may have a calming effect. If you find an approach that calms her, share this information with other team members.

The Meaning of Behavior Problems. All behavior has a meaning. The meaning may not be apparent to you. The resident may not even realize that he or she is demonstrating a behavior that you consider abnormal. This is particularly true if the resident is from a different culture. Behavior that is acceptable in one culture may be considered abnormal by people from other

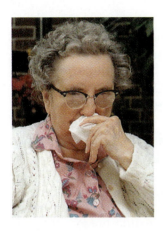

FIGURE 20-1
Residents entering the long-term care facility experience many losses.

TABLE 20-1	ABCs of behavior management
Identify the ABCs	**Definition**
A = Antecedent	The cause or trigger of the behavior
B = Behavior	The behavior itself
C = Consequences	The consequences, effect, or result of the behavior

cultures. Behavior patterns develop throughout a person's lifetime and are affected by heredity, culture, environment, and lifetime experiences.

Normal Coping and Defense Mechanisms. Residents react to losses by using methods they have learned over their lifetime. Residents use coping and defense mechanisms as tools to compensate for losses. Several defense mechanisms are commonly seen. These are:

- Denial, or refusing to admit there is a problem
- **Rationalization,** or providing an acceptable but untrue reason for the illness or behavior
- **Compensation,** or using strength and over-achieving in one area to overcome a weakness in another area of life
- **Projection,** or placing the blame for the situation on someone or something else

The nursing assistant must use good communication and listening skills when dealing with residents who have suffered losses **(Figure 20-1).** Understand that residents are responding to stress when they use coping mechanisms. Do not take angry outbursts or other behavior personally. Although the resident may say he or she is angry with you, this is not always the case. The resident is usually angry because of his or her situation. You may need to modify your behavior. Monitor how the resident responds to you, and adjust your approach to achieve results. Practice empathy. Put yourself in the resident's shoes and try to understand what is happening.

THE ABCs OF BEHAVIOR MANAGEMENT

An effective technique of behavior management is the ABC plan **(Table 20-1).** This plan is useful with both alert and mentally confused residents. The theory behind this program is that if the **an-**tecedent** or **consequences** of the behavior are eliminated or modified, the behavior will change or cease. The antecedent is the event that causes or triggers a behavior. The consequences are the outcome of the behavior.

The Three Steps of Behavior Management

There are three steps in the ABC method of behavior management:

Step 1: Attempt to determine the cause (trigger or antecedent) for the behavior. Does the behavior occur in specific environmental conditions, at a certain time of day, or during a certain activity? Does the presence or absence of other persons trigger the behavior?

Step 2: Eliminate the cause of the behavior. If the cause can be identified and eliminated, the behavior will cease or change.

Step 3: Examine the consequences of the behavior. They may also have to be eliminated or changed in order to change the behavior. Modifying the consequences of behavior requires practice. For example, a mentally confused resident yells and cries. You discover that if you sit and hold the resident's hand, the behavior stops. Sitting and holding her hand serves as a reward for the behavior. To modify the consequences, sit and hold the resident's hand *before* the yelling and crying start. Pay attention to the resident on a regular basis. In this case, modifying the consequences changes the behavior. If the resident's behavior has been rewarded for a long period of time, do not expect to see immediate results. All team members will have to practice the new approach consistently before results are apparent.

Using the ABC Method. Mentally alert residents who use the call signal frequently for minor requests can be distressing to staff. The resident may ask you to turn on the light, position the window blinds, or refill the water glass. Within minutes after you leave the room, the resident signals again. Residents who display this type of behavior are often lonely and scared. They may be using the call signal to get attention. An effective approach is to tell the resident what time you will return when you leave the room. Be sure to return at that time. Keeping your word shows the resident that you can be trusted. Stop in the room and check on the resident as often as you can. When the resident knows he or she can depend on you to check on him or her regularly, unnecessary use of the call signal will decrease.

This simple example shows how the ABCs of behavior management are used effectively. In this case:

A, or the antecedent, is the resident's loneliness and fear.

B, or the behavior, is using the call signal frequently for minor requests.

C, or the consequence, is attention and companionship when you are in the room.

By checking on the resident frequently and keeping your promise to return, you have changed the consequences. You are providing companionship and attention regularly. This eases the resident's loneliness and fear, so there is no reason to continue the behavior.

In these examples, the consequences were modified to change the behavior. Sometimes the antecedent must be changed. For example, a mentally confused resident is quiet all day. She begins to scream every night at bedtime after you have done HS care. You discover that she stops screaming when you enter the room and turn on the light. When you turn the light off, she screams again. The resident is frightened of the dark. Leaving a light on in the room or bathroom will cause the resident to stop screaming.

Role of the Nursing Assistant in Assisting with Behavior Management Programs. If a resident demonstrates a behavior problem, members of the interdisciplinary team will develop a care plan for all team members to use. If you identify a possible cause for the problem behavior, or know of an approach that is effective, inform the nurse. It is very important to include this information in the care plan. The plan will be based on the resident's individual strengths and needs. Behavior management is a form of restorative care, so the principles of restoration

are used. The plan may have to be modified several times, depending on the resident's response. For the plan to be effective, all team members must be **consistent** in their approaches to the resident. For consistency, all care providers use exactly the same approaches in response to the resident.

Implementing the Behavior Management Plan. After the care plan has been developed, become familiar with it and implement the approaches listed. Your objective observations of the resident's response to the plan are important and should be reported to the nurse. The plan may call for you to modify your own behavior in response to the resident's behavior. Appropriate resident behavior is reinforced or rewarded. Residents tend to repeat behavior that is rewarded. Verbal praise, positive feedback, and other signs of approval are rewards. Nonverbal reinforcement such as a hug, smile, or pat on the back may also be used **(Figure 20-2)**. Snacks and privileges are sometimes used as rewards.

The care plan will describe how to reduce the resident's inappropriate behavior. Sometimes this is done by ignoring the behavior, if this can safely be done. The care plan will specify other nonpunitive responses. The goal is not to punish the resident, but to show him or her a more positive way of directing energy.

Your Role in Assisting Residents with Specific Behavior Problems

Making generalizations about behavior management is difficult, because each person is a unique

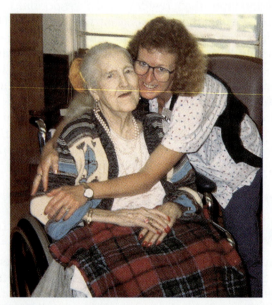

FIGURE 20-2 Residents respond warmly to touch and hugs.

GUIDELINES FOR

Assisting Residents Who Have Behavior Problems

- Follow the approaches listed on the care plan.
- Maintain control of your own responses and reactions.
- Remove the irritant, or cause of the behavior, if known.
- Protect the safety of the resident and others.
- If the care plan calls for you to respond when a resident demonstrates a specific behavior, implement the approaches as soon as the behavior starts. Do not wait for the resident to lose control.
- Use good communication and listening skills.
- Practice empathy.
- Attempt to learn the cause of the behavior, and communicate this information to other team members.

- Communicate effective approaches to other team members.
- Monitor the resident's response to your approaches. Adjust your approach if necessary.
- Discuss family, friends, or other pleasant information with residents. This provides a source of strength, comfort, and support.
- Make certain the resident's physical needs are met.
- Give alert residents as much control as possible. Offer choices in care and routines. Encourage residents to direct their own care.
- Be happy. Smile to communicate caring. Make sure your body language does not send a negative message. Positive behavior is contagious.

individual. However, certain common conditions are seen in residents in long-term care facilities. The general care you provide to residents with these conditions is similar. Always follow the care plan for specific resident information, goals, and approaches. Use common sense.

Depression. Feelings of despair or discouragement, called **depression,** may occur because of stress and loss. Sometimes depression occurs for

unknown reasons. The signs and symptoms of depression vary widely. Decreased concentration, memory loss, fatigue, insomnia, sadness, crying, loss of appetite, overeating, apathy, and loss of self-esteem are all symptoms of depression.

Sleep Disturbances. Sleep problems may be related to physical, emotional, or environmental causes. Some residents complain of being unable to sleep. Others appear to sleep all the time.

GUIDELINES FOR

Assisting the Resident Who Has Depression

- Be honest, supportive, and caring.
- Be a good listener **(Figure 20-3).** Encourage the resident to express feelings.
- Avoid passing judgment or criticizing what the resident feels. Avoid interrupting or changing the subject.
- Give positive feedback on the resident's strengths and successes.
- Acknowledge the resident's feelings.
- Do not make comments like "Cheer up. Things could be worse."
- Encourage physical activity to the extent possible. Exercise reduces stress.
- Encourage the resident to laugh regularly. Laughter is therapeutic and reduces stress. Turn on a funny television program or tell a joke.
- Monitor the resident's appetite and report overeating or undereating to the nurse.
- Report changes in behavior or talk of suicide to the nurse immediately.

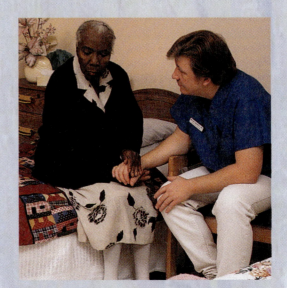

FIGURE 20-3 Allowing the resident to talk and express her feelings shows that you care.

GUIDELINES FOR

Assisting Residents Who Have Problems Sleeping

- Follow the resident's bedtime routine.
- Offer HS care by making the resident comfortable, giving a back rub, controlling room temperature, adjusting the lights, and eliminating noise in the environment.
- If the resident wakes up frightened during the night, provide support and reassurance. Make the resident comfortable.

- If the resident wakes up confused, provide orientation to person, place, and time. Assure the resident that he or she is safe and in the right place.
- If the resident wants to stay awake during the night, provide diversional activities and comfort measures that will not disturb others.
- Warm snacks may be helpful. Avoid beverages containing caffeine.

Look for causes of the sleep disturbance, such as excessive caffeine intake, pain, fear, anxiety, room temperature, or noise.

Complaining or Demanding Behavior. Listening to resident complaints requires a great deal of tact. Sometimes resident complaints are justified, but at times they are not. Listen objectively to what the resident says. Report the information to the nurse objectively. If the complaint is something simple that you can correct, do so immediately.

Yelling and Screaming. Yelling and screaming may be the only way some residents can

GUIDELINES FOR

Assisting the Resident Who Has Complaining or Demanding Behavior

- Reassure the resident that you understand the complaint or problem and will report it to the appropriate person.
- Use good listening skills and support the resident.
- If the complaints are about care given by others, remain neutral and do not criticize other workers. If complaints are about your care, listen, but do not argue or become defensive.

- Attempt to determine the cause of unjustified complaints and correct it if possible.
- Give the resident as much control over daily routines as possible.
- Offer choices to give the resident control, show respect for the resident as a person, and demonstrate that you value his or her opinion.

GUIDELINES FOR

Assisting the Resident Who Is Yelling or Calling Out

- Look for the cause of the behavior. If you can identify it, correct it.
- If the resident is alert, ask what the problem is. Use active listening skills and provide comfort.
- Realize that residents from some cultures scream with pain and grief. This is socially acceptable in the resident's culture.
- Offer the resident something to eat or drink.
- Monitor body language to see if the resident grimaces or shows other signs of pain.

- Try to distract the resident. Redirecting the behavior with a positive activity, such as a walk or looking at a picture album, may be helpful.
- Eliminate or minimize environmental stimulation. Try moving the resident to a quiet area.
- Provide physical comfort measures, such as turning, positioning, or a back rub.
- Take the resident to the bathroom. Some confused residents scream from the discomfort of a full bladder.

GUIDELINES FOR
Assisting the Aggressive Resident

- Attempt to identify the cause of the behavior and eliminate it, if possible.
- Respect the resident's need for personal space.
- Do not back yourself into a room with no way to escape.
- Take physical threats seriously and keep your distance.
- Watch the resident's eyes. They will usually focus on the part of the body to be attacked.
- Remain calm.
- Speak in a soft, low, calm voice.
- Do not make the resident feel trapped or cornered.
- Do not turn your back on the resident.
- Avoid touching the resident, as this may cause further agitation.

- Show that you are interested in what the resident is saying.
- Empathize with the resident and acknowledge that you understand how he or she feels.
- Reassure the resident.
- Praise efforts at self-control.
- Do not argue or try to reason with the resident.
- Make sure your body language is not threatening.
- If aggressive behavior occurs in a public area, move the resident if it is safe to do so. If not, move others out of the way.
- Call for assistance from others, if necessary.

communicate or express displeasure. Most screaming behavior is seen in confused residents, but occasionally alert residents also yell and scream. Dealing with this type of behavior is usually done by trial and error. Remove the irritant, if known. Direct the resident's attention to another activity or try moving to another area, if possible.

Physical or Verbal Aggression.   Physical aggression is hitting, scratching, kicking, biting, or fighting. This is called **combative behavior.** Verbal aggression is arguing, accusing, threatening, or swearing.

Sexual Behavior.   All human beings need sexuality. Sexuality does not diminish with age **(Figure 20-4).** Sexual expression may be physical or psychological. Sexuality is a basic human need, according to Maslow. Always knock before entering a resident's room and wait for a response before entering.

Many health care workers feel that masturbation is inappropriate behavior. Masturbation is satisfying to the resident and is not harmful. It is an acceptable behavior as long as it is done in a private area. If you enter a resident's room and find the resident masturbating, provide privacy and leave the room.

If you enter a room and find two competent, consenting adults engaged in a sexual act, provide privacy and leave. Adults have a legal right to do whatever is pleasing to them, as long as it is not medically contraindicated and both partners are mentally capable of consent. Do not pass judgment on the resident's choice of partner or methods of sexual expression.

Facility staff is responsible for protecting residents who are physically or mentally vulnerable to unwanted sexual contact. Sexual contact with unwilling, alert residents who are physically unable to defend themselves, or confused residents who cannot give full informed consent, is **sexual abuse.** Sexual abuse is a violation of resident rights and is illegal. No health care worker, visitor, or other resident is permitted to sexually abuse others. If sexual abuse occurs, the police are notified. Anyone who sexually harasses or abuses a resident or care provider should be reported to the nurse or other appropriate person according to your facility policy.

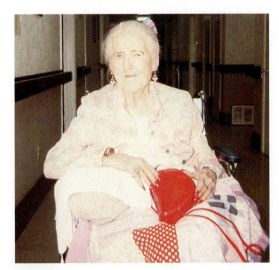

FIGURE 20-4   This resident's appearance is important to her. Assisting her to style her hair and apply makeup, nail polish, and jewelry help her feel attractive and promote a positive self-image.

Sometimes residents may make unwanted sexual advances toward the nursing assistant. Humans have a normal need to express sexuality. The resident's desire for sexuality is normal, but the choice of person is not. If a resident makes sexual advances, do not ridicule or belittle him or her. Be patient and understanding, and speak to the resident in a matter-of-fact manner.

Tactfully inform the resident that the behavior is not acceptable. Follow your facility policy for reporting sexual advances.

Table 20-2 lists types of inappropriate sexual behavior, potential triggers, and ways in which to manage the behavior. **Table 20-3** lists observations to make of resident behaviors. Report your observations to the nurse.

TABLE 20-2 Managing inappropriate sexual behavior

Behavior	Possible Trigger (Antecedent)	Approaches
Sexually suggestive comments, inappropriate sexual behavior (General Guidelines)	• Needs more affection, sense of belonging, need to be touched • As dementia progresses, the need for human contact is often expressed more physically • Environment reminds resident of sex • Fatigue, sensory overload, discomfort, boredom	• Focus on the person, not the behavior • *Remain calm, do not overreact* • *Inform the resident that the behavior is not appropriate* • Redirect the resident calmly and firmly • Involve the resident in an activities program • Do something the resident likes, such as listening to music, taking a walk, or having a snack • Give the resident something else to do • Leave and return later • Change your behavior • Change your physical position or approach • Touch the resident in an appropriate manner, such as by putting lotion on arms and hands • Find ways of incorporating appropriate touch into daily routine • Offer soothing objects to touch, fondle, and hold, such as stuffed animals or dolls • Assist in making the resident look good and feel physically attractive • If the behavior occurs at a certain time of day, keep the resident involved in a purposeful activity during this time • Do an environmental audit. Hot? Cold? Too much stimulation? Too little stimulation? • Offer to take the resident to the bathroom • Move the resident to another location • Encourage and reward appropriate behavior • Be aware of cues indicating unmet intimacy needs
Sexual gestures with staff or inappropriate touching during personal care or ADLs	• Misinterprets caregiver's intention • Resident misinterprets cues, perceives another's touch as sexual, such as touching or sitting next to the resident and touching his or her body with yours • Environment reminds resident of sex • Mistakes caregiver for their partner	• Distract during personal care • Avoid sending the resident mixed sexual messages, even in a joking manner • Ask a caregiver of the same gender (as the resident) to provide personal care • *Remain calm, do not overreact* • *Inform the resident that the behavior is not appropriate* • Respond to the resident in a matter-of-fact manner • Be aware that the behavior is a symptom of the resident's illness • Be aware of your own behavior, body language, and the message you send • Decide ahead of time how you will react if a resident makes inappropriate sexual advances. Advance planning will help you react appropriately when confronted with the situation

Continues

TABLE 20-2	Managing inappropriate sexual behavior, *Continued*	
Behavior	**Possible Trigger (Antecedent)**	**Approaches**
Removing clothes Exposing self Undressing in public Wearing only a shirt	• Too hot in environment • Need to use the bathroom • Clothing uncomfortable • Memory loss, forgets to put on clothes • Unaware of environment; may think he is in his bedroom or getting ready to bathe • Tired, wants to go to bed • Does not remember rules of social behavior	• Check and modify room temperature • Take to bathroom • Make sure clothing fits properly, is comfortable and not too tight • Allow resident to rest in bed • Dress in clothing that opens in back or is difficult to remove (do not put clothing on inside out or backward, use clothing designed to open in back)
Public masturbation or fondling self	• Genital irritation • Reacts to what feels good • No longer has judgment, awareness of appropriate behavior	• Check for irritation at an appropriate time • Remove from public area and provide privacy • Give resident repetitive manual activities to do, such as folding towels
Inappropriate advances toward other residents Sexual behavior with another resident Touching someone else in an inappropriate way	• Other person may remind the resident of a former partner • Other resident may be giving cues that are perceived as sexual advances, such as a woman lifting her skirt • Mistakes other resident for a former partner	• Calmly and firmly inform resident that the behavior is not appropriate • Keep residents separated as much as possible • Monitor helpless residents carefully; protect helpless residents • Seat away from residents of the opposite gender • Have care provided by staff member of same gender as the resident

TABLE 20-3	Behavior observations to make and report
Always report abnormal behavior to the nurse, even if you believe the behavior is "normal for the resident."
Who? Does the behavior involve another person or specific types of people? How are these individuals alike?
What? Describe the behavior. What were the circumstances in which the behavior occurred?
Where? Did the behavior occur in one specific location?
When? What is the time of day? Does the behavior occur at predictable times or in predictable situations, such as during bathing? When the resident is tired, when the resident awakens, or other times?
What were the environmental conditions? Was it light, dark, hot, cold, noisy, quiet?
How do others respond to the resident's behavior? Is there anyone who is never approached by the resident? If so, how does he or she manage or prevent the behavior?
Is there a pattern or clues to the behavior? Can you identify clues or signals that the behavior is about to begin?

COGNITIVE IMPAIRMENT

Cognitive impairment means damaged or impaired thinking. It is not a normal part of aging. It may be caused by disease, trauma, alcohol, street drugs, prescription medications, or anesthesia. Losses of self-care ability are often the first sign of cognitive impairment. Over time, residents become unable to recognize familiar faces, objects, or surroundings. They lose the ability to learn and process new information. The most common symptoms are loss of ability

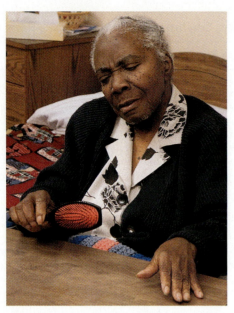

FIGURE 20-5 This resident with dementia has forgotten what the hairbrush is used for.

to make decisions, memory loss, mental confusion, and poor judgment (**Figure 20-5**). In early stages of cognitive loss, the resident usually knows there is a problem. He or she may make up stories and spend a tremendous amount of energy trying to hide the memory loss. If the resident cannot remember something, he or she makes up a story. Avoid judging the resident. Avoid placing too many demands on the resident, which cause stress. Care of residents with cognitive impairment should maintain their quality of life, functional abilities, and dignity. Provide support. Monitor for safety in the environment.

Dementia

Dementia is a mental disorder that causes cognitive impairment. Dementia is not a disease. It can be acute or chronic, and occurs as the result of some diseases and conditions. Dementia is a set of symptoms affecting the resident's thinking, judgment, memory, and ability to reason. In persons with dementia, mental function declines over time. The rights of residents with dementia are the same as those of other residents, but the nursing assistant may need to help residents exercise their rights.

Delirium

Delirium is an acute confusional state. It indicates a treatable illness. There are many causes,

including medications and drugs, fever, isolation, depression, use of restraints, recent relocation, and dehydration. The most common causes are infection, circulatory, respiratory, and metabolic disorders. Often two or three different causes contribute to the delirium. If one cause is eliminated, the delirium will remain until all causes have been discovered and are eliminated. Delirium is characterized by changing states of consciousness, disorganization, behavioral changes, and lack of awareness of the environment. The resident becomes **disoriented,** or loses awareness of person, place, or time. Delirium usually develops quickly, over several hours or several days. Rapid development of symptoms is a key indicator that there is an underlying medical problem. Dementia develops gradually over a much longer period of time. When the medical problem is treated properly, the resident's mental status clears. This may occur quickly, or take several weeks.

Sensory Losses

Sensory loss is difficulty seeing, hearing, smelling, or touching. Loss of sensation may produce signs of cognitive impairment. The problem is worsened if the resident has an existing dementia. If the resident cannot see, hear, feel, or otherwise communicate with others and the environment, he or she may appear cognitively impaired. Besides the inability to communicate with others, the resident may misinterpret noises, people, or other images. The resident may have self-care deficits because he or she cannot see what he or she is doing or hear your instructions. This may cause the resident to have behavior problems. Sometimes simple measures, such as having the eyes examined, putting the resident's glasses on, or using a hearing aid, are enough to improve the condition.

Observing the Resident

Careful assessment and observation by the interdisciplinary team are necessary to differentiate delirium from dementia. Sometimes delirium, medical problems, or sensory losses worsen existing dementia. Because the nursing assistants spend more time with the resident than other team members, their observational skills are very important. Small, seemingly minor changes may be important. Sometimes we think that certain behaviors are "normal for the resident." For example, each night when you give a resident HS care, the resident hits and fights. You accept this

GUIDELINES FOR
Caring for Residents Who Have Dementia

- Approach the resident from the front. Make sure the resident can see or hear you when you approach. Avoid startling the resident.
- Be calm, gentle, and flexible in your approach.
- Control your own body. Avoid sudden, abrupt movement.
- Stay in control of your own responses to the resident. Try to remain calm and soothing when responding to the resident.
- Be creative when responding to the resident. Modify your behavior according to how the resident responds and reacts to you.
- Be matter-of-fact and nondemanding.
- Speak in a "here and now" time frame.
- If the resident is not agitated, use touch to show you care.
- Speak slowly and clearly, using short, simple sentences and words.
- Offer simple choices, but do not overwhelm the resident with options. Best results are obtained if you ask the resident to select one of two choices.
- Break large tasks down into a series of smaller tasks.
- Give the resident familiar, orienting cues for performing ADLs.
- If a resident is combative or agitated, stand at the side when he or she is putting on shoes and socks, to avoid getting kicked.
- Follow the same routine each day.
- If the resident does not understand what you are trying to say, demonstrate. For example, put the brush in the resident's hand. Simulate brushing your hair and tell the resident to imitate you.
- Make eye contact when speaking. Try to be at the resident's eye level whenever possible.
- Make sure your body language matches your words **(Figure 20-6).**
- Keep your voice low and speak calmly.
- Use one-step commands. If the resident does not respond, count to five before repeating. After the resident completes one step, move to the next.
- Avoid rushing the resident. Allow adequate time to complete a task.

- Avoid words such as "don't" or "no" whenever possible. Instead, use words like "do" or "let's."
- Alternate periods of activity with rest.
- Monitor for signs of increasing frustration.
- Accept communication even if it does not make sense. Avoid arguing. For example, the resident tells you that her grandmother ate lunch with her. A good response is, "Are you thinking about your grandmother?"
- Concentrate on what the resident tells you, even if it does not make sense. Respond to what you think the resident is saying.
- Do not argue with the resident about fixed, false beliefs.
- Avoid situations that you know are upsetting to the resident.
- If the resident is upset or agitated, avoid turning your back. Keep your face protected or out of the resident's reach.
- Keep the environment simple and safe. Do not make changes in the environment.
- Provide activities at the time of day the activity would normally be done.
- Reduce excessive noise and stimulation in the environment.

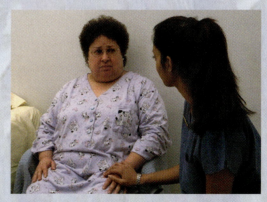

FIGURE 20-6 Your body language should send a caring message.

as normal for the resident, complete your care, and continue your assignment. Because you are the only person in the room with the resident, others may not know of this behavior. The behavior is not normal and may be important. Report your observations of the resident's physical and mental status to the nurse and be alert for changes. Some health care facilities keep a log of behaviors so they can study the time of day, type of behavior, and triggering events. This helps to determine if there is a pattern to the behavior.

ALZHEIMER'S DISEASE

Alzheimer's disease is a disease that causes loss of mental abilities and judgment. It is the most common form of dementia. The cause is unknown, but it is believed that heredity plays a significant role in its development. Most cases of Alzheimer's disease occur in residents over the age of 65, but it can occur in middle-aged individuals. Alzheimer's disease causes physical and chemical changes in the brain. The brain atrophies. In muscles, atrophy is preventable, but this is not true with the brain. The disease progressively worsens and is eventually fatal. However, some individuals may live up to 20 years with the disease. Their physical health may be excellent in the early stages, but declines as the disease progresses. Some medications will improve the symptoms, but there is no cure. Residents with Alzheimer's disease are at high risk for dehydration. The resident may forget to drink, or may lose the sensation of thirst completely. Be aware of the risk and offer fluids frequently.

Three Stages of Alzheimer's Disease

Persons with Alzheimer's disease go through three stages. Physical and mental problems worsen in each stage. Eventually, all cognitive ability is lost. Initially, the resident can perform normal activities of daily living with verbal cues and reminders, but over time the resident becomes totally dependent on others.

Stage I: Mild Dementia. Residents in this stage of Alzheimer's appear normal and can function with minimum assistance and supervision. The changes in this stage are in memory and personality, and include:

- Short-term memory loss; long-term memory remains
- Indifference and apathy
- Resident is not outgoing and is not interested in life
- Decreased concentration and attention span
- Poor judgment
- Unaware of time
- Inability to calculate simple math problems, such as those needed to balance a checkbook
- May forget to eat and drink
- Moodiness
- Blames others for mistakes and problems
- Disorientation to location, inability to remember how to get home
- **Delusions of persecution,** or believing that others are attempting to cause personal harm
- Carelessness
- Unkempt appearance
- Anxiety, agitation, and depression

Stage II: Moderate Dementia. In this stage, short-term memory continues to decline. Long-term memory loss is apparent. All of the symptoms from the first stage continue. The person continues to be in good physical health. Other symptoms are:

- Loss of control over impulses and behavior
- Complete disorientation

- Unable to recognize danger
- Restlessness
- Wandering and pacing
- **Sundowning,** or increased restlessness and wandering in the late afternoon, evening, and night
- Sensory and perceptual changes that cause the person to be unable to differentiate hot, cold, left, right, up, or down
- Loss of ability to recognize common items such as silverware or grooming items
- Loss of ability to perform motor skills, such as eating, dressing, and toileting
- Gradual loss of ability to follow directions
- **Perseveration,** or repetitious behavior, speech, movement, or action
- Difficulty speaking, reading, and writing
- Gradual loss of ability to understand others
- Walking and motor problems; development of a shuffling gait
- Incontinence of bowel and bladder
- **Hallucinations,** or seeing, hearing, smelling, or feeling something that is not real
- **Delusions,** or false beliefs
- **Catastrophic reactions,** or uncontrolled emotional outbursts in response to feeling completely overwhelmed

Stage III: Severe Dementia. The resident in stage III is totally dependent on others for care and develops severe physical problems. The ability to swallow is progressively lost, and the resident is at high risk for choking and aspiration. The resident becomes bedfast and unable to sit in the chair or walk. Seizures may be present. The resident progresses to coma and death. Other signs and symptoms of the third stage of Alzheimer's disease are:

- Complete mental disorientation to time, place, and person
- Loss of ability to communicate
- Inability to recognize family, friends, and facility staff
- Total dependence on others for all care
- Resistance to care
- Refusal to eat
- Sleep disturbances
- Lack of response to activity or environment

COMMUNICATION

Good communication skills are necessary when caring for residents with Alzheimer's disease and other dementias. Try to talk to the resident in an area that is free from distractions. These residents have lost the ability to screen out distractions and noises from the television, radio, or other conversations. Monitor your body language. Make sure it sends the proper message and does not communicate impatience or anger. Begin your conversation socially to win the resident's trust. One way of doing this is to sit and talk before beginning resident care. Always begin your conversation with orienting information. Call the resident by name and tell her who you are. After the resident is relaxed, explain what you are going to do. Make eye contact and be sure you have his or her attention before beginning to speak. Sit at the resident's eye level when you speak whenever possible. If the resident ignores you, wait a minute and try again. Gently touch the resident's arm to get his or her attention. However, avoid startling the resident, which can cause a catastrophic reaction. Speak slowly and clearly, using short, simple sentences. Ask questions that require a yes or no answer. Use concrete terms and familiar words. Keep your tone of voice low and speak in a calm, warm, pleasant manner.

You may have trouble understanding what the resident tells you. Listen actively and carefully. If you do not understand, apologize and ask the resident to repeat. Try to focus on a word or phrase that you understand. Repeat what you do understand and help the resident clarify it. Respond to the resident's emotion. For example, say, "You sound very angry." Remain calm and patient. If the resident repeats certain words, ask family members if they know the meaning. Sometimes people with Alzheimer's disease talk by using code words that close friends and family understand.

Residents with Alzheimer's disease lose the ability to reason. Avoid arguing, which makes the situation worse. Do not tell the resident what he or she can and cannot do. Instead, use distraction. The resident may say "I'm going home to cook dinner for my children." You know the children are grown and live in another state. Instead of arguing with the resident, ask what she likes to cook. Then distract her by asking her to sit with you and look at a magazine. Avoid asking the resident questions that require a good memory. People with dementia often recognize that they have memory loss and are humiliated and frustrated when they cannot remember. Do not talk about residents who have dementia in front of them. We do not know what they understand, and their understanding changes from one moment to the next.

Special Problems

Alzheimer's disease is frustrating for the resident, family, and care provider. The resident is not responsible for the symptoms of the disease. Some residents say unkind things, hit, or act aggressively. The disease has triggered the problem. Because Alzheimer's disease also causes poor impulse control, the resident is powerless to do anything to correct the behavior. Caring for residents with Alzheimer's disease requires patience and understanding.

Catastrophic reactions occur as a result of being startled or in response to overwhelming stimulation. Anger and rage are signs that the resident is feeling loss of control. The resident cannot control the reaction. Catastrophic reactions are noted by increased agitation and physical activity. The resident may talk, yell, or mumble **(Figure 20-7)**. Sometimes the behavior is violent. The best way to deal with catastrophic reactions is to anticipate and prevent them. Monitor the resident's behavior closely and watch for signs of increasing restlessness or agitation. Minimize noise and confusion in the environment. Make sure the resident's physical needs are met. If a catastrophic reaction occurs, avoid trying to reason with the resident. Avoid restraints and use of physical force. Approach the resident using a soft, calm, but firm voice. Touching the resident may make the reaction worse. Remove the resident from the stressful

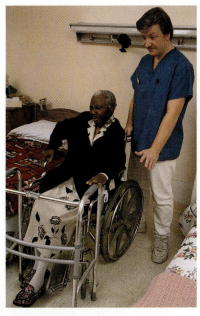

FIGURE 20-7 Recognize early signs of a catastrophic reaction and counteract them whenever possible.

GUIDELINES FOR
Managing Wandering Behavior

- Consider physical causes for the behavior, including illness, the need to use the bathroom, hunger, thirst, and pain. By trial and error, eliminate each cause to see if it reduces the wandering.
- If the resident is wandering trying to find his or her room, place an identifying object on the door to the room. Direct the resident to find the object.
- Decrease noise and stimulation in the environment.
- Remove coats, purses, and other items that the resident associates with going outside.
- Check the resident daily to make sure the identification bracelet is in place.
- Always know what clothing the resident is wearing.
- Distract the resident with a magazine, conversation, activity, food, or drink.
- Give the wanderer a repetitious task, such as folding towels or sorting items.
- Provide a portable radio with a headset. Play the resident's favorite type of music. This simple distraction is often very effective.
- Remind and reassure the resident that he or she is safe and in the right place.
- Make sure that the wanderer gets adequate exercise.
- Avoid trying to reason with a wanderer who is determined to leave. Instead, provide distraction.
- Avoid telling a wanderer "Don't go outside." Thinking and understanding is a complex process. Instructing the resident not to leave will cause him or her to think about going outside. If someone tells you not to think of a green cat, you will think of it.

- Then you will have to unthink it. Saying "stay inside" is a more effective approach with a person who is cognitively impaired.
- Keep toxic substances, chemicals, matches, and other potentially harmful items in locked cupboards.
- Provide adequate lighting. Aging changes in vision make more light necessary to interpret the environment correctly.
- Monitor and respond to exit door alarms.
- Leave a night-light on in the room during the night.
- Make sure the resident is wearing eye glasses and hearing aids, if used. This helps to maintain contact with the environment.
- Post signs and labels on drawers, common rooms, and other items.
- Display familiar items and pictures in the resident's room.
- Consider seating the wanderer in a beanbag chair. They are comfortable but difficult to get out of.
- Know where a current picture of the wanderer is located in case he or she becomes lost.
- Apply a shirt or sweater to the resident and have him wear it for 6 to 8 hours. Remove the garment and place the *unwashed* item in a sealed plastic bag. Mark the resident's name on the bag and put it on the closet shelf. If the wanderer does become lost, the garment can be used by a tracking dog. In the event a tracking garment is not available, the dog may be able to pick up a scent from the pillow.

situation, if possible. Avoid responding with anger and hostility. Distraction may be effective. Reassure the resident by speaking gently. Make every effort to quiet the resident by speaking calmly and listening to what the resident says.

If you feel that your physical safety is threatened during a catastrophic reaction, stand out of the resident's reach. Call for help. Avoid having many care providers approach the resident at one time. Avoid making the resident feel trapped or cornered. Watch the resident's eyes. Residents will usually stare at the person or body part that will be attacked. Protect yourself according to your facility policy.

Wandering

Wandering is a very serious concern for long-term care facilities. Residents who wander within the facility may become lost or injured. Residents who wander outside the facility are in

danger of being hit by a car, overexposed to heat and cold, and placed in other situations that can be harmful or dangerous.

Residents in multi-story facilities often enter the elevator when wandering. Cover the buttons outside the elevator with fabric or duct tape. Staff and visitors will know that they can push the elevator buttons through the fabric, but a confused resident will not. Replace the tape or fabric when it shows signs of wear.

A key to understanding wandering behavior is to realize that there are different types of wanderers. If the type of wandering behavior can be identified, approaches can be planned to keep the resident safe. The types of wanderers are listed in **Table 20-4.**

Allowing residents to wander in a safe area is the best approach to take. Consider physical causes for the wandering, such as pain, thirst, hunger, or looking for the bathroom. Decrease noise levels in the environment. Approach the resident from the front, then walk with the resident by falling in step at her side. If the resident leaves the unit or goes outside, walk with her and circle back in. Distract the resident with food, drink, or activity. Monitor for signs of fatigue and encourage the resident to sit down and get adequate rest. There are many techniques to keep wanderers safe. Most important, wanderers require supervision and understanding. Restraints should be used only as a last resort.

TABLE 20-4 Wanderers

Type of Wanderer	Characteristics	Approaches
Exit seeker/escapist wanderer	• Very high risk for leaving the facility. • The resident may not know where he or she is, but knows that he or she does not want to be there. • May be ambulatory or in a wheelchair. • Resident looks for opportunities to exit and leaves very quickly if presented with an opportunity. • Completely unaware of personal safety. • May not be properly dressed for the outside climate. • Uses very poor judgment. • Probably has a destination in mind.	• Try to determine the resident's intended location in advance. • Avoid arguing or using reality orientation, which agitate the resident. • Use distraction. • This wanderer is usually not looking for a physical location, but instead a state of mind. Try to provide it. If the resident says he or she must go to work, provide the state of mind by talking about the job, responsibilities, and so forth. • Make the resident feel good about himself or herself. • Remove hats, coats, coat rack, purses, shoes, and other items associated with going outside.
Critical/self-stimulation wanderer	• Completely disoriented. • Unaware of safety. • At very high risk of serious injury outside the facility. • Not deliberately trying to leave the facility. • If resident turns a doorknob or pushes the panic bar on the door for stimulation, he or she will exit.	• Close monitoring and supervision. • Diversional activity. • Exercise. • Walking in a small group inside the facility. • Responds well to repetition, structure, predictability, and familiar routines.
Akathisia wanderer	• Resident who has taken psychiatric drugs (chemical restraints) for many years. • Wandering is a side effect of years of drug therapy. • Very restless. • Wanders aimlessly with no apparent purpose. • May cross arms in front of the chest or abdomen when wandering. • Usually does not try to leave the facility.	• Close monitoring and supervision. • Diversional activity. • Exercise. • Walking in a small group inside the facility. • Responds well to repetition, structure, predictability, and familiar routines.
Purposeful wanderer	• Has a specific agenda, but is unable to communicate what it is. • May be looking for the bathroom. • May be bored. • May be overstimulated by noise and other factors in the environment. • May be in pain. • May be hungry or thirsty. • May be stressed and feeling overwhelmed. • May be dehydrated.	• Through trial and error, attempt to learn the resident's agenda and meet it.

Continues

TABLE 20-4 Wanderers, *Continued*

Type of Wanderer	Characteristics	Approaches
Aimless wanderer	• Totally disoriented. May think he or she is in own residence. • Frequently wanders into others' rooms. • May rummage through others' belongings. • Will enter housekeeping closets and unlocked service areas. • Totally unaware of personal safety. • Usually very upsetting to other residents and stressful for facility staff.	• Place cloth shields over doorknobs to change the texture. • Tape paper streamers across doorways. • Post signs that say "Stop," "Do Not Enter," or "Construction Zone." • Provide a dresser or nightstand of items to rummage through in the hallways. • Give the resident a repetitious task, such as folding towels or sorting coins.
Modeling wanderer	• Wander in pairs, usually for stimulation and companionship. • If the first resident exits the facility, the second resident will follow. • Usually completely unaware of safety.	• Provide diversional activities. • Determine the leader's agenda and keep him or her in the facility. • Place dark tile or construction paper on the floor by the doorway. It appears to be a hole, and residents usually will not attempt to cross it.

Problems with ADLs

When performing ADL care, try to focus on familiar skills and tasks. Although the resident cannot learn new tasks, he or she may be able to do familiar ones. Give the resident control by offering one of two choices. Allow enough time for the resident to process the information. If the resident does not understand, repeat the instructions in exactly the same way. Break the task down into small, simple steps. Give only one direction at a time and allow the resident time to complete it before giving the next. Telling the resident to complete an entire task, such as bathing, may be overwhelming. Start by telling the resident to wash his or her face. After the face is washed, instruct the resident in the next step. Sincerely compliment the resident for success.

Problems with Bathing. Resistance to bathing is a common problem in residents with Alzheimer's disease. The resident may have forgotten the purpose of bathing. Residents may be uncomfortable and resist removing their clothing in front of you. Wrapping a towel around the shoulders and pinning it securely may help with modesty problems. Leave the towel in place during the bath. Some residents appear to be fearful of water or afraid of washing. Noises from running water, the whirlpool tub, and heaters in the shower room may frighten the resident. Sound tends to echo in some shower rooms, making the problem worse. Encouraging the resident to sing an old song or playing pleasant music may help. (You may also use a special battery-operated shower radio, or keep the radio plug away from sources of water.)

Because Alzheimer's disease causes problems with sensation, bathing may be uncomfortable. The resident may not be able to feel the water temperature. Bathing is a complex task involving many steps. Taking a bath may simply be too overwhelming for the resident. Residents with Alzheimer's disease may also be sensitive with an unfamiliar nursing assistant.

Maintain a flexible attitude when you are assigned to bathe a cognitively impaired resident. Avoid forcing the resident. If the resident becomes agitated and refuses to bathe, leave and try again later. Before bringing the resident to the tub or shower room, make sure the room is warm and private. Before beginning, ask the resident to feel the water. Say something like "This feels good." Explain what you are going to do and what you want the resident to do, one step at a time. Giving many directions at one time may be overwhelming and will trigger a catastrophic reaction. If you will be giving the resident a complete bath, giving the resident something to hold and occupy the hands may be helpful. Squeezing a sponge or washcloth may distract the resident. Washing the hair may also be frightening. Use the resident's responses to guide your actions. Modify your behavior and care according to the resident's responses to the procedure. Be slow, calm, patient, and reassuring. If you are successful with bathing the resident, share the approaches you used with the nurse and other team members so that the approaches can be added to the care plan.

Dressing Problems. Some residents are resistive to dressing. Others remove their clothing after they are dressed. Keep the morning routine consistent and familiar. Once you start, avoid interruptions, which cause the resident to forget what he or she is supposed to be doing. Make sure the room is warm and private. Ask the resident to select the clothing, if this is not too overwhelming. The clothing should be color-coordinated and appropriate for the resident's age and the season. Lay out clothing in the order in which it will be put on. Break the task down into simple, manageable steps and give the resident easy instructions, one step at a time. Assist with dressing, if needed. Allow the resident to do as much for himself or herself as possible, but do not let the resident become overwhelmed or frustrated. Understand the resident's need for privacy and unwillingness to completely disrobe in front of you. Be sensitive to grooming issues and encourage residents to comb hair, shave, or wear cosmetics and jewelry. Praise the resident and compliment his or her appearance.

OTHER HELPFUL TECHNIQUES

The residents' care plans will list various methods for managing residents who have cognitive impairment or behavior problems. Some of the approaches you will see are described here.

Activities

The activities program has many important functions in the long-term care facility. The activities department plans social and therapeutic programs to meet residents' needs **(Figure 20-8).** Activities meet many resident needs, ranging from socialization to relief of boredom. Many activities meet residents' self-esteem needs. Some activities provide outlets for residents to express feelings. The activity department will post a schedule of daily activities and events. Schedule resident care around the activity programs the residents want to attend. Activities are available to meet the needs of both high-functioning and low-functioning residents. Activities such as parties are enjoyable to all residents.

All residents, including those with behavior problems, will benefit from activities. Some residents will not be able to read the daily schedule. Plan your routine and offer to escort the residents to appropriate activities. The activity department will also provide activities to keep residents occupied on the nursing unit. They will do room visits for residents who are bedfast. They will obtain items such as talking books for residents who have sensory impairments. They plan trips and programs in the community. Special programs, such as music therapy and pet therapy, are enjoyable for many residents. The activity department can be a great source of assistance in the care of residents who have cognitive impairment and behavior problems. Find out what programs and resources are available in your facility, and use them to benefit the residents.

Validation Therapy

Validation therapy is a technique developed by Naomi Feil, who is a social worker, an actress, and a researcher. She describes the therapy as a way to communicate with persons over the age of 75. It is also used for persons with Alzheimer's disease and cognitive impairments **(Figure 20-9).** The program is based on the belief that developmental tasks from earlier years must be resolved. If they were not resolved, they will emerge in old age. The elderly person may display many emotions in trying to conclude them. Feil's research has shown that using validation reduces the need for restraints. It helps residents regain feelings of dignity and self-control. It also increases staff morale. Feil stresses the following concepts:

- Maintaining the identity and dignity of residents is important.
- People with dementia can feel good about themselves.

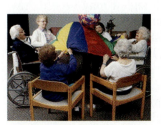

FIGURE 20-8 Activities serve many purposes. This parachute activity is enjoyable, but also provides excellent upper extremity exercise. *(Compliments of Briggs Corporation, Des Moines, IA [800] 247-2343)*

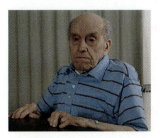

FIGURE 20-9 This cognitively impaired resident was once a child, then an adult. Use validation to reinforce his self-esteem and assist him to complete the developmental tasks of old age.

- All behavior has a purpose. Some disoriented behavior may be acting out of memories.
- The residents' memories and feelings should be acknowledged.
- Cognitively impaired residents have the right to express their feelings.
- Residents must resolve living in order to prepare for dying.
- The elderly have experienced many losses. Many have lost the ability to cope.
- Living in reality is not the only way to live.
- Disoriented residents are worthwhile. Staff can give them joy by allowing them to express their feelings.
- Each person was once a child, then an adult. Residents deserve to be cared for with dignity in their final years of life.

When using validation, allow residents to express their feelings. Reassure them that the feelings are worthwhile. Use a calm, nonthreatening manner. Speak in a loving tone of voice. When the resident describes an emotion, assure him or her that it is okay. A book, videotape, and training program are available for facilities that use this technique.

Reality Orientation

Reality orientation is a technique in which the residents are reoriented to time, place, person, and season. Some facilities do not use reality orientation because they believe it worsens agitation in some residents. The subject is controversial. It is most effective in orienting residents who are delirious. Memory loss in delirium is a temporary condition. After the resident recovers, the confusion clears. Newly admitted residents who are confused by the change in environment may also benefit. A large calendar is placed in the resident's room. Each day is marked off. Large clocks are placed throughout the facility. Signs with large letters label areas, equipment, and personal items **(Figure 20-10).** This enables the resident to find his or her way about the facility.

To be effective, reality orientation must be used by all staff during each resident contact. The goal is to give the resident a sense of identity in time and space. It may decrease anxiety in some residents. When approaching residents, call them by name. Tell them who you are. Do not expect them to remember you.

The principles of reality orientation are to:

- Treat residents as adults
- Treat residents with dignity

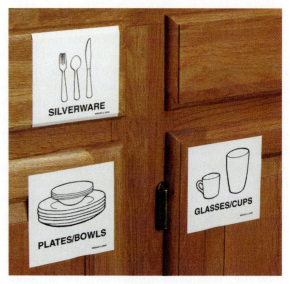

FIGURE 20-10 Using signs to label areas and personal items helps residents to function independently. *(Compliments of Briggs Corporation, Des Moines, IA [800] 247-2343)*

- Speak clearly and directly; avoid speaking loudly
- Use repetition; speak slowly if the resident does not understand
- Allow enough time for the resident to process thoughts and respond
- Keep instructions and responses simple and brief
- Maintain structure in routines
- Make sure residents are wearing hearing aids and glasses
- Promote resident independence
- Frequently provide orientation about the day, date, time, season, and weather
- Avoid making residents feel like you are putting them on the spot or criticizing them
- Answer questions honestly, but avoid information that is upsetting
- Avoid reinforcing the resident's confusion
- Avoid teasing the resident about his or her confusion
- Avoid arguing with residents who are delusional

Although reality orientation is effective in some residents, do not depend on it for keeping residents safe. For example, showing a confused resident how to use the call signal may be effective when you are in the room. Residents with cognitive impairment have short-term memory loss, and will probably forget how to use the call signal as soon as you leave the room. Do not depend on the resident's memory or safety awareness to prevent falls. Use other approaches, such as frequent monitoring or restraint alternatives, for safety.

Reminiscing

Reminiscing is the act of remembering the past **(Figure 20-11A)**. It is a normal activity for all people. One of the developmental tasks of the elderly is a life review. Reminiscence helps residents complete this task. Studies have shown that reminiscence programs can improve cognitive function. A group of women studied had excellent results. Almost everyone enjoys this activity. Reminiscence is an effective one-to-one activity for residents with behavior problems and cognitive impairment. The resident discusses his or her past. You ask questions and make comments. If the resident expresses feelings and emotions, accept them. Reassure the resident that feeling this way is okay. The program can also be done as a group activity. Books, tapes, and kits are available for reminiscence programs **(Figure 20-11B)**. Your activities department may have a formal reminiscence program, but you can also use this approach individually with the residents.

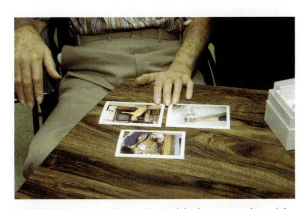

FIGURE 20-11A Discussing old photographs with residents is an excellent way of encouraging reminiscence.

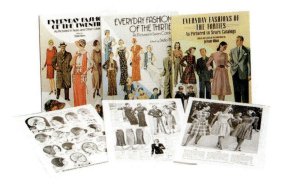

FIGURE 20-11B Looking at pictures of old clothing and furnishings brings back many fond memories. Seeing these items often stimulates residents to tell long-forgotten stories about their past. *(Compliments of Briggs Corporation, Des Moines, IA [800] 247-2343)*

KEY POINTS

- All behavior has meaning, even if the meaning is not evident to you.
- Losses and unmet needs affect residents' behavior.
- Physical and chemical restraints are the treatment of last resort in the management of behavior problems.
- When using the ABC method of behavior management, modifying the antecedent or consequences will change the behavior.
- Consistency is important to the success of a behavior management program.
- Cognitive impairment has many causes, and is not a normal part of aging.
- Safety is a primary concern when caring for residents who have cognitive impairment and dementia.
- Delirium is a reversible condition with medical causes.
- Sensory losses may mimic cognitive impairment or worsen existing dementia.
- Alzheimer's disease causes atrophy of the brain and progressive mental deterioration.
- Wandering is a serious problem in long-term care facilities. The nursing assistant plays an important role in preventing the wanderer from leaving or becoming injured.

REVIEW

A. Multiple Choice

Select the one best answer.

1. Cognitive impairment is
   a. a temporary, reversible condition.
   b. usually caused by infection.
   c. a means of validation.
   d. a decline in intellectual function.

2. A confused resident displays a behavior problem. She yells and screams loudly when she is in bed. A good first step in managing this behavior is
   a. applying a restraint.
   b. asking the nurse to give the resident a tranquilizer.
   c. attempting to learn the cause of the behavior.
   d. isolating the resident.

3. When an alert resident displays a behavior problem, it is most commonly in response to
   a. unmet psychosocial needs.
   b. cognitive impairment.
   c. dementia.
   d. delirium.

4. Defense mechanisms are
   a. means of defending yourself against physical assault.
   b. a response to stress, loss, or unmet needs.
   c. medical problems.
   d. techniques to use when residents are upset.

5. Projection is
   a. refusing to admit there is a problem.
   b. placing the blame for a problem on someone else.
   c. overachieving in one area to overcome a weakness.
   d. making excuses for a problem.

6. According to the ABC method of behavior management,
   a. *A* is an abbreviation for anger.
   b. *A* is an abbreviation for anxiety.
   c. *B* is an abbreviation for behavior.
   d. *C* is an abbreviation for control.

7. When caring for residents who have behavior problems,
   a. adjust your approach to the resident.
   b. leave until the resident calms down.
   c. implement the behavior care plan when the resident becomes upset.
   d. ask the nurse what to do.

8. Masturbation is
   a. acceptable if done in private.
   b. always inappropriate.
   c. harmful to the resident.
   d. an indication that the resident is homosexual.

9. Sexual abuse is
   a. acceptable if done by the resident's spouse.
   b. acceptable if a confused resident consents.
   c. unwanted sexual contact.
   d. appropriate in some situations.

10. Causes of stress and agitation in cognitively impaired residents include
    a. noise and confusion.
    b. validation therapy.
    c. consistent routines.
    d. having a caregiver of the same gender.

11. Dementia
    a. is a disease.
    b. has social causes.
    c. is usually reversible.
    d. is the resident's fault.

12. Delirium is
    a. a mental illness.
    b. caused by reversible medical problems.
    c. a sign of cognitive impairment.
    d. a normal part of aging.

13. Sundowning is
    a. agitation when the resident is put to bed.
    b. restlessness early in the morning.
    c. restlessness in the late afternoon and evening.
    d. a form of combative behavior.

14. Perceptual changes that occur in Alzheimer's disease include
    a. inability to differentiate left from right.
    b. loss of sense of smell.
    c. deterioration in vision.
    d. altered taste of food.

15. Activities are
    a. only for fun and games.
    b. for alert residents only.
    c. planned social and therapeutic events.
    d. always spontaneous and disorganized.

16. Validation is used to
    a. orient confused residents to reality.
    b. punish residents whose behavior is inappropriate.
    c. reverse cognitive impairment.
    d. help residents regain dignity and self-control.

17. Reality orientation works best in residents
    a. with delirium.
    b. with dementia.
    c. who are alert.
    d. who have good short-term memory.

18. Reminiscing is a program that helps
    a. validate the residents' feelings.
    b. the resident remember the past.
    c. orient residents to time, place, person.
    d. residents forget their past problems.

B. True/False Questions

Answer each statement true (T) or false (F).

19. _____ A person's job provides a sense of identity.

20. _____ Residents who are cognitively impaired may display abnormal behavior in response to too much stimulation in the environment.

21. _____ Modifying the behavior changes the antecedent.

22. _____ When managing behavior problems, all care providers should use different approaches with the resident.

23. _____ Cognitive impairment is a normal part of aging.

24. _____ Safety is a primary concern when managing behavior problems and caring for residents who have cognitive impairment and dementia.

25. _____ When caring for residents who have dementia, assume they can do nothing for themselves and provide total care.

26. _____ Residents with Alzheimer's disease may be afraid of being bathed.

27. _____ Residents in the late stage of Alzheimer's disease may lose the ability to swallow.

28. _____ Wanderers should always be restrained for their own safety.

29. _____ Residents with Alzheimer's disease can easily remember something you told them an hour ago.

C. Clinical Application

Answer the following questions.

30. Mrs. Mallory is from a large family. She lived most of her life on a farm. Her husband was in the fields long hours. The resident ran the household and took care of the children. Mrs. Mallory has always been a very controlling person. She has been admitted to your facility for management of her diabetes. The resident is overweight and is unable to walk. The family can no longer care for her at home. Mrs. Mallory is angry with her children and tells you she resents being in the facility. She uses her call signal frequently. Her requests are minor. She asks you to turn the light on or off, add or remove a blanket, bring her ice, pour her a cup of water, and so forth. You are frustrated with her frequent requests. What do you think the cause of the demanding behavior is? How can you best assist this resident?

31. Mrs. Atkins is a confused resident. She wanders about in the facility, but has never attempted to leave. She comes to the nurses' station crying at least once each hour and asks for the location of her room. When she does this, a staff member takes her by the hand, leads her to her room, and gives her a hug. What are the consequences of the resident's behavior? Do you think that the staff is reinforcing the resident's behavior? What can be done to assist Mrs. Atkins?

32. Mr. Morrow sits in a chair in the lounge most of the day watching television. He frequently removes his clothing. What can you do to assist this resident?

33. Mr. Kosmanek immigrated from Poland after World War II. He has Alzheimer's disease and has been admitted to your facility. He sundowns in the evening. When he wakes up in the morning, he routinely asks, "How many did they shoot last night?" You are working the 11 p.m. to 7 a.m. shift. Mr. Kosmanek has tried to leave the nursing home several times. He says, "I must hide so they can't find me." What can the nursing assistant do to keep the resident from leaving the facility and make him feel safe and secure?

34. Mr. Springer, a resident with Alzheimer's disease, frequently refuses to bathe. You are assigned to give him a shower today. The resident has a bad body odor. When you tell him it is time for his shower, he becomes agitated and tells you to leave him alone. He turns and walks rapidly down the hall. What can the nursing assistant do?

CHAPTER 21

Death and Dying

OBJECTIVES

After reading this chapter, you will be able to:

- Spell and define key terms.
- Examine your personal feelings about death, dying, and terminal illness.
- List the five steps in the grieving process and describe what happens in each.
- List 14 signs and symptoms of impending death.
- Describe the care of a dying resident.
- Explain why standard precautions are used when providing postmortem care.
- Demonstrate the procedure related to death and dying.

OBSERVATIONS TO MAKE AND REPORT RELATED TO DEATH AND DYING

Decreasing level of responsiveness

Decreasing movement, muscle tone, and sensation

Relaxation of lower jaw

Mouth falls open

Skin pale, moist, cool to touch; progresses to cold to touch

Skin progresses to blue, gray, or dusky appearance, beginning in the lower extremities and moving upward

Lips, fingernails, and mucous membranes become dusky, gray, or blue

Pulse becomes rapid, weak, or thready

Respirations become slow, labored, irregular, or noisy

Cheyne-Stokes respirations

Blood pressure decreases; blood pressure can no longer be heard at the brachial artery, but the resident remains alive

Mucus collects in the throat, may rattle during respirations

Resident becomes incontinent of urine and feces

Eyes stare and pupils do not respond to light

INTRODUCTION

Health care professionals deal with life and death daily. Caring for residents who are dying and caring for the body after death will probably be part of your responsibility. Death is expected in some residents. Others die suddenly, without warning. The nursing assistant plays an important role in the care of the dying resident. Although you can do nothing to prolong the resi-

dent's life, you will take comfort in the fact that you did all you could to make the resident's last moments on earth as comfortable as possible.

All staff members must be aware of what the resident has been told about his or her condition. In some situations residents are not told of their impending death. This is a medical decision made by the physician. If this is the case, you must respect this decision and abide by it whether you agree or not. In other cases residents are told they are dying and may wish to discuss it. Your listening and communication skills are especially important when caring for the dying resident **(Figure 21-1).**

Resuscitation Orders

Resuscitation is performed on all residents unless the physician has written a **do not resuscitate (DNR) order.** Residents with DNR orders are usually terminally ill and have signed an advance directive indicating that they do not want life-sustaining procedures performed in the event of death. If the resident has a DNR order, no CPR will be performed if the resident's heart stops beating. In the absence of a DNR order, cardiopulmonary resuscitation is performed if a resident shows signs of clinical death. In many facilities, the nursing assistant is trained to perform CPR and may initiate and assist with this procedure.

Each facility has an emergency code designated for resuscitation. Many agencies use the term **code blue** to signify a **cardiac arrest.** A cardiac arrest occurs when the resident's heart and breathing have stopped. Announcing a resuscitation event (or code blue) on the public address system will alert the emergency response team to respond to the unit. CPR and other aggressive measures will be performed to save the resident's life. The ambulance will be called to transport the resident to the hospital. When paramedics arrive, they will use drugs and advanced life support devices to try to save the resident's life.

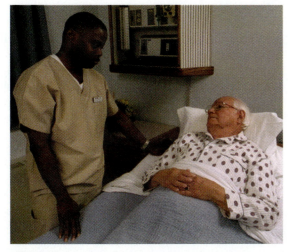

FIGURE 21-1 Active listening is an important communication skill.

EXAMINING YOUR FEELINGS ABOUT DEATH AND DYING

As a whole, society in the United States avoids meaningful discussions about death and dying. As a result, we may be very uncomfortable speaking about this subject. Some people avoid making wills because it reminds them of their own mortality. For some, speaking about death and dying is painful because it reminds them of personal experiences with friends and loved ones. The AIDS epidemic of the 1980s and 1990s has evoked strong feelings about death and dying. Most victims of AIDS were young and in the prime of their lives. Approximately 11% of all new AIDS cases reported to the CDC are in people over age 50. State reporting requirements vary, so people who are HIV positive but have not yet developed AIDS are not necessarily included in this number. Many individuals have not been diagnosed, so the statistics do not accurately reflect the prevalence of HIV disease and AIDS. The incidence of HIV infection and AIDS is increasing. Unfortunately, this age group may not be tested for HIV because they are perceived to have few risk factors. The scientific community is beginning to view AIDS in a new light. We are beginning to see it as a chronic, manageable disease. However, many people are fearful of the disease and continue to see it as a **terminal illness.** A terminal illness is a condition from which the resident is not expected to recover. Young people tend to see themselves as invincible, and receiving a terminal diagnosis is traumatic and painful. A nurse who died of AIDS summed up her feelings about the disease and about dying. She explained that before she developed AIDS, she felt it was a disease for "them." After she became ill, it was difficult for her to accept care given to her by other nurses. As a nurse, she felt she should be giving care, not receiving it. It was embarrassing to lose control of her body functions. She said that the disease caused her to realize that "them is us." There is a great deal of wisdom and insight in this statement. The "them is us" philosophy can be applied to many different diseases in addition to AIDS.

Factors That Influence Your Feelings about Death and Dying

As a nursing assistant, you will care for both young and old residents who are dying. It is never your responsibility to inform them that they are dying. However, once the information has been delivered, you must be prepared to assist the dying resident to meet physical, emotional, psychological, social, and spiritual needs. In some cases, you will also be a source of strength and support for the family.

You may feel that death in infants, children, and young adults is unfair. Health care workers often have different views of death and dying in the elderly, who have lived long lives. Your body begins to age as soon as you are born. Death is a natural extension of life. Your feelings and beliefs about death and dying will affect the care you give. In order to care for dying residents effectively, you must examine and understand your own feelings about death. Sometimes we feel that we have failed in our job if the resident dies. As long as you have done all you can for the dying resident, you have succeeded in your responsibilities. Learn to take comfort in that.

Your age, culture, experiences, religion, values, and personal losses all influence your feelings about death and dying. Sometimes your attitude about death changes because of your personal experiences. As we age, we also may view death differently. Many elderly residents see death as a relief from pain and suffering. Some people fear death. It is a journey into the unknown. They are afraid that it will be lonely and painful. Studies of people who have had near-death experiences have shown that death is not unpleasant or frightening. Residents may also worry about dying alone. Many people worry about unfinished personal business and what will happen to family members and pets after their death.

Hospice. There is no cure for some diseases. Sometimes trauma and injuries to the body are so severe that the resident cannot recover. Some residents do not respond to medical treatment. Some die soon after receiving a terminal diagnosis. Others live for extended periods of time. We cannot predict when death will occur.

A **hospice** is an agency that cares for residents who are dying. Hospice workers are members of an interdisciplinary team who work to meet the resident's and family's physical, emotional, psychological, social, and spiritual needs. Hospice care is delivered in many different settings. Sometimes care is given in a hospital or nursing home. Many individuals use hospice services in their own home. Hospice care is not designed to be aggressive or to prolong life. It is designed to make the resident and family as comfortable as possible as death approaches.

The quality of care given is as good as the care given to all other residents. Family members may participate in resident care if they wish. Hospice care is designed to ensure that the resident dies in comfort, with dignity and respect.

Coping Mechanisms. **Coping mechanisms** are responses to stress that people use to protect their self-esteem. An understanding of some of the coping mechanisms that people use to deal with losses and stress in life will help you understand resident and family reactions to dealing with terminal illness. Coping mechanisms develop throughout a person's life. Success or failure in developing coping skills depends on how well the developmental tasks of earlier life have been mastered. When a person's ability to cope is inadequate, the following reactions may be seen:

- Chronic complaining
- Anger
- Irritability
- Crying and tearfulness
- Agitation
- Restlessness
- Sleep disturbances
- Muscle tension and headaches
- Depression
- Withdrawal
- Weight loss or gain

Residents may criticize and blame you for things that are not your fault. Do not take their comments personally. These residents usually need emotional support. Your understanding of basic human needs, normal developmental tasks, and coping mechanisms will help you provide quality care. The following are other ways you can provide this support:

- Offer choices over routines and as much control as possible.
- Realize that angry outbursts may be the result of feelings of hopelessness, loss, and unmet needs.
- Direct the resident's emotional energy in positive ways.
- Avoid responding to the resident in a negative manner.
- Report any change in the resident's behavior to the nurse.

GRIEVING PROCESS

When we anticipate or experience a loss, we go through a series of emotional changes and behaviors called the **grieving process.** This process was first described by Dr. Elisabeth Kübler-Ross. Loss of someone or something you love is very difficult. The resident, family, friends, and care providers each go through the grieving process, which involves five steps. The grieving process varies with each of us, so all persons do not experience each step. The steps are not always obvious to others. Sometimes we recognize the steps in other people, but fail to recognize them in ourselves. Some people move from one stage to another and back again. It may take a long time to complete all the steps in the grieving process. The resident may die before completing the process. Throughout the grieving process, the nursing assistant must offer honesty, reassurance, understanding, caring, and empathy. Helping a resident die in comfort and dignity is very important. **Table 21-1** gives examples of typical resident reactions and appropriate nursing assistant responses in each stage of the grieving process.

Denial

The first stage in the grieving process is **denial.** This occurs when a person first learns of a terminal diagnosis. The resident may feel that the diagnosis is incorrect. He or she may exhibit false hope, tell untrue stories, and spend a tremendous amount of energy keeping denial alive. The resi-

dent may refuse to participate in his or her care, and may not follow the directions of the physician and other staff. The resident and family need strong emotional support in order to move through this stage. Allow them to express their feelings, but do not provide false hope. Conversations should be based in reality. Spend time with the resident to show that he or she will not be left alone. Later in the denial stage, the resident may isolate himself or herself from others.

Anger

The second stage of the grieving process is **anger.** The resident feels angry with himself or herself, family, staff, the doctor, and God. He or she may use abusive language and refuse care and nutrition. Recognize that the resident is not angry with you personally. Practice empathy and let the resident know you understand how he or she feels.

Bargaining

The third stage of the grieving process is **bargaining.** The resident hopes he or she can live to see a certain event, such as a graduation or birth of a grandchild. Sometimes the resident bargains with God and makes promises, such as attending church every Sunday in return for more time.

TABLE 21-1	Stages of grief
Stages of Grief	**Response of the Nursing Assistant**
Denial	Reflect the resident's statements, but try not to confirm or deny the fact that the resident is dying. *Example: "The lab tests can't be right. I don't have cancer."* *"It must have been difficult for you to learn the results of your tests."*
Anger	Understand the source of the resident's anger. Provide understanding and support. Listen. Try to meet reasonable needs and demands quickly. *Example: "This food is terrible—not fit to eat."* *"Let me see if I can find something that would appeal to you more."*
Bargaining	If it is possible to meet the resident's requests, do so. Listen attentively. *Example: "If only God will spare me this, I'll go to church every week."* *"Would you like a visit from your clergy person?"*
Depression	Avoid clichés that dismiss the resident's depression ("It could be worse. You could be in more pain"). Be caring and supporting. Let the resident know that it is okay to be depressed. *Example: "There just isn't any sense in going on."* *"I understand you are feeling very depressed."*
Acceptance	Do not assume that, because the resident has accepted death, she or he is unafraid, or that she or he does not need emotional support. Listen attentively and be supportive and caring. *Example: "I feel so alone."* *"I am here with you. Would you like to talk?"*

Bargaining is an attempt to postpone the inevitable. This stage is usually short. Realize that the resident still needs time to accept his or her impending death. Spend as much time as you can with the resident to show that you sincerely care.

Depression

Depression (**Figure 21-2**) is the fourth stage in the grieving process. The resident is dealing with the loss of everything that he or she has. The resident's physical ability may decline. He or she is losing his or her home, possessions, loved ones, hopes, and dreams. The resident may also be feeling regrets for things he or she has said or done throughout life. The resident may experience **apathy,** decreased ability to concentrate, insomnia, fatigue, constant crying, poor appetite, and lack of interest in people and the environment. In this stage, the resident is beginning to separate himself or herself from life. Do not attempt to humor or cheer the resident. Allow him or her to express feelings, and be available to sit quietly and provide support.

Acceptance

The final stage in the grieving process is **acceptance.** The resident may feel empty and peaceful. This stage usually brings less emotional pain

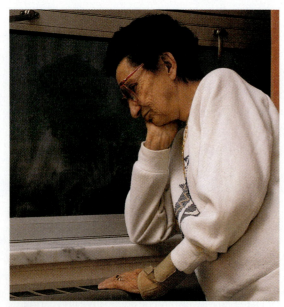

FIGURE 21-2 The depressed resident is beginning to separate herself from life.

and discomfort, and the resident calmly waits for the end. The resident may not want to be alone during this stage. If the resident does not object, allow others with whom he or she is comfortable to assist with care. Allow the resident to express needs in his or her own time and way. Communication may be limited in this stage.

SIGNS OF APPROACHING DEATH

Signs of death may occur slowly or rapidly. Always report changes in the resident's condition to the nurse. Some residents are alert until the moment of death. Others have a period of unconsciousness first. After the resident dies, the physician will examine the resident and pronounce death. In some states, registered nurses may pronounce death. This is never the responsibility of the nursing assistant. The nurse or physician is also responsible for notifying the family after death has been established.

Signs of approaching death are:

- Decreasing level of responsiveness.
- Movement, muscle tone, and sensation decrease until they are eventually lost.
- The lower jaw relaxes and the mouth falls open.
- The skin appears pale and is moist and cool to touch.
- The lips, fingernails, and mucous membranes take on a dusky, gray, or blue color.
- The pulse becomes rapid, weak, or thready.
- Respirations become slow, labored, irregular, or noisy. Cheyne-Stokes respirations may be present. Mucus collects in the throat. This is sometimes called a "death rattle."
- Blood pressure decreases. Sometimes blood pressure can no longer be heard at the brachial artery, but the resident remains alive.
- The resident may become incontinent of urine and feces.
- The eyes stare and pupils do not respond to light (**Figure 21-3**).
- The skin takes on a blue or dusky appearance beginning in the lower extremities, and moving upward. The skin feels cool or cold to touch.

Care of the Dying Resident

Some facilities are now setting aside private rooms for residents who are dying and their families.

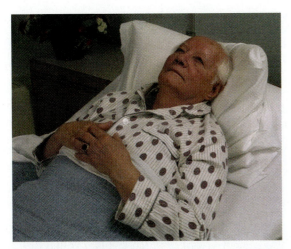

FIGURE 21-3 As death approaches, the eyes stare and the pupils do not respond to light. The resident can still hear, however.

These rooms may be called *hospice rooms*, even though true hospice care is not being provided. This provides a place for the resident and family to spend their last moments together and say their goodbyes without disturbing a roommate. It also avoids upsetting a roommate at the time of the resident's death.

Care of the dying resident is a continuation of care that shows support, dignity, and respect. The Dying Person's Bill of Rights **(Figure 21-4)** provides guidelines and should be used as a basis for care.

The Dying Person's Bill of Rights

- I have the right to be treated as a living human being until I die.
- I have the right to maintain a sense of hopefulness, however changing its focus may be.
- I have the right to be cared for by those who can maintain a sense of hopefulness, however changing this may be.
- I have the right to express my feelings and emotions about my approaching death in my own way.
- I have the right to participate in decisions concerning my care.
- I have the right to expect continuing medical and nursing attention even though "cure" goals must be changed to "comfort" goals.
- I have the right not to die alone.
- I have the right to be free from pain.
- I have the right to have my questions answered honestly.
- I have the right not to be deceived.
- I have the right to have help from and for my family accepting my death.
- I have the right to die in peace and dignity.
- I have the right to retain my individuality and not be judged for my decisions, which may be contrary to the beliefs of others.
- I have the right to discuss and enlarge my religious and/or spiritual experiences, regardless of what they may mean to others.
- I have the right to expect that the sanctity of the human body will be respected after death.
- I have the right to be cared for by caring, sensitive, knowledgeable people who will attempt to understand my needs and will be able to gain some satisfaction in helping me face my death.

FIGURE 21-4 The dying person's bill of rights. *(From Barbus, A. J.: American Journal of Nursing 75(1):99, 1975)*

POSTMORTEM CARE

Your facility will have a policy and procedure for physical care of the body after death. This is called **postmortem care,** and in most cases, the nursing assistant delivers this care. Some facilities have a morgue to which the body is taken. In most facilities the body will be left in the room until it can be transferred to a mortuary. Within two to four hours after death, a condition called **rigor mortis** develops. In this condition, the muscles and limbs of the body become rigid and stiff. Position the body in good alignment before this condition occurs. When circulation stops, the body begins to pull blood into the lowest areas of the body. This process can begin within 20 minutes of death. Over time, this will result in a stained appearance on the back of the body (if the resident is in the supine position). To reduce the risk of staining about the head and neck, elevate the head of the bed 30 degrees, in the semi-Fowler's position. Some facilities do not use ties in the morgue pack to position the body. Follow your facility policies. If used, tie them loosely. If the ties are too tight, they will also cause permanent marks on the body.

Always use standard precautions when providing postmortem care. The body can be infectious after death. Handle the body very gently. Show the same respect and provide the same privacy that you would if the resident were alive. Respect the religious beliefs of the deceased. Spiritual beliefs vary, and people of some faiths have special religious requirements for preparation of the body. **Table 21-2** describes some common religious and cultural beliefs.

GUIDELINES IN

Caring for the Dying Resident

- Practice empathy for the resident, friends, and family.
- Check the care plan for special care instructions.
- Consider and respect the religious beliefs of the resident and family even if they are different from your own.
- Provide privacy when clergy visit **(Figure 21-5)**.
- Learn the resident's cultural and religious practices regarding death.
- Keep the resident clean and comfortable.
- Keep the lips and mouth moist and give frequent oral care.
- Turn the resident every two hours or more. Position with props and pillows for comfort.
- Keep the skin clean. Apply lotion as needed.
- Change the linen immediately if it is wet or soiled. Provide blankets for warmth.
- Provide perineal care after each episode of incontinence.
- The room should be well lighted and as comfortable and pleasant as possible.
- Allow privacy if the family is present, but check on the resident frequently.
- Touch and continue to talk to the resident as you normally would.
- Avoid saying things that you do not want the resident to hear. Explain all procedures before doing them. The resident may appear unconscious, but the sense of hearing may be present. During the dying process, hearing is the last sensation to be lost.
- Support family members. Allow them to be involved in care, if appropriate.
- Make the family as comfortable as possible by providing coffee, pillows, blankets, or other needed items.

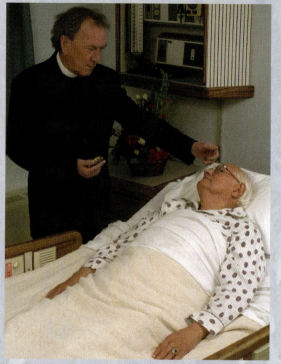

FIGURE 21-5 Respect the resident's religious beliefs. Assist him in preparations for a clergy visit, and provide privacy when religious workers are visiting.

PROCEDURE 86 — Postmortem Care

  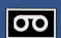

1. Perform your beginning procedure actions.
2. Gather supplies needed: shroud kit or morgue pack **(Figure 21-6)** with gown and identification tags, a basin of warm water, soap, washcloth, towels, swabs for oral care, linen, gloves.
3. Apply gloves.
4. Position the resident on the back with a pillow below the head and shoulders. Elevate the head of the bed 30 degrees.
5. Close the eyes by gently pulling the eyelids down **(Figure 21-7)**.
6. Provide mouth care using moistened oral care swabs or sponges.
7. Close the mouth. A rolled-up washcloth may be placed under the chin to keep the jaw closed.
8. Follow your facility policy for removal of tubing from the body. In most facilities, the nurse will remove tubing. If the death is considered reportable to your coroner's office, the tubing should not be removed.
9. Bathe the body, straighten the arms and legs, and comb the hair.
10. Apply clean dressings to wounds, if necessary. Check with the nurse if dressings are soiled.
11. Place a bed protector or underpad under the buttocks. Urine and stool may continue to seep out after death.
12. Put a gown on the body.
13. Attach identification tags to the body according to facility policy.

Continues

PROCEDURE 86

Postmortem Care, *Continued*

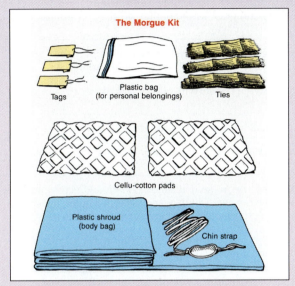

FIGURE 21-6 Standard morgue pack

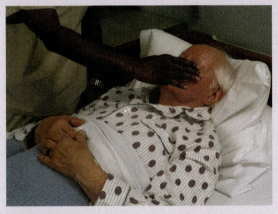

FIGURE 21-7 Gently close the resident's eyes.

14. Replace soiled linen and cover the body to the shoulders with a sheet.
15. Remove gloves and discard according to facility policy.
16. Wash your hands.
17. Straighten the room and remove unnecessary equipment.
18. Wash your hands.
19. Provide privacy and allow family members to be alone with the body.
20. Clean the resident's dentures, and place them in a denture cup. Make sure they are sent to the funeral home with the body.
21. Collect the resident's personal belongings, place them in a bag, and label them correctly. Usually these are given to the family. If no family mem-

bers are present, follow facility policy. Complete and sign the inventory sheet according to your facility policy.
22. After the family leaves, wash your hands and put the **shroud** on the body, if used in your facility. (The shroud is a cloth, paper, or plastic covering used to wrap the body after death.) Wear gloves if contact with blood or body fluid is likely.
23. Remove gloves and discard according to facility policy. Wash your hands.
24. Follow facility policy: either take the body to the morgue or close the door until representatives from the funeral home arrive.
25. Notify the nurse when representatives from the funeral home arrive.
26. Assist the funeral home representatives to move the body if necessary.
27. Strip and clean the unit according to your facility policy after the body has been removed.

TABLE 21-2	Cultural/religious beliefs affecting care at the time of death
Culture/Religion	**Religious Belief**
Adventist (Seventh Day, Church of God)	Some believe in divine healing, anointing with oil, and prayer.
American Indian	There are many different tribes, and beliefs vary with each. Some believe an owl is an omen of death. Some tribes have family members prepare the body for burial. Some tribes will not touch the dead person's belongings after death. Some tribes believe the dead are happy in the spirit world. Others believe the body is an empty shell. Some have extensive preparation of the body and visitation of the deceased. If a member of some tribes dies at home, the house is abandoned forever or may be burned.

Continues

TABLE 21-2 Cultural/religious beliefs affecting care at the time of death, *Continued*

Culture/Religion	Religious Belief
Armenian Church	Holy Communion may be given as a form of last rites; laying-on of hands is practiced.
Baptist	Pastor, resident, and family counsel and pray. Resident may be given Communion. Some practice healing and laying-on of hands.
Black/African American	The deceased is highly respected. Health care providers usually prepare the body. Cremation is usually avoided. May have concerns about organ donation.
Black Muslim	Practices for washing the body, applying the shroud, and funeral rites are carefully prescribed.
Brethren	Anointing with oil is done for physical healing and spiritual guidance.
Buddhist Churches of America	The priest is contacted to provide Last Rites. Chanting may be done at the bedside after death.
Cambodian (Khmer)	Monks recite prayers. Family wants to be present at time of death and may want to care for the resident. Incense may be burned. Death is accepted in a quiet, passive manner. Family and monks may wish to prepare the body. A white cloth is used as a shroud, and mourners wear white.
Central American	Catholics may want a priest to administer Sacrament of the Sick. Candles may be used if oxygen is not in use in room. Family members may wish to prepare the body.
Chinese American	Family may prefer resident not be told of impending death, or may prefer to inform the resident themselves. May not want to talk about the terminal illness with anyone. Some believe that dying at home is bad luck. Others believe that the spirit gets lost if the resident dies in the hospital. Family members may place special cloths and amulets on the body. Some prefer to bathe their own family members after death.
Christian Scientist	A Christian Science practitioner may be called for spiritual support. Have concerns about organ donation.
Church of God	Believe in divine healing through prayer. Speaking in tongues may be used.
Church of Jesus Christ of Latter Day Saints (LDS or Mormon)	Body is dressed in white temple clothing before viewing by family members. Cremation is discouraged. Believe in baptism for others who have died and preaching to deceased.
Colombian	Catholic prayer and anointing of the sick common. Family may practice Catholic prayer at bedside. Family members may cry loudly or become hysterical. All family members may want to see the body before it is taken to the morgue. In Colombia, the deceased are usually buried within 24 to 36 hours. The nurse may need to inform them that in the United States the body may not be buried this quickly.
Cuban	Family may not want resident told of impending death. This varies according to Cuban culture. Family members may stay with resident 24 hours a day during terminal phase of illness.
Eastern Orthodox	Last rites are given. Anointing of the sick is performed as a form of healing with prayer. Cremation is discouraged.
Episcopal	Last Rites are available, but not mandatory. May practice prayer, Communion, and confession.
Ethiopian	Friends are told of death before family so they can be present when family is informed. Female family members are never told first. Great displays of feelings are encouraged at death. They may cry loudly and hysterically. Women may tear their clothing and beat their chests. Men may cry out loud. Some families may want to say goodbye to the deceased before the body is removed from the room.

Continues

TABLE 21-2 Cultural/religious beliefs affecting care at the time of death, *Continued*

Culture/Religion	Religious Belief
Filipino	Head of family is informed away from resident's room. Catholic priest is called to deliver Sacrament of the Sick. DNR decisions may be made by the entire family. Religious objects may be placed around the resident. Family may pray at the bedside when resident is dying. After death, they may cry loudly and hysterically. Family may wish to wash the body. Death is considered a very spiritual event. All family members may say goodbye before body is removed from the room.
Friends (Quaker)	Do not believe in life after death (spiritual afterlife).
Greek Orthodox	The priest should be called while the resident is still conscious. Practice Last Rites and administration of Communion. Believe that life should be preserved until terminated by God.
Gypsy	In general, discussion of death is avoided in this culture. Eldest in authority is informed of death first. A priest may be present for body purification. Family may want the window open at the time of death and afterward so the spirit can leave the room. May ask for special personal items in room at the time of death. An older female relative may remain at the window to keep spirits out of room. The moment of death and the resident's last words are very significant. The body after death may represent a source of spiritual danger to the family. Family may want body embalmed immediately after death to remove blood. They may sit with the body around the clock after death, and will eat and drink at this location.
Haitian	Elaborate rituals after death. When death is imminent, family will cry hysterically and uncontrollably. Family members may bring religious symbols and medallions. They have a deep respect for the dead. Family members may wish to wash the body and participate in postmortem care.
Hindu	Specially prescribed rites. Priest may tie a thread around wrist or neck and place water in mouth. The family washes and dresses the body, and only certain persons may touch the dead. May prefer cremation to burial.
Hmong	Important to wear fine traditional Hmong clothing at the time of death. Family may put amulets on body, which should not be removed. The family usually prepares the body at the funeral home. The body cannot be buried with hard objects, buttons, or zippers against the body.
Iranian	Death is seen as the beginning of a spiritual relationship with God, not the end of life. Family may wish to be present at all times when resident is dying, and may cry and pray at bedside. Families may wish to wash the body.
Islam (Muslim)	Begging forgiveness and confession of sins must be done in presence of family members before death. There are five steps to preparing the body for burial. The first step involves washing of the body by a Muslim of the same gender. May offer special prayers at bedside to ease pain and suffering. Some have spiritual leader give resident holy water to drink prior to death to purify body. After death, arms and legs are straightened and the toes tied together with a bandage. May be opposed to autopsy.
Japanese	Resident and family may be aware of impending death, but will not speak about it. Family may wish to remain at bedside during terminal stage of illness. Cleanliness and dignity of the body are very important.
Jehovah's Witness	Practice baptism and Communion. May be opposed to autopsy.

Continues

TABLE 21-2   Cultural/religious beliefs affecting care at the time of death, *Continued*

Culture/Religion	Religious Belief
Judaism (Orthodox and Conservative)	Jews believe in the sanctity of life. Medical care is generally expected, and there are no medication restrictions. Most surgical procedures are permitted, but body parts that have been removed are traditionally saved for later burial. For most Jews, medical treatment cannot be stopped once it has been started, but members are not required to use extraordinary measures to prolong life. May be opposed to prolonging life if resident has irreversible brain damage. However, active euthanasia is forbidden. Traditional Jews use a burial society to care for the body after death. Society members may or may not be members of the deceased's congregation. They usually prefer no autopsy, but this is permitted if legally required. Embalming is generally discouraged. The resident is buried as soon after death as possible. Cremation is discouraged. For traditional Jews, mourning begins with a seven-day period called *shiva*, in which men do not shave, and family and close friends do not read the newspaper or watch television. Mourning extends over a year. Jewish practices and beliefs can be very different from family to family. Asking the resident or family members about their practices is probably best. Asking is not offensive, and shows that you care about and respect the resident's and family's wishes.
Korean	Chanting, incense, and praying may be used. Family crying and mourning may be extreme. Family may want to spend time alone with the resident after death. Some may wish to wash the body.
Lutheran	Practice prayer. Last Rites optional; the resident may request anointing of the sick.
Methodist	May request donation of body or body parts to medical science.
Mexican American	Entire family may be obligated to visit the sick and dying. Pregnant women may be prohibited from visiting. Spiritual items may be important. May want to die at home because of the fear that the spirit will get lost in the hospital. Crying loudly and wailing is culturally accepted and a sign of respect. A Catholic priest is called for the Sacrament of the Sick. A family member may wish to assist with postmortem care. Family will want time alone with the body before it is removed from the room.
Orthodox Presbyterian	Scripture reading and prayer. Full forgiveness is granted for any illness connected with a sin.
Puerto Rican	If death is imminent, family may stay around the clock. Some believe that all immediate family members must be present at the time of death. Believe that the body must be treated with great respect.
Roman Catholic	Prayer and the rite for anointing of the sick is desired. Resident or family may request anointing if prognosis is poor.
Russian	Family may not want the resident to know of a terminal diagnosis. Depending on religion, family may wish to wash the body and dress it in special clothes.
Russian Orthodox	Practice prayer, Communion, and Last Rites by priest. Many wear a cross necklace, which should not be removed if at all possible. After death the arms are crossed, and fingers set in the form of a cross. Clothing must be a natural fiber so the body changes to ashes sooner. May be opposed to autopsy, embalming, or cremation.
Samoan	Resident and family prefer to be told of terminal diagnosis as early as possible. Family would prefer to care for resident at home, if possible. Family members usually prefer to prepare the body.
Sikh	Believe that the soul remains alive after death. Family washes the body and dresses deceased member in new clothing.
Unitarian Universalist	Cremation may be preferred to burial.

Continues

TABLE 21-2	Cultural/religious beliefs affecting care at the time of death, *Continued*
Culture/Religion	**Religious Belief**
Vietnamese	DNR decisions are made by entire family. For Catholic families, religious items are kept close to resident. For Buddhist families, incense is burned. Families prefer time alone with the deceased before body is moved. The body is highly respected, and the family may prefer to wash it. Some may prefer the body left as it is.
West Indian	When death is near, close family and friends wish to remain at the bedside to pray. Family members may wish to view the body exactly as the resident was at the time of death. Most wish to be alone with the deceased

KEY POINTS

- The nursing assistant is expected to provide care to residents who are dying and to care for the body after death.
- When caring for residents who are dying, the nursing assistant will assist residents and families to meet physical, emotional, psychological, social, and spiritual needs.
- Residents with terminal illness are not expected to recover, but the exact time of death cannot be predicted.
- The nursing assistant's personal beliefs about death and dying will affect the care given to the resident.
- A hospice is an agency that cares for dying residents.
- Hospice care focuses on keeping residents comfortable and allowing them to die with dignity and respect.
- Coping mechanisms are responses to stress and loss that are used to protect self-esteem.
- The five steps in the grieving process are denial, anger, bargaining, depression, and acceptance.
- The resident and family's cultural and religious beliefs about death and dying must be respected.
- Standard precautions are used when caring for the deceased, because the body can be infectious after death.

REVIEW

A. Multiple Choice

Select the one best answer.

1. Our feelings about death and dying are influenced by
   a. residents.
   b. the nurse.
   c. experiences.
   d. doctor's orders.

2. Hospice care is designed to
   a. treat the resident aggressively.
   b. keep the resident comfortable.
   c. prolong life.
   d. care only for the family.

3. Coping mechanisms are
   a. signs of grief.
   b. used to protect self-esteem.
   c. religious rituals.
   d. signs of approaching death.

4. In the first stage of the grieving process, the resident shows signs of
   a. denial.
   b. bargaining.
   c. depression.
   d. acceptance.

5. The resident is trying to separate himself or herself from life during the
   a. denial stage.
   b. anger stage.
   c. depression stage.
   d. bargaining stage.

6. Signs of approaching death include
   a. cooling of the skin, beginning with the lower extremities.
   b. constricted pupils.
   c. steady, slow pulse.
   d. elevated pulse and blood pressure.

7. When caring for the dying resident,
   a. be as quiet as possible and do not speak when providing care.
   b. always explain procedures before doing them.
   c. do not move the resident in bed, as this is painful and disturbing.
   d. keep the room very dark and warm.

8. Which of the following is a true statement about providing postmortem care?
   a. There is no need to provide privacy.
   b. The dentures are always removed from the mouth and given to the family to take home.
   c. Standard precautions are used because the body can be infectious.
   d. The nursing assistant removes all tubes and dressings.

9. The condition in which the muscles become stiff and rigid is
   a. algor mortis.
   b. liver mortis.
   c. muscle mortis.
   d. rigor mortis.

10. When a resident is dying, the room should be
    a. dark and cold.
    b. well lighted and ventilated.
    c. dark and hot.
    d. well lighted and cold.

B. Clinical Applications

Answer the following questions.

11. Mrs. Long has a history of severe depression. She attempted suicide years ago. Mrs. Long's husband has been told that the resident has terminal cancer. Her husband is the resident's legal guardian. He does not want her to know of her terminal diagnosis because he is afraid she will become depressed and attempt suicide again. When you are giving Mrs. Long a bed bath, she asks you if she is dying. How will you respond?

12. You are assigned to care for Mr. Street, a terminally ill resident who is not conscious. The family is in the room. They are discussing how bad the resident looks. What should you do?

13. Mr. Street's daughter tells you that she wants to help you turn the resident on his side. She would like to put lotion on her father's back. What will you do?

14. Mrs. Miles has a terminal diagnosis. When you enter her room to remove her supper tray, you find that she has thrown the food onto the wall. She yells that she is angry with you for giving her poor care. What do you think the problem is? How will you respond?

15. Miss Gantz is an 84-year-old resident who is dying. She tells you she is comfortable because she knows she is going home to be with the Lord. The resident's religious beliefs are not the same as your own. What will you do?

CHAPTER 22

The Nursing Assistant in Home Care

OBJECTIVES

After reading this chapter, you will be able to:

- List the advantages of home health care to the client and family.
- Describe the benefits of working in home health care.
- List at least 10 desirable personal characteristics of the home health nursing assistant.
- Describe the duties of the home health nursing assistant.
- Identify the members of the home health care interdisciplinary team.
- Describe how to maintain a safe home environment.
- Demonstrate food preparation and storage.
- Discuss how to prevent infection in the home.
- Describe documentation, recordkeeping, and reporting in the home care environment.
- List guidelines for time management.
- List at least 10 methods of protecting your personal safety when working as a home care assistant in the community.

OBSERVATIONS TO MAKE AND REPORT RELATED TO THE NURSING ASSISTANT IN HOME CARE

Signs or symptoms of acute illness
Significant changes in client's condition, such as:
    ability to eat independently, or change in
      appetite
    ability to get into or out of bed
    ability to maintain continence or use the toilet

    bathing ability
    dressing ability
New safety problems or falls
Other incidents or injuries
Changes in vital signs

HOME HEALTH CARE: THE CLIENT'S POINT OF VIEW

Individuals have been cared for in their homes for centuries. In the mid-20th century, the trend began moving toward institutional care. Today, we have come full circle, and the trend is moving back toward caring for individuals in their own homes. There are many advantages to home care for the client and family:

- Care is delivered in the comfort and security of one's own home. Most people prefer to be at home instead of in an institution.
- Home care keeps families together, and the client continues to be a full-time member of the family unit.

- Clients state that quality of life is better at home, compared with an institution.
- The psychological benefits, comfort, and security of being at home may promote healing.
- The client has more control over daily routines, and has choices about aspects of daily life, such as the menu, time to get up, time to go to bed, and television shows to watch.
- Institutional risks, such as the risk of infection, are minimized or eliminated.
- Home care promotes continuity of care, and care is more personalized than institutional care.
- Care is usually less expensive than other forms of care.

Clients receiving home care vary widely in age. Many, but not all, are elderly. Some are children with serious illness or disabilities. Some will need temporary care, but others will need lifetime care. New mothers may receive temporary care to assist them with care of the newborn and to learn skills such as bathing an infant. The needs of some clients are complex, placing great demands on family caregivers. Caregiving can be difficult for family members and loved ones. Having caregivers come to the home assists family members to maintain the quality of their own lives, and gives them time to take care of their personal affairs.

INTRODUCTION TO HOME HEALTH CARE

One advantage of being a health care worker is that you can work in a variety of settings **(Figure 22-1).** In many states, nursing assistants may work in home health care upon successful completion of the nursing assistant class and entry into the state registry. In other states, additional education is required to work in home health care. Caring for individuals in their homes can be challenging, but very rewarding. Working in home care is an option that gives autonomy to health care providers. Other benefits of working in home care are:

- Ability to care for one client over a long period of time
- Caring for only one client at a time instead of many
- Independence and ability to make decisions

Most home health care is delivered by home care agencies, which employ an entire interdisciplinary team of home care workers. The home

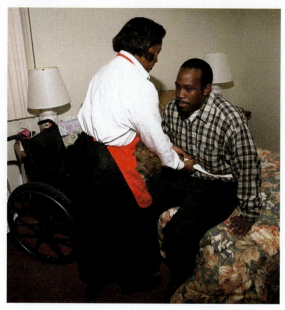

FIGURE 22-1 Your basic nursing assistant skills may be used in many different work settings.

health care agency will orient the workers to their roles, responsibilities, job descriptions, and agency policies and procedures. Other information you will learn in orientation will include:

- Agency philosophy of care
- Rights of clients in home care **(Figure 22-2)**
- Chain of command
- Scope of services provided
- Legal aspects of home health care
- Documentation procedures and forms
- Other services provided by the agency
- Map reading and time keeping
- Safety precautions in the home
- Personal safety
- How to improvise nursing care in the home

As part of your orientation, you will also go into the community with another worker to observe how care is given in the home setting. Your agency may expect you to carry a nursing bag containing items such as gloves, a plastic apron, and equipment for monitoring vital signs.

Assisted Living Facilities. In addition to working in clients' homes, home care workers may also visit residents in assisted living facilities (ALFs). These facilities do not usually provide nursing services. Residents who become ill or injured may need temporary or short-term nursing care. Rather than moving them from their homes in the ALF to a facility that provides

Client's Rights in Home Care

The persons receiving home health care services or their families possess basic rights and responsibilities.
These include:

The right to:
1. be treated with dignity, consideration and respect
2. have their property treated with respect
3. receive a timely response from the agency to requests for service
4. be fully informed on admission of the care and treatment that will be provided, how much it will cost, and how payment will be handled
5. know in advance if you will be responsible for any payment
6. be informed in advance of any changes in your care
7. receive care from professionally trained personnel, to know their names and responsibilities
8. participate in planning care
9. refuse treatment and to be told the consequences of your action
10. expect confidentiality of all information
11. be informed of anticipated termination of service
12. be referred elsewhere if you are denied services solely based on your inability to pay
13. know how to make a complaint or recommend a change in agency policies and services

The responsibility to:
1. remain under a doctor's care while receiving services
2. provide the agency with a complete health history
3. provide the agency all requested insurance and financial information
4. sign the required consents and releases for insurance billing
5. participate in your care by asking questions, expressing concerns, stating if you do not understand
6. provide a safe home environment in which care is given
7. cooperate with your doctor, the staff, and other caregivers
8. accept responsibility for any refusal of treatment
9. abide by agency policies which restrict duties our staff may perform
10. advise agency administration of any dissatisfaction or problems with your care

FIGURE 22-2   The Client's Rights in Home Care

a higher level of care, home health care workers visit the resident in the ALF to provide necessary services. Using home care workers in this manner promotes the "aging in place" philosophy of the assisted living facility and enables residents to remain in a familiar environment while they recover.

Home Health Nursing Assistant Characteristics

Providing home care requires special knowledge and preparation. The nursing assistant who works in the home must:

- Have excellent clinical skills
- Have good observational skills **(Figure 22-3)**
- Be accurate and pay attention to detail

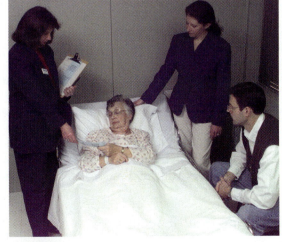

FIGURE 22-3   The nursing assistant must have excellent observational skills to work in home care.

GUIDELINES FOR
Avoiding Personal Liability in Home Health Care

- Make sure you get a job description that lists your duties and responsibilities. Ask questions and clarify if needed. Make sure you understand what is expected.
- Learn and respect the clients' rights.
- Do only those things that you are legally permitted to do.
- Do things the way you were taught; avoid shortcuts.
- Ask for assistance with unfamiliar procedures.
- Think safety at all times **(Figure 22-4)**.
- Monitor the environment for potential hazards.
- Know who to contact in an emergency.
- Contact the supervising nurse promptly to report new information.
- Carefully document your care and observations.
- Participate in client care conferences.
- Attend continuing education classes.

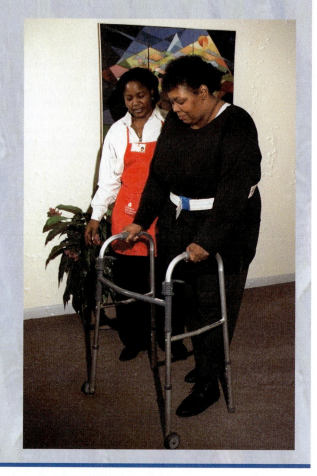

FIGURE 22-4 Use safety precautions in everything you do.

- Be honest, dependable, and trustworthy
- Use good judgment and common sense
- Have good communication skills
- Be self-motivated and self-directed
- Not need intense supervision
- Be flexible and able to solve problems and know when to call for help
- Be well organized, with good time management skills
- Be a team player and get along well with others
- Have dependable transportation
- Have good reporting and recordkeeping skills

The Home Health Team

The home health care team consists of a number of professional and paraprofessional workers **(Figure 22-5)**. The team members will vary according to the clients' needs, but members typically include:

- The client
- The client's family members or primary caregiver
- A physician
- A registered nurse
- Nursing assistants
- A pharmacist
- A dietitian
- Physical, occupational, speech, and respiratory therapists
- A social worker

Each professional member of the team will assess the client's needs related to the professional's discipline, then develop a plan of care to meet those needs. They will also assess the home environment for safety, and estimate a

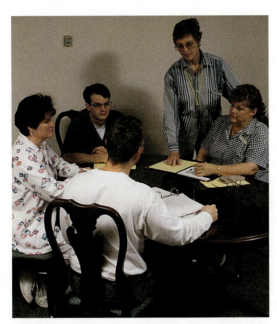

FIGURE 22-5 The home health nursing assistant contributes to the nursing process by participating in care plan meetings.

time frame in which the client can realistically meet the goals. The registered nurse will determine what nursing services are needed, and decide how often the client will need the services of the nursing assistant. The RN will develop the nursing assistant plan of care **(Figure 22-6).** This plan identifies your duties and the care you will be expected to provide. Team members will review the client's plan of care at least monthly, and make revisions when appropriate.

HOME HEALTH ASSISTANT DUTIES

The duties of the home health nursing assistant are planned around client needs and family routines. Your duties may include:

- Assisting the client with bathing, dressing, and other activities of daily living
- Providing special treatments, such as range-of-motion exercises
- Caring for the client's medical equipment, furnishings, and supplies
- Cleaning and disinfecting items used for client care
- Providing comfort measures
- Changing the linen and making the bed
- Washing the client's personal laundry and bed linens

- Doing light housekeeping **(Figure 22-7)**
- Preparing meals
- Shopping for meals **(Figure 22-8)**
- Transporting the client to appointments, as permitted by your agency **(Figure 22-9)**
- Reminding the client to take medications, or supervising self-administration of medications
- Monitoring the client, such as checking the vital signs **(Figure 22-10)**
- Being alert to safety at all times

You will not be expected to:

- Do heavy cleaning, such as waxing floors, yard work, or garden work
- Make decisions about food purchases, unless permitted to do so
- Become involved in family business, disputes, or decisions
- Manage the client's money, unless you receive specific directions from your agency and an accounting is done

Working in the Home Environment

You will be responsible for maintaining a comfortable, safe, and sanitary home environment. Apply the principles of standard precautions and wash your hands frequently, in the same manner as you would in the health care facility. You will need to learn to adapt your nursing assistant skills and available supplies to provide nursing care in the home. For example, many clients have hospital beds at home, but some use a regular bed. You cannot adjust the height of a regular bed to prevent injury to your back, so you may have to squat or kneel to make the bed. The bed may also be raised on wooden blocks, if the client is bedfast and this is not a safety risk. Examples of other potential adaptations are:

- Using a shower curtain or plastic tablecloth under the sheet to protect the mattress if the client is incontinent
- Making equipment using readily available items **(Figure 22-11)**
- Making a cold pack by freezing a wet washcloth, or making an ice pack by placing crushed ice in a zipper bag, then covering it with a towel
- Folding a twin-size sheet to use as a turning sheet or draw sheet
- Using a lightweight cotton blanket or sheet instead of a bath blanket
- Reusing equipment, such as an enema bag, instead of using disposables
- Using plastic bags instead of a linen hamper

Home Health Assistant Care Plan

Client Name: _____ POC Date _____ Client #: _____

Address: _____ Phone: _____

Directions: _____

Family contact: _____ Phone: _____

Diagnosis: _____ Allergies: _____

Frequency and duration of visits: _____

****

RN to complete items below, specify frequency, and provide specific directions.

Assignment	To Do	Instructions	Frequency	Assignment	To Do	Instructions	Frequency
Temperature				Walker/cane			
Pulse and respirations				ROM active/ ROM passive			
Blood pressure				T&R			
Weight				Siderails			
Monitor urine		Obs frequency/ color		Assist medication			
Intake and output				Prepare meals			
Check BM				Serve meals			
Enema				Feed client			
Tub bath/ shower				Wash dishes			
Bed bath				Clean kitchen			
Shampoo				Dust			
Shave				Vacuum			
Comb/brush hair				Change linen			
Catheter care				Make bed			
Nail care				Clean bedroom			
Oral hygiene				Clean bathroom			
Foot care				Shopping/ errand			
OOB in w/c				Transport to appt.			
Assist w/amb				Other			

Special safety and infection control measures: _____

Supplies needed: _____

Special requests: _____

RN signature/date _____ HHA signature/date _____

Change/update/review: _____

RN signature/date _____ HHA signature/date _____

FIGURE 22-6 The home health assistant care plan is completed by the RN and forms the basis for your assignment.

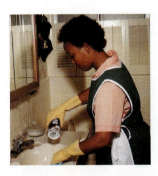

FIGURE 22-7 Light cleaning duties are part of the home care routine.

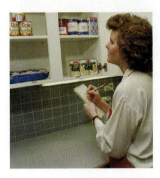

FIGURE 22-8 Your duties may include shopping for groceries. Prepare a list before leaving for the store.

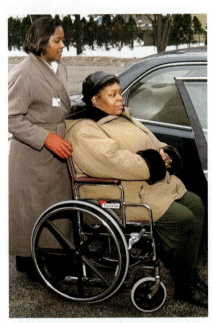

FIGURE 22-9 The home health nursing assistant may be responsible for transporting clients to clinic appointments and therapy.

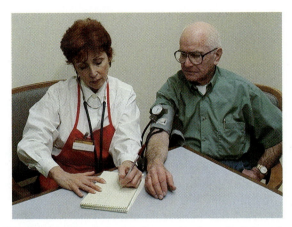

FIGURE 22-10 Accurately monitoring vital signs is an important responsibility.

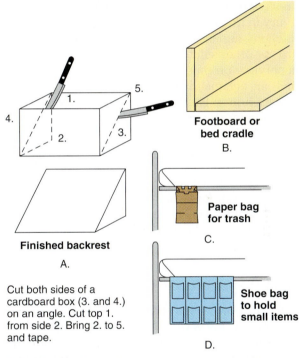

FIGURE 22-11 Make equipment using readily available materials.

Footboard or bed cradle
B.

Finished backrest
A.

Paper bag for trash
C.

Cut both sides of a cardboard box (3. and 4.) on an angle. Cut top 1. from side 2. Bring 2. to 5. and tape.

Shoe bag to hold small items
D.

HOME SAFETY

During your first home visit, check the home for safety problems. If identified, report them to the client's primary caregiver, or the supervising nurse, as appropriate. Become familiar with the location of items in the home, such as smoke detectors, fire extinguishers, a battery-operated radio, flashlight, and other items, as appropriate. Always be alert to unsafe practices, conditions, or situations. Make sure you have a list of emergency contact numbers, such as:

- Police, fire, and ambulance
- Home care agency
- Supervising nurse
- Physician
- Responsible family member, as appropriate

You should find out if the client:

- Uses a medical alert bracelet or necklace.
- Has out-of-hospital code papers or a living will.

- Has a special storage place in the house for important medical information that would be needed in an emergency. Some people keep these in the refrigerator so they can be easily located.

Check for problems that could cause falls or other injuries, such as:

- Clutter or items obstructing the walkway
- Electrical cords or throw rugs that could present a trip hazard
- Chemicals stored in an unsafe or inappropriate manner
- Overloaded electrical outlets
- Unsafe smoking by the client or a family member

Pay close attention to safety risks in the following areas, which are the most common locations of injury in the home: stairs and steps, bathroom(s), kitchens, and basements. If you feel there are hazards or other safety or security risks, inform your supervisor promptly. If the home should be modified, an occupational therapist may be asked to make a home visit to make recommendations. Do not attempt to make mechanical or environmental modifications yourself.

Discuss unsafe conditions with the supervising nurse. Your job is not to rearrange the client's home or routines. You are responsible for maintaining a safe environment. If you think that a client would benefit from special equipment, such as a bedside commode, raised toilet seat, or overbed trapeze, inform the supervising nurse.

Food Preparation

You will plan meals with the client or a family member. If this is your responsibility, plan meals a week in advance **(Figure 22-12)**. Menus should be based on the food guide pyramid and principles of good nutrition. Consider the client's budget and special dietary needs. If you are responsible for shopping, use the client's money wisely, and make sure you can account for everything you spend.

Store fresh food and leftovers in covered, wrapped containers. When preparing food:

- Always wash your hands for at least 15 to 20 seconds before handling food.
- Keep meat and dairy products refrigerated until you are ready to use them.
- Thaw frozen foods in the refrigerator.
- Wash fresh fruits and vegetables.
- Check expiration dates before using food items.

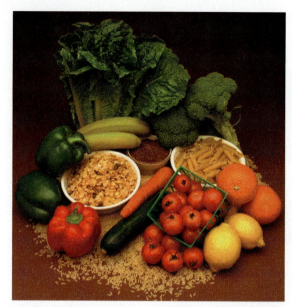

FIGURE 22-12 Clients should eat a well-balanced diet for good health.

- Make sure packages are intact, without bulges or cracks.
- Wash the lids of canned items before opening.
- Cook foods to the proper temperature.
- Keep hot foods hot and cold foods cold.
- Refrigerate leftovers as soon as possible.

Infection Control

Many of your routine tasks involve keeping the environment clean and preventing the spread of infection. For example, you will:

- Wash your hands frequently
- Apply the principles of standard precautions
- Keep the bathroom and kitchen clean **(Figure 22-13)**
- Prepare and store food properly
- Wash dirty dishes

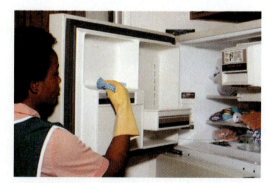

FIGURE 22-13 Clean spills promptly.

- Not allow trash or clutter to accumulate
- Discard tissues and other wastes properly
- Dust daily
- Keep the client's room tidy
- Clean and put away equipment after use
- Put clean clothes away
- Line wastebaskets with plastic bags

Cleaning the Kitchen. The kitchen is a potential source of infection. Handle and store food properly and clean the kitchen after each meal.

- Do not allow dirty dishes or trash to accumulate.
- You may wash dishes by hand, or by using a dishwasher.
- Rinse dishes immediately after use.
- If washing by hand, wash glasses first, then silverware, then dishes.
- Use hot, soapy water.
- Wash pots and pans last.
- Rinse dishes well, then put them in a drainer. Put them away when dry.
- Load the dishwasher with rinsed dishes. Ask the client whether to run the dishwasher or wait until it is full.
- Wash pots and pans by hand. Do not put them in the dishwasher.
- Clean the countertop, sink, and stove.
- Dispose of trash.
- Sweep the floor.
- Keep dishcloths, sponges, and towels clean.

Cleaning the Bathroom. The bathroom is also a great potential source of infection. Carefully and thoroughly clean it each day.

- Use a disinfectant product of the client's (family's) choice.
- Wear utility gloves.
- Clean inside and outside of the sink and wipe the faucets.
- Clean the shower or tub after use.
- Wipe countertops.
- Replace soiled towels and washcloths with clean ones.

Laundry. You may be responsible for washing the client's clothing and bed linen each day. Handle them carefully, and follow washing instructions on labels.

- Ask for instructions before using the washer and dryer.
- Wear gloves when loading the washer or sorting clothing if contact with blood, body fluids, secretions, or excretions is likely.

- Sort clothing, washing lights and darks separately.
- Hang clothes that are drip-dry; dry others in the dryer.
- Use the correct dryer setting.
- Remove clothes from the dryer promptly, and fold or hang.
- Put clean clothes away.
- Provide a clean container for soiled clothes and linen.

TIME MANAGEMENT

You are responsible for planning your assignment and completing it within a designated period of time. You may have several clients to see during your shift. Make good use of your time:

- Make sure you bring everything you need.
- Pack items such as gloves, waterless (alcohol-based) hand cleaner, a stethoscope, and blood pressure cuff in your nursing bag.
- Think about your assignment, and plan your work before arriving at the client's home.
- Organize your supplies and gather everything you will need before beginning.
- Avoid distractions; try to avoid long discussions with family members.
- Call your next client if you are running late.

Time management is somewhat determined by whether you are working an entire shift in one client's home, or if the visit is one of several you will make to various clients during the day. You will have more time and flexibility if you are working an entire shift. However, you should make sure the client's needs are met first, before fulfilling other responsibilities. If you are caring for the client for an entire shift, ask permission to do other things, such as watching television, reading, or doing needlepoint if the client is asleep. Make sure you have taken care of all your duties in the home before you spend time on personal projects. If you are working in the client's home during the night, you should not sleep, even if given permission to do so.

The Client's Family

Family situations are many and varied. Some clients will have other family members living with them in the home. Others may live alone, but have family that live nearby and are involved in their care. Some may have no close family. Although you are responsible for caring for the client, you cannot separate the client from his or her family. However, you must find out if the client wants family members involved in his or her care. You must complete the duties to which you are assigned, and not depend on family members to do them. You must also have the client's permission to release information to family members. The family can be an important source of information for you. They may provide insights that help you give better care. They usually know the client's likes and dislikes.

Remember that you are a guest in the home of the client and family. Do not try to change their routines or lives. Avoid becoming involved in their problems. If there are family issues that may be harmful to the client, inform the supervising nurse.

Be pleasant, courteous, and tactful when dealing with the client's family **(Figure 22-14).** Provide any information that you are permitted to provide, but refer requests for medical information to the nurse. Do not waste time visiting with the family when you are caring for the client. Sometimes family members will ask you to do additional tasks that are not part of your assignment. Whether you can fulfill such a request will depend on:

- The nature of the request
- The time available
- The policies of your agency

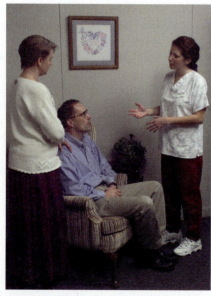

FIGURE 22-14 Treat family members with courtesy, consideration, and tact.

- Whether you are assigned to stay for an entire shift, or if the visit is an intermittent one

If in doubt about a request, consult your agency for further clarification.

REPORTING, DOCUMENTATION, AND RECORDKEEPING

If the client or a family member informs you of new problems with any of the following when no home care worker is on duty, notify your supervisor. Clients with new problems related to these activities require further nursing assessment:

- Eating
- Getting into or out of bed
- Maintaining continence or using the toilet
- Bathing
- Dressing
- Safety

Your agency will provide guidelines for changes in condition that require immediate reporting, such as abnormal vital signs, acute illness, or injuries.

Client Care Records

Client care records (Figure 22-15) are documentation forms that are used for communication and reimbursement purposes. They are a legal record of the care provided. Keeping accurate records is essential. You may not see other home care workers to provide a verbal report, so your written reports provide information about what you did and observations you made. You will be expected to document:

- Care given, such as bathing, positioning, and range-of-motion exercises.
- Observations, such as:
  - vital signs
  - skin condition
  - elimination
  - food and fluid intake
  - incidents
  - changes in condition
  - mental status

Your agency will provide forms and guidelines for documentation.

Time and Travel Records

Time and travel records (Figure 22-16) are reports showing how you spent your time. You will document:

- Time of arrival in the home
- Time of departure

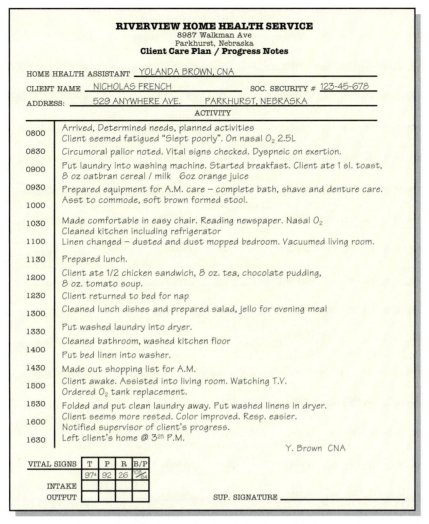

RIVERVIEW HOME HEALTH SERVICE
8987 Walkman Ave
Parkhurst, Nebraska
Client Care Plan / Progress Notes

HOME HEALTH ASSISTANT _YOLANDA BROWN, CNA_

CLIENT NAME _NICHOLAS FRENCH_   SOC. SECURITY # _123-45-678_

ADDRESS: _529 ANYWHERE AVE._   _PARKHURST, NEBRASKA_

ACTIVITY

0800	Arrived, Determined needs, planned activities Client seemed fatigued "Slept poorly". On nasal O_2 2.5L
0830	Circumoral pallor noted. Vital signs checked. Dyspneic on exertion.
0900	Put laundry into washing machine. Started breakfast. Client ate 1 sl. toast, 8 oz oatbran cereal / milk 6oz orange juice
0930	Prepared equipment for A.M. care – complete bath, shave and denture care.
1000	Asst to commode, soft brown formed stool.
1030	Made comfortable in easy chair. Reading newspaper. Nasal O_2 Cleaned kitchen including refrigerator
1100	Linen changed – dusted and dust mopped bedroom. Vacuumed living room.
1130	Prepared lunch.
1200	Client ate 1/2 chicken sandwich, 8 oz. tea, chocolate pudding, 8 oz. tomato soup.
1230	Client returned to bed for nap
1300	Cleaned lunch dishes and prepared salad, jello for evening meal
1330	Put washed laundry into dryer.
1400	Cleaned bathroom, washed kitchen floor Put bed linen into washer.
1430	Made out shopping list for A.M.
1500	Client awake. Assisted into living room. Watching T.V. Ordered O_2 tank replacement.
1530	Folded and put clean laundry away. Put washed linens in dryer.
1600	Client seems more rested. Color improved. Resp. easier. Notified supervisor of client's progress.
1630	Left client's home @ 3^{25} P.M.

Y. Brown CNA

VITAL SIGNS	T	P	R	B/P
	97^4	92	26	108/64
INTAKE				
OUTPUT				SUP. SIGNATURE _____

FIGURE 22-15   A client care record

- Length of time required for specific activities
- Travel time if working in more than one home
- Mileage or transportation costs

Keeping accurate records is very important. Complete the records as you complete each assignment. Do not wait until the end of the day. Your agency may require the client's or family member's signature each day to verify the time and travel record information.

PERSONAL SAFETY

Personal safety is always a concern for home care workers. Before beginning a home care assignment, review the guidelines in Chapter 4 for violence prevention and dealing with violent individuals. Be alert to the conditions and people around you. Inform your employer promptly if you believe unsafe conditions ex-

ist. Thousands of nursing personnel make daily home care visits, and incidents of violence are few. However, you must trust your own instincts. If something does not feel right, it probably isn't.

Auto Insurance

For your own protection and peace of mind, you should insure your vehicle. You should also check with your employer to find out about auto insurance if you are driving your car to and from work, as well as to homes of various clients throughout the work day. You may be surprised to learn that the employer's insurance does not cover you 100% of the time. For example, the policy does not cover you if you have an accident while traveling to or from work and your home. However, it may cover you if you have an accident during the course of your normal work day, when you are

RIVERVIEW HOME HEALTH SERVICE
8987 Walkman Ave
Parkhurst, Nebraska
Time and Travel Log

CARE GIVER NAME _Siadto, Laura CNA_ TITLE _Home Health Assistant_ EMPT. NO. _62718_ DATE _Aug. 29_

CLIENT NAME/ADDRESS (Last, first)	SERVICE PROVIDED	VISIT CODE	NON BILL CODE	TIME IN	TIME OUT	CLIENT CONTACT TIME	ODOMETER READING	MILES
Volheim, Eleonore	Bedbath, Shampoo	4		8^{15}	9^{05}	50 min	From: 45,061 To: 45,068	7 miles
Jaronello, Sharri		1		9^{30}	9^{45}	15 min	From: 45,068 To: 45,083	15 miles
Doyle, Kindra	Enema, bedbath, amb	4		10^{10}	11^{30}	1 hr. 20 min.	From: 45,083 To: 46,001	18 miles
Hammond, Rachel	Ass't c̄ colostomy cath care, bath, ROM	4		11^{50}	1^{20}	1 hr. 30 min.	From: 46,001 To: 46,017	16 miles
Minzey, Aimee		2		1^{30}	1^{35}	—	From: 46,017 To: 46,025	8 miles
Galloway, Rosa		5		1^{50}	2^{00}	10 min	From: 46,025 To: 46,028	3 miles
							From: To:	

Total Visits _6_   Total Mileage _67_   Parking Fees _—_

Visit Code
1 IE Initial Eval & Rx   4 HC Home Care
2 FV Follow Up Visit   5 Hospital/Hospice
3 DV Discharge Visit   6 MC Maternal/Child

Nonbill Code
1. Refused Care
2. Patient Not Home
3. Non-Bill
4. Expired
5. Delivered Supplies

Supervising Nurse: _Bruce Davenport R.N._

FIGURE 22-16 A sample time and travel record

GUIDELINES FOR
Personal Safety

- Wear scrubs or clothing that identifies you as a nursing caregiver.
- Always wear your identification badge.
- Map out the route in advance so you know where you are going.
- Inform the client what time you will be arriving.
- Lock your purse in the trunk of your car at the beginning of your day. Cover it with a blanket so it is not visible. Use a waist belt or fanny pack for essentials such as driver's license and pens.
- Report all real or potential safety problems to your supervisor.
- In potentially dangerous areas, ask your agency if you can make joint visits with a coworker or use an escort.
- If neighbors, relatives, or others become a safety problem, make visits when they are away from the home.
- If a client suggests that a family member escort you, accept the offer if you wish, but never get into someone else's car.
- If the client has a menacing pet, call and ask that it be put away or restrained before your arrival.
- Keep your gas tank full. Keep your vehicle in good condition. Check the tread on the tires frequently.
- Keep your car windows up and doors locked at all times, including when driving.
- Avoid parking on deserted streets or in dark areas.
- Carry your car keys in your hand when you exit the car and when leaving the client's home.
- Carry an extra blanket in the winter and a bottle of water in the summer. Keep a high-protein or nutritious snack, such as peanut butter crackers, in the glove compartment.
- Have your nursing bag or equipment ready to go when you leave the car. Keep an arm free.
- Walk to the home upright, in a professional manner. Be aware of your surroundings. Use common walkways; avoid isolated areas and shortcuts.
- If a dog is threatening, back away. Never turn your back on the animal and run.
- Consider purchasing a cell phone, or carry change for a pay phone in your shoe.
- Attend classes on personal safety and self-defense.

visiting clients' homes. Knowing exactly when your employer's insurance policy covers your automobile is important. You should also find out if you will be expected to transport the client in your personal vehicle. If so, investigate whether your insurance or the employer's insurance will cover the client if you are in an accident. Likewise, find out if you will be expected to drive the client's car. If so, you must learn whose insurance will be responsible in the event of an accident.

KEY POINTS

- Working in home care provides independence and autonomy to health care workers.
- Most home health care is delivered by home care agencies, which employ an entire interdisciplinary team of home care workers.
- Home health care workers may also visit residents in assisted living facilities.
- The home health care nursing assistant's job description lists your duties and responsibilities. Ask questions and clarify if needed. Make sure you understand what is expected.
- The home health care nursing assistant must learn and respect clients' rights.
- The RN will develop the nursing assistant plan of care, describing duties and care that nursing assistants are expected to provide.
- The home health nursing assistant must plan care around client needs and family routines.
- The home health nursing assistant is responsible for maintaining a comfortable, safe, and sanitary home environment.
- Apply the principles of standard precautions and wash your hands frequently.
- The home health nursing assistant must adapt nursing assistant skills and available supplies to provide nursing care in the home.
- Always be alert to unsafe practices, conditions, or situations.
- The home health nursing assistant is responsible for planning his or her assignment and completing it within a designated period of time.
- Think about your assignment, and plan your work before arriving at the client's home.
- The home health nursing assistant is a guest in the client's home.
- Be pleasant, courteous, and tactful when dealing with the client's family.
- If the client or a family member informs you of new problems with eating, getting into or out of bed, maintaining continence or using the bathroom, bathing, dressing, or safety, notify the supervising nurse.
- Client care records are documentation forms that are used for communication and reimbursement purposes.
- Time and travel records are reports showing how you spent your time.
- For personal safety, be alert to the conditions and people around you.

REVIEW

A. Multiple Choice

Select the one best answer.

1. Advantages to working in home health care include
   a. being able to work whenever you want.
   b. the ability to set your own schedule.
   c. the ability to sleep during nighttime assignments.
   d. having independence and the ability to make decisions.

2. The home care nursing assistant is responsible for
   a. doing tasks that are assigned by an RN.
   b. doing whatever he or she thinks should be done.
   c. communicating with the client's physician daily.
   d. advising the client how to run his or her home.

3. Members of the home health care team include all of the following *except*
   a. the client.
   b. a registered nurse.
   c. the client's neighbors.
   d. nursing assistants.

4. Of the areas listed, which is the area in which incidents and injuries most commonly occur?
   a. bathroom
   b. bed
   c. living room
   d. front yard

5. When washing dishes by hand, which item should you wash first?
   a. pots and pans
   b. glasses
   c. silverware
   d. plates

6. If a family member asks you to do an extra task, you should
   a. refuse, because the task is not on your assignment.
   b. always do whatever is asked.
   c. do it, if time is available and agency policies permit.
   d. call the RN supervisor for advice.

7. You will be expected to document all of the following *except*
   a. reasonable family requests.
   b. care given.
   c. food and fluid intake.
   d. mental status.

8. Time and travel records document all of the following *except*
   a. length of time required for specific activities.
   b. time of arrival in the home.
   c. the client's vital signs and appetite.
   d. travel time.

9. When traveling to a home care assignment in an unfamiliar neighborhood, you should
   a. stop at a convenience store or gas station to ask for directions.
   b. map out the route in advance so you know where to go.
   c. drive around the neighborhood until you find the house.
   d. ask the home care agency to provide an escort on the first visit.

10. Protect your personal safety when making home care visits by
    a. carrying essential items in a fanny pack and putting your purse in the car trunk.
    b. wearing street clothes to the client's residence, then changing into your uniform.
    c. asking the client's family to stand outside to watch for your arrival.
    d. asking a friend or relative to accompany you on the home visit.

B. True/False

Answer each statement true (T) or false (F).

11. _____ Inform your employer promptly if you believe that unsafe conditions exist in a home care assignment.

12. _____ If something related to personal safety doesn't feel right, it probably isn't.

13. _____ Frozen meat should be thawed by placing the package on the kitchen counter.

14. _____ Home care workers may also visit residents in assisted living facilities.

15. _____ Refrigerate leftovers within 4 hours of use.

16. _____ The home health nursing assistant is not expected to clean the kitchen or bathroom.

17. _____ Plan your work before arriving at the client's home.

C. Clinical Applications

18. You have been offered a position as a nursing assistant at a long term care facility and a home health care agency. You cannot decide which job to choose. Make a list of the advantages and disadvantages of both jobs that will help you make a decision.

    You care for Mr. Johnson every morning. The client lives alone in an apartment. He is only 46 years old. He had a stroke, and has right hemiplegia. You must prepare his breakfast, assist with his bath, tidy the apartment and do light cleaning, and prepare a light lunch for the client to eat after you leave. Answer the following questions regarding this client.

19. Mr. Johnson tells you he fell last night when he was alone, but was not injured. He was able to get off the floor with the help of a neighbor. He asks you not to report the incident because he fears that his family will find out and have him put in a nursing home. What will you do?

20. Mr. Johnson tells you he has run out of blood pressure pills. He asks you to pick them up at the drug store two blocks away before you leave for the day. This is not on your assignment. What will you do?

CHAPTER 23

Employment Opportunities

OBJECTIVES

After reading this chapter, you will be able to:

- Spell and define key terms.
- List four things you can do to improve your chances of success in finding a job.
- Demonstrate how to prepare a resume.
- List the six components of the resume.
- List nine sources of job leads.
- Describe things you should do to ensure a successful interview.
- List at least eight things you should do after you begin work to demonstrate that you are a responsible employee.

FINDING A POSITION

Many career opportunities are available in long-term care for a qualified nursing assistant. You must choose the setting in which you feel most comfortable working. Long-term care facilities, assisted living centers, subacute units, and other health care facilities hire people with your education and skills.

Finding a job is a full-time job. You must wake up early and set a time to begin looking for work. It may be helpful to list activities to do to look for a job. Apply for jobs early in the day. This makes a good impression and gives you enough time to fill out applications, take tests, or have **interviews.** An interview is a formal meeting in which the employer assesses the qualifications of an applicant and provides information about the job opening. Applying at several facilities in the same area will help you organize your time and save time and travel.

Be prepared when looking for a job. Bring pens and pencils, papers, a map, reference information, and your resume with you. You will also need a photo identification, such as a driver's license, and your social security card. If you have completed the nursing assistant program, bring a copy of your certificate and state certification.

Follow up on all job leads right away. If you hear of a job opening late in the day, call and schedule an appointment for the next day. **Network** with your friends and relatives. Networking involves communicating with people you know who have similar careers, interests, and goals. Tell everyone you know that you are looking for a job. Ask them to tell you about positions they are aware of.

Determining Your Job Skills and Experience

Before looking for a position, make a listing of your background, experience, and job skills **(Figure 23-1).** This includes previous employers, even if you were not employed in the health care field. List names, addresses, and phone numbers of former employers and people you will list as **references.** These are individuals who will recommend you to the employer for the job you are seeking. Before listing a person as a reference, call the person and get permission to use his or her name. Also list work experience you have gained as a homemaker, volunteer, or student, or in hobbies and other personal activities. A **resume** is a summary of your professional or work experience and qualifications. You will use your list to develop a resume, fill out

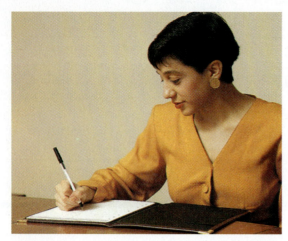

FIGURE 23-1 Your personal assessment will help you develop a resume.

TABLE 23-1	Sample list of interests and aptitudes
Activity or Interest	**Skill, Knowledge, and Talent Required**
Homemaking skills	Manage budgets Manage many priorities at one time Knowledge of human growth and development Child care Cooking Cleaning Laundry
Playing softball	Ability to function as a team player Use of basic math to keep track of scores Physical coordination, strength, and agility Ability to direct and teach others
Teaching Sunday school	Strong moral code Ability to teach and direct others Leadership skills Good reading and writing ability Dependability Ability to honor a commitment Desire to serve others Compassion
Babysitting	Knowledge of human growth and development Food preparation, cooking Cleaning Dependability Knowledge of household management Basic first aid Child care Patience

job applications, and provide information for job interviews.

Interest and Aptitudes. No one is going to see your list but you, so write down everything you can think of. List hobbies, clubs, sports participation, school activities, church activities, volunteer work, and other interests. Then list your personal qualities and special abilities **(Table 23-1).** This list may appear to have nothing to do with job experience, but it will give you an idea of your abilities.

After you have listed your interests and activities, list your full- and part-time work experience. List all work that you have done, including self employment and summer jobs. Next think about the skills it took to do these jobs. Write them down. **Table 23-2** shows you how to turn this list into useful job information.

Education. List all schools you have attended. Begin with your high school. Add any college, military training, vocational education, and on-the-job training. List your degrees, certificates, awards, and honors. List the date you completed your nursing assistant program, the address and phone number of the agency where you took your course, the instructor's name, and a list of skills you are proficient in.

Physical Condition. Ask yourself if you have any physical problems that could interfere with the type of work you do. For example, if you have a back problem, you may not want to work in a care setting that requires frequent, heavy lifting. Some care settings require more strenuous physical ability than others.

Personal Circumstances. Ask yourself what limits you wish to set as to the location or hours of work you will accept. How far are you willing to travel? Do you have a car, or will you depend on public transportation? If you are depending on public transportation, what hours is it available? Do you need a babysitter for your children while you are at work? What time is the babysitter available? Are there any other circumstances in your life that would affect your attendance and dependability at a job?

Career Goals. What kind of work do you want to be doing in 10 years? What type of job will help you reach this goal?

TABLE 23-2 Work Experiences and Skills	
Work Duties	**Skills and Talents**
Picked fruits and vegetables on a farm	Can accept supervision Inspect fruits and vegetables for damage Endurance Ability to bend, stoop, squat, and lift Ability to work with hands Ability to work in extreme temperatures Use of garden tools and small equipment Ability to plant vegetables and fruits Attention to detail
Waitress in a restaurant	Ability to manage many priorities at one time Pleasant personality Ability to keep customers satisfied Desire to serve others Use of basic math skills to calculate restaurant bills Operation of cash register and making change Knowledge of sanitary food service and preparation Ability to bend, lift, and carry heavy trays Ability to stand for long periods of time Ability to follow directions
Cashier in a convenience store	Trustworthiness Honesty Dependability Basic math skills to count money Stocking shelves Maintaining inventory Ability to deal with the public Ability to work with difficult customers Ability to operate cash register and other electrical equipment Ability to stand for long periods of time Ability to bend and lift heavy boxes

Matching your Background and Experience to a Job. Look at the skills, talents, and abilities you listed. Find out what types of jobs match these abilities. Your textbook provides an overview of the responsibilities of the nursing assistant in different settings. You can also find information in the public library. The U.S. Department of Labor publishes books that describe work duties, skills and abilities required, how to enter an occupation, where jobs are located, earnings, work conditions, and future opportunities. Your state employment commission office also has valuable information and free publications about many different jobs and careers. Match your skills, talents, abilities, needs, and interests to the jobs listed. This will give you an idea of the type of job that will best meet your needs.

PREPARING A RESUME

The next step to finding a job is to prepare a resume. Use the list you developed of your talents, abilities, interests, and jobs to help you prepare your resume. A resume should be typed or prepared on a computer **(Figure 23-2)**. There are many computer programs available to assist you. There are also professional services that will prepare your resume for a reasonable cost. Your resume and cover letter should be printed on good quality paper. Avoid listing personal information such as race, age, gender, height, weight, national origin, marital or family status, and religion. Your completed resume should be as concise as possible. One or two pages is best. After you have completed your resume, proofread it for errors and make corrections. Then make one copy of the resume and check the photocopy for stray marks. If the photocopy is clear, print additional copies to distribute to potential employers.

The Seven Components of a Resume

Your resume should be clearly and concisely written. The resume represents you, so you want

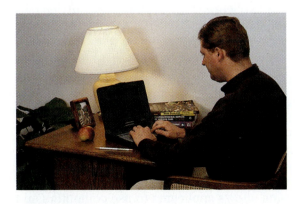

FIGURE 23-2 Use a computer or typewriter to prepare your resume.

it to appear as professional as possible. There are seven components to the resume:

1. The **cover letter** is a business letter of introduction. It should be written in business letter format and be no more than one page long. A cover letter is sent each time you send a resume. The cover letter should state the position you are applying for. Emphasize why your qualifications meet the requirements of the position. In the cover letter, state that you have enclosed your resume and request to schedule an interview.

2. The first section of your resume consists of a section of **personal data.** This includes your name, address, phone number, and professional license or certification number.

3. The next section is the **job objective.** This section of your resume lists the type of position you are seeking and states how your ability and skills qualify you for this position.

4. Next, list your educational background. Begin with high school, and list all education after high school. Include trade or vocational school, college, and continuing education classes. List when and where you went to school and degrees or certificates you earned.

5. **Extracurricular activities** may be listed with your educational background or may be listed separately. These include clubs, hobbies, volunteer work, and other special interests.

6. After you have completed the preliminary information listed above, list your employment. Begin by listing your most recent employer first. This is called **reverse chronological order.** List all employers in this format, even if the job was not in the health care field. Add another page if necessary.

7. After you have listed your previous employers, list at least three references. These should be people who know you well, but who are not relatives. Remember to contact them to ask permission before listing them. List two work-related references and one personal reference.

SEARCHING FOR A JOB

There are many places to get leads for your job search. A good place to begin is with your state job service or employment commission. Many employers list job openings with this agency. There is no cost for employment commission services. In some states, the employment commission allows applicants to use computers and fax machines in their offices to prepare and send resumes. Use all the resources available in your community.

Sources of Job Leads

Leads and referrals for jobs come from many different places. Investigate all the sources listed and others you know of in your community. Some potential sources of job leads are:

- The long-term care facility in which you completed the clinical portion of your nursing assistant class.
- Private employers. Look in the Yellow Pages for employers in your area. Contact employers directly to inquire about employment opportunities. Talk to the person who would supervise you, even if there are no openings now.
- Federal, state, and local government personnel offices list a wide range of employment opportunities in health care facilities operated by the government.
- Public libraries may post job announcements.
- Newspaper ads list many career opportunities. Although the want ads appear in the paper every day, the Sunday edition usually lists the most employment ads.
- Private and temporary employment agencies may have temporary, permanent, or fill-in positions available. Sometimes temporary work through an agency leads to full-time employment.
- Community colleges and trade schools may list employment opportunities on their bulletin board, or may have a job placement office.
- Community organizations, such as clubs, associations, or women's and minority centers may list jobs available in their newsletters or on the bulletin board.
- Community newsletters may list job openings.
- The Internet is a potential source of information. However, never divulge personal data, such as your social security number, to anyone online, including a potential employer.

Completing Job Applications

Call potential employers early in the day. This sends a message that you are up and ready for work. Identify yourself and inquire about available positions. Do not ask about money on the telephone. Many employers will ask you to come to the facility and complete an application.

When you fill out an **application,** take your resume or list with you. An application is the employer's form on which employment information is written. It is acceptable to attach a copy of

Sample Interview Questions
Question: Tell me about yourself.
Answer: Briefly outline your strengths. Concentrate on your education and professional achievements. Avoid discussing marriage, family, and your personal life.
Question: Describe your qualifications for this job.
Answer: Describe your most recent education and experience. List your strongest skills and talents relating to job performance.
Question: Why do you want this job?
Answer: Know something about the employer and say something positive about the company. Avoid using money as the reason you want the position.
Question: Tell me about your last job.
Answer: Describe your duties and responsibilities. Discuss skills that apply to the position for which you are applying.
Question: Why did you leave your last job?
Answer: Be honest, but avoid making negative comments about your previous employer.
Question: Tell me about your goals and ambitions.
Answer: State that you look forward to learning new things, accepting challenges, and taking on new responsibilities. State your career goals.
Question: What are your strengths?
Answer: Describe strong personal qualities such as honesty, dependability, and caring about other people.
Question: What are your weaknesses?
Answer: Mention weaknesses or problems, but state how you have learned and grown from them.

FIGURE 23-3 Have a friend ask you typical interview questions so you can practice your presentation and gain confidence in your answers.

your resume to the form. Having your resume and other information with you will save time and make a good impression on the employer. Read the directions on the application carefully. Fill it out completely in ink. Be neat. A messy application sends a negative message. Avoid leaving blank spaces. Fill out all information. If something on the application does not apply, put *N/A* (not applicable) in the space rather than leaving it blank. List all of your previous employers, even if they were not in health care. If you skip an employer, it looks as if you are hiding something. If a question asks for a narrative answer, plan ahead. Briefly and concisely give the answer. Use only the number of words necessary to fill the space. Check your spelling.

Job Interview

After you have investigated job leads and completed applications, an employer may contact

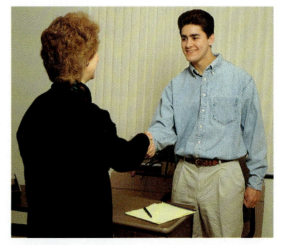

FIGURE 23-4 A firm handshake sends a positive message about you.

you to schedule an interview. You will be given a date and time to meet. The interview is very important. Most hiring decisions are made during the interview. How you present yourself in the interview is as important as your education, experience, and ability to do the job.

Preparing for the Interview. Before the interview, learn as much as you can about the facility, the job available, and how your previous experience and education qualify you for the position. Write down the things you will need to complete an application, if you have not done this already. Have a friend ask you interview questions **(Figure 23-3).** Take a copy of your resume, class certificate, and state certification. You will also need to take your social security card and driver's license, or another picture identification with you. Take your CPR card, if you have one.

Dress correctly for the interview. Your appearance is very important and helps you make a positive first impression. The first impression you make is visual. Be neat, clean, and well groomed. Do not overdress, but avoid looking too casual. Turn off your cell phone or leave it in the car.

The Interview. Go to the interview alone. Arrange for babysitters and transportation ahead of time. Arrive a few minutes early so you have time before the interview to fill out an application and other required information. When you are introduced to the interviewer, shake hands **(Figure 23-4).** Practice shaking hands with your friends so that you have a steady, firm handshake. This sends a message that you have a healthy self-esteem. A weak, limp handshake may send a negative message. Make good eye contact with the interviewer. Your eyes should send a message such as "I like you." Be aware of your posture and the message you are sending through your body language. Stand until you are invited to sit. Try to find common ground with the interviewer. This will make you both more comfortable. Pictures, books, plants, and other items in the interviewer's office make good conversation starters. Express your interest in the job, using the information you gathered when you prepared for the interview. Let the interviewer direct the conversation. Answer questions clearly and concisely. Show how your experience and education will make you a valuable employee. Speak positively of former employers. Making negative comments about a previous employer is not a good practice.

Listen carefully to the interview questions and be sure you understand them before answering. If you do not understand, ask for clarification. Your answers to questions should reflect your positive features. Avoid discussing negative traits unless you are specifically asked to do so. Be honest with the interviewer. It is easier to defend the truth than it is to be caught in a lie. Avoid discussing your personal life or financial problems.

Discussing Salary and Benefits. Discussing salary and benefits can be a sensitive issue. Asking questions about them early in the process gives the employer the impression that you are not interested in working at the facility, but are, instead, shopping for the highest salary available. This sends a negative message. Save discussions about salary and benefits for late in the interview. Let the employer lead into them. If the interviewer has not discussed salary and benefits by the end of the interview, it is appropriate to ask.

Closing the Interview. If the interviewer does not offer you a position or say when a decision will be made, ask when you may call to find out about it. **Figure 23-5** lists reasons employers have given for not hiring applicants. If the interviewer asks you to call back at a certain time or return for another interview, note the date, time, and place. If the job is offered to you, make sure you understand the terms and conditions before accepting it. Do not accept a position if you cannot fulfill the responsibilities. For example, if the employer offers you a position on the 10 p.m. to 6 a.m. shift, and you do not have a babysitter during these hours, arrange for a babysitter before accepting the position. Thank the employer for the interview and reaffirm your interest in the job. Close the interview with a firm handshake.

1. Poor appearance (not dressed properly, poorly groomed).
2. Acting like a know-it-all.
3. Cannot express self clearly; poor voice, diction, grammar.
4. Lack of planning for work—no purpose or goals.
5. Lack of confidence or poise.
6. No interest in or enthusiasm for the job.
7. Not active in school extracurricular programs.
8. Interested only in the best dollar offer.
9. Poor school record (academic, attendance).
10. Unwilling to start at the bottom.
11. Making excuses, hedges on unfavorable record.
12. No tact.
13. Not mature.
14. No curiosity about the job.
15. Critical of past employers.

FIGURE 23-5 Employers listed reasons for not hiring a job applicant. The reasons are listed from 1 (most important reason for not hiring the person) to 15 (least important reason).

After the Interview. Use the interview as a learning experience. Make a list of ways you can improve for your next interview. Have a friend ask you the interview questions again. Practice your answers until you are comfortable. Write the interviewer a short, personal note thanking him or her for the interview.

In some states, employers are required by law to conduct a criminal history check on the background of each applicant. This background check will show if the applicant has ever been arrested. In these states, if an individual has been convicted of certain crimes, he or she cannot work in a long-term care facility.

Many employers require applicants to pass a physical examination and undergo drug testing before hire. An initial tuberculin test may also be performed prior to allowing an individual to work in the long-term care facility.

KEEPING A JOB

After you have accepted a position, remember that honesty and dependability are very important qualities. Arrive for work on time, in proper uniform, and be prepared to work. Punch the time clock in and out on time **(Figure 23-6).** Your paycheck depends on an accurate record of the time worked. Never ask another employee to clock in or out for you. Follow your facility policies and procedures. Maintain a positive attitude and be willing to learn new things. Avoid bringing

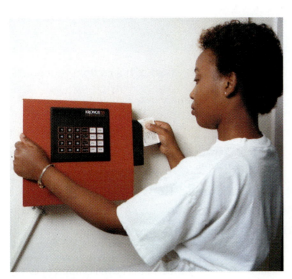

FIGURE 23-6 Clock in and out on time.

your personal problems to work. Be willing to help others and do extra tasks without being asked. Good attendance is very important. Be at work when you are scheduled and avoid calling in sick unless you are ill. If you will be unable to work your next scheduled shift, notify your facility as far in advance as possible so they can find a replacement.

Review the desirable qualities of the nursing assistant, listed in Chapter 1. It may have been several months since you studied these. List each point on a piece of paper and review it daily after you begin employment. The list will serve as a reminder for you of things you should do to become a valuable employee.

Continue to Learn and Grow

Learn all you can about your role and responsibilities. Ask appropriate questions of the nurse, staff development director, and others. Read nursing and medical journals and literature. Medical books are also available from the public library. Attend continuing education classes at your facility and in your community. You must attend at least 12 hours of continuing education classes a year to maintain your nursing assistant certification. Your state may have additional continuing education requirements.

RESIGN PROPERLY

If resignation from your position becomes necessary, always leave on a positive note. Your work record follows you, so you must give proper notice of resignation. Each agency has policies on length of resignation notice. It is generally two weeks, or the length of one pay period. Write a formal letter of resignation to your director of nursing or other supervisor, and list the reasons for your resignation. Even if you are unhappy or dissatisfied, the tone of the letter should be positive. State what your last date of employment will be. (Make sure that you work through that day and avoid calling in sick during the resignation notice.) Thank your nurse manager for the opportunity to learn and grow at the long-term care facility.

KEY POINTS

- There are many employment opportunities for nursing assistants.
- Finding a job is a full-time job.
- The best time to look for a job is early in the day.
- It is helpful to list your skills, activities, background, and experience before preparing your resume.
- Your resume should appear as professional as possible and accurately reflect your education, experience, skills, and interests.
- Information such as race, age, gender, height, weight, national origin, marital and family status, and religion should not be listed on your resume.
- The state employment commission, private employers, government personnel offices, public libraries, newspaper ads, employment agencies, colleges and trade schools, clubs, newsletters, friends, and relatives are all sources of potential job leads.
- Present a professional appearance when you arrive for a job interview.
- Honesty, dependability, and a positive attitude are important characteristics of the nursing assistant.
- This class is just the beginning of your education; you will continue to learn and grow throughout your health care career.
- If resignation is necessary, always give proper notice to the employer.

REVIEW

A. Multiple Choice

Select the one best answer.

1. When searching for a job, you should bring:
   a. phone book.
   b. newspapers.
   c. reference information.
   d. a uniform.

2. Before seeking a job, you must consider
   a. what limits you have as to hours and location of the employer.
   b. only those facilities that pay the most.
   c. the work you are willing to do.
   d. where your friends work.

3. Sources of job information include
   a. magazines.
   b. the state employment commission.
   c. the grapevine.
   d. direct mailings.

4. Your resume should be
   a. neatly written in pencil.
   b. typed or prepared on a computer.
   c. written with carbon copies.
   d. typed in red ink.

5. When mailing your resume to a potential employer, you should include a
   a. self-addressed, stamped envelope.
   b. copy of the want ad in which the job was advertised.
   c. cover letter.
   d. personal note stating why you need a job.

6. The personal data section of your resume should include your
   a. name.
   b. religion.
   c. age.
   d. gender.

7. Which of the following is true about a job interview?
   a. The interviewee should dress very casually.
   b. First impressions are important.
   c. Body language is not important.
   d. A handshake should be weak and limp.

8. When you are invited into the interviewer's office, you should
   a. stand until you are invited to sit.
   b. shake hands with the interviewer only if asked.
   c. avoid eye contact with the interviewer.
   d. ask about salary right away.

9. It is acceptable to ask about salary
   a. on the telephone before making an application with an employer.
   b. at the beginning of the interview.
   c. at the end of the interview.
   d. when the employer calls you to schedule an interview.

10. If it becomes necessary to resign from your position, you should
    a. give proper notice of resignation.
    b. call the employer and tell him or her that you are not coming back.
    c. not return to work.
    d. tell a coworker to inform your employer of your resignation.

B. Clinical Applications

Answer the following questions.

11. You learned how to use the computer when you were in high school. However, you do not have a computer or typewriter on which to prepare your resume. None of your friends have computers or typewriters. Should you write your resume by hand? What other alternatives can you think of?

12. Summerville Care Center has offered you a position available on the 2 p.m. to 10 p.m. shift. You really need a job and would like to work at this facility. You must let the director of nursing know if you will accept the position within the next two days. However, you do not have a babysitter after 6 p.m. What can you do?

13. You have a job interview scheduled at the Meadows Nursing Facility in 30 minutes. When you try to start your car, you find that the battery is dead. You will have to call someone to jump-start your car. You will not be able to make it to the interview on time. What should you do?

14. You are scheduled for your second day of orientation at Brown's Nursing Center. Your daughter has a temperature of 103°F. The day care center will not accept her if she is sick, and you cannot find someone to babysit for her. What will you do?

15. You have worked at Brown's Nursing Center for five months. The director of nursing at Cedars Long-Term Care Facility calls you at home. You interviewed with the director prior to accepting the job at Brown's, but she did not hire you. The director informs you that she now has a position available and offers you $0.15 an hour more than you make at your present job. She tells you that you must start work tomorrow. What will you do?

CHAPTER 24

Surviving a Survey

OBJECTIVES

After reading this chapter, you will be able to:

- Spell and define key terms.
- Describe the types of things that surveyors will observe during a long-term care facility survey.
- Identify what JCAHO surveyors are looking for and describe what is meant by an "outcome oriented" survey.
- List facility policy and procedure information that you should learn about the long-term care facility where you work.
- Describe how to provide resident care that complies with accepted standards of practice.

QUALITY ASSURANCE

All long-term care facilities have a program called **quality assurance (QA).** Some facilities call this program *Continuous Quality Improvement (CQI).* You may be asked to participate on the quality assurance committee. The purpose of quality assurance is to conduct internal reviews to identify problems and find solutions for improvement. The quality assurance committee meets periodically to evaluate care provided and practices in the facility. Restraint use, infections, pressure ulcers, and infection control are some of the areas commonly reviewed. Committee members will audit practices related to these topics on each unit and make recommendations to administration to improve care. Resident care should be continuously reevaluated by the facility and adjusted to meet resident needs. The quality assurance program performs this important function.

OBRA standards state that all nursing assistants must be competent in their responsibilities. The facility is required to periodically evaluate staff competence and maintain a record of these checks. In some facilities, the quality assurance committee participates in evaluating staff competence.

The quality assurance committee is very important to the operation of the facility and success of facility surveys. The committee identifies problems and corrects them. This self-improvement process prevents problems with regulatory agencies and improves the quality of care delivered.

SURVEY PROCESS

Long-term care facilities must meet certain quality standards to operate. A **survey** is a review and evaluation to ensure that facilities are maintaining acceptable standards of practice. Many different agencies establish quality standards for long-term care facilities. Different types of facilities meet different levels of quality inspection standards. The facility holds a state **license,** which permits it to conduct business. Some facilities also possess a **certification.** Certification is necessary to collect Medicare and Medicaid money. Licensure and certification surveys are done by your state health department or human service agency. During a survey, a number of **surveyors** inspect conditions in the facility. Surveyors are representatives of the agency that reviews the long-term care facility, and they make recommendations to that agency.

Sometimes the **Centers for Medicare and Medicaid Services (CMS)** conducts the survey. This agency is a division of the federal government with regulatory authority over health care facilities that receive federal money. Some long-term care facilities are also accredited. **Accreditation** is a voluntary process that health care facilities undergo to ensure that they are meeting high-quality standards. Gaining accreditation is difficult, but very prestigious.

Many different governmental and private agencies survey long-term care facilities. Surveyors review every area of the facility. They observe resident care, staff preparation and education, recordkeeping, infection control, food preparation, and facility cleanliness. They also review facility policies and procedures. The purpose of a survey is to review quality of care, quality of life, and resident rights. Surveys identify specific areas in which care is deficient. Surveyors are instructed not to be consultants to the facility. They are only responsible for identifying deficiencies. The facility is responsible for finding ways to correct the problems.

Survey Preparation

So many agencies survey long-term care facilities that it is impossible to prepare for a survey. Surveyors arrive at the facility unannounced. There are laws that provide for severe penalties or jail terms for individuals who alert the facility to an impending licensure, certification, or OSHA survey. Surveyors want to see resident care and facility routines on a normal day. Knowing this, we must be ready for a survey every day. This means that care is delivered in the manner in which you were taught and that good infection control techniques are practiced routinely. A **deficiency** is a written notice of inadequate care or substandard practices. Infection control problems are a major cause of deficiencies in long-term care facility surveys. Surveyors receive a great deal of education in infection control so they can easily identify deficiencies in this area. The reason that so much emphasis is placed on infection prevention practices is because the spread of infection to residents, visitors, and workers can be very serious.

Type, Frequency, and Length of Long-Term Care Surveys

Long-term care facilities have a regular licensure (and certification, if applicable) visit every 9 to 15 months. Surveyors in some states also visit the facility periodically to evaluate the care that Medicaid recipients receive. This survey is commonly called *inspection of care*. Surveyors return after an annual survey to check to see if corrections have been made. They also visit facilities in response to complaint calls from residents and families. Long-term care facilities are required to post the state complaint line number **(Figure 24-1)** in a visible location so residents and family members can call if they are dissatisfied with care. Because of the many different types of surveys in long-term care, most facilities have two or more surveys a year. Surveyors come to the long-term care facility unannounced and spend up to a week. The length of time spent in the facility is determined by facility size and the nature of deficiencies noted during the first few days of the visit. If the facility is very large or if the nature of deficiencies is severe, the surveyors will remain in the facility for a longer period of time. When surveyors remain in the facility longer than originally anticipated, this is known as an **extended survey.** During an extended survey, surveyors

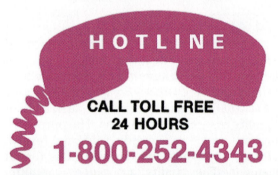

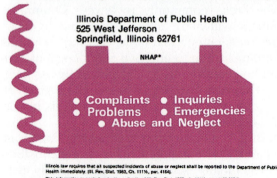

FIGURE 24-1 A state complaint line poster must be posted in a prominent location. (*Courtesy of Illinois Department of Public Health*)

will examine deficient areas in great detail to determine if a danger to residents exists.

TYPICAL LONG–TERM CARE SURVEY

Surveyors have a format that they follow during most surveys, regardless of the type of survey they are conducting. The format may vary slightly depending on the circumstances of the survey, but you can expect the surveyors to do basically the same things each time they visit the facility.

Entrance Conference

When surveyors arrive at the facility, they usually conduct an **entrance conference** with facility administration. During this meeting, surveyors inform management of the reason for the survey and the nature of any complaints received. If the survey is in response to a complaint, they do not identify the person who registered the complaint. One surveyor may conduct the entrance conference while others go directly to the nursing units to make rounds and observe care. Splitting into groups like this prevents staff from correcting problems before the survey begins. Surveyors want to see the care as it is really given on a normal day. There may be very little preparation time from the moment surveyors arrive until they make rounds on the resident units. This is another reason why you should be survey-ready every day.

Initial Facility Tour

During the initial tour of the facility, surveyors will make observations of residents and facility conditions. They write down information, then go back later and examine certain residents and conditions in greater detail. Surveyors will focus on the issues listed in **Table 24-1** and will identify residents for closer evaluation.

The first round has a major impact on the survey process. If conditions are not acceptable or problems are suspected, surveyors will probably go immediately into the extended survey mode. This is an indication that surveyors think conditions in the facility are not up to par. At the very least, the facility will lose the ability to offer nursing assistant education for two full years, even if no major deficiencies are written during the survey. An extended survey always results in the loss of ability to teach nursing assistant classes, so this can have a very negative effect on the operation of the facility.

TABLE 24-1 Survey issues

Quality of Resident Life

- Residents are dressed appropriately
- Residents have appropriate footwear
- The way staff talk to and interact with residents
- How staff respond to resident requests
- Availability and receptiveness of staff to meet resident needs
- Scheduled activities and appropriateness of activities in meeting resident needs

Emotional and Behavioral Conduct of Residents

- How staff respond and react to residents
- How staff meet resident needs
- Resident behavior problems and how these behaviors are addressed by staff
- How promptly staff respond to resident needs

Quality of Resident Care

- Skin condition, including pressure ulcers, rashes, excessive wetness, dry skin
- Skin tears, bruises, or injuries
- Availability of fresh drinking water and assistance with drinking given residents
- Signs and symptoms of dehydration, including dry skin, appearance of urine in drainage bags, dry mucous membranes and lips
- Clinical problems such as edema, contractures, underweight or emaciated appearance, significant weight loss
- Resident positioning, use of pillows, props, handrolls, footboards, and other devices
- Presence and prevalence of all types of infections
- Proper use of standard precautions and good handwashing
- Use of feeding tubes and position of residents when feeding is infusing
- Special care issues, such as ventilators, IV therapy, use of oxygen
- Amputations

Facility Environment and Safety

- Infection control
- Functional, clean, sanitary
- Free from hazards
- Homelike and clean
- Effectiveness of environment in meeting resident needs

Notifications and Interviews

During the long-term care facility survey, a sign is posted on the door advising all who enter that the facility is undergoing a survey. Surveyors will question staff, residents, and families. Anyone who wishes to may speak with the surveyors.

Surveyors will also interview alert residents and conduct a resident council meeting in which they will question residents in detail about facility conditions.

Evaluation of Assessment and Care Planning

The OBRA survey process is designed to ensure favorable resident outcomes. The law requires the facility to complete a comprehensive assessment (MDS) for each resident. Care is planned based on this assessment. Risk factors for changes in condition should be identified, anticipated in advance, and avoided whenever possible. Remember that the OBRA legislation requires long-term care facilities to maintain or improve resident conditions unless medical complications make this impossible. If residents have experienced declines, this may indicate problems in the facility. Surveyors will review assessments, care plans, and preventive practices to ensure that residents' conditions have not declined.

Meal Service

A major emphasis of the survey is focused on meal service and food preparation. The entire survey team will observe food preparation and delivery in different areas of the building. Serving food at the proper temperature and providing adequate mealtime assistance are important. Surveyors will monitor pre- and post-meal grooming and hygiene, sanitary food service practices, food temperature, infection control, and how facility staff care for residents who are incontinent during meals. Surveyors will observe staff feeding residents and will evaluate feeding technique for safety, infection control, and how well staff interact with residents during the meal.

Staff Preparation and Education

Staff preparation, education, and inservice records are reviewed. Surveyors will verify nursing licenses and nursing assistant certifications to make sure they are active and in good standing. They will verify that facility staff have completed the required number of continuing education hours each year.

Other Aspects of the Survey

Surveyors will also evaluate use of restraints, the prevention, development, and treatment of pressure ulcers, resident hygiene and grooming, and correct use of catheters. They will monitor infection control practices, communication skills, and general facility cleanliness.

Surveyors also examine incident reports and evaluate how well the staff protects resident rights. Resident quality of life is reviewed to ensure that the staff is meeting both physical and psychosocial needs. The OBRA legislation requires long-term care facilities to maintain a homelike environment and accommodate resident needs as much as possible. The nursing assistant does a great deal to maintain a homelike quality in the environment and to accommodate resident needs. Surveyors will check to ensure that facilities comply with these requirements. A great emphasis of the survey is an evaluation of how well staff members respect resident rights.

ROLE OF THE NURSING ASSISTANT DURING A SURVEY

The nursing assistant has many important responsibilities in providing direct resident care. View the survey as a positive experience. A survey is an opportunity for you to demonstrate work well done! Surveyors will observe your care and may ask you questions. You would feel terrible if your actions resulted in facility punishment, loss of approval, or fines. The best way to prevent this from happening is to take your responsibilities very seriously, follow all facility policies, and always perform procedures the way you were taught. Using good work practices every day is easier than trying to remember the correct way to do things at the time of a survey. When you know surveyors are in your facility, smile and say hello to them **(Figure 24-2)** if you pass them in the hallway. Surveyors are guests in your facility, and should be treated as such. If a surveyor asks you a particular resident's name, inform the nurse. Asking for the name indicates that surveyors are watching some aspect of that resident's care.

During the long-term care facility survey, you will be observed while you are providing direct resident care. Respecting resident rights is very important. Even if you are nervous, introduce the surveyor to the resident and explain the purpose of the surveyor's visit. Always explain the care you are going to perform and give the resident an opportunity to ask questions, even if the resident is confused. Your documentation of the resident's care on the flow sheets and medical record will be reviewed. This is one of the reasons why accurate daily documentation is so im-

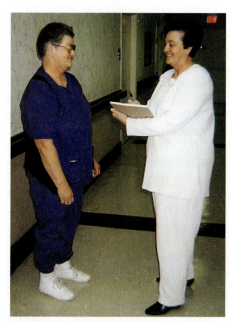

FIGURE 24-2 Speak to the surveyors and treat them as guests in your facility.

portant. You cannot repair incomplete or inadequate documentation at the time of a survey, or any other time. You would be very embarrassed if a surveyor questioned you about incomplete or incorrect documentation, and this can cause your facility to receive a deficiency.

Surveyors will ask you questions about the care you give. They are checking to see if you are following facility policies and procedures. Be proud of your knowledge of the residents, facil-

ity policies, and procedures. When surveyors question you, remain calm and try to figure out why they are asking a particular question. Always be honest, but do not volunteer information unrelated to the question. Surveyors review resident care plans in advance, so they know if the care you provide is in keeping with the care plan. You must be familiar with the goals and approaches listed on each resident's plan of care.

Attendance During a Survey

Having surveyors watch you can be very stressful and frightening. Don't call in sick without reason if you know surveyors are in the facility. Trying to replace staff during a survey is difficult for everyone. Facility administration, your co-workers, and residents are depending on you, and having a full staff is important. If nursing assistants call in sick, care suffers if replacement workers are not available. Short staffing increases everyone's stress, and may cause a negative outcome on the survey.

Survey Completion

Upon completion of a survey, surveyors conduct an **exit conference.** During this conference, facility management is given the survey agency's findings and advised of the nature of deficiencies. A formal written report is mailed to the facility after the survey. This report lists the deficiencies the facility receives. Facilities must post the report in a

GUIDELINES FOR
Surviving a Long-Term Care Facility Survey

- Know your residents well.
- Know what care is stated on the care plan and deliver it.
- Know facility policies and procedures well and practice them daily.
- Practice good handwashing, standard precautions, medical asepsis, and infection control techniques. Remember that infection control is a major area of deficiencies.
- Use gloves when necessary. Dispose of them according to facility policy, and avoid contaminating environmental surfaces with your gloves.
- Make sure to meet the needs of dependent and incontinent residents promptly. Unmet needs are another common area of deficiencies.
- Always try to anticipate problems, such as resident falls, and take measures to prevent them.

- Keep your work area neat and clean at all times.
- Cooperate with your facility quality assurance department in pre-survey reviews and audits.
- Communicate with all residents during care, even if the resident has a cognitive impairment. Always explain procedures before you do them.
- Respect all resident rights.
- Give residents as much control over daily routines as possible.
- Know your facility emergency codes, policies, and procedures.
- Because you can never fully prepare for a survey, make inservice education a part of your life. The more you learn, the better prepared you are.

prominent location. The facility is given a designated amount of time to correct deficiencies. The facility must submit a written **plan of correction** to the survey agency. Surveyors may write two types of deficiencies. Resident-centered deficiencies are violations of requirements that must be met for each resident, such as failure to prevent pressure ulcers, protect dignity, or adequately assess residents. Facility-centered deficiencies are general system problems, such as lack of an adequate infection control program or inadequate staffing. The plan of correction for resident-centered deficiencies must state:

- How the deficiencies identified for specific residents will be corrected
- How the facility will identify other residents having the potential to be affected by the same deficient practice
- What measures will be taken to make sure the deficient practice does not recur
- How the facility will monitor its corrective actions to ensure that the deficient practice does not recur

The plan of correction for facility-centered deficiencies must state:

- What will be done to correct the deficiencies
- Who will make the corrections
- Who will monitor the deficient area
- How similar deficiencies will be prevented in the future

Penalties

If deficiencies are severe, actual harm has occurred to a resident, or the potential for serious harm to residents exists, measures are taken against the facility license, certification, or accreditation. Some agencies fine the facility heavily if care is not up to their standards, or if dangers to residents or employees exist. Survey agencies can also issue a probationary license or even revoke facility approval. The fines can be as high as $10,000 per day in long-term care facilities. Facility payment for Medicare and Medicaid recipients may be withheld. Long-term care facilities can lose their approval to conduct nursing assistant classes because of a survey with a negative outcome. Unfavorable surveys have caused some long-term care facilities to close.

OSHA SURVEYS

In addition to licensure, certification, and accreditation visits, the **Occupational Safety and Health Administration (OSHA)** also surveys long-term care facilities. OSHA is an agency that protects the health and safety of employees. OSHA inspectors review infection control, isolation practices, employee tuberculin testing, material safety data sheets, and other policies and facility practices. The OSHA survey involves interviews with employees and a tour of all areas of the facility. The inspector will ask questions about health and safety practices. OSHA inspectors will make recommendations for correcting unsafe conditions. If the inspector notes dangerous or unsafe conditions during the survey, the agency may receive a **citation** or fine. A citation is a written notice that informs the facility of the violations of OSHA rules. The employer must post the written report of each citation at or near the place the violation occurred for three days, or until the unsafe condition is corrected. OSHA surveys in some facilities have resulted in fines of $100,000 or more.

JOINT COMMISSION SURVEYS

The **Joint Commission on Accreditation of Healthcare Organizations (JCAHO)** is an agency that inspects and accredits hospitals, long-term care facilities, home care providers, medical suppliers, ambulance services, and many other health care agencies. Unlike licensure surveys, JCAHO informs the facility of a scheduled survey several weeks in advance. This is changing, however. JCAHO will begin doing unannounced accreditation surveys in all facilities in 2006. Unannounced surveys will be pilot-tested in volunteer organizations during 2004 and 2005. The JCAHO has planned other significant changes to the survey process as well. The new survey process will be called "Shared Visions—New Pathways." The JCAHO has developed the survey with the expectation that each accredited organization will be in compliance with 100% of the JCAHO standards 100% of the time. The new survey process is bound to bring about many changes as it unfolds.

JCAHO has very high standards. Participation in the accreditation process is voluntary. Some long-term care facilities apply for and receive JCAHO accreditation. Like other survey agencies, JCAHO inspects all departments of the long-term care facility. The discussion here applies to all settings in which resident care is delivered.

The JCAHO survey process does not place as much emphasis on observation of the nursing assistant as other types of surveys. However, the surveyors will check to see that the overall care delivered is in keeping with established standards and infection control guidelines. Maintenance of a safe environment, incident reports, and use of physical and chemical restraints are evaluated to ensure that resident management is in keeping with accepted standards of practice. Emphasis is placed on use of restraint alternatives whenever possible. If residents are in restraints, continuing need for the restraint must be frequently evaluated. Surveyors may question you about emergency fire and disaster codes used in your facility and about your basic job preparation.

Resident Needs

JCAHO surveyors evaluate residents to make sure they receive care according to established standards. Teaching the resident about how to live with and manage his or her medical condition is an important part of the process. Many different care providers are involved in resident teaching. Some teaching is planned by the registered nurse and delivered by the nursing assistant.

Nursing Assistant Qualifications

JCAHO requirements state that nursing assistants should be assigned to care for residents based on identified resident needs and caregiver qualifications, education, and experience. Caregiver qualifications and education are reviewed. Surveyors review the resident's medical record for evidence of assessment, care planning, and quality of services provided. Surveyors will also review age-related competencies for residents on each unit.

JCAHO standards state that all nursing assistants must be competent in their responsibilities. The facility is required to periodically evaluate staff competence and maintain a record of these checks. Staff members must participate in ongoing educational programs. Surveyors will check staff development records to verify attendance and may ask staff how their competency was evaluated. They may also ask you how you would operate a piece of equipment or perform a specific procedure.

Surveyors will review facility policies and procedures and determine whether staff is following them. This part of the survey is outcome-oriented and will be used to evaluate whether the resident has a positive outcome as a result of the internal quality review process. Emphasis is placed on making sure that employees know and

follow facility policies and procedures when caring for residents.

Accreditation

During the JCAHO survey, the survey team evaluates the level of the health care organization's compliance with the commission's standards. Upon survey completion, a report that details areas in which the agency's performance must improve is issued to the facility. Accreditation is granted if the survey is acceptable. If significant problems are identified, accreditation will be awarded upon agreement with administration to correct the problems promptly. If severe deficiencies are identified, JCAHO will follow up with the facility to check progress in making corrections.

HELPFUL INFORMATION

Long-term care facilities perform many different services for residents. The nursing assistant's job description is slightly different in each facility. It is difficult to provide general rules for doing things correctly in a book that is used in a variety of health care settings. Each facility has specific policies and procedures. Different regulatory agencies survey long-term care facilities. Reviewing your facility policy and procedure manual will provide you with valuable information. Good infection control practices are an emphasis in all surveys. Infection control and medical asepsis must be practiced regularly if the facility is to be successful in this area of the survey. Surveyors review infections and other facility practices over the past year. Surveyors are checking to see if there are patterns of nosocomial infections in the facility, which could indicate cross-contamination and inadequate medical asepsis by health care workers. There are many variables. Each nursing assistant should take infection control practices very seriously.

Information You Should Know About Your Long-Term Care Facility

The following is a list of information that can be found in your facility policies, procedures, and orientation information. To deliver resident care in keeping with the standards of the regulatory agencies, follow all policies and learn the answers to these questions in your facility:

- What is the facility's system for resident identification?

- How can you tell the difference between a regular call signal and an emergency signal? How quickly should call signals be answered? Who is responsible for answering signals for residents that are not part of your assignment?
- If you discover a resident in an emergency situation, what is the policy for getting help?
- If you discover a fire, what should you do? How would you prevent smoke from escaping from a room containing a fire? What happens when the fire alarm sounds? Where are the fire extinguishers and emergency exits on your unit? What should you do if you are not on your unit when the fire alarm sounds?
- Where are facility disaster plans located?
- What are the facility codes for fire, disaster, and other emergencies?
- Where are resident care plans located?
- Where are the designated smoking areas, if any, for residents and visitors?
- What is the facility policy for residents with smoking materials in their possession?
- What is the facility policy for supervising residents when they are smoking?
- What are the standard measurements for drinking glasses and other containers in the facility? Where is intake and output recorded? What should you do if the intake or output on your shift appears inadequate?
- How and where do you document what a resident has eaten? What should you do if a resident refuses all or part of a meal?
- In what situations should you complete an incident report?
- What is the proper chain of command in your department?
- What is the facility policy for using restraints? What are the size and application rules for the type of restraints your agency uses?
- What should you do if a resident has signs or symptoms of abuse?
- What are facility policies for separation of clean and soiled items in the resident's room? In other areas of the facility?
- What are the nursing assistant's responsibilities for cleaning utensils, personal care items, and equipment? Where are soiled items cleaned? After cleaning, where are clean items stored?
- What should you do if you find gowns or bed linen that are torn or in poor condition?
- Where is personal protective equipment located **(Figure 24-3)?** How is it discarded after use?
- Where is biohazardous waste discarded?
- What are facility policies for handling contaminated trash and linen?

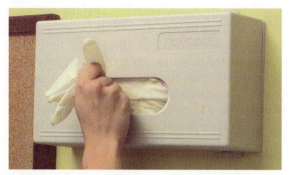

FIGURE 24-3 Apply the principles of standard precautions when caring for all residents.

- Where are the material safety data sheets located?
- Where is the designated eyewash/body wash station?
- What should you do if you discover broken electrical or mechanical equipment?

PROVIDING CARE THAT COMPLIES WITH ACCEPTED STANDARDS OF PRACTICE

Surveyors may or may not evaluate the care you give. Care involves making observations of the resident's specific condition, the environment, and other factors that influence the resident's well-being. To be successful, you must look at the entire picture. Following the guidelines on p. 465 will assist you to provide good resident care every day and ensure that surveyors are satisfied as well.

SURVIVING A SURVEY

Most nursing assistants will tell you that they feel enormous personal stress during facility surveys. This is not necessarily a bad thing. Some stress may help improve your performance. However, feeling overwhelmed with stress is not healthy. Remember, you can only be responsible for yourself and your own actions. You are not responsible for the actions of others. The title of this chapter is "surviving a survey" because it is designed to help you survive. Fear of the unknown is very stressful. Understanding the purpose and methods used during the survey process will help reduce your stress. Participating in and cooperating with your facility quality improvement program will prevent problems from occurring. Developing good work habits

Resident Care and Compliance with Accepted Practice Standards

- Follow all facility policies and procedures for resident care.
- Know the care plan for the residents you are assigned to care for, including the major diagnosis, approaches to problems, and expected outcomes.
- Perform procedures in the way you were taught. Do not perform procedures for which you have not been trained.
- Practice safety in everything you do.
- All residents should have the call signal within reach at all times. Answer call signals promptly.
- Be polite and treat all residents with dignity and respect.
- Always close the door to the room when providing care. Pull the privacy curtain and close the window curtain. This should be done in the care of all residents, whether alert or confused.
- Cover residents completely in bed, chair, or hallways so they are not exposed.
- Always knock on the door before entering a room **(Figure 24-4)** and wait for a response. If you do not get a response, open the door slightly and announce your presence.

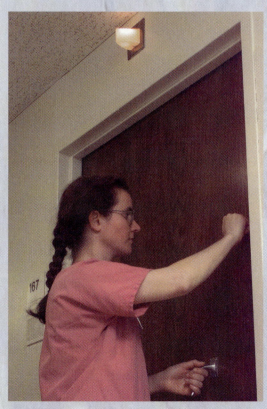

FIGURE 24-4   Knock on the door and wait for a response before entering.

- If the resident's door is open, knock on the door frame or other surface and wait for permission to enter the room.
- Communicate with residents during care and explain procedures before you perform them.
- Know your responsibility for residents who use permanent equipment, such as oxygen, tube feeding, or IV pumps. The flow rate of the pump should match the ordered rate on the care plan. If it does not, notify the nurse. If an alarm sounds on a piece of medical equipment, notify the nurse immediately.
- Comb the resident's hair and tend to grooming needs early in the day so the resident is presentable in appearance for visitors. Assist with grooming needs throughout the day, if necessary.
- Check the resident's fingernails to be sure they are clean and neatly trimmed.
- Use handrolls or other props in the hands of dependent residents, to prevent contractures. Remove the handrolls and clean the palm of the hand daily, or according to facility policy.
- Shave male residents daily. Follow your facility policy for removing facial hair on female residents.
- Give residents oral care three times a day, or according to individual needs.
- Check residents frequently to be sure they are clean and dry. Give incontinent care as necessary.
- All residents should be clean and odor-free.
- Make sure the resident's appearance is presentable at all times. Remove spilled food from clothing, and change the clothing or gown if necessary. Make sure the resident is clean after meals. If food is spilled on bed linen or the floor, replace the linen or remove the food from the floor. When residents are up and dressed during the day, the clothing should be clean, in good repair, color-coordinated, and appropriate for age and season.
- Residents should have footwear appropriate to the floor surface on their feet during transfers. Feet should be covered when a resident is up in the chair so that bare feet are not resting on the floor.
- Pay attention to resident positioning in bed and chair. Preventive mattresses, heel and elbow protectors, and other devices are used if the resident is at risk of skin breakdown. Padding should be used for positioning residents if bony areas will rub against each other or against a firm surface.
- Footboards should be in place for bedfast residents.
- The feet should be supported when residents are up in the chair.
- Residents in wheelchairs should be positioned so that their hips are at the rear of the seat. They should be seated upright and not lean to the side. If you are responsible for residents who move about the facility in wheelchairs, find them and check on them periodically to be sure their needs are met.

Continues

GUIDELINES FOR

Resident Care and Compliance with Accepted Practice Standards, *Continued*

- If the resident has edema of the hands or feet, the edematous area should be elevated. Report the edema to the nurse.
- Avoid the use of restraints whenever possible. If restraints are used, apply them only according to manufacturer's directions.
- Release restraints every 2 hours for 10 full minutes for ambulation and exercise. Visually check residents who are in restraints at least every 30 minutes, or according to facility policy.
- Follow facility safety precautions and post signs if oxygen is in use.
- Clean and soiled equipment should be separated by one room's width in the hallway. For example, the housekeeping cart and soiled linen hamper are soiled. They are separated from the clean linen cart and food cart by one room's width or more, if this is your facility policy **(Figure 24-5)**.
- Remove housekeeping carts and soiled linen hampers from the hallway when meals are being served, if this is your facility policy.
- Items in the refrigerator should be covered, labeled, and dated. The refrigerator should have a thermometer. The temperature should be below 45°F, or according to facility policy. Food and beverages should not be stored in the same refrigerator with medications or laboratory specimens.
- Follow your facility policy for storage of chemicals and other potentially toxic items.
- Apply the principles of standard precautions consistently in the care of all residents.
- Wash your hands before and after caring for each resident, and before and after using gloves.

- Avoid contaminating the environment with soiled gloves. Remove one glove or use a paper towel under your hand if environmental contact is necessary.
- Discard gloves and other personal protective equipment according to facility policy.
- Hold both clean and soiled linen away from your uniform.
- Avoid placing soiled linen on the floor.
- Keep clean linen carts covered when not in use.
- Avoid stacking linen in resident rooms; take only needed linen into the room.
- Avoid overfilling linen hampers and barrels. The lid should fit tightly.
- Be sure each resident has fresh water. The water pitcher must always be covered with a lid. If the lid is missing, replace the pitcher.
- Store bedpans and urinals properly. Follow facility policies for covering them during transport.
- Monitor the position of the catheter tubing and bag. The tubing should be secured to the leg and not obstructed or bent. The bag must be below the level of the bladder, but should never touch the floor. Avoid attaching the bag to the side rails.
- Personal care items such as combs, toothbrushes, and hygienic supplies should be covered if necessary, and stored or labeled so that they are used by only one resident.
- Follow facility policies for routine cleaning tasks, and for dating and labeling clean items.
- Disinfect bathtubs, shower chairs, and pieces of permanent equipment before and after each use.
- Clean and soiled items should be separated in the bedside stand.
- Cover food and beverages when you carry them in the hallway.
- When you are passing ice, keep the ice scoop covered when not in use. Follow your facility policy for preventing contamination of the ice chest or dispenser.
- Pass meal trays immediately when they arrive on the unit to maintain food temperature. Cut meat, butter bread, open cartons, put condiments on food, and assist residents with meals as necessary.
- Pass all clean trays before returning soiled trays to the food cart.
- Monitor resident position when eating. Residents should be upright. They should be as close to the table as possible. Table height should not be so high that the resident has to reach up for the food. The resident's feet should be supported on a footstool or other device if they do not reach the floor.
- Prompt or assist residents who are not eating.
- Offer substitutes if the resident does not eat the meat or vegetable, or follow your facility policy for replacing uneaten food.

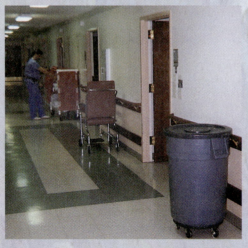

FIGURE 24-5 Separate clean and soiled items in the hallway by one room's width.

Continues

GUIDELINES FOR

Resident Care and Compliance with Accepted Practice Standards, *Continued*

- When feeding residents, sit at eye level and maintain a conversation, even if the resident is confused.
- Alternate liquids with solids when feeding.
- Change incontinent residents promptly. Provide perineal care after each incontinent episode.
- Always notify the nurse of a change in the resident's condition, even if it seems insignificant.
- Notify the nurse immediately of red or open areas on a resident's skin.

- Document your care completely and accurately. Do not leave blank spaces in flow sheets. Read what you are signing on flow sheets before signing your initials to them. Surveyors review what you have documented. Inadequate documentation can adversely affect the survey. Your documentation is a permanent, legal record of the care provided, and you may have to defend it in court.

---

and organizational skills, and using them every day, will help reduce your stress during surveys.

Surveyors learn a great deal about the facility before arriving to do a survey. Many of the issues reviewed are cumulative issues. This means they develop over a period of time, such as occurrence of pressure ulcers, weight loss, and having many resident falls and injuries. Being at peak performance only during survey times will not prevent the cumulative problems. However, doing your best each day will prevent many of these problems from occurring. The review of cumulative outcomes is a central issue. However, it is not the only issue reviewed. The atmosphere and conditions in the facility during the first four hours of the survey often set the tone for the remainder of the survey. Everyone hopes that the tone will be positive. You will be observed providing normal daily care for the residents. If you make an error when a surveyor is watching you, correct it immediately. Surveyors realize that their observing you is likely to cause nervousness. By correcting the error, you are showing that you are aware of the problem and know the proper way to perform the activity.

The survey verifies the level and quality of health care provided to residents. It also reviews the environmental conditions in the facility.

Surveyors look for positive outcomes. They observe residents to see if the facility is providing care and services to maintain and improve residents' conditions and prevent declines whenever possible. Your performance at the time of the survey is important. Knowing your job; organizing your work; being kind, compassionate, and respectful to the residents; and being confident in your ability are work habits and tools that you develop over time. These tools will also help you survive the survey.

Learn to view the survey as a routine daily event. Think about it. Someone *is* evaluating health care workers' performance every day of the year. Your performance is evaluated by nurses and facility managers, residents, and family members. In a way, their evaluations of your performance are more critical than those of the state surveyors. These individuals determine who will work at the facility. They determine whether resident care is satisfactory every day. They make decisions regarding whether residents will remain in the facility or move elsewhere. Having the everyday support of these individuals is helpful when surveyors visit the facility. In any event, the stress you feel during a formal facility survey will be reduced once you realize that you are actually being evaluated every day.

KEY POINTS

- Long-term care facilities must meet quality standards to operate.
- Licensure is a process in which the facility is inspected for a state license to operate.
- Certification is necessary if long-term care facilities accept Medicare and/or Medicaid money as reimbursement for resident care.
- Accreditation is a voluntary process in which facilities are inspected to ensure that they meet high-quality standards of resident care.

- OSHA inspects long-term care facilities to monitor infection control and safety practices that affect employees.
- Many agencies survey health care facilities, so the facility must be survey-ready every day.
- Most surveys are unannounced.
- Long-term care facility surveyors usually observe the nursing assistant giving direct resident care.
- Infection control practices are a very important part of all surveys.
- The nursing assistant is responsible for learning and following the policies and procedures of the long-term care facility.
- Following facility policies and doing things the way you were taught will prevent problems during surveys.
- The nursing assistant is responsible for providing care that complies with accepted standards of practice for health care providers.

REVIEW

A. Multiple Choice

Select the one best answer.

1. Licensure, certification, and accreditation surveys are done to
   a. ensure that facilities deliver quality care.
   b. punish the long-term care facility.
   c. check for compliance with OSHA standards.
   d. check for Medicare fraud and abuse.

2. OSHA is
   a. a governmental agency responsible for resident safety.
   b. a federal agency that studies infections and makes recommendations.
   c. an agency responsible for developing and enforcing job safety standards.
   d. a federal agency that regulates safety of food, drugs, and medical devices.

3. Long-term care surveyors evaluate
   a. quality of care.
   b. facility census.
   c. staff attendance.
   d. policies to make sure they are current.

4. Most long-term care facility surveys are
   a. announced 24 hours before the survey.
   b. anticipated by administration.
   c. unannounced.
   d. conducted in private.

5. To prepare for a survey, you should
   a. provide care in the manner in which you were taught.
   b. begin preparing when surveyors arrive.
   c. tell residents to behave themselves.
   d. work slowly so you get more help.

6. When you pass surveyors in the hallway, you should
   a. ignore them.
   b. smile and say hello.
   c. ask them what their findings are.
   d. find out the purpose of their visit.

7. The Joint Commission cn Accreditation of Healthcare Organizations survey is
   a. a voluntary process.
   b. mandated by the government.
   c. part of the certification survey.
   d. required for licensure.

8. Surveyors will check to be sure that
   a. care providers are clean and well groomed.
   b. sterile technique is used routinely in resident care.
   c. workers follow facility policies and procedures.
   d. all scheduled staff are on duty.

9. Surveyors will monitor
   a. the staff locker room.
   b. break times.
   c. food service and preparation.
   d. residents' personal affairs.

10. When providing care according to accepted standards of practice, you should
    a. practice safety.
    b. answer emergency call signals for only your assigned residents.
    c. knock on the door before entering the room of alert residents only.
    d. do your documentation at least weekly.

B. Clinical Applications

Answer the following questions.

11. The nurse informs you that surveyors have just arrived at the facility for the annual survey. The residents you are assigned to care for are all eating breakfast. What will you do first?

12. The nurse informs you that a surveyor will observe you giving Mr. Harrison his bed bath and morning care. Mr. Harrison is a confused resident who does not communicate. In addition to bathing technique, what are some other things that the surveyor will be watching for?

13. When the surveyor observes you caring for Mr. Harrison, she asks you his medical diagnosis. You do not know the answer. What will you tell her?

14. While you are bathing Mr. Harrison, the surveyor asks you what you would do if the fire alarm sounded during the resident's bath. How will you respond?

15. After you bathe Mr. Harrison, the surveyor tells you she would like to observe you emptying the resident's catheter bag. You are very nervous and accidentally spill some urine on the floor. The resident is on intake and output. What should you do?

Appendix

PROCEDURES FOR CARDIAC AND RESPIRATORY EMERGENCIES

Cardiopulmonary resuscitation (CPR) is a procedure used to maintain blood circulation throughout the body until the emergency medical services (EMS) respond to the facility. *You must never perform these procedures until you have completed an approved course, taught by an American Heart Association or American Red Cross approved instructor. The information in this book is not intended to take the place of an approved course.*

Text continued on page 472

PROCEDURE
A1 — Head-Tilt, Chin-Lift Maneuver

1. Place one hand on the forehead. Place the fingers of the opposite hand below the center of the jawbone, directly under the chin.
2. Tilt the head back gently.
3. With your fingertips, lift the lower jaw forward. The lower teeth should almost touch the upper teeth. Avoid pressing on the neck, which may worsen an airway obstruction.
4. Keep the resident's mouth open. If necessary, pull the resident's lower lip forward. Avoid inserting your fingers into the mouth.
5. If the resident cannot maintain this position, maintain the airway manually, by holding your hands in place if necessary.
6. As soon as the resident is safe, and the nurse or other professionals have assumed responsibility for care, wash your hands well.

PROCEDURE
A2 — Jaw-Thrust Maneuver

1. Move the resident into the supine position as a single unit. Avoid twisting the neck, back, or spine during movement.
2. Pull the head of the bed away from the wall.
3. Position yourself above the resident's head.
4. Position your elbows on the mattress.
5. Using your forearms, stabilize the sides of the head to prevent movement.
6. Place one hand on each side of the lower jaw, just below the ears.
7. Use the tips of your index fingers to push the lower jaw forward.
8. Keep the resident's mouth open. If necessary, pull the resident's lower lip forward. Avoid inserting your fingers into the mouth.

Continues

PROCEDURE	Jaw-Thrust Maneuver,		
A2	*Continued*	OBRA	

9. If the resident cannot maintain this position, maintain the airway manually, by holding your hands in place if necessary.

10. As soon as the resident is safe, and the nurse or other professionals have assumed responsibility for care, wash your hands well.

PROCEDURE	Mouth-to-Mask Ventilation		
A3		OBRA	

Note: Follow your facility policy for mouth-to-mouth ventilation. To prevent the transmission of disease, standard precautions should be used. This means that gloves are worn for the finger sweep. A ventilation barrier mask with a valve that prevents the backflow of secretions (called an anti-reflux or one-way valve), or resuscitation face shield should be placed between your mouth and the resident's mouth for ventilations. Familiarize yourself with the devices used in your facility. CPR classes are offered to teach you how to use ventilation devices correctly. Attending a CPR class will benefit you personally and professionally.

Supplies needed:
- Disposable exam gloves
- Pocket mask with anti-reflux (one-way) valve

1. Pull the head of the bed away from the wall.
2. Apply gloves.
3. Open the resident's airway using the head-tilt, chin-lift method, or jaw-thrust maneuver.
4. Position yourself at the resident's head.
5. Position the mask on the resident's face with the small end over the bridge of the nose, and the wide end on the resident's chin. The ventilation port should be centered over the resident's mouth.
6. Seal the mask to the resident's face by positioning your thumbs on the top of the mask and fingers at the sides. Hold the airway in the open position.
7. Take a deep breath, then seal your mouth over the ventilation port, exhaling into the mask. The ventilation should take 1 to 1½ seconds for infants and children, and 2 seconds for adults. During the ventilation, look at the resident's chest. It should rise as you blow air in.
8. Remove your mouth from the mask, and allow the resident to exhale passively. Continue to breathe into the mask once every 4 to 5 seconds.

PROCEDURE	Adult CPR, One Rescuer		
A4		OBRA	

Supplies needed:
- Gloves
- Pocket mask with anti-reflux (one-way) valve

1. Gently shake the resident and ask, "Are you okay?" Call the resident's name if you know it.
2. Call for help. If someone responds, send her to activate the EMS system. If no one responds, quickly call EMS yourself, then return to the resident as soon as possible.
3. Turn the resident on his or her back as a unit. For CPR to be effective, the resident must by lying on a hard surface, such as the floor.
4. Open the airway, using the head-tilt, chin-lift method.
5. Kneel near the resident, so you can observe the chest. Listen and feel for breath sounds on your cheek and ear, while simultaneously looking to see if the chest is rising and falling.
6. If the resident is breathing, maintain an open airway and monitor breathing.

Continues

7. If the resident is not breathing, seal the nose and mouth with a barrier ventilation device, such as a pocket mask. The technique used is determined by the equipment available.
8. Take a deep breath, then seal your mouth over the ventilation port, exhaling into the mask. The ventilation should take 1 to 1½ seconds for infants and children, and 2 seconds for adults. During the ventilation, look at the resident's chest. It should rise as you blow air in.
9. Remove your mouth from the mask, and allow the resident to exhale passively.
10. Check for the presence of a pulse, using the carotid pulse in the neck. Maintain the open airway with one hand. Use the other hand to feel for the pulse, by sliding the tips of your index and second finger into the groove in the large muscle on the side of the neck. Check for the pulse on the same side on which you are kneeling. Avoid crossing over the neck or applying pressure to the throat. Check for the pulse for a full 5 to 10 seconds. If there is a pulse, but no respirations, continue to ventilate once every 5 seconds (12 times a minute). Check the pulse periodically.
11. If no pulse is present, locate the "landmark" hand position. Run your fingers up the lower margins of the ribs, and locate the xiphoid process. Hold your index and middle fingers over the xiphoid process to keep your place. Proper hand placement is very important to prevent injury. Place the heel of your other hand on the chest next to your fingers. Next, place the landmark hand on top of the other hand, interlacing the fingers. Lock your elbows.
12. Keeping your elbows straight, compress straight down to a depth of 1½ to 2 inches at a rate of 100 compressions per minute. (This is *not 100 actual*

compressions a minute, but rather a *rate of 100 per minute*, meaning more than one compression per second).
- Downward pressure should be on the sternum only. Avoid pressing on the ribs with your fingers.
- Keep the fingers interlaced and slightly elevated from the chest.
- Compressions should be smooth and rhythmic.
- Completely release pressure, but maintain hand contact with the chest between each compression. The release in pressure allows the heart to refill with blood.
- Count out loud during compressions: "One and, two and, three and, —."
13. Do 2 ventilations at the end of each set of 15 compressions.
14. Do 4 cycles of 15 compressions and 2 ventilations.
- Monitor to make sure the chest rises and falls with each ventilation.
15. At the end of four cycles, feel for the carotid pulse. If there is no pulse, give two more ventilations. Continue CPR with cycles of 15 compressions and 2 ventilations. Feel for the pulse again every few minutes.
16. If the resident begins breathing, is still unconscious, and has no evidence of trauma, place her in the recovery position.
17. If the heart is beating, but there are no ventilations, continue rescue breathing once every 5 seconds (12 times per minute).
18. Do not stop CPR unless the resident's pulse returns, you are given further instructions by a licensed health professional, or you are exhausted and unable to continue.

Supplies needed:
- Disposable exam gloves
- Pocket mask with anti-reflux (one-way) valve

The technique for two-rescuer CPR is exactly the same as for one-rescuer CPR. The two rescuers should be on opposite sides of the resident, if possible. The compression-ventilation ratio is 15:2 at a rate of 100 a minute. Pause compressions briefly after every 15th compression so the ventilator can give 2 ventilations. The rescuer at the head will monitor for return of spon-

taneous pulse and respirations. This persons should also monitor the pulse during compressions to ensure that circulation is effective. At the end of one minute, stop for no more than 10 seconds to evaluate pulse and respirations. Stop every few minutes thereafter.

1. If a second rescuer arrives:
- The second rescuer identifies herself by saying, "I know CPR; can I help?"
- Send the second rescuer to call EMS, if this has not been done.

A5 · Adult CPR, Two Rescuers, *Continued*

- When the second rescuer returns, she checks the carotid pulse for five seconds, then says, "Stop CPR." She checks for the spontaneous return of the pulse when no compressions are performed. If the pulse is absent, she says, "No pulse," then gives two ventilations.
2. The compressor gives 15 compressions at the rate of 100 a minute, then pauses briefly, keeping the hands in place on the chest. The ventilator gives two ventilations. The cycle resumes with 15 compressions to 2 ventilations and repeats indefinitely until further help arrives, the victim regains consciousness, or the rescuers are exhausted and unable to continue.
   - The ventilator is responsible for reassessing the resident. Palpate the carotid pulse during the other rescuer's chest compressions. You will feel a pulse if the compressions are effective. Signal the compressor periodically to pause for

five seconds for a reassessment of pulse and respirations.
3. When the compressor becomes fatigued, the rescuers should change positions with minimal interruption. The best time to do this is at the end of a cycle of 15 compressions. The compressor moves to the head and checks the pulse. The ventilator moves to the chest and locates the landmark. If the pulse is absent, the ventilator says, "No pulse," then gives two ventilations.
4. After the ventilations are given, the person at the chest begins compressions again. He counts out loud so the ventilator can anticipate when to give ventilations.
5. Continue CPR until a licensed health care provider arrives and gives further directions, the resident's pulse or respirations resume spontaneously, or both rescuers are exhausted and unable to continue.

Learn your facility's system for identifying residents on whom CPR should be performed. Learn the procedures for getting help and beginning CPR. Learn your emergency response codes. In the long-term care facility, you must know whether CPR is to be initiated. A resident who is very old or has a terminal illness may not wish to be resuscitated if cardiac arrest occurs. If this is the case, the resident will complete an advance directive, and the physician will write a

"do not resuscitate" (DNR) order. If there is no DNR order, full life support measures will be provided for cardiac arrest.

THE RECOVERY POSITION

If the resident is unresponsive, but is breathing and has a pulse, he or she should be positioned in the recovery position to prevent complica-

A6 · Positioning the Resident in the Recovery Position

1. Kneel beside the resident and straighten the legs.
2. Place the arm nearest you above the resident's head with the palm up and the elbow bent slightly.
3. Position the opposite arm across the chest.
4. Place your lower hand on the resident's thigh on the far side of the body. Pull the thigh up slightly, closer to the center of the resident's body.
5. Place your upper hand on the resident's shoulder on the opposite side of the body.
6. With one hand on the thigh and the other on the shoulder, roll the resident on the side facing you.

7. Move the resident's upper hand close to the cheek, bending the elbow. This hand should be close to the face, but not under the body. Adjust the upper body so that the hip and knee are at right angles.
8. Tilt the resident's head back slightly to keep the airway open. Now place the upper hand, palm facing down, under the cheek to maintain the head position.
9. Continue to monitor the resident closely for adequate breathing.

PROCEDURE A7 — CARDIAC EMERGENCIES AND USE OF AN ELEVATOR

OBRA

Note: The following is an actual long-term care facility policy for managing a cardiac arrest in a multistory facility with one elevator. If an emergency occurs on an upper floor, the elevator must be available for ambulance arrival. Likewise, the elevator must be available for EMS personnel to remove the resident from the building promptly. In an emergency, seconds count, and workers must synchronize their activities. Your facility will have a similar policy and procedure for ensuring that the elevator is available.

1. In an cardiac or respiratory arrest, a nursing assistant from the unit will be instructed to use the intercom to page, "Stat code, _____ floor." Each nurse will assign a nursing assistant from his or her floor to monitor the elevator until the emergency ends. If residents or visitors wish to use the elevator, ask them to refrain from pushing the button until the "all clear" is announced. You may tape a sign over the elevator buttons stating: "do not use the elevator."
2. One nursing assistant from the unit on which the emergency occurs will call the elevator, then bring it to the first floor. He or she will lock the elevator, then remain in place until the ambulance arrives.
3. Upon ambulance arrival, the nursing assistant will escort the ambulance personnel to the floor on which the emergency occurred. Direct ambulance personnel to the resident's room. Lock the elevator, remaining with it.
4. When the ambulance is ready to depart, escort the EMS personnel to the first floor.
5. After the resident has been unloaded, return to the unit, leaving the elevator unlocked. Announce, "Stat code all clear" over the intercom, at which time normal elevator use will resume.
6. In the event the elevator is needed to transport emergency equipment or supplies from one floor to the next during the emergency, announce over the intercom, "Release the elevator to _____ floor for equipment transport." The nursing assistant who is operating the elevator will remain in the elevator and go at once to the floor requesting transport. Personnel from that floor will transport equipment to the specific room where the stat situation has occurred. He or she returns to the original unit by way of the stairs. The nursing assistant who is assigned to the elevator locks the elevator and remains with it at all times.
7. All departments on all levels of the facility are expected to cooperate with this procedure. Remember, a life hangs in the balance, and this is the most critical of all emergencies.
8. All personnel remaining on their units are expected to keep residents away from elevator doors so there is a clear path for equipment, ambulance personnel, and facility staff responding to the emergency. Avoid pressing the buttons to call the elevator to another floor when it is locked off during the emergency. Doing this will cause the EMS personnel to stop at each floor on their way out of the facility, delaying the resident's departure. Seconds count, and getting the resident to the hospital rapidly is of utmost importance.

PROCEDURE A8 — Measuring Blood Pressure (One-Step Procedure)

OBRA

Note: The one-step blood pressure procedure is provided here for schools that teach this method. The guidelines and reportable values for this procedure vary slightly from state to state, and from one facility to another. Your instructor will inform you if the guidelines or reportable values in your state or facility differ from those listed here. Know and follow the required guidelines for your state and facility.

1. Assemble your equipment:
   - sphygmomanometer (blood pressure cuff)
   - stethoscope
   - alcohol sponges
   - notepad
   - pen
2. Wipe the ear pieces and diaphragm of the stethoscope with alcohol pads.
3. Perform your beginning procedure actions. The resident may be lying down or seated in a chair for this procedure.
4. Push the sleeve up at least five inches above the elbow.
5. Extend the resident's arm and rest it on the arm of the chair, the bed, or the resident's lap, with the palm upward.
6. Unroll the cuff and open the valve on the bulb. Squeeze the cuff to deflate the cuff completely.
7. Locate the brachial artery, on the thumb side of

Continues

the inner elbow, by palpating with two or three fingers.

8. Wrap the cuff snugly around the arm, centering the bladder over the brachial artery. The cuff should be one inch above the artery in the antecubital space, in front of the elbow.

9. Position the gauge so you can see the numbers clearly.

10. Confirm the location of the brachial artery.

11. Place the ear pieces of the stethoscope in your ears. Position the diaphragm to the stethoscope over the brachial artery. The diaphragm should not be touching the blood pressure cuff. Hold the diaphragm in place with the fingers of your nondominant hand.

12. With your dominant hand, tighten the thumbscrew on the valve (turn clockwise) to close it. Do not tighten it so much that you will have difficulty releasing it.

13. Pump the bulb to inflate the cuff until the gauge reaches 160, or according to facility policy.

14. Slowly open the valve by turning the thumbscrew counterclockwise. Allow the air to escape slowly.

15. Listen for the sound of the pulse in the stethoscope. A few seconds will pass without sound. If you hear pulse sounds immediately, deflate the cuff. Wait a minute, then repeat the procedure, this time inflating the cuff to 200.

16. Note the number on the gauge when you hear the first sound. This is the systolic blood pressure.

17. Continue listening as the air escapes slowly from the cuff. You will hear a continuous pulse sound. Note the number on the gauge when the sounds disappear completely. This is the diastolic blood pressure.

18. After the sounds disappear completely, open the thumbscrew completely to deflate the cuff.

19. Remove the stethoscope from your ears.

20. Remove the cuff from the resident's arm.

21. Record the blood pressure on your notepad. Blood pressure is recorded as a fraction, with the systolic reading first, followed by the diastolic reading, such as 120/80.

22. Roll the blood pressure cuff over the gauge and return it to the case.

23. Wipe the ear pieces and diaphragm of the stethoscope with an alcohol sponge. If the stethoscope tubing has contacted the bed linen, wipe it as well.

24. Perform your procedure completion actions.

25. Report blood pressures over 140/90 or under 100/60 to the nurse immediately, or according to facility policy.

---

tions. The recovery position is a modified lateral position. The resident's position must:

- Be stable
- Avoid pressure on the chest
- Avoid pressure on the lower arm
- Allow the airway to remain open

Continue to monitor the resident according to facility policy to ensure that the pulse and respirations remain adequate. Take vital signs according to the nurse's instructions.

DOCUMENTING PERCENTAGE OF MEALS CONSUMED

Several methods are used for documenting percentage of meals consumed. Documenting appetite is more than eyeballing the food tray and estimating how much food was eaten. You must document the percentage of the significant food items on the tray.

Some facilities record percentages of each food item on the tray for residents with weight loss, or when accurate intake recording is essential. Two alternate methods of recording meal intake are listed in Tables A-1 and A-2.

GUIDELINES FOR HAND HYGIENE

Introduction

In 2002, the Centers for Disease Control (CDC) published the results of extensive handwashing studies, as well as new recommendations for cleansing hands. Each recommendation is categorized on the basis of existing scientific data, theoretical rationale, applicability, and economic impact. The CDC system for categorizing recommendations is:

Category IA. Strongly recommended for implementation and strongly supported by well-

TABLE A-1 Alternate method of documenting meal intake	
Breakfast	
Egg, cheese or cottage cheese	50%
Hot or cold cereal	30%
Bread	10%
Bacon, ham or sausage	10%
Total	100%

Occasionally, a resident will request no protein foods (eggs, meat, cheese, cottage cheese) at breakfast. Please reassign the percentages to the other items on the tray and document accordingly.

Lunch and Supper	
Meat, egg, cheese, or cottage cheese	40%
Starchy vegetable	20%
Vegetable or salad	20%
Bread	10%
Dessert	10%
Total	100%

The meat and starchy vegetables may be combined in some dishes, such as casseroles. If so, add the point values for these items to total 60%. Sandwiches are also 60% because the two bread slices are the starchy vegetable. An additional bread item such as crackers may also be served at the meal.

TABLE A-2 Alternate method of documenting meal intake

	Food Item	Percentage of Meal
Breakfast		
	eggs	35%
	eggs and bacon	40%
	eggs and sausage	45%
	toast *or* cereal	30%
	milk	20%
	fruit juice	15%
Dinner and Supper	meat group, including eggs, main dish, legumes	50%
	fruit group, including dessert items	15%
	bread or cereal group	10%
	vegetable group	15%
	fluids	10%

designed experimental, clinical, or epidemiological studies.

Category IB. Strongly recommended for implementation and supported by certain experimental, clinical, or epidemiological studies and a strong theoretical rationale.

Category IC. Required for implementation, as mandated by federal or state regulation or standard.

Category II. Suggested for implementation and supported by suggestive clinical or epidemiological studies or a theoretical rationale.

No recommendation. Unresolved issue; practices for which insufficient evidence or no consensus regarding efficacy exist.

Recommendations

1. Indications for handwashing and hand antisepsis
   - When hands are visibly dirty or contaminated with proteinaceous material or are visibly soiled with blood or other body fluids, wash hands with either a non-antimicrobial soap and water or an antimicrobial soap and water (IA).
   - If hands are not visibly soiled, use an alcohol-based hand rub for routinely decontaminating hands in all other clinical situations described in items (IA).
   - Alternatively, wash hands with an antimicrobial soap and water in all clinical situations (IB).
   - Wash hands before having direct contact with patients (IB).
   - Wash hands before donning sterile gloves when inserting a central intravascular catheter (IB).
   - Cleanse hands before inserting indwelling urinary catheters, peripheral vascular catheters, or other invasive devices that do not require a surgical procedure (IB).
   - Cleanse hands after contact with a patient's intact skin (e.g., when taking a pulse or blood pressure, and lifting a patient) (IB).
   - Wash hands after contact with body fluids or excretions, mucous membranes, nonintact skin, and wound dressings if hands are not visibly soiled (IA).
   - Cleanse hands if moving from a contaminated body site to a clean body site during patient care (II).

- Cleanse hands after contact with inanimate objects (including medical equipment) in the immediate vicinity of the patient (II).
- Wash hands after removing gloves (IB).
- Before eating and after using a restroom, wash hands with a non-antimicrobial soap and water or with an antimicrobial soap and water (IB).
- Antimicrobial-impregnated wipes (i.e., towelettes) may be considered as an alternative to washing hands with non-antimicrobial soap and water. Because they are not as effective as alcohol-based hand rubs or washing hands with an antimicrobial soap and water for reducing bacterial counts on the hands of health care workers, they are not a substitute for using an alcohol-based hand rub or antimicrobial soap (IB).
- Wash hands with non-antimicrobial soap and water or with antimicrobial soap and water if exposure to Bacillus anthracis [anthrax] is suspected or proven. The physical action of washing and rinsing hands under such circumstances is recommended because alcohols, chlorhexidine, iodophors, and other antiseptic agents have poor activity against spores (II).
- No recommendation can be made regarding the routine use of nonalcohol-based hand rubs for hand hygiene in health care settings. Unresolved issue.

2. Hand-hygiene technique
- When cleansing hands with an alcohol-based hand rub, apply product to palm of one hand and rub hands together, covering all surfaces of hands and fingers, until hands are dry (IB).
- Follow the manufacturer's recommendations regarding the volume of product to use.
- When washing hands with soap and water, wet hands first with water, apply an amount of product recommended by the manufacturer to hands, and rub hands together vigorously for at least 15 seconds, covering all surfaces of the hands and fingers. Rinse hands with water and dry thoroughly with a disposable towel. Use towel to turn off the faucet (IB).
- Avoid using hot water, because repeated exposure to hot water may increase the risk of dermatitis (IB).
- Liquid, bar, leaflet or powdered forms of plain soap are acceptable when washing hands with a non-antimicrobial soap and water. When bar soap is used, soap racks that facilitate drainage and small bars of soap should be used (II).
- Multiple-use cloth towels of the hanging or roll type are not recommended for use in health care settings (II).

3. Other recommendations
- Do not add soap to a partially empty soap dispenser. This practice of "topping off" dispensers can lead to bacterial contamination of soap (IA).
- Provide workers with hand lotions or creams to minimize the occurrence of irritant contact dermatitis associated with hand antisepsis or handwashing (IA).
- Do not wear artificial fingernails or extenders when having direct contact with patients at high risk (e.g., those in intensive care units or operating rooms) (IA).
- Keep natural nail tips less than 1/4-inch long (II).
- Wear gloves when contact with blood or other potentially infectious materials, mucous membranes, and nonintact skin could occur (IC).
- Remove gloves after caring for a patient. Do not wear the same pair of gloves for the care of more than one patient, and do not wash gloves between uses with different patients (IB).
- Change gloves during patient care if moving from a contaminated body site to a clean body site (II).
- No recommendation can be made regarding the wearing of rings in health care settings. Unresolved issue.
- Monitor workers' adherence to recommended hand-hygiene practices and provide personnel with information regarding their performance (IA).
- Encourage patients and their families to remind workers to decontaminate their hands (II).
- Store supplies of alcohol-based hand rubs in cabinets or areas approved for flammable materials (IC).

LATEX ALLERGY

Health care workers are at risk for developing latex allergy because they frequently use latex gloves. Many of the products used in patient care contain latex, as do many household and personal items. Persons who have hayfever, hand dermatitis, and allergies to foods such as bananas, avocados, kiwi fruits, and chestnuts are at increased risk of latex allergy. The amount and type of exposure needed to cause latex sensitivity are not known, although it is believed that wearing latex gloves when a rash is present on the hands increases the risk. A skin rash is often the first sign that a worker is becoming sensitive to latex.

Three types of reactions can occur in persons who use latex products:

1. Irritant contact dermatitis—contact dermatitis; the development of dry, itchy, irritated areas on the skin, usually the hands. However, this problem may have many other causes as well, so one should not assume that a latex sensitivity is present without further diagnostic testing. *Irritant contact dermatitis is not a true allergy.*
2. Allergic contact dermatitis (delayed hypersensitivity)—a sensitivity to the chemicals used during the manufacturing process. The reaction is similar to the symptoms of poison ivy.
3. Latex allergy is a serious reaction to latex. This type of allergy is diagnosed with a blood or skin test. Even low exposure to latex can cause sensitive individuals to react. Reactions usually begin shortly after exposure to latex, but they can occur hours later. Mild reactions cause hives, itching, and skin redness. More severe reactions cause respiratory symptoms, including runny nose, sneezing, itchy eyes, difficulty breathing, and wheezing. Shock is the most severe reaction. This type of shock is similar to that experienced by persons who are allergic to bee stings.

Preventing Latex Allergy

Many health care facilities have latex-free carts. Some facilities are becoming completely latex-free. Health care workers should take the following steps to protect themselves from latex exposure and allergy in the workplace:

- Use nonlatex gloves for activities that are not likely to involve contact with infectious materials (food preparation, routine housekeeping, maintenance, etc.). If latex gloves are used, avoid powdered gloves, which increase sensi-

tivity through inhalation of latex proteins when gloves are removed.

- Use barrier protection as necessary when handling known or potentially infectious materials. If you use latex gloves, use powder-free gloves. Hypoallergenic latex gloves do not reduce the risk of latex allergy. However, they may reduce reactions to chemical additives in the latex (allergic contact dermatitis). *Cloth stethoscope covers provide an excellent barrier against latex exposure, but can be a potential source of contamination to patients. Make sure your stethoscope cover is laundered regularly to reduce the potential risk of transmission.*
- Avoid oil-based hand creams or lotions (which can cause glove deterioration) unless they have been shown to reduce latex-related problems and maintain glove barrier protection.
- After removing latex gloves, wash hands with a mild soap and dry thoroughly.
- Attend educational classes about latex exposure provided by your employer:
- Become familiar with procedures for preventing latex allergy.
- Learn to recognize the symptoms of latex allergy: skin rashes; hives; flushing; itching; nasal, eye, or sinus symptoms; asthma; and shock.
- If you develop symptoms of latex allergy, avoid direct contact with latex gloves and other latex-containing products until you can see a physician who is experienced in treating latex allergy.
- If you have latex allergy, consult your physician regarding precautions to use, such as:
  - Avoiding contact with latex gloves and other latex-containing products
  - Avoiding areas where you might inhale the powder from latex gloves worn by other workers
  - Informing your employer and your health care providers (physicians, nurses, dentists, etc.) that you have latex allergy
  - Wearing a medical alert bracelet
- Carefully follow your physician's instructions for dealing with allergic reactions to latex.

Glossary

abandonment leaving or walking off the premises before another worker has been assigned to care for your residents

abbreviation a shortened form of a word or term

abdominal distention enlargement of the abdomen due to excess gas, fecal matter, or urinary retention

abdominal pacemaker *See* pacemaker

abduction moving an extremity away from the body

abduction pillow a special pillow used to keep the legs apart for a resident who has had hip replacement surgery

abrasion a scrape or injury that rubs off the surface of the skin

abuse the willful infliction of injury, unreasonable confinement, intimidation, or punishment that results in physical harm, pain, or mental anguish

acceptance the final stage in the grieving process in which the resident calmly waits for death

accident an unexpected, undesirable event that commonly results in injury

accreditation a process in which health care facilities voluntarily participate to ensure that high standards of care are maintained

acquired immune deficiency syndrome (AIDS) a progressively fatal disease caused by the HIV virus and spread by contact with blood or moist body fluids

active assistive range of motion exercises that are started or completed by the resident with some assistance from the care provider

active range of motion moving all joints through their normal movements independently

activities of daily living (ADLs) personal care activities people do each day to meet their human needs

acute illness illness that develops suddenly and last for a short time

adaptive devices pieces of equipment used to help a resident perform a task independently

adduction moving an extremity toward the body

ADLs *See* activities of daily living

admission the procedure for checking the resident into the health care facility and getting him or her settled

advance directive a document that designates the resident's wishes in the event that the resident is unable to speak for himself or herself

AED *See* automatic external defibrillator

afternoon care routine care that is given after lunch

AIDS *See* acquired immune deficiency syndrome

airborne method of transmission in which very small germs suspended in dust and moisture in the air are inhaled by a susceptible host

airborne precautions practices that health care workers use to protect themselves from airborne pathogens

ALF *See* assisted living facility

AM care routine care given to prepare the resident for breakfast

ambulation the act of walking or moving from one place to another

analgesic pain-relieving medication

aneroid gauge a gauge that operates with a spring-loaded dial

aneurysm a ballooning of the wall of an artery due to a structural weakness

anger the second step in the grieving process, in which the resident is angry because of a terminal diagnosis

antecedent an event that causes or triggers a behavior

antecubital space the space in front of the elbow

antibiotics medications used to eliminate pathogens from the body

antiembolism stockings elastic hosiery used on some residents to relieve edema and prevent blood clots

antiseptic chemical agent designed to cleanse the skin

anus the outlet of the intestines at the rectum, from which waste products are eliminated

apathy indifference; lack of feeling or emotion

aphasia a condition in which the speech center in the brain has been damaged

apical pulse the pulse taken at the apex of the heart

apnea absence of respiration

appliance a plastic collection device used to contain the excretions from an ostomy

application the form on which employment information is written and a request for employment is made

arteries blood vessels that carry freshly oxygenated blood to body parts

arthritis a chronic condition that causes a range of problems from mild discomfort to severe joint pain, deformities, and disability

aseptic technique practices used that are free of all microbes

aspiration inhaling food, fluid, or other objects into the lungs

assess to gather information and facts so as to identify the resident's problems and needs

assisted living facility (ALF) a senior housing option that provides housing and personal care support services in a residential setting

ataxic uncoordinated; poorly or defectively coordinated

ataxic gait an uncoordinated gait caused by neurological disease, in which the resident keeps the legs farther apart to maintain balance

atrophy weakness and muscle wasting from lack of use

attending behavior behaviors used to improve the transfer of verbal communication

attitude the outer reflection of feelings

aura a sensation, smell, or a bright light that precedes the onset of a seizure

aural temperature also called *tympanic temperature;* the temperature taken at the tympanic membrane inside the ear

autoimmune disorder a condition in which the individual makes antibodies that work against his or her own body

automatic external defibrillator (AED) a computerized device used when a resident is unresponsive, not breathing, and pulseless. When attached to the chest, the unit determines if an electrical shock is necessary to reestablish or regulate the heartbeat

axilla the area under the arm; the armpit

axillary temperature the temperature taken in the armpit

bacteria one-celled microorganisms that can cause disease

bargaining the third stage in the grieving process, in which the resident attempts to buy more time

barrier something that interferes with communication

bath blanket a soft cotton or flannel blanket used to protect resident privacy and provide warmth during procedures in which the body is exposed

bed bath the bathing procedure used for a resident who is unable to get out of bed

bed cradle a metal or plastic frame suspended over the hospital bed to keep the weight of the linen off the resident's body

bed rest a medically prescribed treatment in which the resident is not allowed out of bed

bedpan a device used for elimination in bed

bedside stand the nightstand used to store personal possessions, grooming, and hygiene items

bedsore *See* pressure ulcer

belt restraint a safety device that encircles the resident's waist and serves as a reminder to prevent rising

biohazardous waste disposable items that are contaminated with blood or body fluids

bioterrorism the use of biological agents, such as pathogenic organisms or agricultural pests, for terrorist purposes

bladder a hollow muscle in which urine is stored until it is eliminated from the body

bland diet a diet containing foods that are low in residue, with limited or no seasoning

blood pressure measurement of the force of the blood on the walls of the arteries

bloodborne pathogens microbes that cause diseases that are spread through contact with blood or body fluid

BM *See* bowel movement

body mechanics correct use of the body to lift or move heavy objects or residents

bony prominences places where the bones are close to the surface of the skin

bowel movement (BM) solid waste eliminated from the digestive system

brachial artery the artery in the antecubital space, in front of the elbow

bradycardia slow pulse rate, usually less than 60 beats per minute

bronchi the two large branches of the trachea through which air passes to the lungs

bruise injury to the skin caused by hitting or striking; the area turns black and blue

burnout complete physical, mental, or emotional fatigue or exhaustion

calorie-controlled diet a diet that restricts the total number of calories served to the resident; usually served to overweight residents

cannula a plastic or metal tube inserted into a tracheostomy to keep the stoma open

CAPD *See* continuous ambulatory peritoneal dialysis

carbohydrates foods that produce heat and energy in the body

cardiac arrest a condition that occurs when the heartbeat and respirations cease

care plan a plan developed by the interdisciplinary health care team that describes the goals and approaches to be used by all team members when caring for the resident

carrier a person who can give a disease to others; the person may not know of the infection

catastrophic reactions uncontrolled emotional outbursts in response to feeling completely overwhelmed or fearful; may include crying, sudden mood changes, anger, and combative behavior

catheter a hollow tube used to drain secretions from the body

causative agent a pathogen that causes disease

CDC *See* Centers for Disease Control and Prevention

Celsius (centigrade) scale a scale for measuring temperature in which the boiling point of water is 100

Centers for Disease Control and Prevention (CDC) a federal agency that studies diseases and makes recommendations on protective measures

Centers for Medicare and Medicaid Services (CMS) a governmental agency that sets policy and administers Medicare and Medicaid payments to health care facilities

centigrade scale *See* Celsius scale

cerebrovascular accident (CVA) also called a *stroke* or *brain attack;* a condition caused by a sudden interruption of blood to the brain, commonly a blood clot or breakage of a small blood vessel, may cause hemiparesis, hemiplegia, and/or speech, vision, emotional, and perception problems

certification an inspection process for facilities that accept state or federal funds as payment for health care

chain of command the lines of authority in each department

chain of infection a description of the factors necessary for an infection to spread

chairfast confined to a chair

chart the notebook or binder containing the resident's medical record

chemical restraint a medication or drug used to alter behavior for staff convenience, and not required to treat a resident's medical symptoms

chemicals substances that may be harmful if they touch the skin or mucous membranes, and are usually dangerous if swallowed

chemotherapy the treatment of cancer using specific chemical agents or drugs that destroy cancer cells

Cheyne-Stokes respirations periods of dyspnea alternating with periods of apnea

chorea abnormal, erratic, involuntary movements seen in Huntington's disease

chronic illness an illness or disease that lasts for a long time

circumduction circular movement of a joint, such as the thumb or wrist

citation a written notice that informs the health care agency or facility of alleged violations of OSHA rules and the time frame in which the conditions must be corrected

clean-catch (midstream) specimen a urine specimen collected from the middle of the urinary stream

cleansing enema introduction of fluid into the lower bowel to remove solid waste

clear-liquid diet a diet that is high in water and carbohydrates, with little nutritive value

clergy a minister of the gospel, a pastor, priest, or rabbi

client the person being cared for in the home

client care records documentation forms used for communication and reimbursement in home health care

closed drainage system a drainage bag and tubing connected to a catheter that is not opened

CMS *See* Centers for Medicare and Medicaid Services

coccyx the bone at the base of the spine

code blue an emergency designation to alert staff and summon help when a cardiac arrest occurs

cognitive impairment a decline in intellectual functioning

colostomy a surgical procedure in which the colon is attached to the outside of the body and waste is eliminated into a plastic bag attached to the skin

combative hitting or fighting the care provider

combative behavior physically aggressive behavior; hitting, kicking, scratching, biting

comfort a state of physical and emotional well-being in which the resident is calm and relaxed, and not in pain or upset

commercially prepared enema an enema solution prepackaged in a small dispenser

common vehicle food, water, or other items in which pathogens can live and multiply

compassionate kind and merciful

compensation using strength and overachieving in one area to overcome a weakness in another area of life

complete bath washing the entire body of a resident

condom catheter an external catheter applied to the penis of an incontinent male

confidentiality keeping personal information about the resident private; not revealing it to unauthorized persons

consent permission to perform care, treatments, and procedures

consequences the outcome of a behavior

consistent the same, uniform; describes approaches to care that are used and performed the same by all care providers

constipation passage of hard, dry stool from the lower bowel

constrict to make smaller

contact precautions a category of transmission-based precautions used when caring for residents who have infections that can be spread by skin and wound drainage, secretions, excretions, blood, body fluids, or contact with mucous membranes

continuity of care all staff working on the same goals and providing the same approaches to the resident 24 hours a day

continuous ambulatory peritoneal dialysis (CAPD) A type of peritoneal dialysis that needs no machine. The dialysis solution passes from a plastic bag through a catheter and into the abdomen. After several hours, the solution is drained into a disposable bag. The nurse refills the abdomen with fresh solution, to begin the cleaning process again. With this type of dialysis, the resident has the freedom of continuing with normal daily activities and routines with minimal interruption.

contractures permanent shortening and deformity of muscles from lack of use

contraindicated not indicated, inappropriate

coping mechanisms responses to stress and loss that people use to protect feelings of self-esteem

cover letter a letter of introduction sent to a prospective employer with a resume

cubic centimeter (cc) a metric unit of measure used in health care facilities; equal to one milliliter (30 cc equals 1 ounce)

cues brief verbal hints to tell the resident what you want him or her to do

culture the pattern or lifestyle of an individual or group

cumulative trauma disorders injuries to nerves, tissues, tendons, and joints that occur over a period of months to years

CVA *See* cerebrovascular accident

cyanosis a dark bluish or purplish discoloration of the skin and mucous membranes caused by inadequate oxygen in the blood

dangling sitting on the side of the bed with the legs over the edge of the mattress

decline worsening or deterioration in the resident's physical or mental condition

decubiti more than one pressure ulcer

decubitus ulcer *See* pressure ulcer

defamation of character making false or damaging statements about another person

defecation elimination of solid waste from the lower bowel

defibrillation a method of treatment that uses an electric shock to reverse disorganized activity in the heart during cardiac arrest

deficiency a written notice of inadequate care or a substandard practice

deformity disfigurement of the body

degenerative changes deterioration of a body part or system due to age or disease

dehydration a serious condition resulting from inadequate water in the body

delirium an acute confusional state that is an indication of a treatable illness

delusions false beliefs

delusions of persecution thinking that others are trying to cause personal harm

dementia a set of symptoms affecting the resident's thinking, judgment, memory, and ability to reason

denial refusing to accept something as the truth; also, the first stage in the grieving process, in which the resident denies the terminal diagnosis

dentures artificial teeth

dependable being trustworthy and able to be relied on

dependent unable to care for oneself

depression feelings of despair and discouragement; also, the fourth stage in the grieving process, in which the resident is trying to deal with loss

dermis the thicker, inner layer of the skin

developmental disability a severe physical and/or mental impairment that is apparent before the age of 22 and is likely to continue indefinitely

developmental tasks intellectual, social, and emotional skills that a person must accomplish at a certain age level

diabetes a chronic disease caused by a disorder of carbohydrate metabolism

diabetic diet a diet calculated by the dietitian to meet the needs of a resident with diabetes mellitus; the diet limits free sugar and some other foods

diagnosis the term describing the resident's disease or condition; determination of what is wrong with the resident

dialysis a process of removing waste products from the blood; used for residents with kidney disease

diarrhea passage of loose, watery, liquid stools

diastolic blood pressure the last sound heard when taking the blood pressure; taken during the relaxation phase of the heart cycle

dilate to become larger

direct contact the spread of infection by touching

disability inability to function normally because of a physical or mental problem

discharge the procedure by which the resident leaves the health care agency

discharge planner a social worker who is responsible for helping the resident make the transition between the long-term care facility and the community

disinfection a cleaning process that destroys most microorganisms; a chemical is usually used to disinfect reusable items

disoriented unaware of person, place, or time

distal situated farthest away from the center of the resident's body

distended enlarged

DNR *See* do not resuscitate order

do not resuscitate (DNR) order a physician's order indicating that no CPR or life-sustaining measures will be performed

dorsiflexion (dorsal flexion) pulling the foot upward toward the head

drainage bag a bag connected to a catheter to collect urine or other body waste

draw sheet a small sheet placed horizontally across the center of the hospital bed

droplet method of transmission in which germs are spread by secretions produced during laughing, talking, singing, sneezing, or coughing; these germs are large and usually do not spread more than three feet in the air

droplet precautions the type of isolation used for infections that are transmitted in respiratory secretions; the pathogens that cause infections requiring droplet precautions are usually confined to an area within three feet of the resident

durable power of attorney for health care a document that designates another individual to make medical decisions on behalf of the resident

dysarthria a condition often caused by a head injury or stroke, in which the resident has weakness or paralysis of the lips, tongue, or throat

dysphagia difficulty swallowing food and liquids

dysrhythmia an abnormal heart rhythm

dyspnea difficulty breathing, labored respirations

E. coli 0157:H7 a strain of Escherichia coli that is found in the intestines of some cattle; it is most commonly transmitted to humans in undercooked ground meat. This dangerous strain can cause renal failure and death

ecchymosis a bruise; an injury caused by bleeding under the skin

edema swelling

emesis basin a kidney-shaped basin used for oral care procedures and vomiting

empathetic able to understand how someone else feels

empathy understanding how someone else feels

EMS (emergency medical services) usually an ambulance or fire department

enabler a device that empowers residents and allows them to function independently

enema introduction of fluid into the lower bowel

entrance conference a meeting between surveyors and facility administration to discuss the purpose of a survey; the entrance conference is conducted at the beginning of a survey

environmental services department the housekeeping department; the department responsible for cleanliness and sanitation in most health care facilities

epidermis the thinner, outer layer of the skin

epiglottis a muscular flap that covers the trachea during swallowing

ergonomics adapting the job and the workplace to the worker's needs

Escherichia coli a type of bacteria that normally resides in the intestines

esophagus the tube through which food passes from the back of the throat to the stomach

evaluation the determination of how the resident's plan of care is working

eversion turning a joint outward

exacerbation a time in the course of a disease when signs and symptoms worsen

excretions human waste products eliminated from the body

exhalation breathing air out of the lungs

exit conference a meeting between surveyors and facility administration upon completion of a survey to discuss the surveyors' findings and the nature of any deficiencies

expiration breathing air out of the lungs

exposure control plan a written program that the employer is required to have that describes what to do if an employee accidently contacts blood or body fluids

expressive aphasia a condition in which the speech center in the brain has been damaged; residents with this condition have difficulty saying what they want to say. They may also have trouble with gestures and writing

extended survey a survey that lasts longer than originally anticipated so surveyors can examine resident care and facility practices in greater detail

extension straightening a joint

external catheter a catheter applied to the outside of the penis of an incontinent male

external genitalia the reproductive organs on the outside of the body

external rotation turning a joint outward, away from the median line

extracurricular activities clubs, hobbies, volunteer work, and special interests

extremity restraint a safety device that encircles the arm or leg and prevents movement

factual something that you know to be true

Fahrenheit scale a scale commonly used for measuring temperature

false imprisonment holding or restraining a resident against his or her will

fats nutrients, found in food products such as butter and oil, that are used for heat and energy production in the body

fecal impaction a large, hard, dry mass of stool that the resident is unable to pass

fecal material solid waste eliminated from the digestive system

feces solid waste eliminated from the digestive system

fetal position a position in which the resident is turned on the side with the head tucked down and knees drawn up

fistula a method of suturing a vein to an artery for the purpose of performing hemodialysis

flammable combustible; burns readily

flank the area of the back immediately above the waist where the kidneys are located

flatus gas expelled from the digestive tract

flexion bending at a joint

flora microbes that inhabit the internal and external surfaces of healthy individuals

fluid restrictions limiting the total amount of fluid the resident can have in a 24-hour period

fomites linen, equipment, and other items contaminated with microbes

food pyramid a U.S. Department of Agriculture diagram that provides a guide to eating a well-balanced diet

foot board a piece of wood or plastic placed at the end of the hospital bed and used for positioning the resident's feet

force energy, strength, or power

force fluids an order to encourage the resident to drink as much liquid as possible

foreskin the loose tissue at the tip of the penis

Fowler's position a semi-sitting position in bed

fracture a broken bone

friction force created by rubbing the skin; for example, against bed linen

full-liquid diet a temporary diet used for residents with digestive disorders; includes clear and milk-based liquids

functional incontinence inability to control the passage of urine due to physical inability to get to the toilet

gait the way a person walks

gait belt a heavy canvas belt used to assist the resident with ambulation

gastrostomy a surgical procedure in which a feeding tube is placed directly into the resident's stomach, with the end extending through the abdominal skin

gastrostomy tube also called *G-tube*; the feeding tube used in a resident who has had a gastrostomy

gatch handles handles at the foot of a bed that raise and lower the head, knee, and height of the bed

generalized spread throughout the entire body

generalized application applied to the resident's entire body

genital area the area of the body where the external reproductive organs are located

geriatrics care of the elderly

global aphasia inability to speak or understand

Good Samaritan laws laws that protect health care workers who provide emergency care outside the place of employment

graduate a measuring device with markings on the side

graft a method of connecting an artery and a vein with a tube for the purpose of performing hemodialysis

grievance a complaint

grieving process five steps that people go through when they anticipate or suffer a loss

habit training a type of bladder management program used for mentally confused residents who urinate at the same time each day

hallucination seeing, hearing, smelling, or feeling something that is not real

handroll prop that is placed in the hand to prevent contractures

hantavirus a virus that is spread by contact with rodents (rats and mice) or their excretions, including urine and feces

HD *See* Huntington's disease

head lice human parasites that feed on blood; they cannot be contracted from contact with pets or other animals

health care proxy an individual who has been legally designated to make medical decisions on behalf of the resident

Health Insurance Portability and Accountability Act (HIPAA) a law that applies to resident privacy, confidentiality, and medical records. The HIPAA regulations protect all individually identifiable health information in any form. The rules apply to paper, verbal, and electronic documentation, billing records, and clinical records. Staff members are provided with only the information needed to carry out their duties

health maintenance organization (HMO) a group of health care providers and hospitals paid by insurance companies to care for residents for a monthly fee

hemiparesis weakness on one side of the body

hemiplegia paralysis on one side of the body

hemodialysis removal of waste products from the body done by cleansing the resident's blood; this procedure must be performed at a special dialysis center

hemorrhage excessive bleeding

HEPA *See* high efficiency particulate air respirator

hepatitis B an infection of the liver caused by a virus; it can cause liver cancer and death

hepatitis C an infection of the liver caused by a virus; it can be spread through contact with blood or body fluids

herpes zoster *See* shingles

high efficiency particulate air (HEPA) respirator mask/respirator used to protect employees working in rooms of residents who have diseases spread by the airborne method of transmission

HIPAA *See* Health Insurance Portability and Accountability Act

HIV *See* human immunodeficiency virus disease

HMO *See* health maintenance organization

holistically focusing care on the whole person as an individual with many complex, interrelated strengths and needs

hormones chemical messengers of the body that originate in organs and glands of the body

hospice an organization that cares for dying residents

hospice care physical, psychological, and spiritual care provided to residents who have limited life expectancy and their families

hospital institution that cares for people with acute illnesses

host the place where a disease-causing germ can grow

HS care routine care given at bedtime to prepare the resident for sleep

human immune deficiency virus (HIV) disease the disease caused by the human immune deficiency virus that may progress to AIDS; it is spread by direct or indirect contact with blood and body fluids

humidifier a device that attaches to the oxygen supply to add moisture before oxygen is delivered to the resident

Huntington's disease (HD) a hereditary disease that causes choreiform movements, anxiety, and dementia

hygiene personal cleanliness

hyperalimentation a method of feeding a resident total nutrition intravenously, to allow the gastrointestinal system to rest and heal

hyperextension gentle, excessive extension of a joint, slightly past the point of resistance

hyperglycemia an abnormally high concentration of glucose (sugar) in the blood

hypertension high blood pressure, usually 140/90 or above

hypoglycemia an abnormally low concentration of glucose (sugar) in the blood

hypotension low blood pressure, usually 100/60 or below

hypothermia abnormally low body temperature (below 95°F)

I & O *See* intake and output

identification band a plastic bracelet, usually worn on the wrist or ankle, that contains the resident's name and other identifying information

immobility being motionless and unable to move

immobilize to support or restrain in a way that prevents movement

immune system part of the circulatory system that recognizes invading germs and works to eliminate them from the body

immunization administration of drugs that stimulate the immune system to protect against certain diseases

implementation the process of carrying out a plan of care

inactivity being still, quiet, sedentary, or immobile

incident an occurrence or event that interrupts normal procedures or causes a crisis

incident report a special form that is completed for each accident or unusual occurrence in a long-term care facility; the incident report describes what happened and contains other important information

incision a cut in the skin made with a knife

incontinence management program a routine in which the resident is taken to the toilet at regular intervals

incontinent unable to control the passage of urine from the bladder, or stool from the bowel, or both

incoordination uncoordinated, irregular voluntary muscle movement

independent self reliant, able to care for self

indirect contact touching objects, equipment, or dishes contaminated with harmful microorganisms

indwelling catheter a hollow tube inserted into the bladder to remove urine; the catheter remains in the body for a period of time

infection a state of sickness or disease caused by pathogens in the body

infection control medical asepsis; methods used in health care facilities to prevent the spread of infection

infusion site the site where an intravenous needle is inserted into the body

inhalation breathing air into the lungs

inspiration breathing air into the lungs

instantaneous injuries injuries that occur suddenly and without warning, usually as a result of an accident

insulin a hormone secreted by the pancreas that regulates glucose metabolism

intake and output (I & O) an estimated measurement of all the liquid the resident takes in and all the fluid lost in a 24-hour period

interdisciplinary team a group of caregivers who work together for the good of the patient, resident, or client

intermittent catheter a catheter that is inserted into the bladder for the purpose of obtaining a specimen, or for emptying the bladder, and is then withdrawn

internal rotation turning a joint inward, toward the median line

interview a formal meeting in which the employer assesses the qualifications of an applicant and provides information about a job opening

intravenous (IV) feeding administering sterile liquid and nutrients into a vein with a needle

inversion turning a joint inward

involuntary seclusion isolating a resident as a form of punishment

isolation measures used when a resident has an infectious disease; it is used to prevent the spread of pathogens to others

IV standard a metal pole used to hang an IV bag, bottle, or pump above the infusion site

jaundice a yellow color of the skin seen in hepatitis and some other diseases

JCAHO *See* Joint Commission on Accreditation of Healthcare Organizations

job objective the section of your resume that lists the type of position you are seeking and states how your abilities and skills qualify you for this position

Joint Commission on Accreditation of Healthcare Organizations (JCAHO) an organization that inspects and accredits health care agencies that meet high quality standards

Kegel exercises exercises used to make the muscles around the bladder stronger

Kelly a special clamp used to close tubes quickly

kidneys the organs that filter waste products from the blood and produce urine

labia majora two large, hair covered structures on the external female genitalia

labia minora two small, liplike structures inside the labia majora on the external female genitalia

laboratory requisition a document with identifying resident information that specifies the type of lab test to be performed on a specimen

large intestine the lower part of the bowel

larynx the voice box

lateral position lying on the left or right side

leg drainage bag a bag attached to a catheter to collect urine; it is secured to the leg with an elastic or rubber strap

lethargy abnormal drowsiness or sleepiness

level of consciousness the degree of awareness or alertness, which ranges from fully awake and alert to confusion and unconsciousness

libel making false statements about another person in writing

license a state permit allowing the long-term care facility to operate

licensed practical nurse (LPN) a nurse who has completed one to two years of nursing school and passed a state licensing examination

licensed vocational nurse (LVN) a licensed practical nurse

living will a document that specifies the resident's wishes in the event that the resident is in a terminal condition

localized confined to a specific area of the body

localized application applied to a specific area of a resident's body

lockout-tagout placing a locking tag on a broken piece of equipment so that the equipment cannot be used

long-term care facility health care institution that cares for residents with chronic diseases and personal care needs

low bed a bed in which the frame is four to six inches from the floor to the top of the frame deck; such beds reduce the risk of injury if the resident falls from the bed

low-cholesterol diet a diet that is low in fat and cholesterol; used for residents with heart, blood vessel, liver, and gallbladder disease

lowfat diet a diet that is low in fats; used for residents with heart, blood vessel, liver, and gallbladder disease

LPN *See* licensed practical nurse

LVN *See* licensed vocational nurse

malnutrition inadequate nutrition due to poor diet or inability to absorb nutrients

malpractice negligence that results in harm to the resident

Maslow's hierarchy of needs a chart based on a widely accepted theory of physical and psychological needs of all human beings

material safety data sheets (MSDS) information sheets on chemicals used in the workplace that list the health hazards, safe use, and emergency procedures for chemical exposure

MDS *See* Minimum Data Set 2.0

mechanical soft diet a diet that is finely ground or chopped; used for residents who have chewing or swallowing problems

mechanically altered diets a diet that is altered in texture to meet the needs of residents who have chewing, swallowing, or digestive problems

medial pertaining to or situated toward the midline of the body

median situated in the median plane or in the midline of the body

Medicaid a program funded by the state and federal governments that pays for health care for individuals with a low income

medical asepsis practices used in health care facilities to prevent the spread of infection

medical record a record of the resident's true condition and a record of progress and care

Medicare a program administered by the federal government that helps the elderly and disabled pay for care in a hospital, long-term care facility, and/or home health care setting

mentally retarded lower-than-average intellectual development; retardation ranges from mild to severe

metabolism rate the rate at which the body uses energy

methicillin-resistant Staphylococcus aureus (MRSA) a pathogen commonly seen in health care facilities that causes illness or infection; the pathogen resists treatment with most antibiotics

microorganisms living germs that cannot be seen with the naked eye

micturition the act of eliminating urine from the body

midstream (clean-catch) specimen a urine specimen collected from the middle of the urinary stream

milliliter (mL) a metric unit of measure used in health care facilities; 30 mL equal one ounce; one milliliter is the same as one cubic centimeter

minerals inorganic compounds in food used to build body tissues

Minimum Data Set 2.0 (MDS) the assessment tool upon which the care plan is based; completed upon admission and quarterly for all residents of long-term care facilities

misappropriation of property theft

mite a tiny parasite that cannot be seen with the naked eye

miter to tuck a sheet in by forming a 45° angle perpendicular to the mattress

mixed incontinence inability to control passage of both liquid and solid waste from the body

mobility the ability to move about

mode of transmission the way in which a disease-causing pathogen is spread

morning care routine care that is given after breakfast

MRSA *See* methicillin-resistant Staphylococcus aureus

MS *See* multiple sclerosis

MSDS *See* material safety data sheet

mucous membranes tissues of the body that secrete mucus; these areas open to the outside of the body

multiple sclerosis (MS) a progressive neurological disorder that causes a degeneration of the nervous system, which interferes with conduction of nerve impulses

multiskilled workers nursing assistants who have received additional education to enable them to perform tasks and procedures that are not taught in the original, basic NA program

musculoskeletal system the name commonly used to refer to the muscular and skeletal systems

myths commonly accepted beliefs that are not true

N95 respirator a mask with very small pores that may be worn when caring for residents in airborne precautions

nasogastric tube a tube inserted into the nose and threaded through the esophagus into the stomach; it can be used for feeding or medical procedures

negative pressure environment a description of the ventilation system used in an airborne precautions room; the room air is drawn upward into the ventilation system and is either specially filtered or exhausted directly to the outside of the building

neglect failing to provide services to residents to prevent physical harm or mental anguish

negligence failing to provide services to a resident in the same manner as a reasonably prudent person would do

network to communicate with people you know who have similar careers, goals, and interests

neurogenic bladder a condition in which the resident cannot feel the sensation of urine in the bladder, causing it to become very full and retain urine

NIC *See* Nursing Interventions Classification

nits the eggs left by lice; if untreated, the eggs will hatch into more lice

no concentrated sweets diet a regular diet that is not calorie restricted; however, free sugar, fruit in sugary syrup, and most regular desserts are not served on this diet

NOC *See* Nursing Outcomes Classification

nonintact skin skin that is broken, chapped, or cracked

nonrapid eye movement (NREM) sleep the part of the sleep cycle that begins when the resident first falls asleep. As he or she progresses through the cycle, arousal becomes more difficult and sleep becomes deeper

normal flora microorganisms that are healthful and necessary for the body to function correctly; they are not harmful in the area in which they reside, but can cause infection if spread to other parts of the body

nosocomial infection an infection acquired by a resident in a health care facility

Nursing Interventions Classification (NIC) a comprehensive, standardized language describing treatments that nursing personnel perform; this method was established by nurse researchers at the University of Iowa in 1987

Nursing Outcomes Classification (NOC) a method of measuring how well the resident is meeting care plan goals; this method was established by nurse researchers at the University of Iowa in 1991

nursing process the four-step process of assessment, planning, implementation, and evaluation of the resident and care provided to meet the resident's needs

nutrients chemical substances in food that are necessary for life

objective observations made by seeing, hearing, feeling, touching, and smelling

OBRA (Omnibus Budget Reconciliation Act of 1987) legislation that called for sweeping reforms of the long-term care industry; describes requirements for nursing assistant education

obstructed airway food or a foreign body blocking the trachea or windpipe, making it impossible to breathe

Occupational Safety and Health Administration (OSHA) a governmental agency responsible for developing and enforcing job safety and health standards to protect employees

occupied bedmaking procedure for making the bed with the resident in the bed

ombudsman a resident advocate; he or she can provide information on how to find a facility and get quality care, can help in solving problems, and can assist residents to file grievances, if requested

opposition touching each of the fingers against the thumb

oral temperature temperature taken by placing the thermometer in the resident's mouth

orthotic a device that restores or improves function and prevents deformity

OSHA *See* Occupational Safety and Health Administration

osteoporosis a decrease in bone mass that leads to fractures with minimal or no trauma

ostomy a surgically created opening into the body

ovaries glands in the female that produce eggs and are responsible for hormone production

overbed table a narrow table on wheels used to hold the resident's water, meal trays, and clean items

overflow incontinence the escape of urine that occurs when the bladder is very full and can hold no more urine

pacemaker a surgically implanted device that regulates the rate of the heartbeat. Most commonly, the pacemaker is implanted in the chest, but occasionally it is placed in the abdomen

pain a state of discomfort that is unpleasant for the resident; it is always a warning that something is wrong

palmar flexion the act of bending the hand down toward the palm

paraphrasing a method of restating the message communicated to you in clear, simple terms

paraplegic a person who has permanent loss of sensation and movement below the waist

parasites tiny animals that survive by feeding off another human or animal

Parkinson's disease (PD) a neurological disease that causes tremors, shuffling gait, and dementia

partial bath washing the face, hands, underarms, back, and genital area

passive range of motion joint exercises performed on the resident by the care provider

pathogen a microorganism that causes disease

patient a person who is cared for in a hospital

PD *See* Parkinson's disease

penis the external male organ used for sex and elimination

peri-care *See* perineal care

perineal care washing the genital and anal areas of the body

perineum the area between the anus and vagina in the female; the area between the anus and scrotum in the male

peripherally inserted central catheter (PICC) an intravenous line that is inserted in the arm and threaded through the venous system to the superior vena cava; used for long-term intravenous therapy and TPN

peristalsis muscular contractions of the digestive tract that move food and waste products through the intestines

peritoneal dialysis dialysis done by inserting solution through a cannula into the resident's abdominal cavity

perseveration repetitious behavior, movements, or actions

personal data the section of your resume that lists your name, address, phone number, and professional license or certification number

personal protective equipment (PPE) equipment worn to protect the health care worker and the resident from contact with disease-causing pathogens

personal space a comfortable distance in which to communicate with others

petechiae small purplish spots on the body surface, caused by minute hemorrhages

PFR95 respirator a mask with very small pores that may be worn when caring for residents in airborne precautions

pharynx the throat

physical restraints physical, manual, or mechanical devices attached or adjacent to the resident's body that the resident cannot remove easily and prevent access to the body

PICC *See* peripherally inserted central catheter

plan of correction a written plan submitted by the health care agency in response to deficient survey findings; the plan will list what corrections will be made, by whom, who will monitor the correction, and what will be done to prevent similar deficiencies in the future

planning deciding what to do with information gathered in an assessment

plantar flexion bending the foot downward, away from the body

plaque an acidic, decay-causing substance in the mouth

portal of entry the place where a pathogen enters the body

portal of exit the way pathogens leave the body. This may be in excretions, secretions, or body fluids, such as urine, feces, saliva, tears, drainage from open wounds, blood, mucus, or respiratory fluids

post polio syndrome (PPS) a neurologic condition marked by increased weakness and abnormal muscle fatigue in persons who had polio many years earlier

postmortem care physical care of the body after death

postoperative care care given to residents after surgical procedures

postural support a device that maintains good body alignment and posture

PPE *See* personal protective equipment

PPO *See* preferred provider organization

PPS *See* post polio syndrome

preferred provider organization (PPO) a list of physicians and health care facilities/agencies that contract with insurance companies to provide health care to insurance company subscribers

prefix the word element at the beginning of a word

prehypertension blood pressure between 120/80 and 139/89; persons with this condition are likely to develop high blood pressure in the future and should take steps to decrease their risk

pressure sore *See* pressure ulcer

pressure ulcer also called *bedsore, decubitus ulcer, pressure sore;* an ulcer that forms on the skin over a bony prominence as the result of pressure

priorities things that are very important that must be taken care of first

probe the attachment to an electronic thermometer used to measure temperature

probe cover the plastic, disposable cover or sheath used on the thermometer probe when taking a resident's temperature

professional a skilled practitioner who is capable, competent, and efficient

professional boundaries unspoken limits on physical and emotional relationships with residents; boundaries limit and define how a health care worker acts with residents

projection placing the blame for the illness or situation on someone or something else

prompted voiding a bladder management program used for residents who know that the bladder is full, but do not communicate the need to use the toilet

pronation moving a joint to face downward

prone position lying on the abdomen with the head turned to one side

prostate gland a gland in the male that encircles the urethra just below the bladder and secretes a fluid which forms part of the semen

prosthesis an artificial body part

prosthetic refers to a device that takes the place of a body part

protective isolation also called *reverse isolation;* used in some health care facilities to protect residents who have weakened immune systems from contacting pathogens in the environment

proteins nutrients in food that build and repair tissues

pseudomembranous colitis a very serious condition in which severe diarrhea is caused by a bacterium called Clostridium difficile (C. difficile); it commonly develops in residents who have been on antibiotic therapy

pulse the expansion and contraction of an artery that can be felt on the outside surface of the body

pulse oximeter a device that measures the oxygen in the arterial blood

pulse points locations on the body where the pulse can be felt

pulse pressure the difference between the systolic and diastolic blood pressure

pulse rate the number of pulse beats per minute

pureed diet a diet blenderized to a smooth consistency

QA *See* quality assurance

quad cane a cane with four feet; the most stable type of cane

quality assurance (QA) an internal review made by facility staff to identify problems and find solutions for improvement

RACE System the steps that should be followed in case of fire

radial deviation turning the wrist inward toward the radius

radial pulse the pulse felt on the thumb side of the wrist

radiation therapy a type of cancer treatment in which the skin is exposed to high doses of radiation

range of motion normal joint movements

rapid eye movement (REM) sleep the part of the sleep cycle that restores mental function; the part of the sleep cycle in which dreams occur

rationalization providing an acceptable, but untrue reason for an illness or behavior

reality orientation a technique in which a resident is reoriented to time, place, person, and season

reasonable accommodation considering the resident's likes, dislikes, needs, and preferences when providing care and services

receptive aphasia a condition in which the speech center in the brain has been damaged; residents with this condition have trouble understanding spoken language, and may also have trouble reading and understanding gestures

rectal temperature the temperature taken by inserting the thermometer into the anus

rectum the last six to eight inches of the large intestine, where fecal material is stored until it is eliminated from the body through the anus

references individuals who know you will who will recommend you to the prospective employer for the job you are seeking

reflex incontinence a loss of urine that occurs without awareness in residents who are paralyzed or have other neurologic problems

reflexes unconscious or involuntary movements

registered nurse (RN) a nurse who has completed two to four years of nursing school and has passed a state licensure examination

regular diet a normal diet based on the five food groups in the food pyramid

rehabilitation program(s) designed by a therapist to help a resident regain lost skills or to teach new skills

reimburse to repay an institution for the cost of services provided

reminiscing the act of remembering the past

remission a time period when a chronic disease appears stable and relatively symptom-free

reprisal retaliation

reservoir host; the person who has an infection

resident the person who is cared for in a long-term care facility

Resident's Bill of Rights a legal document listing the rights of residents in long-term care facilities

resolved through, over, completed

respiration the act of breathing in and out

responsible behavior behavior that is dependable and trustworthy

rest a state of mental and physical comfort, calmness, and relaxation

restoration basic nursing care measures designed to maintain or improve a resident's function and assist the resident to return to self-care

restorative care nursing care designed to assist the resident to attain and maintain the highest level of function possible

restorative environment an environment that has been modified so the resident can function as independently as possible

restraints physical, manual, or mechanical devices attached or adjacent to the resident's body that the resident cannot remove easily and prevent access to the resident's body

resume a summary of your professional or work experience and qualifications

retention enema introduction of fluid into the lower bowel to soften, lubricate, and remove solid waste

retraction drawing back, away from the body

reverse chronological order the order in which your previous jobs are listed on your resume, beginning with most recent job first

reverse isolation *See* protective isolation

rhythm a recurring action or movement

rigor mortis a condition that occurs two to four hours after death, in which the muscles and limbs become stiff

risk factor condition that has the potential to cause the resident's health to worsen; condition indicating that a problem may develop or predisposing the resident to development of a problem

RN *See* registered nurse

root the element that gives meaning to a medical word

rotation moving a joint in, out, and around

scabies a skin condition caused by a mite; it causes a rash and severe itching and is highly contagious

scheduled toileting a bladder management program used for residents who cannot use the bathroom without physical help; the resident is taken to the bathroom on a fixed schedule developed by the nurse

scrotum the sac-like structure containing the testes on the male genitalia

secretions drainage, discharge, or seeping from the body

seizure a convulsion or condition characterized by severe shaking and jerking of the body

self-actualization the realization of one's full potential

self-care deficit inability to perform an activity of daily living

self-esteem your opinion of yourself

semiprone position a modified prone position in which the body is supported on pillows to relieve pressure from most of the bony prominences

semisupine position a modified side-lying position in which the body is supported on pillows to relieve pressure from most of the bony prominences

senile purpura dark purple bruises on the forearms and backs of hands in the elderly

sensory loss difficulty seeing, hearing, smelling, or touching

sepsis systemic poisoning of the body caused by bacteria; a serious infection

septic infected; poisoned

sexual abuse forcing a resident to perform a sexual act

shearing moving the resident so the skin is stretched between the bone inside and the surface (such as a sheet) outside, causing skin damage

sheath a cover for a probe or instrument

shingles (herpes zoster) a condition that occurs only in people who have had chickenpox; the resident develops blister-like lesions on the torso that follow the nerve pathways, and are extremely painful; the condition is infectious through the airborne and contact routes until all lesions crust over

shock the result of blood loss that causes inadequate blood flow to the vital organs

shroud a cloth, paper, or plastic covering used to wrap the body after death

shunt a passage between two blood vessels, commonly under the forearm skin in residents who are receiving hemodialysis

signs conditions of the resident that can be seen or observed by others

Sims' position a side-lying position in which the resident is placed on the left side with the right leg flexed and bent; used for rectal examinations and treatments

skin tears injuries in which the epidermis is torn

slander making false statements about another person

sleep a period of continuous or intermittent unconsciousness in which physical movements are decreased and allows the mind and body to rest; sleep is a basic need

sleep deprivation prolonged sleep loss (inadequate quality or quantity of REM or NREM sleep)

sliding technique a technique used for transfers when the resident cannot bear weight; the resident is moved on a sheet

small intestine the part of the digestive system that receives food from the stomach and completes digestion, absorbing nutrients from the food into the bloodstream

sodium-restricted diet a diet that is prepared with no sodium (salt) or limited sodium

soft diet a diet containing foods that are low in residue, with limited or no seasoning

source causative agent; a pathogen that causes disease

spasticity sudden, frequent, involuntary muscle contractions that impair function

sperm reproductive secretion from the testes in the male

sphygmomanometer the instrument used to measure blood pressure

splint a device used to maintain the position of an extremity or joint

standard precautions measures that health care workers use to prevent the spread of infection to themselves and others

standards of care common health care practices based on current information about health care and facility policies

stereotyping fixed images or beliefs that categorize an individual or group

sterile free from all pathogens

sterilization processes used to kill all germs

stethoscope the instrument used to listen to sounds inside the body

stoma the opening of an ostomy to the outside of the body

stool feces; solid waste eliminated from the digestive system

strain injury to a muscle or muscles from stretching or overuse

stress physical or emotional strain and tension

stress incontinence inability to control the passage of urine due to muscular weakness

strict I & O an accurate measurement of all the liquid the resident takes in and all the fluid the resident loses in a 24-hour period

stump sock a stocking that is placed over an amputated extremity before the prosthesis is applied

subacute a level of care for the resident who has complex care needs but is not critically ill

subcutaneous tissue the fatty layer below the epidermis

subjective describes observations based on what you think, or what the resident tells you; may or may not be factual

suffix the word element at the end of a word

sundowning increased restlessness and confusion in the late afternoon, evening, and night

supination moving a joint so it faces upward

supine position lying on the back; face up

supplemental feedings nourishments given to the resident in addition to meals, to meet special nutritional needs

suprapubic catheter a hollow tube surgically inserted into the bladder through the abdomen

survey a review and evaluation to ensure that a long-term care facility is maintaining acceptable standards of practice, quality of care, and quality of life for residents

surveyor a representative of a private or governmental agency who reviews long-term care facility policies, procedures, and practices for quality of care

susceptibility the ability of the body to resist disease

susceptible host a person who can become infected with a disease-causing pathogen

sympathy feeling very sorry for someone because of their physical condition or situation; sympathy is not healthy for you or the resident; feeling sympathetic can cause you to cross professional boundaries and enter the relationship danger zone

symptoms an indication of a disease or disorder that is noticed by the resident, but cannot be observed by others

syncope fainting

systolic blood pressure the first sound heard when taking the blood pressure; taken during the contraction phase of the heart cycle

tachycardia rapid pulse rate, usually more than 100 beats per minute

tact the ability to speak and act without offending others

tactful considerate, polite, and thoughtful

tagout *See* lockout-tagout

task analysis analyzing the steps of a procedure and determining which steps the resident can complete independently

TB *See* tuberculosis

temperature measurement of heat within the body

tepid lukewarm

terminal illness an illness for which there is no cure

testes the egg-shaped reproductive glands located in the scrotum in the male

therapeutic diet a special or modified diet prepared to treat a resident's individual nutritional needs

thermal burn an injury to the skin caused by contact with flame, steam, hot water, or hot object

thermometer the instrument used to measure temperature

TIA *See* transient ischemic attack

time and travel records reports showing how the nursing assistant spent his or her time when working in home health care

toe pleat a fold in the top linen near the end of the bed that provides extra space and keeps the linen from pressing or pulling the feet downward

tornado warning a state of alert that occurs when a tornado is in the area

tornado watch a state of alert suggesting that conditions are right for a tornado to develop

total parenteral nutrition (TPN) a method of feeding a resident total nutrition intravenously, to allow the gastrointestinal system to rest and heal

TPN *See* total parenteral nutrition

trachea the upper windpipe extending from the larynx to the bronchus

tracheostomy an opening into the trachea through which the resident breathes

transfer moving the resident from one place, unit, or facility to another

transfer belt a heavy canvas belt used to move a resident from one location to another

transient ischemic attack (TIA) a period of temporarily diminished blood flow to the brain; occurs suddenly and commonly lasts from 2 to 15 minutes

transmission-based precautions isolation categories designed to interrupt the mode of transmission so the pathogen cannot spread

transport bag a sealed plastic bag labeled with a biohazard emblem; used to contain laboratory specimens during transport to the lab

tremors involuntary shaking

trochanter roll a rolled bath blanket used for bedfast residents to prevent external rotation of the hips

tuberculosis (TB) a contagious disease that is spread by airborne contact; it commonly affects the lungs, but can cause illness in other parts of the body

turgor elasticity of skin; skin that stretches and tents when pinched is an indication of dehydration

tympanic temperature also called *aural temperature;* the temperature taken at the tympanic membrane inside the ear

tympanic thermometer the thermometer used to measure temperature inside the ear

ulnar deviation turning the wrist outward toward the ulna

unit the resident's personal space in the facility; includes a bed, chair, overbed table, nightstand, dresser, wastebasket, and closet

universal choking sign one or both hands on the throat

ureters the tubes that carry urine from the kidneys to the bladder

urethra the hollow tube leading from the bladder to the outside of the body

urge incontinence inability to control the passage of urine in which the need to urinate is very strong and sudden, preventing the resident from getting to the toilet on time

urinal a container used for urinary elimination in the male resident

urinary meatus the external opening to the urethra where urine leaves the body

urinary retention inability to empty the bladder completely

urination the act of passing liquid waste to the outside of the body

uterus the internal organ in the female in which a baby develops and receives nourishment

vagina the canal in the female extending from the external genitalia to the uterus

validation therapy a technique that validates feelings, helps residents resolve developmental tasks, and enhances feelings of dignity and self-control

Vancomycin-resistant Enterococcus (VRE) a drug-resistant pathogen seen in health care facilities that commonly causes infections

vector an insect, rodent, or small animal that spreads disease

veins blood vessels that carry blood from the body parts back to the heart

ventilator a device used to assist or control breathing

vest restraint a safety device applied to the resident's upper body to limit movement and prevent rising

viruses tiny pathogens that cause disease; antibiotics will not eliminate them

vital signs temperature, pulse, respiration, and blood pressure

vitamins organic substances in food that are necessary for normal body function

voiding urination; the act of passing liquid waste to the outside of the body

VRE *See* Vancomycin-resistant Enterococcus

vulva the external genitalia in the female

waterless bathing a prepackaged bathing system in which a package of moistened washcloths is used instead of a water basin and soap

Index